Introduction to Quantitative EEG and Neurofeedback: Advanced Theory and Applications

Second Edition

Introduction to Quantitative EEG and Neurofeedback: Advanced Theory and Applications

Second Edition

Thomas H. Budzynski, PhD
Department of Psychosocial and Community Health
University of Washington School of Nursing
Poulsbo, Washington

Helen Kogan Budzynski, PhD, RN
Department of Psychosocial and Community Health
University of Washington School of Nursing
Poulsbo, Washington

James R. Evans, PhD
Department of Psychology
University of South Carolina
Columbia, South Carolina

Andrew Abarbanel, MD
Soquel, California

AMSTERDAM • BOSTON • HEIDELBERG • LONDON • NEW YORK • OXFORD
PARIS • SAN DIEGO • SAN FRANCISCO • SINGAPORE • SYDNEY • TOKYO
Academic Press is an imprint of Elsevier

Academic Press is an imprint of Elsevier
30 Corporate Drive, Suite 400, Burlington, MA 01803, USA
32 Jamestown Road, London NW1 7BY, UK
525 B Street, Suite 1900, San Diego, CA 92101-4495, USA
360 Park Avenue South, New York, NY 10010-1710, USA

First edition 1999
Second edition 2009

Library of Congress Cataloging-in-Publication Data
A catalog record for this book is available from the Library of Congress

British Library Cataloguing in Publication Data
A catalogue record for this book is available from the British Library

ISBN: 978-0-12-374534-7

For information on all Academic Press publications
visit our website at www.elsevierdirect.com

Typeset by Charon Tec Ltd., A Macmillan Company. (www.macmillansolutions.com)

Printed and bound by CPI Group (UK) Ltd, Croydon, CR0 4YY

Transferred to Digital Printing, 2013

Contents

PART 1

QEEG and Neurofeedback: Basics and New Theory

1   Neuromodulation technologies: An attempt at classification   3

Siegfried Othmer, Ph.D.

2 *History of the scientific standards of QEEG normative databases*   *29*

Robert W. Thatcher, Ph.D. and Joel F. Lubar, Ph.D.

PART 2

Advancing Neurofeedback Practice

**Thomas F. Collura, Ph.D., Robert W. Thatcher, Ph.D., Mark
Llewellyn Smith, L.C.S.W., William A. Lambos, Ph.D., BCIA-EEG,
and Charles R. Stark, M.D., BCIA-EEG**

Nancy E. White, Ph.D. and Leonard M. Richards, Th.D.

PART 3

Alternative Treatment Approaches to Neurofeedback

7 *Hemoencephalography: Photon-based blood flow neurofeedback*   *169*

Hershel Toomim, Ph.D. and Jeffrey Carmen, Ph.D.

PART 4

Recent Clinical Applications of Neurofeedback

12 Neurofeedback for the treatment of depression: Current status of theoretical issues and clinical research   295

D. Corydon Hammond, Ph.D., ECNS, QEEG-D, BCIA-EEG and Elsa Baehr, Ph.D.

13 Neurofeedback and attachment disorder: Theory and practice   315

Sebern F. Fisher, M.A., BCIA

14 QEEG and neurofeedback for assessment and effective intervention with attention deficit hyperactivity disorder (ADHD) 337

Lynda Thompson, Ph.D. and Michael Thompson, M.D.

15 Asperger's syndrome intervention: combining neurofeedback, biofeedback and metacognition 365

Michael Thompson, M.D. and Lynda Thompson, Ph.D.

16 *Neurofeedback in pain management*   *417*

**Victoria L. Ibric, M.D., Ph.D. BCIAC and Liviu
G. Dragomirescu, Ph.D.**

17 *Anxiety, EEG patterns and neurofeedback*   *453*
Jane Price, M.A. and Thomas Budzynski, Ph.D.

PART 5

Ethical/Legal Issues

18 *Ethics in neurofeedback practice*   *475*
Sebastian Striefel, Ph.D.

Contributors

Numbers in parentheses indicate the pages on which the authors contributions begin

Elsa Baehr (295)
Baehr & Baehr Ltd, Chicago, Illinois, USA

Thomas Budzynski (453)
University of Washington, Washington,
  USA

Rex L. Cannon (239)
University of Tennessee, Knoxville,
  Tennessee, USA

David S. Cantor (63)
Psychological Sciences Institute, PC,
  Duluth, Georgia, USA

Jeffrey Carmen (169)
Clinical psychology practice, Manlius,
  New York, USA

Liviu G. Dragomirescu (417)
Department of Ecology, University of
  Bucharest, Romania

Thomas F. Collura (103, 195)
BrainMaster Technologies, Inc., Oakwood,
  Ohio, USA

James R. Evans (225)
Professor Emeritus, University of South
  Carolina, South Carolina, USA.

Sebern F. Fisher (315)
Private practice, Northampton,
  Massachusetts, USA

D. Corydon Hammond (295)
University of Utah School of Medicine,
  Salt Lake City, Utah, USA

Victoria L. Ibric (417)
President, Neurofeedback and
  Neuro Rehab Institute, Inc., Pasadena,
  California, USA.

William A. Lambos (103)
Cognitive Neuro Sciences, Inc. and
  University of South Florida, Florida,
  USA

Mark Llewellyn Smith (103)
Private practice, New York, USA

Joel F. Lubar (29)
Brain Research and
  Neuropsychology Lab., University of
  Tennessee, Knoxville, Tennessee, USA

Galina Mindlin (225)
Columbia, Univ. College of Physicians
  and Surgeons, New York, USA

Siegfried Othmer (3)
EEG Institute, Woodland Hills,
  California, USA

Jane Price (453)
Sterlingworth Center, Greenville,
  South Carolina, USA

Leonard M. Richards (143)
The Enhancement Institute, Houston
  Texas, USA

Leslie H. Sherlin (83)
Nova Tech EEG, Inc., Mesa, Arizona, USA

David Siever (195)
Mind Alive Inc., Edmonton, Alberta,
  Canada

Tato M. Sokhadze (239)
Department of Psychiatry and Behavioral
  Sciences, University of Louisville School
  of Medicine, Louisville, Kentucky, USA

Charles R. Stark (103)
Cognitive Neuro Sciences, Inc., Melbourne,
  Florida, USA.

Sebastian Striefel (475)
Professor Emeritus, Utah State University,
  Logan, Utah, USA

Robert W. Thatcher (29, 103, 269)
EEG and NeuroImaging Laboratory,
  Applied Neuroscience, Inc.,
  St. Petersburg, and Professor, Department
  of Neurology, University of South Florida,
  Florida, USA

Lynda Thompson (337, 365)
ADD Centre and Biofeedback Institute of
  Toronto, Mississauga, Ontario, Canada

Michael Thompson (337, 365)
ADD Centre and Biofeedback Institute of
  Toronto, Mississauga, Ontario, Canada

Hershel Toomim (169)
Biocomp Research Institute, Los Angeles,
  California, USA

David L. Trudeau (239)
University of Minnesota, School of Health
  Sciences, Department of Family Medicine
  and Community Health, Minneapolis,
  Minnesota, USA

Nancy E. White (143)
The Enhancement Institute, Houston,
  Texas, USA

Preface

When the first edition of *Introduction to Quantitative EEG and Neurofeedback* was published in 1999, it was the only book available providing a broad overview of the field of neurofeedback (NF) and the use of quantitative EEG (QEEG) in relationship to that field. Although since then at least three other texts have been published which deal in depth with neurofeedback (and, to some degree, with QEEG), the many recent advances in neurofeedback-related areas warrant an updated second edition. Since the basics of QEEG and neurofeedback are available elsewhere, the chapters in this edition emphasize recent thinking regarding mechanisms of efficacy of NF, advances in QEEG and its application to NF, advances in use of neurofeedback with many disorders covered in the first edition as well as new clinical applications, current status of auditory-visual entrainment (AVE) and other procedures often used in conjunction with traditional NF, and an update on ethical concerns in the practice of NF. As with the first edition, chapters are authored by current leaders in the field, many of whom are among the early "pioneers."

The last ten years have seen a rapid growth of the field of NF both in the US and internationally. Practitioners can be found in at least 27 countries, and membership of the International Society for Neurofeedback and Research (ISNR) has grown by 51% during the past five years. Keeping pace with this growth has been the evolution of clinical practice and research. New QEEG databases have been developed, and older ones refined with the addition of new measures of potential clinical relevance (e.g. phase reset, co-modulation). Older and newer QEEG measures of neural connectivity have received increasing attention, and improved methods of determining cortical and sub-cortical areas of dysfunction from the EEG (e.g. LORETA) are now available.

Major developments at the interface of QEEG and NF include LORETA-based feedback, and NF training involving rewarding of "live" (ongoing; immediate) approximations to normalcy of single or multiple QEEG measures based on database norms (i.e. Z-score training). Use of NF with ADHD, anxiety and mood disorders has been refined in conjunction with new knowledge about such disorders (e.g. discovery of several sub-types of ADHD). Recent clinical experience has indicated the value of NF with various other conditions, including reactive attachment disorder, autistic spectrum disorders, and pain. The use of adjunctive and alternative methods of intervention such as auditory-visual entrainment and brain-music treatment, alone or in conjunction with NF, has expanded to create interesting new types of NF. These developments, and more, are covered in the chapters of this book.

Although the QEEG and NF fields have experienced rapid expansion, some aspects have remained relatively static. While there has been some high quality research concerning the clinical value of QEEG and NF, the fields are still regularly dismissed by much of mainstream medicine, education and psychology as lacking in research support. It could be debated: How much of this is due to honestly perceived limits of related research, or to lack of adequate marketing, or to fears of competition by entrenched interest groups? But, even within the ranks of neurotherapists who have no doubt about the many therapeutic benefits of NF, there remain questions about such topics as which specific methods among the many touted as "best" by their advocates are likely to be most effective with their particular clients and why. They, too, would like research-based answers. Questions continue to exist on such topics as why there sometimes are no changes in targeted QEEG abnormalities following successful NF treatment. Acceptable answers need to be found if the field is to maintain (or gain) credibility regarding one of its basic premises, i.e. that changing EEG via NF is what primarily accounts for desired behavioral change.

Having been involved in editing both editions of this book, the writer is led to wonder what the contents of a third edition a decade or so from now might be. Hopefully, a chapter would provide research-based information on exact mechanisms through which NF achieves positive results. Specific possibilities might include oscillatory entrainment, selective activation/inhibition of neuronal assemblies, facilitation of new neuronal pathways, increased blood flow and/or neurochemical changes. This type of knowledge, along with developments in QEEG such as norms for larger frequency ranges and more electrode sites, should enable greater precision in developing individualized NF training protocols. A chapter, possibly emanating from work such as that on EEG phenotypes, might describe a taxonomy of behavior-related abnormalities, both undesirable and desirable, based on objective, replicable EEG patterns rather than on subjective behavioral observations as presently is the case. Surely, there would again be chapters on successful use of NF with clinical disorders but, hopefully, backed by results of well-funded, large-scale, controlled research. Specific populations where such research is very much needed include prisons and Veterans Administration facilities.

There is little doubt that NF will continue to grow. If it does so in conjunction with high quality research and development, there might even be third edition chapters with titles such as "QEEG-based Neurofeedback Drastically Lowers Criminal Recidivism Rate", or "Neurofeedback as the Treatment of Choice for Traumatic Brain Injury". NF may be finally widely recognized as the safe, highly effective treatment modality the editors and chapter authors of this book consider it to be. Pleasant dreams!

Jim Evans

Introduction

The neurofeedback paradigm: by watching and listening to real-time multimedia representations of its own electrical activity, the brain can improve its functionality and even its structure.

No medications or surgical interventions at all! Because this paradigm runs counter to long-existing medical and scientific doctrine as taught in most of our medical and academic institutions of higher learning, such a new paradigm is considered an anathema and deserves to be ignored if not actually scorned by most health care power brokers in these institutions. Thomas Kuhn, the scientist philosopher, is said to have noted that before a new paradigm is accepted, most of the adherents of the older paradigm must have died. Neurofeedback, despite being 40 years of age, is still in the stage of development as a new paradigm and the health care establishment is somewhat focused on keeping it that way. I am old enough to remember that in the early 70s we established "biofeedbackers" and felt that the personal computers would never replace the sturdy, reliable "stand-alone" biofeedback units. Who could know how incredibly fast the science and development of computer technology would progress.

Over the past 30 years other new developments have been taking place. Statistics are being used in the social sciences as they had been in the "hard sciences" for some years. Physiological measurements are becoming more accurate and being judged against standards and databases which themselves are rapidly developing in specificity and comparability. Now these measures can be statistically quantified. Are measurements average, below, or above, and by how much? Not too many years ago the electrical signals generated by the brain and appearing on the scalp were considered to be too small, too random, and too meaningless to be considered seriously as a diagnostic indicator of brain activity. However, with the advent of such breakthroughs as miniaturized electronic circuits, the Fast Fourier Transform chip, complex filtering, very high impedance preamps, low noise biological amplifiers, and accurate analog to digital converters, computers can now be programed to process the EEG data in ways limited only by the creativity of the programers and hardware designers.

Equations derived from very abstract levels of mathematics can now be programed into the neurofeedback computer software to operate on the basic EEG signals as they come off the scalp. Fast evolving EEG database information can now become an integral part of the neurofeedback protocols as it is programed into the software. In real time the client's own EEG parameters can be compared to database norms and the differences projected immediately onto the multimedia computer screen and speakers. The chapters on QEEG and Z-Score feedback will inform you of some of these amazing creative efforts in the development of the databases, and the protocols which compare the actual measures with these database norms as they feed back to the clients information that will transform their lives. One chapter will enlighten the reader about the unique LORETA (Low Resolution Electromagnetic Tomography) which enables researchers and clinicians to "look" deep into the brain and define dysfunctional areas. Consider this. If the LORETA can peer into deeper brain structures to find disordered areas as they change in real time, could it not be used for feedback? Yes it can. The chapter by Sherlin will touch on this very new application.

This relatively new neurofeedback paradigm has also attracted some of the very best clinicians who are willing to invest their time and funds in becoming proficient at this craft and in so doing are helping to "push the envelope"—benefiting the clients, the designers of new neurofeedback equipment and the researchers. Using these high tech computers with their innovative software, this new breed of clinician combines a knowledge of these systems together with specialized brain physiology, psychophysiology, psychotherapy and physical therapy skills as well. We have included in this book a number of chapters by these innovative clinicians who detail their own augmented neurotherapy approaches in such areas as RAD (Reactive Attachment Disorder), OCD (Obsessive Compulsion Disorder), Asperger's Disorder, chronic pain, depression, PTSD and ADHD among others.

Most of these clinicians have risked their livelihoods and reputations to follow a path that is strewn with obstacles as is the case with all new paradigms. They do this because they fervently believe that these neurotherapy approaches really do help clients overcome seriously disordered lives, and without relying on medications or long-term psychotherapy in most cases. In this book we could only include the thoughts and efforts of a small percent of the researchers, equipment developers, programers, mathematicians and clinicians who have combined their multitude of talents to build this exciting field. We hope this text will serve not only as a source of valuable information to all professionals interested in helping individuals with these problems, but also as a tribute to those with the courage and foresight to follow along this path.

PART 1

QEEG and Neurofeedback: Basics and New Theory

Neuromodulation technologies: An attempt at classification

Siegfried Othmer, Ph.D.

EEG Institute, Woodland Hills, California, USA

I. INTRODUCTION

This chapter addresses the question of how to classify the neuromodulation effects resulting from widely differing neurofeedback approaches developed over the last four decades. We have seen a proliferation of targets and objectives to which attention is directed in the training. With regard to clinical outcomes, however, one encounters a broad zone of commonality. Why is it that the premises and technological approaches within the neurofeedback network of scholars and clinicians are so disparate, yet they largely achieve common clinical goals? This in-depth analysis may lead us closer to the "essence" of neurofeedback and provide focus for further development efforts.

In its most common applications, EEG feedback typically combines two challenges—one directed to the frequency-based organization of brain communication and one that targets inappropriate state transitions. These two challenges lead to very different rules of engagement. As such rules are unearthed, they must be understood in terms of an appropriate model of brain function. At a more philosophical level, an understanding of this whole process also takes us to the very cusp of the mind–body problem, the neural network relations that provide the nexus where our thoughts are encoded and interact directly and inseparably with network representations of psychophysiological states.

This chapter will attempt to appraise the "state of the field" at this moment. The objective is to discern the commonalities among the various approaches on the one hand, and among the clinical findings on the other. This will lead to a codification of a "minimal set of claims" that could serve to cover the commonalities among the techniques, and it will lead to a simple classification scheme for the various clinical findings. The evidence in favor of such a minimal set of claims will be adduced largely by reference. Further, the classification of the various

3

clinical findings will serve the objective of a more appropriate or natural language for the field of neurotherapy than is provided in the formalism of the Diagnostic and Statistical Manual of Mental Disorders (DSM-IV, APA, 1994).

II.   TRACING THE HISTORICAL THREADS OF NEUROFEEDBACK

A.   The alpha rhythm and "felt states"

The field of neurofeedback began in two threads of research that concerned themselves with one or another of the primary resting rhythms of the EEG. Here the local synchrony of the neuronal assemblies was such that the EEG amplitude would episodically rise above the ambient into dominant spindle-burst activity. In the case of the alpha rhythm, the feature was so obvious in the record that it became the first identified signature of the EEG in the original discovery of Hans Berger (1929). Joe Kamiya then first studied it in relation to our felt states, the question addressed being whether the human subject is able to have any kind of awareness regarding his own alpha activity (Kamiya, 1968). An affirmative finding eventually led to active reinforcement on alpha spindle incidence getting under-way (Hardt and Kamiya, 1976). The preoccupation with subjective states of aware-ness and of feeling, however, was not consonant with the prevailing Zeitgeist, and Kamiya's research found little resonance in the broader field of psychology.

B.   The sensorimotor rhythm and behavioral state

The work of Maurice Barry Sterman very consciously took a different tack. First of all, the work utilized animal subjects, so there was no question of inquiring into felt states, but that would not have been Sterman's inclination in any event. The thrust was to connect the realm of the EEG with that of overt behavior and of behavioral states. The focus became the sensorimotor rhythm, spindle-burst EEG activity localized to the cat sensorimotor cortex that was observable even in the waking state during periods of motoric stillness. It was observed that training the behavior in order to manifest the SMR spindle was not as efficient as rewarding the animal for the appear-ance of the SMR spindle and having behavioral stillness as the concomitant. Either way, however, the phenomena were coupled (Sterman et al., 1969). (For a review of this early research that ties into later neurofeedback, see Othmer et al., 1999.)

When attention later turned to the use of this simple reinforcement technique for the suppression of seizure susceptibility in humans, the training had to be done under circumstances in which the EEG was often not well-behaved as it had been in the cats. Sterman was the first to install inhibit functions on this account, but the intent was simply to assure that inappropriate triggers of a reward were suppressed.

Significantly, the focus of the work remained entirely on the elicitation of an SMR bursting response. A second issue was that the human waking EEG did not manifest SMR spindles that clearly rose above the background activity, as was the case for cats. But the training philosophy carried over, as only extreme SMR amplitude excursions were rewarded. This was expected to either end up in skewing the SMR amplitude distribution or perhaps in moving the entire distribution to higher amplitudes. The focus on seizure management placed this method within the domain of neurology, but it was unlikely then (and remains unlikely now) that the field of neurology would look favorably upon behavioral interventions. (For a review, see Sterman, 2000.)

C. EEG operant feedback and normalcy patterns

Joel Lubar was the first to employ inhibit functions with the overt objective of training toward more normal distributions. This proscriptive aspect of the training imposed its own rules on the training task, and also made for a non-prescriptive appeal to the brain that differed considerably from what was involved in the reward-based training. It also elevated the issue of EEG normalcy as a guiding principle to EEG reinforcement protocols, with profound implications for the emerging field. (For a review of this early work, see Nash, 2000.)

D. Stimulation-based treatment

Paralleling the above developments were various stimulation-based approaches to brain-state alteration, mainly using audio-visual modes. Indeed this work had its earliest precursors in the work of Adrian and Matthews (1934), who evaluated optical stimulation in their replication of Berger's rhythm. It therefore preceded EEG feedback by some three decades. But audio-visual stimulation had suffered the same fate as Kamiya's work of being taken up by a variety of enthusiasts over the years, which then spoiled it for the attentions of academic researchers. Stimulation-based techniques have since come to be seen as competitive with reward-based feedback in terms of clinical efficacy, and must therefore be included in any comprehensive appraisal of the field. The evidence for this is strongest for ADHD (Siever, 2007). In order to accommodate both neurofeedback and stimulation the more inclusive term of neuromodulation will be used below.

The development of the field subsequent to the early initiatives by Kamiya, Sterman, and Lubar has been modestly evolutionary, but the essential character of the work was laid down during the early days of the field, and threads of continuity carry through to this day. Only the stimulation-based work requires a separate treatment. The subsequent discussion is conducted more at the conceptual level rather than being constructed strictly upon the established empirical basis. Of course empirical data drive the discussion, but it would be premature to make fine distinctions on the basis of the available evidence, or to be too judgmental at this point, for example with respect to the relative efficacy of the various techniques.

Most if not all of the approaches remain in a state of both technical and tactical immaturity. Moreover, the clinical world is not restricted to using only one mode but will likely see the emergence of a multiplicity of techniques and combinations of techniques for synergistic effects. The question of which is best therefore does not even merit a response at this time. And by the time the question can be answered well, it will hopefully no longer be relevant.

III.   A CLASSIFICATION OF NEUROMODULATION TECHNOLOGIES

At the top level we may partition the field into volitional and non-volitional approaches, with feedback techniques generally falling into the former category and stimulation-based techniques into the latter. This is in line with the traditional focus on "voluntary controls" in the biofeedback literature, and with the emphasis on recruitment of the individual's efforts and intentions in the service of better self-regulation in traditional biofeedback. Clinical experience with neurofeedback, however, calls even this facile partitioning into question. Neurofeedback training "works," after all, with extremely cognitively compromised infants (e.g., victims of near-drowning) who cannot possibly have any awareness of the objective of the training. Even neurofeedback must therefore be understandable at the brain level, without any assumptions about "higher-level" engagement with the process.

Paraphrasing Robert Bly, one might argue that the "brain is here to seek its own joy," and that it will be attracted to anything that engages it, intrigues it, plays with it, or mirrors it. Given that rather unobjectionable assumption, one might argue that overt instructions to "succeed" may be optional even in the feedback paradigm. Feedback may be sufficiently rewarding intrinsically to mobilize the process even in the compromised brain. One might additionally inquire about the role of volition in Sterman's cat research (Sterman et al., 1969). Certainly the cats were strategizing to get food. When one of them happened to trigger food reward while engaged in an elaborate stretch movement, she subsequently repeated the same movement time and again in the hopes of repeating her success. The strategy might well have been counter-productive in the end. But no matter. It was rewarding enough to be sustained. Beyond experiencing food as a reward, for which no special provision needs to be made, nothing more appears to be required. It seems that we cannot give volition an essential or even an exalted role in EEG feedback.

On the other hand, perhaps not much is lost, as the following anecdote illustrates. A person undergoing training with NeuroCarePro software (see www.zengar.com) expressed his satisfaction with the experience at the end of the session, but could not help voicing his irritation with the fact that the CD he was listening to kept interrupting the flow of the music: "I feel much better, sleeping well, but can you ask her to use a new CD that doesn't have skips?"

He had clearly not even been aware that the skips were the bearers of information relevant to his brain—in fact the only ones his brain was receiving—and yet the process clearly influenced him. Not only was he annoyed with the discontinuities in the music, but his brain was also. And the brain had more information to work with than he did. It did not take that exquisite correlation engine long to figure out that it was part of an interactive system in which it was playing an active role. And just as the brain will incorporate a tennis racket as an extension of the arm as soon as it is picked up, the brain will rapidly appropriate the feedback loop as part of its sphere of influence. Clearly we must understand neurofeedback at the brain level. Once that task is accomplished, we can readmit the role of volition to the discussion, as it can strongly enrich the feedback process in most real-world situations.

A less ambiguous distinction may lie in the recognition that feedback is cognitively mediated and stimulation-based approaches are more directly brain-mediated. In nearly all of conventional neurofeedback, the feedback signal is processed as "information," whereas stimulation is experienced by the brain as a direct perturbation of its activity. The feedback signal is processed along with all other news from the environment, and it is appraised similarly. In time, a correlation becomes apparent to the CNS between some feature of the information stream and some aspect of its own internal activity. By contrast, in frequency-based stimulation techniques we are simply creating excess (or in some instances reduced) neuronal synchrony, which then has implications for brain function downstream to which the CNS in turn reacts.

In the feedback case, the work is subject to all of our cognitive and attentional limitations, our susceptibility to distractions, and to the vote of our emotions as to whether we are actually committed to the process. In the stimulation case, the brain has no option but to respond. Repetitively pulsed light sources will ineluctably impose their periodicity on visual cortex, from whence they are propagated throughout cortex. Given the simplicity involved in stimulation-based methods, one might well ask why conventional neurofeedback has not already been largely displaced. A rather general observation appears to hold for neuromodulation technologies, namely that newly emerging techniques don't really displace older ones but rather add to them. It seems that old protocols never die.

A different question therefore needs to be asked, which is why is there so much speciation occurring in EEG feedback at all? What are the evolutionary niches that allow all of the techniques to survive unto the present day? Perhaps we are just in an early proliferation phase, with consolidation to follow later. This issue will hopefully be clarified in what follows. At any rate, our present task of simply classifying the various techniques is challenged by all of the diversity that is already extant.

A simple classification based on the above considerations is that of "active" versus "passive" techniques. We are not writing on a blank page, however, and past usage has tended to regard stimulation techniques as active interventions, and neurofeedback as passive. A more organic view of the matter would hold that the point of reference should be the client, who is the passive recipient of the stimulation and the potentially active participant in feedback.

Focusing then on the "active" technique of feedback, a major division could be established on the basis of whether the success criterion is defined very narrowly or broadly. The former may be referred to as *prescriptive* and the latter as *non-prescriptive*. Reward-based training targeting a particular EEG frequency band would be considered prescriptive. Success can only be had if an amplitude objective is met within a narrow band of frequencies. Inhibit-based training is an example of non-prescriptive training. The brain is simply being alerted to an adverse state of affairs, and it is given no particular hint as to how to remedy the problem.

The same partitioning could also be labeled "prescriptive" and "proscriptive" training. In the latter, the brain is simply being notified of some transgression or another with respect to certain established bounds of EEG phenomenology. Deviation (in EEG terms) is deemed to index deviance (in behavioral terms) or dysregulation (in neurophysiological terms). The CNS is left to its own devices to sort things out. At the present state of maturity of our field, prescriptive training tends to be frequency-based, and proscriptive training tends to be event-based. If the dysregulation status of the person is found to have worsened beyond some threshold value, by one or more EEG criteria, then attention is drawn to the event and rewards are withheld for the duration.

A.   Slow cortical potential training

Where does Slow Cortical Potential training fit into this picture? This is the technique, developed by the Tübingen group led by Niels Birbaumer, in which the trainee is asked to alter his or her low-frequency EEG transiently by several microvolts within an 8-second window (Strehl *et al.*, 2006). The rewarded change can be either positive or negative, depending on the assigned goal in a particular trial. Acquisition of control is the principal objective here. The main applications to date have been to locked-in syndrome (for communication purposes), to seizure management, and to ADHD. The impression one gets is that the technique is just as diagnostically non-specific as frequency-based reinforcement. The work has been helpful for the abatement of migraines, for example (Kropp *et al.*, 2002). We have here a case of event-based training that is prescriptive in the prescriptive/proscriptive partitioning while being non-prescriptive in the prescriptive vs. non-prescriptive division. That is to say, the CNS is left to sort out how the training objective is to be met.

B.   Stimulation-based technologies

How do stimulation-based technologies fit into these categories? Standard audio-visual entrainment has tended toward stimulation of particular EEG frequencies, and as such falls into the category of prescriptive modes of neuromodulation. More recently, however, the technologies have added swept modes of operation, with the general goal of stimulation without a specific target in terms of frequency. These modes of operation come closer to being in the non-prescriptive category.

The derivative technologies of the ROSHI and the LENS, on the other hand, use entrainment techniques effectively for the purpose of disentrainment. The original ROSHI design would pick out the dominant EEG activity in the low-frequency regime and apply a stimulation that was out of phase with the ongoing signal, and thus bring about its dephasing and disruption (Ibric and Davis, 2007). The LENS effectively does the same thing by means of electromagnetic stimulation with a carrier frequency in the megaHertz region, modulated by the EEG signal of interest (Ochs, 2006). In this case, however, the disruption is achieved with a frequency shift rather than a phase shift. Over short time intervals, a frequency shift and a phase shift amount effectively to the same thing.

The particulars probably don't matter nearly as much as ROSHI and LENS practitioners may be inclined to believe. It is the process of disruption that matters. That being the case, these techniques should be lumped into the bin of non-prescriptive modes. The techniques are applied identically regardless of the diagnostic presentation. Once a training site has been selected, these techniques are referenced entirely to the instantaneous behavior of the EEG. Consequently, an understanding of these methods should be possible largely with reference to EEG phenomenology itself. It is true that adjustments in clinical approach (i.e., with respect to site selection and hierarchy of targeting) may be made on the basis of the response to the training. But that is only as it should be, and it does not gainsay the observation that the training is driven entirely by the instantaneous EEG.

The LENS in particular has undergone a developmental pathway that is highly instructive for our more general purposes. Len Ochs observed over the years that the response to the stimulation was far greater than most practitioners were expecting. Already in feedback practitioners were encountering negative effects associated with lingering too long with a protocol that retrospectively can be judged non-optimal. The same was true for the stimulation techniques, only possibly more so. In response, Ochs trimmed back the stimulus duration farther and farther, each time finding that the clinical effectiveness remained robust while the probability of an adverse outcome diminished. The latter never declined to zero, however.

One had the impression that if prescriptive neurofeedback were a rifle that we are increasingly learning how to aim, then LENS would be a cannon whose aim remained ambiguous. The technique in essence remains non-prescriptive, and in application of such a powerful technique to a severely dysregulated nervous system, the outcome must of necessity remain somewhat unpredictable.

The development of the ROSHI was even more overtly in the direction of non-prescriptive training. With the personal ROSHI, the stimulus was provided over a range of EEG frequencies pseudo-randomly selected, and delivered over brief intervals. The principle underlying this approach was that of stochastic resonance. A finite probability exists that the stimulus at any given time would have the right frequency and phase properties to effect the desired disentrainment that in the original ROSHI had been so carefully engineered. At worst one suffers a loss in clinical efficiency, which is not relevant in the personal use applications for which the device was mainly intended.

There are other aspects to the ROSHI design that remain proprietary, and I will honor the wishes of the designer and refrain from bringing these elements into the discussion. Significantly, the personal ROSHI stimulates both hemispheres differentially, thus introducing a phase disparity with which the brain must come to terms. This challenge in the phase domain is intrinsic to its design, and probably accounts for its broad efficacy.

One might reasonably object that a finite probability also exists that the stimulus phase would be such as to induce entrainment rather than disentrainment. It turns out that this does not really matter! When formal attention was finally given to the audio-visual entrainment technique some years ago by Lubar's group, it was found that after the stimulus period was over, the EEG would tend to show disentrainment effects (Frederick et al., 1999). The implications are obvious: When the brain is subjected to the interference we call entrainment, it yields to the stimulus but also mounts a defense. The defense is the learned response, and that is what lingers after the stimulus is over. Fortuitously, we are presented with the delightful paradox that the right outcome does not depend strongly on the particulars of the stimulus. It is the disruption itself that matters. So, if standard neurofeedback is the rifle, and the LENS is the cannon, then the ROSHI is the shotgun.

IV. THE EVOLUTION OF STANDARD REWARD AND INHIBIT-BASED NEUROFEEDBACK

The exciting developments over the years with the ROSHI and the LENS leave one with the impression that a significant advance over standard neurofeedback practice may have been achieved. Certainly these techniques have added significantly to the clinical arsenal. But in the meantime neurofeedback has seen its own evolution. To complete the picture, these developments also need to be discussed.

The rise of quantitative EEG analysis within the field of neurofeedback that took place in the early nineties had a significant influence on the subsequent development of clinical neurofeedback, as well as determining how the whole process was to be understood. The mandate of quantitative analysis of the EEG is to establish the stationary properties of the system, furnishing measures that will hopefully be valid even the day, the week, and the month after the data are acquired. This focus on the steady-state properties of the EEG already was fraught with implications that were not appreciated generally at the time.

QEEG information is acquired using either Fourier transform or other similar transform techniques (e.g., Gabor). Here a sufficiently long time sample is converted into its constituent frequencies. "Sufficiently long" means that the time window must accommodate the lowest frequencies of interest without compromise. Typically 0.5 Hz is taken as the low end of the range of interest, and at least a half cycle needs to fit comfortably within the window in order to be represented properly. A windowing function is usually installed to minimize aliasing effects, which further narrows the effective length of the time window. A proper representation of 0.5 Hz therefore mandates a time window greater than one second.

Now, it will be recalled that Sterman's original interest was in recognizing individual spindle-burst activity in the cat, and the same objective was later translated to human subjects. The steady-state amplitude of the EEG in the SMR-band was never of interest at all. So the question arises: How well do transform-based systems do when the task is to recognize brief transients? The answer is that they don't do well at all. This should be no surprise. The whole intent is to furnish data on the steady-state properties of the EEG, and an analysis scheme oriented to that task cannot be expected also to do well with transient data. In the real EEG one might see several SMR/beta spindles over the course of one sampling window of nominally 1 sec. These are averaged over in the spectral calculation, and individuality is lost (Fig. 1.1).

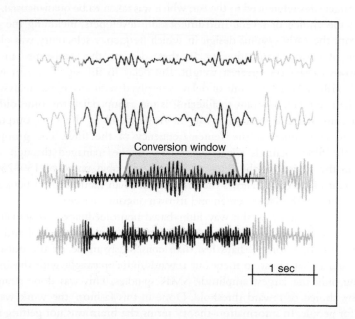

FIGURE 1.1   The data sampling process for transformation from the time to the frequency domain is represented. A finite conversion window, with the windowing function shown as shaded, illustrates the uneasy compromise that needs to be made between the conflicting demands of reporting EEG change promptly and of representing steady-state values. From top to bottom, the graphs reflect the spectral bands of 0–30 Hz; 4–7 Hz; 15–18 Hz; and 22–30 Hz. Gains have been individually adjusted for readability.

Consider further what happens when a lonely spindle-burst of high amplitude, the very thing Sterman was targeting for success, comes along in the signal stream. First it encounters the windowing function, which means that its full expression in the transform is delayed (hence delaying the issuing of a reward). Some time later it leaves the sampling window (in a subsequent time sample), causing the signal amplitude to decline as it does so. But this decline in signal amplitude does not reflect what is happening at that moment, as one would wish; instead it reflects what happened a second ago. So, we have the disagreeable situation that what enters the window as signal inevitably exits the window as artifact some time later. The simple expedient of moving toward transform-based analysis has cut the signal-to-noise ratio in half for highly dynamic signals such as the EEG (unless an asymmetric windowing function is employed).

A second change that accompanied the transition to QEEG-driven training was the conversion to referential placement from the bipolar montages that Sterman and Lubar had used in their initial research. If the QEEG measures were going to inform neurofeedback then the montages had best be compatible. The localization of brain events that was becoming possible led to a conceptual change in how neurofeedback was to be done, with an increased emphasis on the training of steady-state amplitudes at single target sites referenced to the ear, which was taken to be quasi-neutral.

It was the choice of several instrumentation developers, including the author, to stay with the early systems design in which frequency selectivity was obtained by means of narrow-band filtering. In these designs, the "real-time" incoming signal always carries the greatest weight. But delay in the signal stream was not thereby banished. Some amount of delay is involved with any signal analysis technique. The parameter relevant to filtering is the group delay, the time difference between comparable signatures in the raw signal and in the filter output. This quantity is determined at the center frequency of the filter. The group delay through the filter chain is a parameter that can be managed through suitable choices in the design of the filter to be in a tolerable range of 150–250 msec. This amount of delay still allows the brain to make an identification between the emerging data on the video screen and its own ongoing activity.

A significant change in the way filter-based neurofeedback was actually conducted occurred over a period of years. The change was incremental and cumulative, and was therefore perhaps less than consciously made. At the outset both Sterman and Lubar chose to mete out rewards quite sparingly, with the intent of rewarding only the largest amplitude SMR spindles. This was done straightforwardly by choice of reward threshold. Done in this fashion, the work was quite tedious for people. In information-theory terms, the brain was not getting a lot of information to work with.

The simple expedient of increasing the reward incidence made the training much more lively, engaging, and rewarding. The payoff in clinical efficiency was dramatic. But over time this success was taken to what appeared to be ridiculous extremes. Thresholds were being set so that the reward incidence was at the 70–85% and even

90% levels. One was reminded of modern American schooling where nearly every-body gets an A. The clinical results were holding up, but what was being discriminated here if 90% of what was happening in the reward band garnered passing marks?

The game had in fact changed underfoot in a manner that was probably not fully appreciated at the time. Typically, the discrete rewards were limited in incidence to a rate of two per second. With the rewards now plentiful, they were arriving in a regular cadence to which the brain rapidly accommodated. With the rewards having become the expectation, the attended event became the occasional dropout of the rewards. (This is reminiscent of the odd-ball design in evoked potential research, in which the occasional odd-ball stimulus evokes the attentional resources as reflected in increased P300 amplitudes.) Effectively, the discrete rewards had come to perform a function we associate with inhibits! In the meantime, the role of the reward had been assumed by the analog signal in the reward band, which was being continuously displayed on the video screen.

The CNS was now in continuous engagement with the analytical representation of its own activity on the screen. The reward here is intrinsic to the process, and is entirely independent of threshold. Given a chance to engage with its own activity, the brain will quite naturally be inclined to do so. The problem of boredom is resolved by the simple expedient of enlarging the size, the continuity, the promptness, and the salience of the signal stream. The brain will not fail to be interested in its own activity.

In consequence of the above developments, clinical practice then followed the strengths of the respective methods of signal analysis. The relative strength of the filter-based approach was in tracking the dynamics in the reward band, so the preoccupation of filter-based systems has remained with reward-based training. The relative strength of the transform-based systems was in discerning change in ambient band amplitudes with slightly longer effective integration times, and thus the focus of QEEG-based training has been increasingly on the inhibit strategy, with reliance on amplitude-based training.

V. RESONANT-FREQUENCY TRAINING

Although reward-based training has largely been performed under the rubric of SMR/beta training, it has been clear for many years now that people respond quite variedly to the standard protocols. This turns out to be largely a matter of reward frequency, so that the response can be tuned by the mere expedient of adjusting the reward frequency. This diminishes the special role that SMR-band reinforcement has played in our clinical work and in our conceptions. In practice, of course, standard SMR-band training has remained prominent within the field, but that is largely because most practitioners feel obligated to maintain standardization of protocols to the extent possible, and in consequence they have not yet investigated the frequency optimization hypothesis.

It is the responsiveness to optimized-frequency training that makes this training approach practical. The immediate response of the reinforcement is in terms of state shifts in the arousal, attentional, and affective domains. These state shifts are readily perceived within a matter of a minute or two or three by anyone who responds sensitively to this training. Reports on perceived state change are elicited by the therapist, and on this basis the reward frequency is adjusted on the timescale of minutes. As the optimum reward frequency is approached, the trainee achieves a more optimal state in terms of arousal, vigilance, alertness, and euthymia. At the same time, the strength of the training increases perceptibly. For those familiar with the theory of resonant systems, this maps out a conventional resonance curve, and it is our impression that the person's felt states and the responsivity to reinforcement map out essentially the same curve.

This frequency-dependent behavior is shown in terms of a standard resonance curve in Fig. 1.2. This curve traces out the frequency response of the "real" component of the resonant system. Both positive feeling states and response to training are thought to be reflected in this single curve, as sketched in Fig. 1.3. In any physical resonant system, however, there is also the "imaginary" component to consider, and this is mapped out as well in Fig. 1.2. We have some tantalizing evidence that this quadrature component shows up in terms of an enhanced sensitivity near the resonant frequency, and may be experienced in terms of adverse feeling states. A crude analogy may have to serve us here: the relative calm at the resonant frequency may be like the eye of the hurricane, but turbulence is maximized in the vicinity of that eye.

Since this behavior can be observed in different people across the entire frequency band from 0.01 Hz to 45 Hz, it is likely that the same general organizing principles apply for every part of the band. That is to say, all spindle-burst activity must be organized as resonant systems, even down to the lowest frequency we have characterized. On the other hand, in each person who is sensitive to this training, one frequency band appears to stand out above all others in terms of its relevance to training self-regulation in that individual. The original finding that training one particular band, namely the SMR band, has quite broad (i.e., non-specific) implications for self-regulation status now stands on a more solid foundation, albeit with the proviso that the particular frequency is unique to the individual. The SMR band has just lost its special status in this approach.

VI.   AN ATTEMPT TO ACHIEVE SYNTHESIS

The EEG is organized to a level of detail and precision that is difficult to discern with our conventional measurement tools. Regardless of what elements of the signal we choose to focus on, yet others must remain out of focus or off-screen entirely. If one chooses to view the EEG with high-frequency resolution, for example, the segregation into distinct, narrow, rigorously demarcated frequency

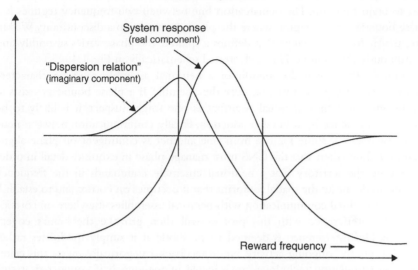

FIGURE 1.2   A response curve is shown for a resonant system. It is assumed that spindle-burst formation in the EEG exhibits the properties of a resonant system. The real and imaginary components of the system response are plotted vertically. The feedback challenge is sufficiently frequency-specific that in sensitive responders an opportunity presents itself to map out the resonance curve for an individual. One EEG frequency clearly dominates the response in such individuals.

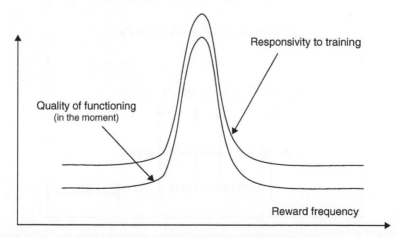

FIGURE 1.3   Both the responsiveness to the reinforcement (responsivity) and the subjective quality of functioning of the individual appear to map out the real component of a resonance curve as the reinforcement frequency is incremented episodically through the band. These dependences are observed on highly sensitive responders, but are likely to hold more generally.

bands is quite striking. Since this cannot be trivial to arrange, it must be important to brain function. The demarcation line between two frequency regimes is a phase boundary, i.e., a region where the phase can undergo a discontinuity. Within a particular frequency range that defines a spindle, the phase varies smoothly and continuously throughout. This is illustrated schematically in Fig. 1.4.

Similarly, the spatial distribution of a neuronal assembly must be characterized by a smooth phase variation over the assembly. If a phase boundary exists at the margins of such a neuronal assembly, as one might suspect, it is likely to be obscured in practice by volume conduction. Finally, communication between neuronal assemblies at some remove from one another is contingent on phase alignment. It follows, then, that the CNS must manage phase in exquisite detail in order to regulate the territory that a neuronal ensemble commands in the frequency domain, to delineate the spatial footprint that it occupies on cortex, and to establish and maintain distal communication with neuronal assemblies elsewhere on cortex.

Subtle interference with this process will then provoke the brain's cogent response. The interference is deemed to be subtle if it simply modulates rather than disrupts the ongoing activity. Neurofeedback categorically meets this criterion, and stimulation techniques are capable of meeting it if conducted at sufficiently low drive levels. Both feedback and stimulation techniques are strongest

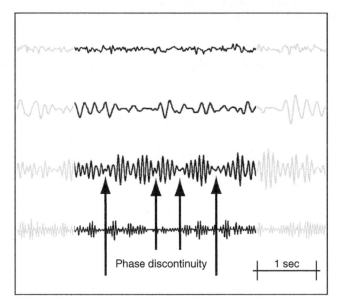

FIGURE 1.4   The phase discontinuities observed between spindle-bursts in the 15–18 Hz band make the case that these spindle-bursts represent functionally independent cortical events. Under that assumption, it makes sense to target the individual bursts that are under active management by the brain, as opposed to targeting averages over independent events. This calls for a highly responsive feedback system with the largest possible signal bandwidth.

if they impinge upon the aspect of brain function that is under the immediate management of the brain, and that is the relative phase or, equivalently, the instantaneous frequency of the packet.

This model for neuromodulation accounts for the power of the LENS and ROSHI approaches, and for the power of the optimized reward frequency training in feedback. It also accounts for the observation in QEEG-based work that coherence training appears stronger than amplitude-based training. In LENS, the stimulus provides the phase reference. In the case of the ROSHI, the stimulus phase differs between the two hemispheres. In the frequency-optimized feedback, which is typically conducted with a single channel in bipolar montage, the one site is the reference for the other. The same holds true in coherence training with two-channel montage: one site represents the phase reference for the other.

In EEG training with a bipolar montage, the net reward signal is a strong function of the relative phase. This is an essential point, and it is not an obvious one. The reader is referred to a detailed treatment of this topic in Putman and Othmer (2006). By virtue of common-mode rejection in the differential amplifier, activity that is synchronous between the two sites is not seen at the output, and therefore cannot ever be rewarded. And if it cannot be rewarded, then with respect to everything else it is effectively being inhibited. The net effect is to reward differentiation of activity between the two sites, which is the real take-away message. The approach was first investigated with inter-hemispheric placements at homotopic sites, which we used rather exclusively for some years (Othmer and Othmer, 2007). Clinical results in terms of continuous performance tests have been published for this method, demonstrating improved outcomes with respect to earlier data (Putman et al., 2005).

Looked at in the above way, even this very specifically targeted reward-based training can be seen as having a proscriptive rather than a prescriptive aspect: the state of synchrony, of phase conformity, is proscribed. Conversely, the technique rewards "everything but the condition of synchrony." And since the only thing precluded from success is the synchrony condition, with respect to the broad remaining phase domain the technique can even be seen as having a non-prescriptive aspect as well: the phase relationship is not being tightly constrained.

The training itself amounts to a subtle, continuous challenge that lies largely in the phase domain. It must be acknowledged at this point that the dominance of phase is not obvious from the mathematics. Indeed, amplitude differences between the two sites play just as strongly into the net reward. Since the relative role of amplitude and phase in real-life situations is not obvious, their respective roles can be clarified with a Monte Carlo calculation in which the experimental situation is simulated in all of its natural variability. This has been done with the assumption of randomness in relative phase and in the amplitude at the two sites (Putman and Othmer, 2006). A nearly complete exclusion of rewards is found for relative phase less than 40 degrees in this simulation. In real EEGs there will be some finite correlation in amplitudes, and that only serves to strengthen the posited phase dependence. (If the variance in the amplitude ratio is pinned, then the actual variance must be accounted for in the phase.)

Looking carefully at real EEGs also makes it clear that phase is often the more dynamic variable of the two. The sequential independent spindle-bursts one sees with a fixed narrow-band filter (as shown in Fig. 1.1) may represent neuronal assemblies of slowly varying amplitude that are simply migrating in frequency through the filter band. Others undulate back and forth within the filter pass-band. What really makes the difference is that our experimental situation is so arranged as to highlight phase variations, with the result that these will come to the fore in the reward schema. The argument goes as follows: A narrow-band filter can be seen for our purposes as a transducer of frequency fluctuations into amplitude fluctuations. Frequency variation and phase fluctuations are obviously directly related. Dynamic, continuous reward-based training using narrow-band filters attempts to shape the EEG frequency distribution toward the middle of the resonance curve, with often immediate and sometimes trenchant consequences for the person's state. These factors are in play even in ostensibly single-site amplitude training with referential placement (because references are not silent).

Bipolar montage then further augments the role of narrow-band filters as phase discriminants because the amplitudes at the two sites are now more correlated than in referential montage, which shifts the burden of variability more onto the phase. In typical application, the bipolar montage will be deployed either at near-neighbor sites or at homotopic sites. In these cases, the correlation of amplitudes (i.e., comodulation) is typically enhanced with respect to arbitrary site combinations.

Of course we aren't looking at normal EEGs in the usual clinical situation. In the presence of dysregulation, we typically see enhanced EEG amplitudes, particularly in the low-frequency regime. Enhanced amplitudes can be modeled equivalently as excess local synchrony. Bipolar training in the midst of such activity can then be seen as disruptive of that activity, tending us toward better function. The fear about bipolar training under such adverse circumstances is entirely misplaced. In practice, it is all a question of finding the optimum response frequency. Ironically, that criterion enforces an even tighter constraint: *All reward frequencies may conceivably be contraindicated, or at least disfavored—except for the narrow band that is favored.*

Sometimes, of course, QEEG data reveal deficits in connectivity between sites rather than excesses. Would the standard bipolar training be a mistake under such circumstances, in that promotion of desynchronization is not called for? There is no evidence yet that this presents a problem. Just as the sign of the phase challenge is a secondary issue in LENS, so we believe it to be in feedback as well. Efficacy lies in the subtle challenge to the system, often surprisingly indifferent to the particulars. The intent is to normalize the pathways of communication, and this can be done by challenging them in one way or another. The brain will take it from there. Any kind of response by the brain to the provocation is likely to go in the direction of improved regulation. We don't have to make the pearl. We only have to provide the grain of sand.

The above argument has made the case that clinical efficacy is broadly available in neurofeedback. Clinical efficiency, however, is an entirely different matter.

As already implied in the discussion of optimized frequency training, the greatest clinical efficiency may be highly constrained in terms of protocol.

The implication of findings with LENS, with ROSHI, with frequency-optimized bipolar training, and with coherence-based training is that phase-based targeting is more responsive, and more availing, than amplitude-based training. To be effective, the feedback signal must provide information on the relevant timescale, and in that regard we have three timescales to consider. There is first the timescale of the conversion interval in Fast Fourier transform analysis on which QEEG-based training is based. This approach was first featured in the Lexicor unit and is currently used in NeuroCarePro (Gabor transform). Secondly, there is the timescale of individual spindle-burst on which most dynamic training using filtering functions operates. This is on the order of a third to half a second. Thirdly, there is the timescale of as little as a single cycle of the EEG at the relevant frequency—the timescale on which the LENS can operate. At a typical application frequency in the theta range of frequencies, the timescale may be only a fourth to a seventh of a second.

There has been an overall trend toward dynamic training and away from the QEEG-driven focus on reinforcing band amplitudes. This trend has even asserted itself in inhibit-based training, which has been the strength of QEEG-guided training. Over the years there has been a gradual shift from the use of fixed thresholds to dynamic or adaptive thresholding. This was initially driven by a need to keep the level of difficulty within bounds. Software was reworked so as to maintain the level of difficulty fairly constant. The thresholds "breathed" with the ebb and flow of things on longer timescales.

In NeuroCarePro this idea was taken even further. By making the thresholds even more dynamic, inhibit-based training in that system became more like transient detection that zeroes in on inappropriate state shifts. This is shown in Fig. 1.5. Effectively we have a slope detector, or derivative detector, which calls attention to unusual excursions in variability. Once again, it is more important to alert the brain immediately to its incipient transgression than to merely inform it as to levels of EEG amplitudes. The brain does not react as well to old news. So in NeuroCarePro the inhibits have become a matter of event detection. One expects that elevated EEG amplitudes are correlated with elevated variability as well. But even if that is not the case, elevated variability makes the better target in any event because it focuses on the present moment.

The nearly universal trend within the field has clearly been from stationary properties of the EEG to EEG dynamics, from discrete rewards to continuous reinforcement, from static to dynamic thresholds, from amplitude-based training to phase-based training. The considerations for effective training have become increasingly referenced to the EEG itself, and in that regard we have moved to feedback "at the speed of thought," operating with the highest response speed of which the signal analysis routines are capable. The emphasis has been on the ongoing dynamics within the reward band (which can be anywhere) and on how the brain handles state transitions. This sounds rather far removed from where we

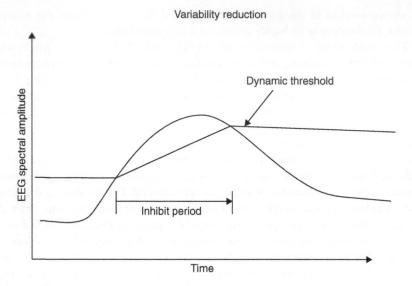

FIGURE 1.5   The process of dynamic thresholding is illustrated for a large excursion in EEG spectral amplitude in the inhibit band. Since the percentage of time over which the inhibit may be engaged is kept fixed, a triggered inhibit will immediately cause an adjustment in the instantaneous threshold. The result is that actual inhibit periods will always be finite. Effectively, we have a transient detector that alerts us to the initiation of an excursion into dysregulation.

started, which was with a concern with the resting states of the system, the alpha rhythm and the sensorimotor rhythm. The story is not complete, however. We have in fact omitted from the discussion one basic approach that has been with us since the beginning of the field, and that is Alpha/Theta and alpha synchrony training.

VII.   ALPHA/THETA AND SYNCHRONY TRAINING

Alpha/Theta training, which involves reinforcement in both the alpha and theta bands—typically under eyes-closed conditions—has not been drawn into the discussion up to this point because the implicit focus thus far has been on the application of neuromodulation to the enhancement of brain function. The principal objective in Alpha/Theta training is instead to facilitate certain psychological states that promote healing from trauma reactions, recovery from addiction, etc. (For application to addiction recovery, see Scott *et al.*, 2005.) Inevitably, however, subjecting someone to these reinforcements for hours on end may also have a residual training component. For yet others, the mere exposure to these reinforcements may steep them back into their prior pathology. This is particularly the case for those who exhibit alpha intrusion into their sleep EEG, and those with a history of minor traumatic brain injury.

The promotion of alpha and theta amplitudes effectively enhances local synchrony. Unfortunately, elevated synchrony also characterizes much of the severe pathology that we encounter in clinical practice. For many who could in principle benefit from Alpha/Theta training, the reinforcement of alpha and theta bands is a somewhat hazardous terrain. It is also for this reason that the bias of bipolar training toward desynchronization of the EEG makes it preferable as a starting protocol. The bipolar training is always done first, with the result that even vulnerable individuals may then tolerate the Alpha/Theta training later.

Whereas this cautionary tone reflects our own experience over the last 20 years, it is also true that long-term practitioners such as Lester Fehmi have used alpha training routinely in their practice to good effect with a clinical population for many years—more than 30 in the case of Les Fehmi. From the early days, however, Fehmi has used a different approach, which may account for his success on the one hand, and the absence of adverse reports on the other: multi-channel synchrony training (Fehmi, 2007). He was not alone in this. The work of Jim Hardt has also relied on multi-channel synchrony since the early days (Hardt, 1978). And the very first commercially viable computerized instrument to do EEG feedback was developed by Adam Crane on the principle of four-channel synchrony. In fact the first clinical practice in EEG feedback on any significant commercial scale consisted almost entirely of four-channel synchrony training performed on American Biotec's Capscan Prism 5 (Crane, 2007).

Just how is it, then, that enhancing synchrony using straightforward alpha reinforcement with a single channel can be troublesome, whereas promoting even greater synchrony with multiple channels is not similarly fraught with hazards? Most likely it is an issue of control. The precision of control that is required to garner rewards in four- and five-channel synchrony training is simply not available to the injured brain. Facilitating local synchrony with a single-channel setup does not discriminate against the unruly alpha and theta that we observe in the dysregulated brain. Multi-channel synchrony training, on the other hand, promotes global synchrony, which represents a much more specific challenge that is difficult for the dysfunctional brain to organize.

In the final analysis, then, alpha synchrony training makes the same case that has just been made for SMR/beta training and its progeny. Single-channel training of band amplitudes is trumped by multi-site training that focuses on the training of phase relationships. And when such a highly specific phase challenge is mounted, the consequences are not only for enhanced experiences of deep states in the moment but also for improved self-regulation as a learned response.

Another point of similarity is that the training is event-based. The question is one of enhancing phase conformity whenever an alpha spindle is observed in cortex. It is not a matter of training up ambient alpha amplitudes. The analogies go further. Self-regulation is enhanced broadly with reinforcement at only a single frequency, with a technique that uses standard placements and rises above issues of localization of function. In this case, moreover, there isn't much question about the optimum reinforcement frequency. In practice, it is to be found within ± 1 Hz of 10.5 Hz in nearly everyone.

In Les Fehmi's mechanization of synchrony training, the reinforcement is delivered with every cycle of the alpha rhythm that meets criterion. It turns out that the timing of the delivery of the reward signal with respect to the underlying alpha signal is crucial. With the phase delay optimized, the reward pulse serves to augment the next cycle of the alpha spindle. This is firstly another demonstration that "phase matters." Secondly, we have here a stimulation aspect to what is fundamentally a feedback paradigm.

In pursuit of the hypothesis that synchrony training may represent a natural complement to bipolar training, we have begun an investigation into the clinical utility of simple two-channel synchrony training of the resting rhythms of the brain, alpha and SMR. For some years already, we have been doing Alpha/ Theta training with two-channel synchrony at P3 and P4, with results that clearly exceed the prior work with single-channel training at Pz. Synchrony training in the alpha band may additionally have its own rationale in the context of awake-state training, as distinct from the induction of deep states in Alpha/Theta.

SMR synchrony training has been evaluated at C3 and C4, with results that have been rewarding in a number of clients. The training tends to be optimized at 14 Hz ± 0.5 Hz, but the sample so far has been small. This may be seen as a derivative of Lubar's and Tansey's reinforcement of SMR at Cz. Driven forward by such success, we have also looked at synchrony training at frontal sites, where frontal midline theta presents an inviting target. Jay Gunkelman has been recommending frontal midline theta rewards for some years now, and that kindled our interest. Indeed, synchrony training at 7 Hz using F3 and F4 placement has had salutary effects in some clients.

It is with synchrony training that the "standard bands" may find their full clinical utility. With bipolar training promoting engagement and activation, synchrony training moves in the direction of disengagement and of resting states. Access to both is required for good brain function. The preliminary findings with SMR synchrony training may (if confirmed) lead to a reinterpretation of Sterman's early results with seizure management. Clinical effectiveness may be attributable more to the desynchronization of the EEG from the use of bipolar placement at C3–T3 than to the focus on the SMR frequency specifically. Moreover, Sterman's current emphasis on keeping rewards relatively rare, and mandating a refractory period after the reward, may be seen as an attempt to promote transient local SMR synchrony with a single-channel referential montage. The rewarded event must be clearly distinguishable from the ambient background.

VIII. GENERAL SELF-REGULATION AND SPECIFIC DYSFUNCTIONS

Neurofeedback had to assert itself early on in a distinctly inhospitable environment. In response, researchers attempted to accommodate by being exceedingly conservative in their claims. Meanwhile, evidence was proliferating even then that the standard protocols were not specific treatments for either ADHD or seizure disorder but instead improved brain function in considerable generality. As feedback researchers were already being hounded by the placebo ghost, it would not serve to mention that neurofeedback was starting to look like a panacea as well. However, the refinement of protocol-based training discussed in this chapter has continued to enlarge the clinical scope of the work. Protocol-based neurofeedback was becoming a generalized approach toward improved self-regulation. The complementary approach of QEEG-based training appeared, for most applications, to be an unnecessary complication.

In many cases, specific functional deficits largely resolved even with the standard approaches. The first priority therefore was to do the best possible job with general self-regulation training. And in the sequencing of training objectives it is prudent to put the deepest and most basic dysregulations first, and to attend to more specific dysfunctions later, if indeed any are left to attend to. In conventional biofeedback, the recent finding that heart rate variability training is more effective in resolving myofascial pain syndrome and asthma susceptibility than more targeted approaches is yet another confirming instance of general self-regulation training trumping the more specific biofeedback approaches.

But sometimes specific deficits remain to be attended to, and QEEG analysis has been shown to be worthwhile in identifying suitable targets for training. In the refinement of QEEG-based approaches over the years there has been a gradual movement from amplitude-based training to the normalization of coherence relationships. This approach has been researched most thoroughly by Kirt Thornton, with a principal focus on specific learning disabilities and on traumatic brain injury. The general thrust of his approach is to work specific linkages that are identified with QEEG measurement under challenge conditions. Remediation is achieved predominantly with coherence up-training in the high-frequency regime (Thornton, 2006).

The Thornton method is nicely complementary to the other techniques so far discussed, which nearly all tend to have their greatest strengths at low EEG frequencies. A partitioning suggests itself that the low EEG frequencies govern the regulation of persistent states, whereas the high-frequency training impinges upon functions that are only episodically engaged in cognitive or other activity. The basic regulatory functions include arousal regulation; affect regulation; autonomic set-point and balance; motor system excitability; interoception; attentional repertoire and executive function; and working memory. The higher frequency training impinges more on the sensorium and on cognitive processes.

The principal hazard at low EEG frequencies is excessive coherence in the injured, the traumatized, the genetically disadvantaged, or the otherwise dysregulated brain. Such excess coherence at low frequency is often associated with brain instability, and hence with gross mental dysfunction, the more intractable psychopathologies, and behavioral volatility. By contrast, the principal hazard at high frequency is lack of task engagement, characterized by dropout of the expected coherence dynamics under challenge. This failure to function is often detrimental only to the affected person, and may be benign as far as the rest of the world is concerned. Hence it may be missed by caregivers, school personnel, mental health practitioners, and even by the person at issue.

Unsurprisingly, then, what populates mental health practices are the problems of general dysregulation, and these should indeed command our primary attentions. But a thorough-going application of all the tools of neuroregulation would include the more specific approaches deployed by Thornton and others.

Finally, coherence-normalization training is also used prominently by clinicians such as Jonathan Walker and Robert Coben (Walker *et al.*, 2007; Coben and Padolsky, 2007; see also Chapter 5 in this volume). The work was pioneered by the late Joe Horvat (2007). Significantly, however, the focus here is typically on the largest deviations observed in baseline coherence measures, which tend to show up at low EEG frequencies. In contrast to the work of Thornton, the outcomes here are best described as improved self-regulation in considerable generality. Highly specific targeting, just as in resonant frequency training, does not imply narrowly targeted outcomes. The approaches of Horvat, Walker, and Coben therefore belong with nearly everything else in the bin of general self-regulation training, leaving Kirt Thornton's approach as the unique departure into the domain of localized dysfunction.

IX. SUMMARY AND CONCLUSION

Whereas the modes of neuromodulation have undergone considerable proliferation over the years, there are unmistakable trends toward commonalities at a more basic level. From the original model of specific mechanisms-based protocols for limited diagnostic conditions, the field has moved toward a more systems-based approach relying ever more heavily on the EEG itself to establish training objectives. From a focus on steady-state properties of the EEG there has been a shift to the brain's organization of transient, episodic states; from a focus on localized phenomena there has been a shift toward multi-site relationships; and from a focus on amplitude and comodulation disparities there has been a shift toward phase and coherence relationships. Effectively there has been a shift from the use of a basic set of static protocols with fixed thresholds to dynamic, open-ended training with adaptive thresholding and multiple targeting. Even more generally, a shift of emphasis from prescriptive to non-prescriptive training has been underway, and the shift in the balance is continuing from prescriptive toward proscriptive training.

Although different technologies and training philosophies each have their particular areas of strength, the overriding impression is one of considerable commonality in outcomes, irrespective of mode and only secondarily dependent on the particulars of targeting. This implies that our appeal is to a highly integrated regulation regime with procedures that mobilize global reorganization fairly generally. It is the integrated nature of neural network functioning and its hierarchical organization that allow such varied challenges to achieve clinical success (see Othmer, 2007).

The story is not complete, however, without reference to the precise targeting of deficits observed under challenge, an approach that has shown itself uniquely efficacious for specific cognitive deficits. Whereas most of our clinical applications involve more general enhancement of the client's self-regulation status for which a variety of methods may be availing, this targeted approach offers relief for more localized, more specifically cerebral deficits. As such, it also offers the most definitive evidence of specific results traceable to a specific intervention, filling a need in this era of evidence-based therapies.

The broad range of applicability of modes of neuromodulation suggests that good brain function depends on tight constraints in the timing of neuronal information transport, and that the failure of such precision in the domain of timing and frequency represents the dominant failure mode of the central nervous system, accounting for much of mental dysfunction. The remedy offered by the neuromodulation technologies ultimately offers the best evidence for the posited causal mechanism.

The minimal set of claims that support neurofeedback efficacy may be articulated as follows: Any sufficiently subtle disturbance of brain function, with respect to a variable that is under active management by the CNS, will evoke a response by the CNS that attempts to restore the desired setpoint. The repetition of such a challenge will likely lead in time to improved self-regulatory capacity as a learned response. The evidence at hand suggests that the relative phase prevailing between two sites on the scalp represents a particularly attractive target for neurofeedback intervention because of its criticality to good brain communication, its dynamic features, and its ready accessibility.

The implication of the above is that neurofeedback training can be accomplished in an endless variety of ways, which makes it only too likely that the field will have to contend with continuing proliferation of methods. Nevertheless, the emerging techniques and procedures should still yield to simple ordering and classification. At this point there appears to be no single approach that covers all of the clinical bases. And in order to cover all of the bases, two requirements at least must be met in the prevailing state of the art. There must be some appeal in the frequency domain to the temporal organization of neuronal assemblies, and there must be some means in the time domain to recognize inappropriate changes of state, as these are revealed in the frequency-domain properties of the EEG. The first of these is some kind of narrowly prescriptive reward-based training, and the second is some kind of inhibit-based (i.e., proscriptive) detection scheme for inappropriate state shifts.

The latter of these can be considered a kind of error-correction scheme. The transient, sudden nature of this intervention implies that the brain is restricted here to its already existing resources. That is to say, the brain can only move toward states that are accessible to it, that are already available in state space. This is a necessary constituent of feedback for many conditions, but it is not sufficient by itself to restore optimum brain function for all. There must also be the opportunity for the brain to acquire new patterns of functioning, capacities that are gained incrementally and cumulatively over longer exposure times in training as the state space itself evolves under persistent challenge. This is accomplished by a targeted appeal to specific EEG frequencies. We are only at the beginning of the process of learning how to do this well.

REFERENCES

Adrian, E. D. and Matthews, B. H. C. (1934). The Berger rhythm: potential changes from the occipital lobes in man. *Brain*, **57**, 355–384.

American Psychiatric Association (1994). *Diagnostic and Statistical Manual of Mental Disorders*, 4th edition.

Berger, H. (1929). Über das Elektroenkephalogramm des Menschen. *Arch. Psychiatr. Nervenkr.*, **87**, 527–570.

Coben, R. and Podolsky, I. (2007). Assessment-Guided Neurofeedback for Autistic Spectrum Disorder. *J. Neurotherapy*, **11(1)**, 5–23.

Crane, R. A. (2007). Infinite Potential: A Neurofeedback Pioneer Looks Back and Ahead. In *Handbook of Neurofeedback* (J. R. Evans, ed.), pp. 3–21. The Haworth Press.

Fehmi, L. G. (2007). Multichannel EEG Phase Synchrony Training and Verbally Guided Attention Training for Disorders of Attention. In *Handbook of Neurofeedback* (J. R. Evans, ed.), pp. 301–314. Haworth Press.

Frederick, J. A., Lubar, J. F. and Rasey, H. W. (1999). Effects of 18.5 Hz auditory and visual stimulation on EEG amplitude at the vertex. *J. Neurotherapy*, **3(3/4)**, 23–28.

Hardt, J. V. (1978). A Dedicated Microcomputer for Multi-Channel, Multi-Subject Biofeedback. In *Proceedings of the 9th Annual Meeting of the Biofeedback Society of America*, pp. 6–8.

Hardt, J. V. and Kamiya, J. (1976). Anxiety change through Coherence and the Quirks of Coherence/ Phase training: A Clinical Perspective electroencephalographic alpha feedback seen only in high anxiety subjects. *Science*, **201**, 79–81.

Horvat, J. J. (2007). Coherence and the Quirks of Coherence/Phase training: A Clinical Perspective. In *Handbook of Neurofeedback* (J. R. Evans, ed.), pp. 213–227. Haworth Press.

Ibric, V. L. and Davis, C. J. (2007). The ROSHI in Neurofeedback. In *Handbook of Neurofeedback* (J.R. Evans, ed), pp. 185–211. The Haworth Press.

Kamiya, J. (1968). Conscious control of brain waves. *Psychology Today*, **1**, 56–60. (November).

Kropp, P., Siniatchkin, M. and Gerber, W.-D. (2002). On the Pathophysiology of Migraine—Links for "Empirically Based Treatment" with Neurofeedback. *Applied Psychophysiology and Biofeedback*, **27(3)**, 203–213.

Nash, J. K. (2000). Treatment of Attention Deficit Hyperactivity Disorder with Neurotherapy. *Clinical Electroencephalography*, **31(1)**, 30–37.

Ochs, L. (2006). The Low Energy Neurofeedback System (LENS): Theory, Background, and Introduction. *J. Neurotherapy*, **10(2/3)**, 5–40.

Othmer, S. (2007). Implications of Network Models for Neurofeedback. In *Handbook of Neurofeedback* (J. R. Evans, ed.), pp. 25–60. The Haworth Press.

Othmer, S. F. and Othmer, S. (2007). Interhemispheric EEG training: Clinical Experience and Conceptual Models. In *Handbook of Neurofeedback* (J. R. Evans, ed.), pp. 109–136. The Haworth Press.

Othmer, S., Othmer, S. F. and Kaiser, D. A. (1999). EEG Biofeedback: An Emerging Model for Its Global Efficacy. In *Introduction to Quantitative EEG and Neurofeedback* (J. R. Evans and A. Abarbanel, eds), pp. 243–310. San Diego: Academic Press.

Putman, J. A. and Othmer, S. (2006). Phase Sensitivity of Bipolar EEG Training Protocols. *J. Neurotherapy*, **10(1)**, 73–79.

Putman, J. A., Othmer, S. F., Othmer, S. and Pollock, V. E. (2005). TOVA Results Following Inter-Hemispheric Bipolar Training. *J. Neurotherapy*, **9(1)**, 27–36.

Scott, W. C., Kaiser, D. A., Othmer, S. and Sideroff, S. I. (2005). Effects of an EEG Biofeedback Protocol on a Mixed Substance Abusing Population. *American Journal of Drug and Alcohol Abuse*, **31(3)**, 455–469.

Siever, D. (2007). Audio-Visual Entrainment: History, Physiology, and Clinical Studies. In *Handbook of Neurofeedback* (J. R. Evans, ed.), pp. 155–183. The Haworth Press.

Sterman, M. B. (2000). Basic Concepts and Clinical Findings in the Treatment of Seizure Disorders with EEG Operant Conditioning. *Clinical Electroencephalography*, **31(1)**, 45–55.

Sterman, M. B., Wyrwicka, W. and Howe, R. (1969). Behavioral and neurophysiological studies of the sensorimotor rhythm in the cat. *Electroencephalography and Clinical Neurophysiology*, **27**, 678–679.

Strehl, U., Leins, U. and Goth, G. (2006). Self-regulation of slow cortical potentials: a new treatment for children with attention-deficit/hyperactivity disorder. *Pediatrics*, **118**, 1530–1540.

Thornton, K. E. (2006). No Child Left Behind Goals (and more) are obtainable with the NeuroCognitive Approach, Vol. 1. BookSurge Publishing Co.

Walker, J. E., Kozlowski, G. P. and Lawson, R. (2007). A Modular Activation/Coherence Approach to Evaluating Clinical/QEEG Correlations and for Guiding Neurofeedback Training: Modular Insufficiencies, Modular Excesses, Disconnections, and Hyperconnections. *J. Neurotherapy*, **11(1)**, 25–44.

CHAPTER 2

History of the scientific standards of QEEG normative databases

Robert W. Thatcher[1], Ph.D. and Joel F. Lubar[2], Ph.D.

[1]*EEG and NeuroImaging Laboratory, Applied Neuroscience, Inc.,*
St. Petersburg, FL, USA
[2]*Brain Research and Neuropsychology Lab., University of Tennessee,*
Knoxville, TN, USA

I. INTRODUCTION

Normative reference databases serve a vital and important function in modern clinical science and patient evaluation. There are numerous clinical normative databases that aid in the evaluation of a wide range of clinical disorders; for example, blood constituent normative databases; MRI, fMRI and Positron Emission Tomography (PET) normative databases; ocular and retinal normative databases; blood pressure normative databases; nerve conduction velocity normative databases; postural databases; bone density normative databases; ultra sound normative databases; genetic normative databases; and motor development databases, to name a few. A comprehensive survey of existing clinical normative databases can be obtained by searching the National Library of Medicine's database using the search terms "Normative Databases" at http://www.ncbi.nlm.nih.gov/sites/entrez.

All clinically applied normative databases share a common set of statistical and scientific standards that have evolved over the years. The standards include peer reviewed publications, disclosure of the inclusion/exclusion criteria, tests of statistical validity, tests of reliability, cross-validation tests, adequate sample sizes for different age groups, etc. Normative databases are distinct from non–clinical control groups in their scope, and their sampling restriction to clinically normal or otherwise healthy individuals for the purpose of comparison. Another distinguishing characteristic of normative databases is the ability to compare a single individual to a population of "normal" individuals in order to identify the measures that are deviant from normal, and the magnitude of deviation. Normative databases themselves do not diagnose a patient's clinical problem. Rather, a trained professional first evaluates the patient's clinical history, and clinical symptoms and complaints, and then uses the results of normative database comparisons in order to aid in the development of an accurate clinical diagnosis.

Introduction to QEEG and Neurofeedback, Second Edition
ISBN: 978-0-12-374534-7

29

As mentioned previously, the age range, the number of samples per age group, the mixture of gender and socio-economic status, geographical distribution and thus a "representative" population are also distinguishing characteristics of a "normative" database because an individual is compared to a group of subjects comprising a reference normative database. In the case of QEEG, matching of amplifier frequency characteristics when a patient's EEG was acquired by a different amplifier than the database amplifier is also critical for normative databases but rarely important for standard "control group" studies. Cultural and ethnic factors and day-to-day variance and random environmental factors are typically factored into "normative" databases as "random control" factors; in contrast, a more limited sampling process is often used in non-clinical "control groups."

The adequacy of the sample size of any database is related to the "effect size" and the statistical power, and thus sample size, varies depending on these factors (Cohen, 1977). In general, sample size is less important than careful calibration, elimination of artifact, accepted standards during the collection of data and accepted standards for the analysis of data and approximation to a Gaussian distribution. Peer reviewed publications are essential for all databases because high standards are required by anonymous reviewers and scientifically sub-standard databases will either not be published or if they are then the limitations are made public. To not publish a normative database in a peer reviewed journal is unacceptable and is a non-starter when a clinician considers the database that they are going to use to evaluate a patient. State licensing agencies and other authorities should be notified when sub-standard databases are used to evaluate a clinical patient, and, certainly, signed informed consent informing the patient that they are being evaluated using an unpublished and/or sub-standard database is necessary to protect the public.

II.   DEFINITIONS OF DIGITAL EEG AND QUANTITATIVE EEG (QEEG)

Nuwer (1997) defined digital EEG as ". . . the paperless acquisition and recording of the EEG via computer-based instrumentation, with waveform storage in a digital format on electronic media, and waveform display on an electronic monitor or other computer output device." The primary purposes of digital EEG is for efficiency of storage, the saving of paper, and for the purposes of visual examination of the EEG tracings. An attempt was made to distinguish digital EEG from quantitative EEG by defining quantitative EEG (QEEG or qEEG) as "the mathematical processing of digitally recorded EEG in order to highlight specific waveform components, transform the EEG into a format or domain that elucidates relevant information, or associate numerical results with the EEG data for subsequent review or comparison." (Nuwer, 1997, p. 278).

The reality is that there is no clear distinction between digital EEG and quantitative EEG because both involve mathematical transformations. For example, the process of analog-to-digital conversion involves transforms by analog and digital filtering as well as amplification, sample and hold of the electrical scalp potentials, remontaging and reformatting the EEG. Clearly, digital EEG involves mathematical and transformational processing using a computer, and therefore the distinction between quantitative EEG and digital EEG is weak and artificial.

III.   SIMULTANEOUS DIGITAL EEG TRACINGS AND QUANTITATIVE EEG

Figure 2.1 illustrates a common modern quantitative EEG analysis where EEG traces are viewed and examined at the same time that quantitative analyses are displayed, so as to facilitate and extend analytical power. Common sense dictates that the digital EEG and QEEG, when simultaneously available, facilitate rapid, accurate and reliable evaluation of the electroencephalograpm. Since 1929, when the human EEG was first measured (Berger, 1929), modern science has learned an enormous amount about the current sources of the EEG, and the manner in

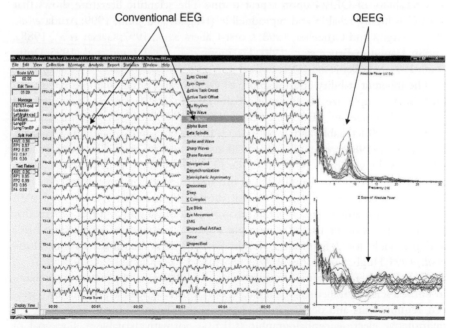

Conventional EEG   QEEG

FIGURE 2.1   Example of conventional digital EEG (left) and QEEG (right) on the same screen at the same time. The conventional EEG includes examination and marking of EEG traces and events. The QEEG (right) includes the Fast Fourier Transform (top right) and normative database Z-scores (bottom right).

which ensembles of synaptic generators are synchronously organized. It is known that short distance local generators are connected by white matter axons to other local generators that can be many centimeters distant. The interplay and coordination of short distance local generators with the longer distant white matter connections has been mathematically modeled, and shown to be essential for our understanding of the genesis of the EEG (Nunez, 1981, 1995; Thatcher and John, 1977; Thatcher et al., 1986).

The first QEEG study was by Hans Berger (1932, 1934) when he used the Fourier transform to spectrally analyze the EEG, as he recognized the importance of quantification and objectivity in the evaluation of the electroencephalogram (EEG). The relevance of quantitative EEG (QEEG) to the diagnosis and prognosis of brain dysfunction stems directly from the quantitative EEG's ability to reliably and objectively evaluate the distribution of brain electrical energies, and to compare different EEG measures to a normative database.

IV. TEST–RETEST RELIABILITY OF QEEG

The clinical sensitivity and specificity of QEEG is directly related to the stability and reliability of QEEG upon repeat testing. The scientific literature shows that QEEG is highly reliable and reproducible (Hughes and John, 1999; Aruda et al., 1996; Burgess and Gruzelier, 1993; Corsi-Cabera et al., 1997; Gasser et al., 1988a, 1988b; Hamilton-Bruce et al., 1991; Harmony et al., 1993; Lund et al., 1995; Duffy et al., 1994; Salinsky et al., 1991; Pollock et al., 1991).

The inherent stability and reliability of QEEG can even be demonstrated with quite small sample sizes. For example, Salinsky et al. (1991) reported that repeated 20-second samples of EEG were about 82% reliable, at 40 seconds the samples were about 90% reliable and at 60 seconds they were approximately 92% reliable. Gasser et al. (1985) concluded that: "20 sec. of activity are sufficient to reduce adequately the variability inherent in the EEG" and Hamilton-Bruce et al., (1991) found statistically high reliability when the same EEG was independently analyzed by three different individuals. Although the QEEG is highly reliable even with relatively short sample sizes, it is the recommendation of most QEEG experts that larger samples sizes be used; for example, at least 60 seconds of artifact-free EEG, and preferably for 2–5 minutes, should be used in a clinical evaluation (Duffy et al., 1994; Hughes and John, 1999).

Although there are common purposes and applications of normative databases in clinical science, nonetheless, each type of normative database poses its own special requirements and details. In the sections to follow we focus exclusively on quantitative electroencephalographic (QEEG) normative databases. The goal of this chapter is to present the history of the application of scientific standards as they apply to QEEG, and to provide a practical guide for the understanding and evaluation of QEEG normative databases.

V. HISTORY OF STANDARDS OF QEEG NORMATIVE DATABASES

The earliest quantitative EEG (QEEG) reference normative database was developed in the 1950s at UCLA as part of the NASA study and selection of astronaughts for purposes of space travel (Adey *et al.*, 1961, 1964a and 1964b). The UCLA database involved several hundred carefully selected subjects who were candidates for the burgeoning NASA space exploration program, as well as UCLA faculty and students. Careful clinical inclusion and exclusion criteria were not used because there was no intended clinical application of this early QEEG reference normative database. Instead, the essential quantitative foundations of QEEG normative databases were tested such as the calculation of means and standard deviations, and measures of Gaussianity, complex demodulation, Fourier spectral analysis and basic statistical parameters necessary for any reference normative database.

Predictive accuracy and error rates depend on the data that make up a given EEG database as well as the statistical methods used to produce and compare QEEG normative databases. Historically, many of the statistical standards of normative databases were first applied by two Swedish Neurologists—Dr. Milos Matousek and Dr. Ingemar Petersen—in 1973 in the first peer reviewed publication of a normative database (Matousek and Petersen, 1973a; 1973b). Matousek and Petersen set the standards of peer reviewed publications, clinical inclusion/exclusion criteria, and parametric statistical standards for future QEEG normative databases. The cultural validity and reliability of the Matousek and Petersen 1973 database were established by E. Roy John and colleagues in 1975 when they successfully replicated, by independent cross-validation, the Matousek and Petersen Swedish database after collecting EEG from carefully screened 9- to 11-year-old Harlem black children who were performing at grade level and had no history of neurological disorders (John, 1977; John *et al.*, 1977, 1987).

VI. HISTORY OF INCLUSION/EXCLUSION CRITERIA AND "REPRESENTATIVE SAMPLES"

Matousek and Petersen (Matousek and Petersen, 1973a, 1973b) measured QEEG in 401 subjects (218 females) ranging in age from 2 months to 22 years and living in Stockholm, Sweden—all without any negative clinical histories and performing at grade level. The sample sizes varied from 18 to 49 per one-year age groupings. Similar inclusion/exclusion criteria were later used in the construction of the NYU normative database (John, 1977; John *et al.*, 1977, 1987), the University of Maryland (UM) database (Thatcher, 1988; Thatcher *et al.*, 1983, 1986, 1987, 2003, 2005a, 2005b) and Gordon and colleagues (2005) in the development of independent QEEG normative databases. Careful screening of the subjects that comprise a normative database is critical so that representative samples of healthy and otherwise normally functioning individuals are selected, and individuals with a history of neurological problems, psychiatric problems, school failure and other deviant behaviors are excluded.

Representative sampling means a demographically balanced sample of different genders, different ethnic backgrounds, different socio-economic status, and different ages. This is important in evaluating a QEEG normative database because the database is a "reference" in which many demographic factors must be included in order to minimize sampling bias.

VII.   HISTORY OF ARTIFACT-FREE DATA AND RELIABILITY MEASURES

Sample adequacy in a QEEG normative database requires strict removal of artifact and measures of high test–retest reliability. Historically, multiple trained individuals visually examined the EEG samples from each and every subject that was to be included in the database. Removal of artifact by visual examination is necessary regardless of any digital signal processing methods that may be used to remove artifact. Split-half reliability and test–retest reliability measures with values >0.9 are also important in order to provide a quantitative measure of the internal consistency and reliability of the normative database (John, 1977; John et al., 1987; Thatcher, 1998; Thatcher et al., 2003; Duffy et al., 1994).

Caution should be exercised when using reconstruction methods such as Independent Components Analysis (ICA) or Principal Component Analysis (PCA) to compute a QEEG normative database. In general, these methods should be avoided because they will invalidate the computation of coherence and phase differences because the regression and reconstruction affect the raw digital samples themselves and distort coherence and phase. The best method of eliminating artifact is by making sure that high standards of recording are met, and that the patient's EEG is monitored during recording so that artifact can be minimized. Elimination of artifact after recording should involve the deletion of the artifact from the analysis and not by regression and/or reconstruction using methods such as ICA or PCA.

VIII.   HISTORY OF SAMPLE SIZE PER AGE GROUP

There is no absolute sample size that is best for a QEEG database because, statistically, sample size is related to the "effect size" and "power" (Hayes, 1973; Winer, 1971). The smaller the effect size the larger the sample size necessary to detect that effect. The power of a statistical measure varies as a function of sample size and the effect size (Cohen, 1977). Another issue related to sample size is the degree to which a sample approximates a Gaussian distribution. As explained in the section below, increased sample size is often necessary in order to achieve closer approximations to Gaussian, which in turn is related to the accuracy of cross-validation. Thus, the sample size is one of several inter-related issues in all normative databases, and the sample size should not be singled out as being the most important factor in a QEEG normative database. It is best to refer to "adequate" sample size as measured by the extent to which the samples are Gaussian, and the degree of cross-validation accuracy (John et al., 1987; Thatcher et al., 2003). The term *adequate* is related to the effect size, which in the case of human development is critical because different rates of maturation occur at different ages.

As mentioned previously, the Matousek and Petersen (1973a, 1973b) normative QEEG database had a total sample size of 401 in children ranging in age from 1 month to 22 years. It was known that there are rapid changes in EEG measures during early childhood, and for this reason Matousek and Petersen (1973a) and Hagne et al. (1973) emphasized using relatively large sample sizes during the period of time when the brain is changing most rapidly. For example, Hagne et al. (1973) used a sample size of N = 29 for infants from three weeks of age to 1 year of age. In step with this fact were the subsequent QEEG normative databases at NYU (John et al., 1977, 1987) and UM (Thatcher, 1998; Thatcher et al., 1987, 2003) in which the preferential increase in sample size during early childhood was emphasized as well as during old age when potential rapid declines in neural function may occur.

IX.   HISTORY OF AGE STRATIFICATION VS. AGE REGRESSION

There are two general approaches that deal with the issue of sample size per age group:

- age stratification, and
- age regression.

Age stratification involves computing means and standard deviations of age groupings of the subjects (Matousek and Petersen, 1973a; John, 1977; Thatcher et al., 1987, 2003). The grouping of subjects, and thus the number of subjects per age group, depends on the age of the sample and the relative rate of maturation. Matousek and Petersen (1973a, 1973b) used one-year age groupings, Thatcher et al. (1987) (University of Maryland database) used one-year age groupings as well as two- and five-year age groupings (Thatcher et al., 2003, 2005a, 2005b). A simple method to increase stability and sample size is to use "sliding" averages for the age stratification. For example, Thatcher et al. (2003) used one-year age groups with 0.75 year overlapping to produce a series of sliding averages, and more recently used two-year age groupings with 0.75-year overlapping. Which method is chosen depends on the accuracy of cross-validation and age resolution, with careful examination of validation at different ages of the subjects.

The second method called *age regression* was first used by John et al. (1977, 1980) in which a least squares regression was used to fit a straight line to the EEG data samples over the entire age range of the subjects. Once the intercepts and coefficients are computed then one simply evaluates the polynomial equation using the age of the subject in order to produce the expected mean and standard deviation for that particular subject. A Z-score is then computed by the standard method $Z = X - x/sd$. An important consideration when using an age regression method is the order of the polynomial, and the amount of variance accounted for by a polynomial. If there are rapid maturational changes in the brain, thus producing a "growth spurt", then a simple linear regression is likely to miss the growth spurt. A quadratic or cubic polynomial which will account for more of the variance over age will likely detect growth spurts better than a simple linear regression.

X.   HISTORY OF GAUSSIAN DISTRIBUTION APPROXIMATION AND CROSS-VALIDATION

The statistics of replication and independent cross-validation of normative QEEG databases was first applied by E. Roy John and collaborators in 1974 to 1977 (John, 1977; John et al., 1977, 1987). As mentioned previously, the first independent cross-validation of a normative QEEG database was by John and colleagues in which the EEG from a sample of New York Harlem black children were compared to the Matousek and Petersen (5, 6) norms with correlations >0.8 in many instances and statistically significant correlations for the majority of the measures (John, 1977).

The importance of approximation to a Gaussian distribution was emphasized by both Dr. E. Roy John and Dr. Frank Duffy, a Harvard Neurologist, in the 1970s and 1980s. In 1994 the American EEG Association produced a position paper in which the statistical standards of replication, cross-validation, reliability and Gaussian approximation were iterated as acceptable basic standards to be met by any normative QEEG database (Duffy et al., 1994). The American EEG Society included the same standards. From 1980 into the 1990s Dr. John and colleagues continued to evaluate and analyze the statistical properties of normative QEEG databases, including EEG samples obtained from different laboratories in non USA locations in the world. Gaussian approximations and reliability, and cross-validation statistical standards for QEEG databases were applied to all of these databases by John and Colleagues (John et al., 1987, 1980; Prichep, 2005) and as well as by other QEEG normative databases, for example, Gasser et al. (1988a, 1988b) and Thatcher and colleagues (1983, 1986, 1987, 2003, 2005a, 2005b).

Figure 2.2 shows examples of approximate Gaussian distributions and the sensitivity as calculated in Fig. 2.3. Table 2.1 is an example of a standard table of sensitivities for different age groups in the University of Maryland QEEG normative database (Thatcher et al., 2003).

Figure 2.3 shows an example of Gaussian approximation and cross-validation of a QEEG normative database. It shows an illustrative bell-shaped curve showing the ideal Gaussian and the average cross-validation values of the database by which estimates of

Cross-Validation Birth to 82 Year EEG Normative Database

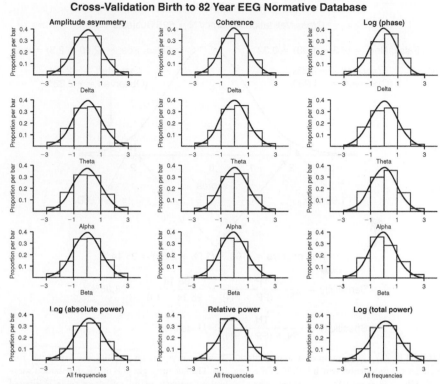

FIGURE 2.2   Histograms of the Z-Score Gaussian distributions and cross-validation for all ages (adapted from Thatcher *et al.*, 2003).

statistical sensitivity can be derived. True positives equal the percentage of Z-scores that lay within the tails of the Gaussian distribution. False negatives (FN) equal the percentage of Z-scores that fall outside of the tails of the Gaussian distribution. The error rates or the statistical sensitivity of a quantitative electroencephalogram (QEEG) normative database are directly related to the deviation from a Gaussian distribution. Fig. 2.3 depicts a mathematical method of estimating the statistical sensitivity of a normative EEG database in terms of the deviation from Gaussian.

XI.   HISTORY OF THE USE OF THE Z-SCORE AND QEEG NORMATIVE DATABASES

Matousek and Petersen (1973a, 1973b) computed means and standard deviations in one-year age groups, and were the first to use T-tests and Z-scores to compare an individual to the normative database means and standard deviations. The T-test is defined as the ratio of the difference between values divided by the standard deviation. The Z statistic is defined as the difference between the value from an

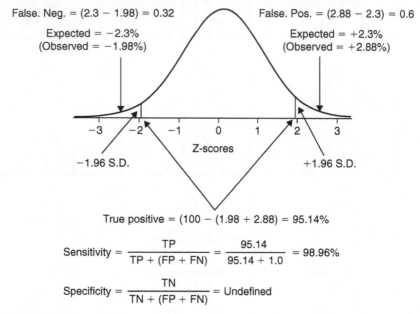

Sensitivity Based on Deviation from Gaussian

Cross-Validation Accuracy N = 625 Subjects

False. Neg. = (2.3 − 1.98) = 0.32

Expected = −2.3%
(Observed = −1.98%)

False. Pos. = (2.88 − 2.3) = 0.6

Expected = +2.3%
(Observed = +2.88%)

−1.96 S.D.   +1.96 S.D.

Z-scores

True positive = (100 − (1.98 + 2.88) = 95.14%

$$\text{Sensitivity} = \frac{TP}{TP + (FP + FN)} = \frac{95.14}{95.14 + 1.0} = 98.96\%$$

$$\text{Specificity} = \frac{TN}{TN + (FP + FN)} = \text{Undefined}$$

FIGURE 2.3   An example of a normal or Gaussian curve showing values of Z (±1.96) that includes the proportion which is 0.95 of the total area. The left and right tails of the distribution show probability values of 0.025 (one-tailed). The classification accuracy of any sample of subjects is based on the assumption that a normal distribution can be compared. The probability of finding an observed EEG value in a given range of any population can be determined, and then the sensitivity of the sample can be tested by cross-validation (adapted from Thatcher *et al.*, 2003).

individual and the mean of the population divided by the standard deviation of the population or

$$Z = \frac{x_i - \overline{X}}{SD}.$$

John and colleagues (John, 1977; John *et al.*, 1977, 1987) expanded on the use of the Z-score for clinical evaluation including the use of multivariate measures such as the Mahalanobis distance metric (Cooley and Lohnes, 1971; John *et al.*, 1987; John *et al.*, 1988). A direct normalization of the Gaussian distribution using Z-scores is useful in comparing individuals to a QEEG normative database (Thatcher, 1998; Thatcher *et al.*, 2003). That is, the standard score form of the Gaussian is where the mean = 0 and standard deviation = 1 or, by substitution into the Gaussian equation for a bell shaped curve, then

$$Y = \frac{1}{\sqrt{2\pi}} e^{-z2/2}$$

TABLE 2.1   Example of cross-validation and sensitivity tests of a normative database
using the procedures described in Figure 2. (Adapted from Thatcher *et al.*, 2003.)

FFT Normative Database Sensitivities			
2 STDEVs AGES	CALC SENSITIVITY: FP = TP/(TP + FP) or FN = TP/(TP + FN)		
	(+/−2 SD)	(>=2 SD)	(<=−2 SD)	
0–5.99	0.95448265	0.9771774	0.97730526	
6–9.99	0.95440363	0.9772031	0.97720054	+/−2 Std. Dev.
10–12.99	0.9543997	0.97724346	0.97715624	
13–15.99	0.95440512	0.97723601	0.97716911	
16–ADULT	0.9543945	0.97718143	0.97721307	
ALL	0.95442375	0.97720714	0.97721661	
3 STDEVs AGES	CALC SENSITIVITY: FP = TP/(TP + FP) or FN = TP/(TP + FN)		
	(+/−3 SD)	(>=3 SD)	(<=−3 SD)	
0–5.99	0.99743898	0.99871123	0.99872774	
6–9.99	0.99744112	0.99871611	0.99872501	+/−3 Std. Dev.
10–12.99	0.99744688	0.99873171	0.99871518	
13–15.99	0.99743186	0.99871951	0.99871234	
16–ADULT	0.99743835	0.99870216	0.99873619	
ALL	0.99744002	0.99871716	0.99872286	

where Y = Gaussian distribution and the Z-score is a deviation in standard deviation units measured along the baseline of the Gaussian curve from a mean of 0,
and a standard deviation = 1 with deviations to the right of the mean being positive and those to the left negative. By substituting different values of Z then different values of Y can be calculated. For example, when $Z = 0, Y = 0.3989$ or,
in other words, the height of the curve at the mean of the normal distribution
in standard-score form is given by the number 0.3989. For purposes of assessing
deviation from normal, the values of Z above and below the mean, which include
95% of the area of the Gaussian are often used as a level of confidence necessary
to minimize Type I and Type II errors (Hayes, 1973). The standard-score equation
is also used to cross-validate a normative database, which again emphasizes the
importance of approximation to a Gaussian for any normative QEEG database.

XII.   CROSS-VALIDATIONS OF NORMATIVE
DATABASES: NEW YORK UNIVERSITY AND
UNIVERSITY OF MARYLAND

As described previously, cross-validation is critical in determining the sensitivity
and false positives and false negatives of a normative database. Due to the expense
to acquire independent data, most cross-validations are computed using a leave-
one-out cross-validation procedure (John *et al.*, 1977, 1987; Thatcher *et al.*, 2003,
2005a, 2005b). A completely independent cross-validation using different subjects is

TABLE 2.2   Correlation coefficients from an independent cross-validation of NYU vs. UM normative EEG databases (reprinted by permission of CNS Response, Inc.)

	Absolute power	Absolute power	Relative power	Relative power	Coherence	Coherence	Amp. asym	Amp. asym
	Anterior	Posterior	Anterior	Posterior	Anterior	Posterior	Anterior	Posterior
Delta	0.815	0.880	0.854	0.925	0.804	0.935	0.854	0.820
Theta	0.926	0.940	0.877	0.895	0.853	0.914	0.902	0.816
Alpha	0.951	0.958	0.901	0.887	0.873	0.946	0.899	0.979
Beta	0.820	0.882	0.757	0.784	0.848	0.900	0.846	0.876

the best method of cross-validation although it is, as previously stated, more expensive and difficult and, accordingly, no independent cross-validations of two different normative databases have been conducted in the last 30 years, until recently.

In 2007 an independent cross-validation of the New York University and the University of Maryland databases was conducted. The study was conducted because a company had collected raw digital EEG from several hundred clinical patients, and had computed Z-scores using the New York University (NYU) normative database (John, 1977; John et al., 1977, 1987, 1988). The question was: does the University of Maryland (UM) normative database produce similar Z-scores as the NYU database using the same exact raw digital data? The correlation coefficients from the independent cross-validation between the NYU and UM normative databases are shown in Table 2.2. The analysis included 332 psychiatric patients and an age range from 6.2 years to 84.9 years. Anterior includes electrodes Fp1/2, Fz, F3/4, F7/8, T3/4, C3/4 and Cz. Posterior includes electrodes O1/2, P3/4, T5/6 and Pz. The correlations ranged from 0.757 to 0.979. The high degree of cross-validation accuracy in this study is emphasized by the fact that at 331 degrees of freedom a correlation of 0.142 is significant at $P < 0.01$.

Figure 2.4 shows bar graphs of the correlation coefficients from the independent cross-validation comparison between the NYU and the UM Z-scores. This study is important because it demonstrates a high degree of cross-correlation and cross-validation between two independent QEEG normative databases. Both the NYU and UM databases were constructed in medical centers with government grants and oversight, and both have been clinically validated in peer reviewed publications (John et al., 1977, 1987, 1988; Thatcher et al., 1986, 1987, 2003, 2005b) as well has having FDA registration.

XIII.   HISTORY OF AMPLIFIER MATCHING AND QEEG NORMATIVE DATABASES

Surprisingly, this particular standard was largely neglected during much of the history of QEEG normative databases. E. Roy John and colleagues (from 1982 to 1988)

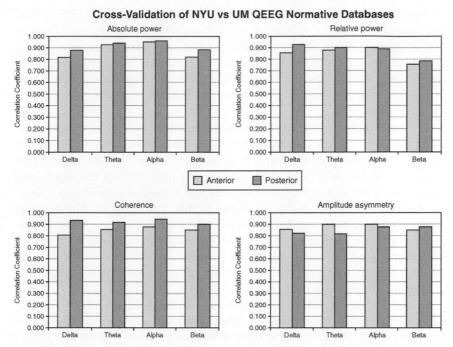

Cross-Validation of NYU vs UM QEEG Normative Databases

FIGURE 2.4   Results of an independent cross-validation comparison of Z-scores from 332 psychiatric patients ranging in age from 6.2 years to 84.9 years using the New York University (NYU) and University of Maryland (UM) normative databases. Anterior and posterior refer to the anterior and posterior location of electrodes. Highly significant independent cross-validation was observed, which shows the high degree of consistency between two peer reviewed and clinically validated QEEG normative databases. (Reprinted with permission from CNS Response, Inc.)

formed a consortium of universities and medical schools that were using QEEG. The consortium met several times over a few years and was one of the supporters of the edited volume by John titled *Machinery of the Mind* (John, 1990).

One of the important issues consistently raised at the consortium meetings was the need for "standardization." In the 1980s it was technically difficult to match different EEG systems because of the infantile development of analysis software. This history forced most QEEG users to use relative power because absolute power was not comparable between different EEG machines. There was no frequency response standardization between different EEG machines, and thus there was no cross-platform standardization of QEEG. It was not until the mid 1990s that computer speed and software development made amplifier matching and normative database amplifier equilibration a possibility.

The first use of standardized matching of amplifiers was to the University of Maryland (UM) database. The procedure involved injecting microvolt calibration sine waves into the input of amplifiers of different EEG machines, and then injecting the same microvolt signals into the normative database amplifiers thus obtaining two frequency response curves (Thatcher *et al.*, 2003). Equilibration of a normative QEEG database to different EEG machines is the ratio of the frequency response curves of the two amplifiers that are then used as amplitude scaling coefficients in the power spectral analysis. This was an important step because suddenly absolute power Z-scores and normative database comparisons became possible.

Relative power is a last resort type of measure to be used when there is no equilibration of absolute amplitude because relative power always distorts the spectrum, and relative power depends on absolute power in order to interpret relative power. This is because relative power is a percentage of the whole, and thus an increase in mid "beta," e.g., 14–18 Hz will be seen as a decrease in "theta," e.g., 4–7 Hz when in fact there is no change in theta and vice versa. The frequencies in absolute power are independent of each other and are not distorted. It is always best to use absolute values whenever possible, and not relative values or even ratios. A ratio can change due to the denominator or the numerator, and one cannot determine which has changed without evaluating the absolute values used to compute the ratios.

As illustrated in Fig. 2.5, a simple method of amplifier equilibration to exactly match the frequency characteristics of different amplifiers is to calibrate the amplifiers using microvolt sine waves at discrete frequencies from 1–30 Hz and injecting the sine waves into the inputs of the EEG amplifiers. Then take the ratio of the microvolt values at each frequency and use the ratios to exactly equate the spectral output values to the normative database amplifiers. This method creates a universal equilibration process so that microvolts in a given amplifier are equal to

Normative Database Amplifier Matching—Microvolt Sine Waves 0–40 Hz Equilibration Ratios to Match Frequency Responses

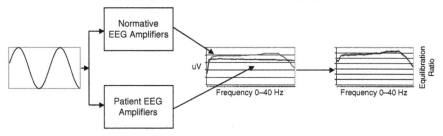

FIGURE 2.5   Flow chart of the amplifier standardization procedure. Micro-volt (uV) sine waves are injected into the input of amplifiers, and the frequency responses are calculated. The frequency response of the normative database amplifiers and the frequency response of the Deymed amplifier are in the middle graph. As shown in the right graph, EEG amplifier systems are then equated as the ratio of the two amplifier frequency response curves and the spectral analysis is adjusted based on the equilibration ratios so that there is a standardized import and matching of amplifier systems, with the common unit being microvolts (uV).

microvolts in all other amplifiers including the normative database amplifiers. By equilibrating amplifiers, then direct comparisons between a given patient's EEG and the normative database means and standard deviations are valid and meaningful. If amplifier matching is not accomplished, all normative database comparisons are potentially invalid and caution should be exercised not to use a normative database when amplifiers have not been equilibrated.

We have found that amplifiers differ primarily from 0–2 Hz, and in order to accurately match to the normative database amplifiers one can filter at 1 Hz, thus avoiding mismatches at less than 1 Hz. There is a wide variety of different frequency response curves for different amplifiers and there is no one "gold standard" for EEG amplifiers. For older amplifiers that have a more limited frequency response, e.g., the NYU and University of Maryland amplifiers and Biologic, then the match of frequencies is limited to the frequency range that is common between the two amplifier systems. For example, Deymed has a nearly flat response from 0.5 Hz to 70 Hz, and thus the match to the NYU and UM amplifiers is only from 0.5 Hz to 30 Hz because the latter amplifiers used cut-off filters at approximately 30 Hz. Many amplifiers currently in use also have cut-off frequencies of around 30 Hz but there is still a lot of information in the EEG from 0.5 Hz to 30 Hz, and equilibration is necessary to optimally use these amplifiers in a normative database comparison.

XIV. CONTENT VALIDITY OF QEEG NORMATIVE DATABASES

A. Neuropsychological correlations

Content validity is defined by the extent to which an empirical measurement reflects a specific domain of content (Nunnally, 1978). For example, a test in arithmetic operations would not be content valid if the test problems focused only on addition, thus neglecting subtraction, multiplication and division. By the same token, a content-valid measure of cognitive decline following a stroke should include measures of memory capacity, attention and executive function, etc.

There are many examples of the clinical content validity of QEEG and normative databases in ADD, ADHD, schizophrenia, compulsive disorders, depression, epilepsy, TBI (Thatcher et al., 1998a, 1998b) and a wide number of clinical groupings of patients as reviewed by Hughes and John (1999). There are over 250 citations in the review by Hughes and John, and there are approximately 23 citations to peer reviewed journal articles in which a normal reference database was used. Another recent review of QEEG normative databases and the clinical application of QEEG to psychiatric disorders cited 169 publications (Coburn et al., 2006). An Internet search of the National Library of Medicine will give citations to more QEEG and content-validity peer-reviewed studies using a reference normal group

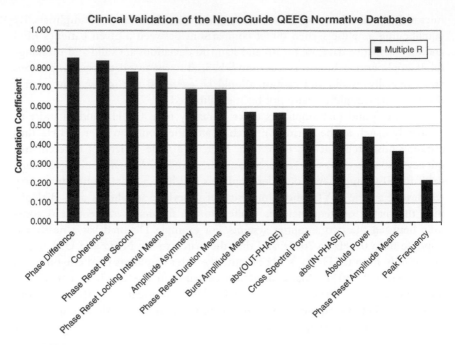

FIGURE 2.6 Correlations between QEEG measures and full-scale I.Q. (WISC-R). N = 332 subjects from the University of Maryland QEEG normative database (see Table 1.3). The highest correlations between QEEG and I.Q. are phase differences and coherence (47). The x-axis shows different QEEG measures, and the y-axis the correlation coefficient in a multivariate regression analysis with full-scale I.Q. as the dependent variable. Phase Reset and Burst Metrics are new measures which also exhibit high clinical correlations and clinical validation.

than were included in the Hughes and John review or the Coburn *et al.* (2006) review. Finally, for a recent review that emphasizes clinical correlations and clinical validation of a normative database see Gordon *et al.* (2005).

Figure 2.6 and Table 2.3 show an example of the range of clinical correlations to full-scale I.Q. in 373 normal individuals from 5 to 55 years of age.

It can be seen in Figure 2.6 that relative high correlations with I.Q. (0.859) are achievable when using a normative database and multiple regression of different variable types, and that different QEEG measures exhibit different magnitudes of correlation. The multiple regression prediction of I.Q. is not intended to replace neuropsychological tests. However, an advantage of a QEEG normative database prediction of I.Q. is that it can be repeated without confounding by learning, and it can be given to untestable patients such as stroke, paralysis and uncooperative individuals. Also, QEEG predictions of intelligence provide an insight into which aspects of neural functioning, such as location and connectivity, contribute to the prediction of intelligence, thus providing a deeper understanding of intelligence in an individual subject.

TABLE 2.3   List of correlations between full-scale I.Q. and QEEG
measures from 373 normal subjects aged 5–55 years (47)

QEEG measure	Correlation coefficient—QEEG and full-scale I.Q. (Wisc-R)
Phase Difference	0.859
Coherence	0.842
Phase Reset per Second	0.785
Phase Reset Locking Interval Means	0.780
Amplitude Asymmetry	0.691
Phase Reset Duration Means	0.688
Burst Amplitude Means	0.574
Out-of-Phase Cross-Spectral Power	0.570
Cross Spectral Power	0.485
In-Phase Cross-Spectral Power	0.481
Absolute Power	0.443
Phase Reset Amplitude Means	0.372
Peak Frequency	0.218

B. Example for traumatic brain injury

There are numerous peer reviewed journal articles showing high correlations between Z-scores involving the UM and NYU and other normative databases over the last 20 years (see review by Hughes and John, 1999). It is beyond the scope of this chapter to attempt to review all of these studies. Instead, we will focus on one of the many clinical correlation sub-groups, namely, traumatic brain injury.

The National Library of Medicine lists 1,672 peer reviewed journal articles on the subject of EEG and traumatic brain injury. The vast majority of these studies involved quantitative analyses and, in general, the scientific literature presents a consistent and common quantitative EEG pattern correlated with TBI. Namely, reduced amplitude of the alpha and beta and gamma frequency bands of EEG (8–12 Hz, 13–25 Hz and 30–40 Hz) (Mas et al., 1993; von Bierbrauer et al., 1993; Ruijs et al., 1994; Korn et al., 2005; Hellstrom-Westas and Rosen, 2005; Thompson et al., 2005; Tebano et al., 1988; Thatcher et al., 1998a, 2001a; Roche et al., 2004; Slewa-Younan, 2002; Slobounov et al., 2002) and changes in EEG coherence and phase delays in frontal and temporal relations (Thatcher et al., 1989, 1991, 1998b, 2001a, 2001b; Hoffman et al., 1995, 1996; Trudeau et al., 1998). The reduced amplitude of EEG is believed to be due to a reduced number of synaptic generators and/or reduced integrity of the protein/lipid membranes of neurons (Thatcher et al., 1997, 1998a, 2001b).

EEG coherence is a measure of the amount of shared electrical activity at a particular frequency, and is analogous to a cross-correlation coefficient. EEG coherence is amplitude independent and reflects the amount of functional connectivity between distant EEG generators (Nunez, 1981, 1994; Thatcher et al., 1986). EEG phase delays between distant regions of the cortex are mediated in part by the conduction velocity of the cerebral white matter, which is a likely reason that EEG phase delays are often distorted following a traumatic brain injury (Thatcher *et al.*, 1989, 2001a). In general, the more severe the traumatic brain injury, the more deviant the QEEG measures (Thatcher *et al.*, 2001a, 2001b).

Quantitative EEG studies of the diagnosis of TBI typically show quite high sensitivity and specificity, even for mild head injuries. For example, a study of 608 mild TBI patients and 103 age matched control subjects demonstrated discriminant sensitivity = 96.59%; Specificity = 89.15%, Positive Predictive Value (PPV) = 93.6% (Average of Tables 2.2, 2.3, 2.5) and Negative Predictive Value (NPV) = 97.4% (Average of Tables 2.3, 2.4, 2.5) in four independent cross-validations. A similar sensitivity and specificity for QEEG diagnosis of TBI was published by Trudeau *et al.* (1998) and Thatcher *et al.* (2001a). All of these studies met most of the American Academy of Neurology's criteria for diagnostic medical tests of:

1. The "criteria for test abnormality was defined explicitly and clearly"
2. Control groups were "different from those originally used to derive the test's normal limits"
3. "test–retest reliability was high"
4. The test was more sensitive than "routine EEG" or "neuroimaging tests", and
5. The study occurred in an essentially "blinded" design (i.e., objectively and without ability to influence or bias the results).

XV.   HISTORY OF THREE-DIMENSIONAL CURRENT SOURCE NORMATIVE DATABASES

Parametric statistics that rely upon a Gaussian distribution have been successfully used in studies of Low Resolution Electromagnetic Tomography or LORETA (Thatcher *et al.*, 2005a, 2005b; Huizenga *et al.*, 2002; Hori and He, 2001; Waldorp *et al.*, 2001; Bosch-Bayard *et al.*, 2001; Machado *et al.*, 2004). Bosch-Bayard *et al.* (2001) created a Z-score normative database that exhibited high sensitivity and specificity using a variation of LORETA called VARETA.

A subsequent study by Machado *et al.* (2004) extended these analyses again using VARETA. Thatcher *et al.* (2005a) also showed that LORETA current values in wide frequency bands approximate a normal distribution after transforms with reasonable sensitivity. This same paper compared Z-scores to non-parametric statistical procedures, and showed that Z-scores were more accurate than non-parametric statistics (2005a). Lubar *et al.* (2003) used non-parametric statistics in an experimental control study with similar levels of significance as reported by Thatcher *et al.* (2005a). Fig. 2.7 shows an example of how a log transform can move a non-gaussian distribution toward a better approximation of a Gaussian when using LORETA (Thatcher *et al.*, 2005a, 2005b).

LORETA three-dimensional current source normative databases have also been cross-validated, and the sensitivity computed using the same methods as for the surface EEG (Thatcher *et al.*, 2005b). Figure 2.8 shows an example of localization accuracy of a LORETA normative database in the evaluation of confirmed neural pathologies.

LORETA Norms Histogram Distributions

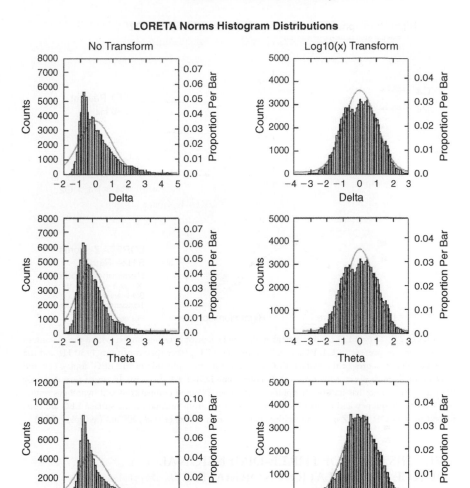

FIGURE 2.7   Shows the distribution of current source densities before (left) and after (right) $\log_{10}$ transform for the delta, theta and alpha frequencies. It can be seen that reasonable approximation to Gaussian was achieved by the $\log_{10}$ transform. (From Thatcher *et al.*, 2005a.)

All of these studies demonstrated that when proper statistical standards are applied to EEG measures, whether they are surface EEG or three-dimensional source localization, then high cross-validation accuracy can be achieved. Recently, Hoffman (2006) confirmed that high accuracy can be achieved using a LORETA Z-score normative database to evaluate patients with confirmed pathologies (e.g., left temporal lobe epilepsy and focal brain damage) using the University of Maryland normative database (Thatcher *et al.*, 2003) and the University of Tennessee normative database (Lubar *et al.*, 2003).

Right Hemisphere Hematoma—Maximal in C4 > P4 > O2

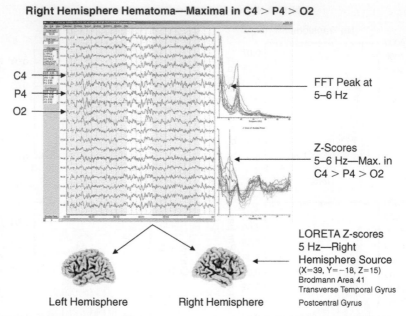

FIGURE 2.8   The EEG from a patient with a right hemisphere hematoma where the maximum shows waves are present in C4, P4 and O2 (Top). The FFT power spectrum from 1–30 Hz and the corresponding Z-scores of the surface EEG are shown in the right side of the EEG display. Left and right hemisphere displays of the maximal Z-scores using LORETA (Bottom). It can be seen that only the right hemisphere has statistically significant Z values. Planned comparisons and hypothesis testing based on the frequency and location of maximal deviation from normal on the surface EEG are confirmed by the LORETA Z-score normative analysis. (From Thatcher *et al.*, 2005b.) (see color plate.)

XVI. HISTORY OF THREE-DIMENSIONAL SOURCE CORRELATION NORMATIVE DATABASES

Thatcher *et al.* (1994), Thatcher (1995) and Hoechstetter *et al.* (2004) used a multiple dipole source solution for scalp EEG electrical potentials. They then used coherence to compute the correlation between the three-dimensional current sources, and demonstrated changes in the correlation between current sources related to different tasks. Pascual-Marqui *et al.* (2001) used low resolution electromagnetic tomography (LORETA) to compute current sources, and then used a Pearson Product correlation coefficient to explore differences in source correlations between a normal control group and a group of schizophrenic patients. Recently, high statistical standards were applied to LORETA three-dimenional source correlations in a QEEG normative database (Thatcher *et al.*, 2007a). All of these studies revealed interesting and reproducible relations between current sources and network connectivity that provide a deeper understanding of the surface EEG dynamics.

The same statistical standards as enumerated previously were applied to the LORETA source correlation normative database, i.e., peer reviewed publication, gaussian approximation, removal of artifact, high reliability and cross-validation. The LORETA normative database studies prove that nearly any measure can be used in a normative database as long as the appropriate statistical and scientific standards are met.

XVII.   HISTORY OF REAL-TIME Z-SCORE NORMATIVE DATABASES

As mentioned above, many different normative databases can be constructed and validated as long as the basic scientific standards of gaussianity, cross-validation, amplifier matching and peer reviewed publications are met. A recent example of a new application of a normative database is the use of complex demodulation as a joint-time-frequency-analysis (JTFA) for the purposes of real-time biofeedback (Thatcher, 1998, 2000a, 2000b; Thatcher et al., 1987, 2003). This method has recently been implemented in EEG biofeedback systems and used to compute statistical Z-scores in real-time. Complex demodulation is an analytic technique that multiplies a time series by a sine wave and a cosine wave, and then applies a low pass filter (Granger et al., 1964; Otnes and Enochson, 1977; Thatcher et al., 2007b). This results in mapping of the time series to the unit circle or "complex plane" whereby instantaneous power and instantaneous phase differences and coherence are computed.

Unlike the Fourier transform which depends on windowing and integration over an interval of time, complex demodulation computes the instantaneous power and phase at each time point, and thus an instantaneous Z-score necessarily includes the within subject variance of instantaneous electrical activity as well as the between subject variance for subjects of a given age. The summation of instantaneous Z-scores is Gaussian distributed and has high cross-validation (Thatcher et al., 2003), however the individual time point by time point Z-score is always smaller than the summation due to within subject variance. The use of within subject variance results in a more "conservative" estimate of deviation from normal, solely for the purposes of instantaneous biofeedback methods. A standard FFT normative database analysis should first be computed in order to identify the electrode locations and EEG features that are most deviant from normal which can be linked to the patient's symptoms and complaints.

Linking a subject's symptoms and complaints, e.g., PTSD, Depression, Schizophrenia, TBI, etc. to functional localization of the brain is an important objective of those who use a normative database. Similar to a blood bank analysis, the list of deviant or normal measures is given to the clinician as one test among many that are used to help render a diagnosis. It is important that linking deregulation of neural activity in localized regions of the brain to known

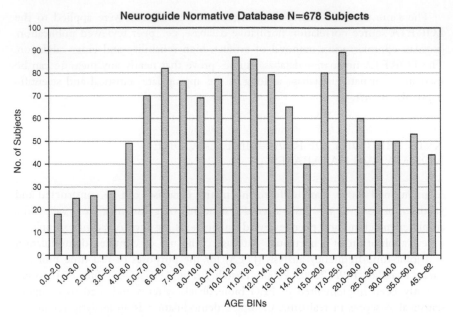

FIGURE 2.9 The number of subjects per age group in the Z-score Lifespan EEG reference normative database. The database is a "lifespan" database with 2 months of age being the youngest subject and 82.3 years of age being the oldest subject. Two-year means were computed using a sliding average with 6-month overlap of subjects. This produced a more stable and higher age resolution normative database, and a total of 21 different age groups. The 21 age groups and age ranges, and number of subjects per age group, are shown in the bar graph. (Adapted from Thatcher *et al.*, 2003.)

functional localization, for example left parietal lobe and dyslexia, right frontal and depression, cingulate gyrus and attention deficit, occipital lobes and vision problems, etc. is done by a trained clinician. Textbooks on functional localization in neurology and psychiatry are available to aid the clinician in learning about the link between a patient's symptoms and different brain regions (Heilman and Valenstein, 1993; Brazis *et al.*, 2007). A link of the anatomical locations and patterns of a patient's deviant Z-scores is important in order to derive clinical meaning from the QEEG.

Once a QEEG normative database analysis is completed, then one can use a Z-score biofeedback program to train patients to move their instantaneous Z-scores toward zero or the norm. The absolute value and range of the instantaneous Z-scores, while smaller than those obtained using the offline QEEG normative database, are nonetheless valid and capable of being minimized toward zero. An advantage of a Z-score biofeedback program is simplification by reducing diverse measures to a single metric, i.e., the metric of a Z-score. Thus, there is greater standardization and less guesswork about whether to reinforce or suppress coherence or phase differences or power, etc. at a particular location and particular frequency band.

Figure 2.9 shows the number of subjects per year in the normative EEG lifespan database, N = 625, that spans an age range from 2 months to 82 years of age. It can be seen that the largest number of subjects is in the younger ages (e.g., 1 to 14 years, N = 470) when the EEG is changing most rapidly. A proportionately smaller number of subjects represents the adult age range from 14–82 years (N = 155). In order to increase the time resolution of age, sliding averages were used for age stratification of the instantaneous Z-scores for purposes of EEG biofeedback. Two-year means were computed using a sliding average with 6-month overlap of subjects. This produced a more stable and higher age resolution normative database and a total of 21 different age groups. The 21 age groups and age ranges, and number of subjects per age group, are shown in the bar graph in Figure 2.9.

XVIII.   ACTIVE TASKS VS. EYES CLOSED AND EYES OPEN QEEG DATABASES

An active task refers to the recording of EEG and/or evoked potentials (EPs) while a subject performs some kind of perceptual or cognitive task. Many EEG, EP and event-related potential (ERP) studies have reported reproducible changes in brain dynamics which are task dependent. Such studies are important for understanding normal and pathological brain processes responsible for perceptual and cognitive function. In contrast, an eyes closed or eyes open EEG state involves an alert subject simply sitting quietly and not moving. The eyes closed and/or eyes open conditions are commonly used as reference normative EEG databases because of the simplicity and relative uniformity of EEG recording conditions. Such databases can be compared across laboratories and populations with relatively high reliability. Active tasks, on the other hand, are dependent on the intensity of stimuli, the background noise of the room, the distance between the subject and the stimuli, the subject's understanding of the task instructions, the subject's motivation, etc. These are very difficult to control across experimenters or across clinics for the purposes of constructing a "reference" normative EEG database.

One of the most carefully constructed active task normative database is by Brain Resources, Inc. in Australia (Gordon *et al.*, 2005). The BRC database does require replication of specific task conditions using a Neuroscan, Inc. EEG amplifier system. The relative sensitivity and specificity of resting eyes open and eyes closed EEG versus an active task normative database has not been published to our knowledge. Another well constructed and tested active task normative database is the go no-go task developed by Russian scientists (Kropotov *et al.*, 2005) with medium to high sensitivity and accuracy in the evaluation of attention deficits and other disorders. We were unable to find any peer reviewed journal articles of EEG databases produced by Dr. Kropotov and therefore there is no information on the sensitivity, cross-validation, amplifier matching and other standards for EEG databases.

It should be kept in mind that the alert eyes closed EEG state is very much an active state, e.g., there is still about 20% glucose metabolism of the whole body occurring in the brain of an eyes closed subject (Herscovitch, 1994; Raichle, 2002). During the eyes closed state, there is dynamic circulation of neural activity in connected cortical, reticular and thalamo-cortical loops (Thatcher and John, 1977; Nunez, 1995). The allocation of neural resource is simply different from when the subject is directing his or her attention to an experimentally controlled situation. Active tasks are very important because they reflect the switching and dynamic allocation of neural resource, which also has clinical importance. However, a scientifically sound and stable resting EEG normative database can enhance and also facilitate the understanding of the underlying neural dynamics and clinical condition of a patient during an active task. For example, comparison to a resting baseline normative database during different active task conditions may help reveal anatomical localization of neural processes and network dynamics without the need for a comparison to an exactly matching active task.

XIX. SUMMARY OF NORMATIVE DATABASE VALIDATION AND SENSITIVITY TESTS

Figure 2.10 is an illustration of a step-by-step procedure by which any normative EEG database can be validated and sensitivities calculated. The left side of the figure is the edited and artifact clean and reliable digital EEG time series, which may be re-referenced or re-montaged, that is then analyzed in either the time domain or the frequency domain.

The selected normal subjects are grouped by age with a sufficiently large sample size. The means and standard deviations of the EEG time series and/or frequency domain analyses are computed for each age group. Transforms are applied to approximate a Gaussian distribution of the EEG measures that comprise the means. Once approximation to Gaussian is completed, Z-scores are computed for each subject in the database and leave one out Gaussian cross-validation is computed in order to arrive at optimum Gaussian cross-validation sensitivity. Finally, the Gaussian validated norms are subjected to content and predictive validation procedures such as correlation with neuropsychological test scores and intelligence, etc. and also discriminant analyses and neural networks and outcome statistics, etc. The content validations are with respect to clinical measures such as intelligence, neuropsychological test scores, school achievement and other clinical measures. The predictive validations are with respect to the discriminative, statistical or neural network clinical classification accuracy. Both parametric and non-parametric statistics are used to determine the content and predictive validity of a normative EEG database.

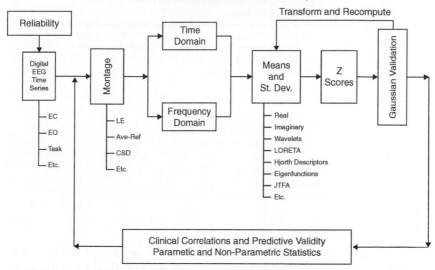

FIGURE 2.10   Illustration of the steps involved in developing a normative QEEG database. The left is the start of the process with data acquisition, amplifier matching, artifact rejection and quality control. Approximation to a Gaussian is followed by cross-validation, and then finally clinical correlations. (From 11.)

XX.   GOLD STANDARD CHECK LIST FOR A NORMATIVE QEEG DATABASE

Table 2.4 is a "Gold Standard" check list which summarizes the minimal standards of QEEG normative databases that were discussed previously. Those clinicians interested in using a QEEG normative database are encouraged to enter a check for each of the standards that a given database has met. The more standards that are met the better.

XXI.   PROBLEMS IN COMBINING SUB-STANDARD QEEG DATABASES WITH SCIENTIFICALLY ACCEPTABLE DATABASES

Often an EEG data sample from a patient is sent to a laboratory or QEEG service, and the data is compared to multiple databases including sub-standard databases. As expected, the results are often conflicting, contradictory and confusing. There is an assumption that somehow multiple comparisons to multiple databases is better than comparing a patient's EEG to a single well-published database that has met high statistical and scientific standards. This assumption is wrong and potentially

TABLE 2.4   List of "gold standards" by which to judge
QEEG normative databases

	Standards	Yes	No
1	Amplifier matching		
2	Peer reviewed publications		
3	Artifact rejection		
4	Test–retest reliability		
5	Inclusion/exclusion criteria		
6	Adequate sample size per age group		
7	Approximation to a Gaussian		
8	Cross-validation		
9	Clinical correlation		
10	FDA registered		

dangerous to unsuspecting patients and clinicians who are provided with multiple comparisons. If a patient or a clinician receives multiple database comparisons involving unmatched amplifier characteristics then they should ask the provider of the normative database for the methods of amplifier equilibration, and for a list of the scientific standards of the normative databases.

It is the responsibility of users of normative databases to know the scientific standards of the database that they are comparing their patients to, and to provide informed consent to patients in situations where the patient's EEG samples are compared to a non peer-reviewed database, and/or unknown number of subjects per year database, and/or unknown inclusion/exclusion criteria database, and/or no statistical validation test database, and/or a non-FDA registered database, etc. State law and the FDA and IRBs require wording in an informed consent form that is clear and unambiguous in which the patient is informed that their EEG data will be compared to an unpublished or otherwise unknown QEEG normative database. Hopefully the "Gold Standards" check list in Table 2.4 will help in this process.

XXII.   FUTURE STANDARDIZATION OF QEEG NORMATIVE DATABASES

The post-Newtonian period of European history (1685–1850s) is marked by an emphasis on standards and rules as an outgrowth of Newtonian mathematics in the 1600s. It was recognized that standards were a prerequisite for the future industrial revolution involving mass production and efficient engineering and growth of new knowledge. A similar need for standardization of QEEG normative databases is present today. Amplifier equilibration and standardization has long been an elusive goal as mentioned previously. However, new technologies are available that provide for simple and inexpensive standardization of EEG amplifiers for purposes of comparison.

In the future the essential standard will be to equate the microvolt measurement of the electrical energies of the human brain recorded at different frequencies from different amplifiers using accepted statistical tests and standards of validation and verification as listed in rows 2 to 10 in Table 2.4.

REFERENCES

Adey, W. R., Walter, D. O. and Hendrix, C. E. (1961). Computer techniques in correlation and spectral analyses of cerebral slow waves during discriminative behavior. *Exp Neurol.*, 3, 501–524.

Adey, W. R. (1964a). Data acquisition and analysis techniques in a Brain Research Institute. *Ann N Y Acad Sci.*, 31(115), 844–866.

Adey, W. R. (1964b). Biological instrumentation, electrophysiological recording and analytic techniques. *Physiologist.*, 72, 65–68.

Arruda, J. E., Weiler, M. D., Valentino, D., Willis, W. G., Rossi, J. S., Stern, R. A., Gold, S. M. and Costa, L. (1996). A guide for applying principal-components analysis and confirmatory factor analysis to quantitative electroencephalogram data. *Int J Psychophysiol.*, 23(1–2), 63–81.

Berger, H. (1929). Uber das Electrenkephalogramm des Menschen. *Archiv. Fur. Psychiatrie und Neverkrankheiten*, 87, 527–570.

Berger, H. (1932). Uber das Electrenkephalogramm des Menschen. Vierte Mitteilungj. *Archiv. Fur. Psychiatrie und Neverkrankheiten,* 97, 6–26.

Berger, H. (1934). Uber das Electrenkephalogramm des Menschen. Neunte Mitteilungj. *Archiv. Fur. Psychiatrie und Neverkrankheiten*, 102, 538–557.

Brazis, P. W., Masdeu, J. C. and Biller, J. (2007). *Localization in Clinical Neurology*. Philadelphia, PA: Lippincott Williams and Wilkins.

Bosch-Bayard, J., Valdes-Sosa, P., Virues-Alba, T., *et al.* (2001). 3D statistical parametric mapping of EEG source spectra by means of variable resolution electromagnetic tomography (VARETA). *Clinical Electroencephalogr.*, 32(2), 47–61.

Burgess, A. and Gruzelier, J. (1993). Individual reliability of amplitude distribution in topographical mapping of EEG. *Electroencephalogr Clinical Neurophysiol.*, 86(4), 219–223.

Coburn, K. L., Lauterback, E. C., Boutros, N. N., Black, K. J., Arciniegas, D. B. and Coffey, C. E. (2006). The value of quantitative electroencephalography in clinical psychiatry: A report by the committee on research of the American Neuropsychiatric Association. *J. Neuropsychiat. and Clin. Neurosci.*, 18, 460–500.

Cohen, J. (1977). *Statistical power analysis for the behavioral sciences.* New York: Academic Press.

Cooley, W. W. and Lohnes, P. R. (1971). *Multivariate Data Analysis.* New York: John Wiley & Sons.

Corsi-Cabrera, M., Solis-Ortiz, S. and Guevara, M. A. (1997). Stability of EEG inter- and intrahemispheric correlation in women. *Electroencephalogr Clin Neurophysiol*, 102(3), 248–255.

Duffy, F., Hughes, J. R., Miranda, F., Bernad, P. and Cook, P. (1994). Status of quantitative EEG (QEEG) in clinical practice. *Clinical Electroencephalography*, 25(4), vi–vixxii.

Gasser, T., Verleger, R., Bacher, P. and Sroka, L. (1988a). Development of the EEG of school-age children and adolescents. *I. Analysis of band power. Electroencephalography and Clinical Neurophysiology,*, 69(2), 91–99.

Gasser, T., Jennen-Steinmetz, C., Sroka, L., Verleger, R. and Mocks, J. (1988b). Development of the EEG of school-age children and adolescents. *II: Topography. Electroencephalography Clinical Neurophysiology,*, 69(2), 100–109.

Gordon, E., Cooper, N., Rennie, C., Hermens, D. and Williams, L. M. (2005). Integrative neuroscience: The role of a standardized database. *Clin. EEG and Neurosci.*, 36(2), 64–75.

Granger, C. W. J. and Hatanka, M. (1964). *Spectral Analysis of Economic Time Series*. New Jersey: Princeton University Press.

Hagne, I., Persson, J., Magnusson, R. and Petersen, I. (1973). Spectral analysis via fast Fourier transform of waking EEG in normal infants. In *Automation of clinical electroencephalography* (P. Kellaway and I. Petersen, eds), pp. 103–143. New York: Raven Press.

Hamilton-Bruce, M. A., Boundy, K. L. and Purdie, G. H. (1991). Interoperator variability in quantitative electroencephalography. *Clin Exp Neurol.*, **28**, 219–224.

Harmony, T., Fernandez, T., Rodriguez, M., Reyes, A., Marosi, E. and Bernal, J. (1993). Test–retest reliability of EEG spectral parameters during cognitive tasks: II. Coherence. *Int J. Neuroscience,*, **68(3–4)**, 263–271.

Hayes, W. L. (1973). *Statistics for the social sciences*. New York: Holt, Rhinehart and Winston.

Heilman, K. M. and Valenstein, E. (1993). *Clinical Neuropsychology*, 3rd edition. New York: Oxford University Press.

Hellstrom-Westas, L. and Rosen, I. (2005). Electroencephalography and brain damage in preterm infants. *Early Hum Dev.*, **81(3)**, 255–261.

Herscovitch, P. (1994). Radiotracer techniques for functional neuroimaging with positron emission tomography. In *Functional Neuroimaging: Technical Foundations* (R. W. Thatcher, M. Halletr, T. Zeffro, E. R. John and M. Huerta, eds), pp. 29–46. San Diego: Academic Press.

Hoechstetter, K., Bornfleth, H., Weckesser, D., Ille, N., Berg, P. and Scherg, M. (2004). BESA source coherence: A new method to study cortical oscillatory coupling. *Brain Topography*, **16**, 233–238.

Hoffman, D. A., Stockdale, S., Hicks, L., *et al.* (1995). Diagnosis and treatment of head injury. *Journal of Neurotherapy.*, **1(1)**, 14–21.

Hoffman, D. A., Stockdale, S., Van Egren, L., *et al.* (1996). Symptom changes in the treatment of mild traumatic brain injury using EEG neurofeedback. *Clinical Electroencephalography (Abstract)*, **27(3)**, 164.

Hoffman, D. (2006). LORETA: An attempt at a simple answer to a complex controversy. *J. Neurotherapy*, **10(1)**, 57–72.

Hori, J. and He, B. (2001). Equivalent dipole source imaging of brain electric activity by means of parametric projection filter. *Ann Biomed Eng.*, **29(5)**, 436–445.

Huizenga, H. M., de Munck, J. C., Waldorp, L. J. and Grasman, R. P. (2002). Spatiotemporal EEG/MEG source analysis based on a parametric noise covariance model. *IEEE Trans Biomed Eng.*, **49(6)**, 533–539.

Hughes, J. R. and John, E. R. (1999). Conventional and quantitative electroencephalography in psychiatry. *Neuropsychiatry*, **11**, 190–208.

John, E. R. (1990). *Machinery of the Mind: Data, theory, and speculations about higher brain function*. Boston: Birkhauser.

John, E. R. (1977). Neurometrics: Quantitative Electrophysiological Analyses. In *Functional Neuroscience* (E. R. John and R. W. Thatcher, eds) **II**, New Jersey: L. Erlbaum Assoc.

John, E. R., Karmel, B., Corning, W., *et al.* (1977). Neurometrics: Numerical taxonomy identifies different profiles of brain functions within groups of behaviorally similar people. *Science*, **196**, 1393–1410.

John, E. R., Ahn, H., Prichep, L. S., Trepetin, M., Brown, D. and Kaye, H. (1980). Developmental equations for the electroencephalogram. *Science*, **210**, 1255–1258.

John, E. R., Prichep, L. S. and Easton, P. (1987). Normative data banks and neurometrics: Basic concepts, methods and results of norm construction. In *Handbook of electroencephalography and clinical neurophysiology: III. Computer analysis of the EEG and other neurophysiological signals* (A. Remond, ed.), pp. 449–495. Amsterdam: Elsevier.

John, E. R., Prichep, L. S., Fridman, J. and Easton, P. (1988). Neurometrics: Computer assisted differential diagnosis of brain dysfunctions. *Science*, **293**, 162–169.

Korn, A., Golan, H., Melamed, I., Pascual-Marqui, R. and Friedman, A. (2005). Focal cortical dysfunction and blood-brain barrier disruption in patients with Postconcussion syndrome. *Journal of Clinical Neurophysiology*, **22(1)**, 1–9.

Kropotov, J. D., Grin-Yatsenko, V. A., Ponomarev, V. A., Chutko, L. S., Yakovenko, E. A. and Nikishena, I. S. (2005). ERPs correlates of EEG relative beta training in ADHD children. *Int. J. Psychophysiol.*, **55(1)**, 23–34.

Lubar, J. F., Congedo, M. and Askew, J. (2003). Low-resolution electromagnetic tomography (LORETA) of cerebral activity in chronic depressive disorder. *International Journal of Psychophysiology*, 49, 175–185.

Lund, T. R., Sponheim, S. R., Iacono, W. G. and Clementz, B. A. (1995). Internal consistency reliability of resting EEG power spectra in schizophrenic and normal subjects. *Psychophysiology*, 32(1), 66–71.

Machado, C., Cuspineda, E., Valdes, P., *et al.* (2004). Assessing acute middle cerebral artery ischemic stroke by quantitative electric tomography. *Clin. EEG and Neurosci.*, 35(2), 116–124.

Mas, F., Prichep, L. S. and Alper, K. (1993). Treatment resistant depression in a case of minor head injury: an electrophysiological hypothesis. *Clinical Electroencephalography*, 24(3), 118–122.

Matousek, M. and Petersen, I. (1973a). Automatic evaluation of background activity by means of age-dependent EEG quotients. *EEG & Clin. Neurophysiol.*, 35, 603–612.

Matousek, M. and Petersen, I. (1973b). Frequency analysis of the EEG background activity by means of age-dependent EEG quotients. In *Automation of clinical electroencephalography* (P. Kellaway and I. Petersen, eds), pp. 75 Otnes, R. K. and Enochson, L. (1972). *Digital time series analysis*. New York: John Wiley and Sons.

102. New York: Raven Press.

Nunez, P. (1981). *Electrical Fields of the Brain*. New York: Oxford University Press.

Nunez, P. (1995). *Neocortical dynamics and human EEG rhythms*. New York: Oxford University Press.

Nunnally, J. C. (1978). *Psychometric theory*. New York: McGraw-Hill.

Nuwer, M. R. (1997). Assessment of digital EEG, quantitative EEG and EEG brain mapping report of the American Academy of Neurology and the American Clinical Neurophysiology Society. *Neurology*, 49, 277–292.

Otnes, R. K. and Enochson, L. (1972). *Digital time series analysis*. New York: John Wiley and Sons.

Pascual-Marqui, R. D., Koukkou, M., Lehmann, D. and Kochi, K. (2001). Functional localization and functional connectivity with LORETA comparison of normal controls and first episode drug naïve schizophrenics. *J. of Neurotherapy*, 4(4), 35–37.

Pollock, V. E., Schneider, L. S. and Lyness, S. A. (1991). Reliability of topographic quantitative EEG amplitude in healthy late-middle-aged and elderly subjects. *Electroencephalogr Clinical Neurophysiology*, 79(1), 20–26.

Prichep, L. S. (2005). Use of normative databases and statistical methods in demonstrating clinical utility of QEEG: Importance and cautions. *Clin. EEG and Neurosci.*, 36(2), 82–87.

Raichle, M. (2002). Appraising the brain's energy budget. *PNAS*, 99(16), 10237–10239.

Roche, R. A., Dockree, P. M., Garavan, H., Foxe, J. J., Robertson, I. H. and O'Mara, S. M. (2004). EEG alpha power changes reflect response inhibition deficits after traumatic brain injury (TBI) in humans. *Neurosci Lett.*, 13 362(1), 1–5.

Ruijs, M. B., Gabreels, F. J. and Thijssen, H. M. (1994). The utility of electroencephalography and cerebral computed tomography in children with mild and moderately severe closed head injuries. *Neuropediatrics*, 25(2), 73–77.

Salinsky, M. C., Oken, B. S. and Morehead, L. (1991). Test–retest reliability in EEG frequency analysis. *Electroencephalogr Clinical Neurophysiology*, 79(5), 382–392.

Slewa-Younan, S., Green, A. M., Baguley, I. J., Felmingham, K. L., Haig, A. R. and Gordon, E. (2002). Is 'gamma' (40 Hz) synchronous activity disturbed in patients with traumatic brain injury?. *Clin Neurophysiol.*, 113(10), 1640–1646.

Slobounov, S., Sebastianelli, W. and Simon, R. (2002). Neurophysiological and behavioral concomitants of mild brain injury in collegiate athletes. *Clin Neurophysiol.*, 113(2), 185–193.

Tebano, M. T., Cameroni, M., Gallozzi, G., *et al.* (1988). EEG spectral analysis after minor head injury in man. *EEG and Clinical Neurophysiology*, 70, 185–189.

Thatcher, R. W. (1995). Tomographic EEG/MEG. *Journal of Neuroimaging*, 5, 35–45.

Thatcher, R. W. (1998). EEG normative databases and EEG biofeedback. *Journal of Neurotherapy*, 2(4), 8–39.

Thatcher, R. W. (2000a). EEG Operant Conditioning (Biofeedback) and Traumatic Brain Injury. *Clinical EEG*, 31(1), 38–44.

Thatcher, R. W. (2000b). *An EEG Least Action Model of Biofeedback*. 8th Annual ISNR conference, St. Paul, MN, September.

Thatcher, R. W. and Collura, T. F. (2006). Z-Score EEG Biofeedback. *Int. Soc. for Neuronal Regulation*, Atlanta, G. A., Sept. 2006.

Thatcher, R. W. and John, E. R. (1977). Functional Neuroscience. In *Foundations of Cognitive Processes* (E. R. John and R. W. Thatcher, eds) 1. New York: L. Erlbaum Assoc. Academic Press.

Thatcher, R. W., McAlaster, R., Lester, M. L., Horst, R. L. and Cantor, D. S. (1983). Hemispheric EEG Asymmetries Related to Cognitive Functioning in Children. In *Cognitive Processing in the Right Hemisphere* (A. Perecuman, ed.), New York: Academic Press.

Thatcher, R. W., Krause, P. and Hrybyk, M. (1986). Corticocortical Association Fibers and EEG Coherence: A Two Compartmental Model. *Electroencephalog. Clinical Neurophysiol.*, **64**, 123–143.

Thatcher, R. W., Walker, R. A. and Guidice, S. (1987). Human cerebral hemispheres develop at different rates and ages. *Science*, **236**, 1110–1113.

Thatcher, R. W., Walker, R. A., Gerson, I. and Geisler, F. (1989). EEG discriminant analyses of mild head trauma. *EEG and Clin. Neurophysiol.*, **73**, 93–106.

Thatcher, R. W., Cantor, D. S., McAlaster, R., Geisler, F. and Krause, P. (1991). Comprehensive predictions of outcome in closed head injury: The development of prognostic equations. *Annals New York Academy of Sciences*, **620**, 82–104.

Thatcher, R., Wang, B., Toro, C. and Hallett, M. (1994). Human Neural Network Dynamics Using Multimodal Registration of EEG, PET and MRI. In *Functional Neuroimaging: Technical Foundations* (R. Thatcher, M. Hallett, T. Zeffiro, E. John and M. Huerta, eds), pp. 269–279, New York: Academic Press.

Thatcher, R. W., Camacho, M., Salazar, A., Linden, C., Biver, C. and Clarke, L. (1997). Quantitative MRI of the gray-white matter distribution in traumatic brain injury. *J. Neurotrauma*, **14**, 1–14.

Thatcher, R. W. (1998). EEG normative databases and EEG biofeedback. *Journal of Neurotherapy*, **2(4)**, 8–39.

Thatcher, R. W., Biver, C., McAlaster, R. and Salazar, A. M. (1998a). Biophysical linkage between MRI and EEG coherence in traumatic brain injury. *NeuroImage*, **8(4)**, 307–326.

Thatcher, R. W., Biver, C., Camacho, M., McAlaster, R. and Salazar, A. M. (1998b). Biophysical linkage between MRI and EEG amplitude in traumatic brain injury. *NeuroImage*, **7**, 352–367.

Thatcher, R. W., North, D., Curtin, R., *et al.* (2001a). An EEG Severity Index of Traumatic Brain Injury, *J. Neuropsychiatry and Clinical Neuroscience*, **13(1)**, 77–87.

Thatcher, R. W., Biver, C. L., Gomez-Molina, J. F., *et al.* (2001b). Estimation of the EEG Power Spectrum by MRI T2 Relaxation Time in Traumatic Brain Injury. *Clinical Neurophysiology*, **112**, 1729–1745.

Thatcher, R. W., Walker, R. A., Biver, C., North, D. and Curtin, R. (2003). Quantitative EEG Normative databases: Validation and Clinical Correlation. *J. Neurotherapy*, **7 (No. ¼)**, 87–122.

Thatcher, R. W., North, D. and Biver, C. (2005a). EEG inverse solutions and parametric vs. nonparametric statistics of Low Resolution Electromagnetic Tomography (LORETA). *Clin. EEG and Neuroscience*, **36(1)**, 1–9.

Thatcher, R. W., North, D. and Biver, C. (2005b). Evaluation and Validity of a LORETA normative EEG database. *Clin. EEG and Neuroscience*, **36(2)**, 116–122.

Thatcher, R. W., North, D. and Biver, C. (2005c). EEG and Intelligence: Univariate and Multivariate Comparisons Between EEG Coherence, EEG Phase Delay and Power. *Clinical Neurophysiology*, **116(9)**, 2129–2141.

Thatcher, R. W., Biver, C. J. and North, D. (2007a). Spatial-temporal current source correlations and cortical connectivity. *Clin. EEG and Neuroscience*, **38(1)**, 35–48.

Thatcher, R. W., North, D. and Biver, C. (2007b). Self-organized criticality and the development of EEG phase reset. *Human Brain Mapping*, (in press, 2007).

Thompson, J., Sebastianelli, W. and Slobounov, S. (2005). EEG and postural correlates of mild traumatic brain injury in athletes. *Neuroscience Letters*, **377(3)**, 158–163.

Trudeau, D. L., Anderson, J., Hansen, L. M., *et al.* (1998). Findings of mild traumatic brain injury in combat veterans with PTSD and a history of blast concussion. *J. Neuropsychiatry Clin Neurosci.*, **10(3)**, 308–313.

von Bierbrauer, A., Weissenborn, K., Hinrichs, H., Scholz, M. and Kunkel, H. (1993). Automatic (computer-assisted) EEG analysis in comparison with visual EEG analysis in patients following minor cranio-cerebral trauma (a follow-up study). *EEG EMG Z Elektroenzephalogr Elektromyogr Verwandte Geb.*, **23(3)**, 151–157.

Waldorp, L. J., Huizenga, H. M., Dolan, C. V. and Molenaar, P. C. (2001). Estimated generalized least squares electromagnetic source analysis based on a parametric noise covariance model. *IEEE Trans Biomed Eng.*, **48(6)**, 737–741.

Winer, B. J. (1971). *Statistical Principles in Experimental Design*. New York: McGraw-Hill.

PART 2

Advancing Neurofeedback Practice

CHAPTER 3

Applying advanced methods in clinical practice

David S. Cantor, Ph.D.

Psychological Sciences Institute,
PC, Duluth, GA, USA

QEEG has come a long way in its relatively short life in terms of use in clinical practice. Now, as we clinicians become aware of the scientific basis and power of using parametrically based measures of QEEG to assess an individual against age-matched populations, we find new ways to employ this technique. Neurofeedback clinicians are realizing the utility of defining deviations from normal, of clarifying syndromes, and finding heretofore unrecognized etiology as ways of guiding therapeutic interventions. This chapter presents some recent advanced techniques combined with QEEG, which can produce powerful results. The case studies illustrate the methods and some results which can be achieved through use of these multiple applications.

There are literally thousands of univariate electrophysiological measures that can be derived, transformed, and normed into Z-scores, to be used to indicate degrees of deviations from normal. The problem confronting the clinician is to realize the meaningfulness of these deviations. How are we, as clinicians, able to define these deviations in terms of behavior syndromes and specific functional impairments? Further, with so many variables available, can we recognize how these variables are inter-correlated and, thus, how they represent sets of information redundancy? One of the advantages of statistical measurement approaches with parametric data is the ability to reduce redundancies by methods of multivariate analyses. This exponentially increases the capacity for discriminative sensitivity in defining behavioral syndromes of specific functional clusters. This is a gigantic step forward in understanding the functional pathology of the patients facing us and, as we gain experiences, will transform the practice of neurofeedback training.

I. DIAGNOSTIC CONSIDERATIONS—UNIVARIATE VERSUS MULTIVARIATE MEASURES

QEEG offers a powerful application tool as a method for providing convergent evidence in the identification of clinical syndromes for individuals. Over the years,

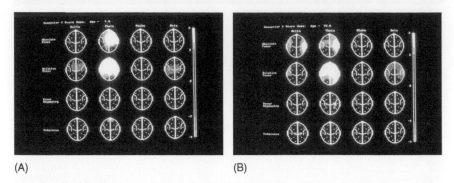

(A)   (B)

FIGURE 3.1A AND B   Common univariate feature Z-score sets across two very cases with a different diagnosis.

various clinicians using QEEG have attempted to establish "brain maps" to correspond with specific disorders such as learning disorders, attention deficit hyperactivity disorders (ADHD), chronic alcoholism, depression, etc. While certain features may be associated with general types of impairment, the utilization of univariate sets of features have, to date, been unable to provide unique solutions in defining specific psychiatric disorders (Coburn *et al.*, 2006). This is illustrated in Fig. 3.1.

As noted in Fig. 3.1A and B above, the two maps exhibit two patients with diffuse theta as the primary univariate set characterizing their deviance from age-expected norms. The two patients, however, have two very different diagnostic categorizations. Fig. 3.1A represents a set of maps for a 7-year-old child with significant learning disabilities whereas Fig. 3.1B represents a set of maps for a patient diagnosed has having advance Alzheimer's Disease. While these two patients have similar problems in as far as they have difficulty with learning new information and short-term memory, there are likely more subtle "feature" sets which would discriminate these two individuals. Univariate maps of data sets lack the specificity and statistical discriminability in defining these disorders. Table 3.1 illustrates this point.

Looking at only the univariate features without recognizing the full "space" of all deviant measures, one may not realize the particular cluster of measure that may contribute to specific disorders with distinct features. Multivariate statistical measurement sets encompass the "space" of regions by measurement, yielding distinctive complex patterns which yield greater sensitivity in discriminability. Table 3.2 shows an example of the "discriminant" accuracy in classifying groups of patients into specific psychiatric disorders as described by the Diagnostic and Statistical Manual of the American Psychiatric Association (2000).

In Table 3.2, two-way discriminants are illustrated (comparing two groups against each other) showing the accuracy on the initial discriminant set of measures, and the replicability when this same equation is applied to an independent comparison of the same groups including different samples from the same populations. For example, on the first line, the initial discriminant accuracy comparing "Normals" versus

TABLE 3.1　Schematic showing the matrix of abnormal neurometric values (marked with an X) for a theoretical patient with Disorder 1. Rows of the matrix are extracted Z transformed features, and columns are brain regions (taken from Prichep and John, 1992)

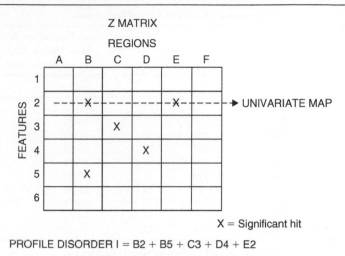

Z MATRIX

REGIONS

X = Significant hit

PROFILE DISORDER I = B2 + B5 + C3 + D4 + E2

"Depressives" was accurate in identifying normals as normal 88% of the time, and the depressives as depressive 86% of the time on creation of the initial discriminant. In an independent test of the discriminant function, 83% of the "Normals" were correctly identified as "normal" whereas 93% of the "Depressives" were identified as "depressive." The lower portion of the table shows the power of these discriminant functions when making three- and four-way comparisons. The real power of these findings is realized when the discriminability is this high, based on electrophysiology. At this point in time, it is not recommended that psychiatric diagnosis should be made on these measurement sets alone, but rather, as indicated previously, they can add much in the form of convergent validation when employing other tools in the process of clinical evaluation.

In psychiatry the implications of more accurate diagnostic classification for a given patient are significant, when considering the therapeutic pathways to be applied to the patient. For example, suppose a 60-year-old male approaches a psychiatrist with the vague symptoms of forgetfulness, some dysphoria, and anxiety about his concerns over his changing functional abilities. A psychiatrist is faced with deciding if the patient may have an early stage Alzheimer's disorder causing the problems with memory, with secondary problems of reactive anxiety and depression over his abilities, OR if he has developed a major affective disorder with typical associated anxiety and is having secondary effects of forgetfulness because of the dysphoria and malaise. Distinction of these two possibilities is critical since

TABLE 3.2 Table showing two group and three group discriminant comparisons with diagnostic accuracy including cases in predicting medication response (taken from Prichep & John, 1992)

Neurometric QEEG Two Group Discriminants						
Groups			n		Mean Discriminant Accuracy (%) (Initial Discrim./Independent Replication)	
I	vs.	II	I	II	I	II
N	vs.	Dep	95	111	88/86	83/93
Uni	vs.	Bip	65	32	84/87	88/94
N	vs.	MHI	150	52	91/84	89/92
N	vs.	Sz	149	57	96/99	90/82
Dep	vs.	Sz	103	46	84/88	85/85**
N	vs.	Alc	120	30	95/95	75/90*
Abn	vs.	Alc	32–97	30	91/88	96/93*
N	vs.	LD	158	175	89/79	72/71
Vas Dem	vs.	Dem	93	13	94/82	92/85*
RitResp	vs.	NonResp	16	12	81/81*	83/83*

Neurometric QEEG Multiple Group Discriminants											
Groups				n				Mean Discriminant Accuracy (%) (Initial Discrim,/Independent Replication)			
I	vs. II	vs. III	vs. IV	I	II	III	IV	I	II	III	IV
N	vs. Dep	vs. Dem		85	87	125		84/85	84/80	84/71	–
N	vs. Dep	vs. Alc	vs. Dem	120	103	30	125	77/75	72/85	80/80	79/77

*Jack-knifed replication
**Med. Group used for replication
Group codes are as follows: N = Normal; Dep = Major Affective Disorder, Depression, Uni = Unipolar Depression; Bip = Bipolar Depression; MHI = Mild Head Injury; Sz = Chronic Schizophrenia; Abn = Abnormal groups combined; Alc = Alcoholic; LD = Learning Disabled; RitResp = Responders to Ritalin; NonResp = Nonresponders to Ritalin; Dem = Dementia (SDAT); Vas Dem = Dementia of vascular etiology.

two different classes of medications are typical first line treatment considerations for these respective disorders. The alternative is that the psychiatrist may choose to use a "mixture" of medications in the hopes that such a compound will sufficiently treat "all" symptoms of the patient without undue side effects of using a more complex psychotropic approach. Defining this patient as more likely an Alzheimer's disorder will not only target a more specific set of psychotropic medications to consider but, also, such a conclusion has other prognostic considerations for the long-term care of the patient.

Recently, research showing the correspondence of QEEG profiles to specified pharmacological approaches has been demonstrated. This validates evidence based medicine (EBM) for psychiatric conditions, which shows brain physiological profiles to be more accurate rather than a nominal level classifications system such as the Diagnostic and Statistical Manual currently used as a guide for diagnosis and hypothetically selecting the treatment (Suffin and Emory, 1995). With the recent paradigm shift toward EBM as the new standard for defining health care, this is an important consideration.

Most recently, work by John *et al.* (2007) has demonstrated that six primary clusters of cluster functions made up of combinations of univariate and multivariate measures of brain function can account for more than 95% of *all* psychiatric disorders. This finding suggests that distinctive brain profile "signatures" may be more important, not only in confirming the presence of a brain dysfunctional patterning consistent with a psychiatric condition but, more critically, in testing and tracking treatment paradigms. It can be used to distinctively and optimally treat each profile. Such an approach may yield distinctive pathways for treatment based on the underlying physiological systems contributing to the behavior patterns. This would replace the current tendency of making idiocyncratic choices for treatment based on clinician intutiton or trial and error, neither of which has a strong probability of clinical improvement.

II.   PHARMACO-EEG

For the same reasons that QEEG measures are sensitive enough to be affected by medications, QEEG measure offers the possibility of establishing specific biomarkers for successful treatment (Suffin and Emory, 1995; Hunter *et al.*, 2007; Bares *et al.*, 2007; Saletu *et al.*, 2006; Hansen *et al.*, 2003; Fogelson *et al.*, 2003; Galderisi, 2002). For example, in a study by Clemens *et al.* 2006, quantitative EEG (QEEG) effects of therapeutic doses of carbamazepine (CBZ), oxcarbazepine (OXC), valproate (VA) and lamotrigine (LA) monotherapy were investigated in patients with the beginnings of epilepsy. Baseline waking EEG (EEG1) was recorded in the untreated state; the second EEG (EEG2) was done after 8 weeks of reaching the therapeutic dose. Left occipital data were used for analysis. QEEG target parameters were absolute band-power (delta: AD, theta: AT, alpha: AA, beta: AB), and alpha mean frequency (AMF). Group effects (untreated versus treated condition in the CBZ, VA, OXC, LA groups) were computed for each target parameter. One group with benign rolandic epilepsy remained untreated for clinical reasons and served to estimate the QEEG test–retest differences. In addition, the individual QEEG response to each drug was calculated as (EEG2-EEG1).

The results noted statistically significant ($p < 0.05$) group differences indicated by the QEEG domain systematically affected by the drugs. More specifically, CBZ caused AT increase and AMF decrease while OXC caused AMF decrease. VA and LA did not decrease AMF (LA even increased it), but reduced broad-band power. Individual power and AMF changes showed considerable variability in each group. A greater than 0.5 Hz AMF decrease (that was reported to predict cognitive impairment in prior studies) occurred in 10/41 patients in the CBZ group but never in the OXC, VA, LA groups. Much of the literature to date on the relationship of QEEG and pharmacotherapeutic applications has noted that, in general, several QEEG studies on early predictors of treatment response to first generation antipsychotics have produced consistent findings, but have thus far produced no clinical impact. For other psychotropic drug classes few and inconsistent reports have appeared (Mucci et al., 2006).

In addition to predicting effects of medication in psychiatric conditions at large, QEEG offers a methodology for tracking changes in brain function to establish treatment efficacy in individual cases, especially when a progressive disorder is present such as forms of dementias (Sneddon et al., 2006; Goforth et al., 2004; Rodriquez et al., 2002) or in disorders in which the nature of the disorder is assumed to be static such is in ADHD (Song et al., 2005). While space is limited here, the reader is directed to a proposed model that helps in understanding the evaluation of underlying brain dysfunction in psychiatric disorders and a selection of pharmacotherapeutic agents (John and Prichep, 2006). Perhaps the most important research to be done in this area is to predict potential side effects or adverse reactions. Identifying agents which *may do more harm* than good in treatment on a case-by-case basis using QEEG has significant ramifications in the context of emergent empirically based medicine (EBM) protocols for treatment (Hunter et al., 2005).

III.   QEEG—THERAPEUTIC APPLICATIONS IN NEUROFEEDBACK

The power in being able to define deviations of brain function within a normally distributed measurement set is that one can target deviant measures to "normalize" by a variety of intervention modalities with the premise that as one normalizes functioning of the brain, so should there be consequential changes in behavior that become more "normalized." The correlation of Neurometric QEEG measures to parameters of behavior is implicit in the manner in which populations defined for the inclusion typically meet criteria of normal functioning and behavior. Thus, it stands to reason that deviations in brain function will likely have a correlated change in some aspect of function and behavior. In this context, QEEG lends itself well to be used as a monitoring tool to "measure" treatment efficacy, and may in fact have predictive value for treatment efficacy for profiles of brain function.

The evolution of protocol development of neurofeedback protocols to be used in clinical cases has evolved to use QEEG as a guideline for defining what brain regions and measures are to be targeted to train in order to achieve a corresponding change in functional performance and behavior. In general, the thought is that by delineating which aspects of brain function are "deviant" from normal, and by correcting such measures by EEG neurofeedback training, there is a facilitation for functional performance which should be achieved. Other than examining functional disruptions through the QEEG alone, another alternative means of diagnosis is through source location methods. The following case illustrates how QEEG components can be used in conjunction with other diagnostic techniques. To further the illustration, the discussion of the LORETA, a source utilization method, will be presented next.

IV. DIAGNOSTICS—UTILIZATION SOURCE LOCALIZATION METHODS

A discussion of source localization methods with spectral EEG data could be a chapter within itself, so the reader is directed to examine a number of some of the more recent techniques that illustrate methods of source localization (see Alberta, L. et al., 2008; Hallez, H. et al., 2007; Russell, J. P. and Koles, Z. J., 2006; Pascual-Marqui, R. et al., 2002).

LORETA is a functional imaging technique where the cortex is modeled as a collection of volume elements (voxels) in the digitized Talariach atlas provided by the Brain Imaging Center of the Montreal Neurological Institute. The LORETA inverse solution corresponds to the three-dimensional distribution of electric activity that has a maximum similarity (i.e., maximum synchronization) in terms of orientation and strength, between neighboring neuronal populations.

The empirical validity of LORETA has been established under diverse physiological conditions. Clinically, using a narrow band QEEG analysis, a point of maximal deviation from normal can be identified by examining Z-score deviation in the spectra and then using the LORETA solution at that frequency. In this manner, the maximal source of deviant activity can be identified in three-dimensional neuroanatomic space. Often this source localization method for maximal deviation of function can be validated by neuropsychological techniques measuring performance and/or historic or other examination information. An example of this technique is illustrated below.

V. CASE SAMPLE EMPLOYING UNIVARIATE, MULTIVARIATE AND SOURCE LOCALIZATION METHODS TO "DIAGNOSIS" OF THE NATURE OF PRESENTING SYMPTOMS

A. Case DS

As an adult, this patient has received medical treatment for cancer, cardiac problems (pacemaker installed 9/2005), and hypertension (past 5 years). He has been treated by his neurologist for cognitive and behavioral problems related to progressive memory loss over 5 years. His problems were reportedly somewhat exacerbated by involvement in a motor vehicle accident (11/18/2005) in which his body was struck by an SUV in a drug store parking lot resulting in Post Concussive Syndrome. His medical history is complicated by having a pacemaker, thus inhibiting the use of an MRI. CT scans and EEG are negative. Memory problems are reportedly for recall and recognition of names rather than for visual events. He denied having any untreated physical problems that he felt should receive medical attention. He is a nonsmoker. He has no prior history of cigarette smoking. Use of alcohol was reported to be occasional.

Neuropsychological testing revealed that he is functioning in the average range for age in intellectual functioning with a relative weakness or deficit in both immediate and delayed memory. His scores on other learning/memory subtests indicated varied attention, and generally poor memory abilities for age in learning and recalling an auditory and visually presented stimuli. His language/communication abilities (including expressive and receptive vocabulary skills) were generally lower than expectations for his age, yet consistent with his estimated verbal IQ on the WAIS-III. His skills to read quickly and comprehend the information immediately were significantly weaker and in the Below Average for age range. A QEEG data analysis was conducted, collecting digitized EEG from 19 locations of the International 10–20 System, and deriving age-corrected functional deviations in hundreds of brain measures as collected from scalp recording. The brain map shown in Fig. 3.2 indicated only limited measures with Z-scores (SDs from normal).

A multivariate discriminant function was mathematically conducted to compare this individual to populations of individuals with resulting functional effects from Post Concussive Syndrome ($p < 0.025$). A narrow band (0.3 Hz) spectral analysis was used to derive points of maximal deviation from age-matched normal population. Note that maximal measure reflects muscle artifact at T3. Thus, other maxima were used to submit to source localization. Using a maximal deviation at 8.64 Hz, sLORETA[1], which in this case was also corrected for age, the following structures were identified (Fig. 3.3).

Functional analyses of EEG activity indicates profile features implicating cortical and subcortical dysfunction which is statistically consistent with residual effects from Post Concussive Syndrome, exacerbating a previously identified Dementia NOS. Functional neuroimaging indicated primary posterior cortical dysfunction which may account for problems with reading, and which is notably more deviant in the right posterior quadrant which may be associated with reported mood liability. Basal structures including hypophysis, amygdala, and hippocampal dysfunction are indicated particularly by the sLORETA analysis, and this is consistent with possible dysregulation, especially after being treated with Effexor, of

---

[1]"sLORETA" is an updated revised version of the earlier LORETTA.

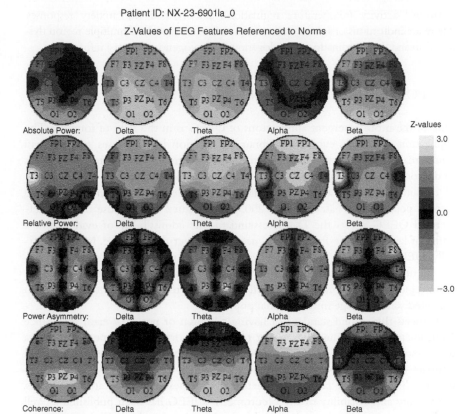

Patient ID: NX-23-6901la_0

Z-Values of EEG Features Referenced to Norms

FIGURE 3.2   Univariate Z-scores measures for Case DS (see color plate).

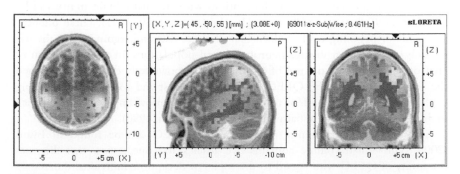

FIGURE 3.3   sLORETA source localization for Case DS at 8.64 Hz (see color plate).

hormonal activity (temperature regulation), anxiety, and fear/anxiety responses. There are indications of sensory integration deficits as a result of multiple region dysfunction and dyscoordination of endogenous and exogenous sensory information.

VI. FORENSIC APPLICATIONS

One of the more emergent applications of QEEG is in the field of forensics. The application of QEEG evidence of brain dysfunction in civil cases such as head injury make implicit sense since the primary objective of using such evidence is to demonstrate the region and severity of brain dysfunction, with a certain degree of certainty that such a finding would exceed expectations of an age-matched normal population. Thatcher *et al.* (2003) have argued that the use of norm referenced QEEG meets the Daubert standards for admissibility of evidence in a court of law. There are four criteria needed to meet this standard. More specifically, QEEG meets the standard of *hypothesis testing* in that because the measures can be fit to normal distribution, one can test whether or not function in a given brain region or across brain regions differs in a statistically significant manner from expected values for age in the normal population.

It meets the second standard of having a known or potential error rate. Since Neurometric QEEG measures are fit to a normal distribution, one can derive a direct estimate of standard error around any measure within the distribution, and estimate error rates depending on where within the normal distribution a given measure lies. The third criteria of meeting peer review and publication standards, the validity and reliability of the Neurometric QEEG has been published as well as illustrations of QEEG in thousands of publications in the behavioral sciences and neurology.

Finally, the fourth standard of general acceptance pertains to clinical consensus of usefulness in various clinical arenas. A most recent review of QEEG utilization of the diagnosis and treatment of psychiatric disorders is provided by Coburn *et al.*, 2006, and discussion in its applications with traumatic brain injury can be found in Duff (2004) as well as in Thatcher, *et al*, (1989, 1991). These publications and forthcoming works will further illustrate data and arguments for the use of such techniques in various neurobehavioral populations. In the application of civil or criminal cases, the use of QEEG is most powerfully demonstrated when the features noted in the QEEG profile can correspond to structural imaging evidence such as MRI and/or to functional assessment of impaired performance such as neuropsychological batteries (Prichep and John, 1990).

Studies illustrating forensic applications of QEEG can be found in Evans (2006). This edited volume contains five articles and one review that discusses the utility of QEEG with regard to the topics of deception, individual differences in convicted murderers and using QEEG guided neurotherapy in forensic cases. Many aspects of this general theme will be reflected in the ensuing chapters of

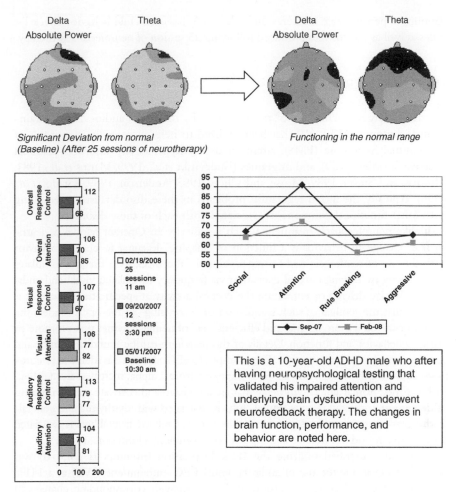

FIGURE 3.4   Electrophysiological, performance, and behavior rating measures before and after neurofeedback therapy (see color plate).

this book. However, a simple illustration of this principal is outlined in the form of a clinical case study.

A.   Case JR

This case was referred by his parents for this evaluation regarding problems with academic performance and possible attention deficits. Neuropsychological testing validated that he had an attention deficit hyperactivity disorder—combined type. After conducting a QEEG analysis, excessive delta and theta absolute power was identified. Fig. 3.4 illustrates baseline QEEG measures, integrated visual and auditory (IVA) continuous performance measures, and selected Achenbach child behavior check list scales as well as the changes produced following 25 session of neurofeedback therapy.

VII. AVE THERAPY

Another emergent technique to "train" EEG is by the use of audio-visual entrainment techniques (AVE). AVE has been utilized to help decrease the symptoms of Premenstual Syndrome (PMS), attention deficit hyperactivity disorders, seasonal affective disorder (SAD), and migraines (Budzynski et al., 1999, Manns et al., 1981, Thomas, and Siever, 1989, Morse and Chow, 1993, Anderson, 1989, Kuano et al., 1996). Typically, the mood regulation problems in these disorders improved along with other functional components associated with each of these disorders.

Unlike neurofeedback treatment which is basically an Operant Model of learning, i.e., change in behavior is a function of "shaping" learning to change behavior with the use of reinforcers tied to target values of the EEG, AVE therapy stimulates EEG activity by driving cortical excitation via frequency modulated visual and auditory events. By driving or entraining the cortical activity at specific frequencies, it is thought that the residual of such stimulation or "exercising" of the brain renders the brain to establish a more normal and efficient "set" of neural activities that promote or improve behavior and function. Details of this paradigm can be found in Cantor and Stevens (unpublished manuscript). For example, QEEG research has identified neurophysiological indicators in the EEG of increased frontal alpha, increased frontal beta, and increased frontal alpha asymmetry that are associated and correlate with symptoms of depression. Increased relative frontal alpha is associated with dysthymia and generalized depression or unipolar depression while increased relative frontal beta is associated more with a mood disturbance and bipolar symptomology (John et al., 1988).

The study described utilizing the Beck Depression Inventory-II (BDI-II) was designed to examine the use of auditory-visual EEG entrainment (AVE) at a 14 Hz beta frequency to decrease symptoms of depression with corresponding changes in underlying abnormal neurophysiology. The subjects (N = 16) ranged in age from 21–54, and were screened utilizing the BDI-II and broken into two groups (N = 8): simulated and AVE treatment with a crossover design. Both groups were given the BDI-II and QEEG testing at baseline, 4 weeks following either AVE or simulated treatment, and then again after an additional 4 weeks after a switch in treatment in the crossover design. Results revealed significant changes in reduction of depression only after the 4 weeks of AVE therapy (p > 0.01) using an impendent group T–test of the BDI-II scores. QEEG scores adjusted for normal age deviations demonstrate significant change scores over time in cortical regions noted for mood regulation. The changes in total depression scores from the BDI-II are shown in Fig. 3.5. In this figure, group 1 represents the group receiving AVE therapy in the first 4 weeks followed by 4 weeks of a simulated procedure, whereas group 2 represents the group receiving a simulated procedure in the first 4 weeks followed by AVE therapy in the next 4 weeks.

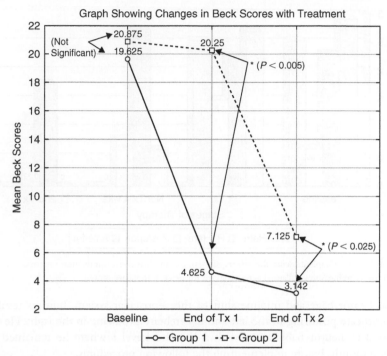

FIGURE 3.5   Changes in the Total Depression score for the BDI-II in a double crossover design treatment study.

Other adaptations of this technique have been explored with stimulating brain functional systems in coma patients suffering from traumatic brain injury, with resultant significant changes in patient level of responsiveness corresponding to brain activity changes produced by AVE therapy when all other methods of coma stimulation failed (Johnston, *et al.*, 1992). The use of AVE therapy and its clinical effectiveness is still being researched but offers promising benefits, particularly in patients that are not able to utilize the Operant Learning nature of Neurofeedback protocols (for example, very young children, coma patients, and patients that are otherwise non-responsive to other forms of intervention).

The following case illustration is another variant use of the AVE type of therapy employing information from QEEG, and from both brainstem and cortical evoked response measures.

A. Case BM

BM is a 25-year-old male who was working on the side of the road as a construction worker when he was struck by a motor vehicle at 65 mph and thrown 100 feet. He registered with an initial Glasgow coma score of 4 on admission to a subacute coma care center. A CT scan indicated right hemisphere swelling with right

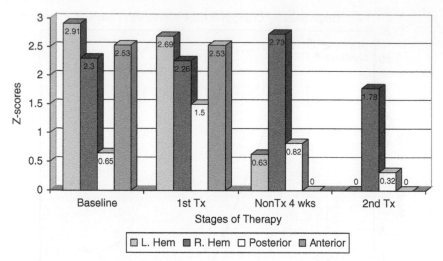

FIGURE 3.6   Graph showing the effects of e-stim of median nerve stimulation on cortical recovery. Multivariate measures collapsed across regions for delta + theta are shown.

frontal hemorrhage and midline shift of the ventricular system. Injuries resulted in decorticate posturing in the left and decerebrate posturing in the right. He was admitted to neurorehabilitation with a Rancho Level I where he remained for nearly 6 months before implementing the following procedures.

Neurometric QEEG testing indicated widespread cortical dysfunction with right more deviant than left except in the temporal regions. Visual evoked responses to light stimulation indicated intact but slow responses to stimulation, with the right hemisphere worse than the left. Somatosensory evoked responses to left median nerve stimulation was normal but not for the right. Although some mild cortical improvement occurred in the absence of stimulation during the previous 6 months, he remained at a Rancho Level I with eyes closed virtually all the time.

Based on these findings, a program of electrical stimulation to the left median (Cantor, *et al.*, 1994) nerve was undertaken using a functional electro stimulation (FES) every 20 sec of every minute 6 hours/day for 4 weeks. A 4-week period without stimulation followed and 4 weeks of treatment again followed after the non-stimulation period. Following successful "wakening" from this stimulation along an intact pathway from the left median nerve, protocols were changed to provide stimulation of the right median nerve and monitor changes in brainstem responses over a period of time. The protocols applied to the right median nerve yielded successful results. QEEG multivariate measures of bipolar delta + theta were used to evaluate changes in deviation from normal starting from the first baseline, over the beginning to the ending of treatment and 4 weeks post-treatment (Fig. 3.6). During this period, eye-opening behaviors and spontaneous motor activity increased significantly.

Behavioral scoring procedures showed significant improvement in sustained eye-opening throughout the day. As a result of increased eye-opening, engagement

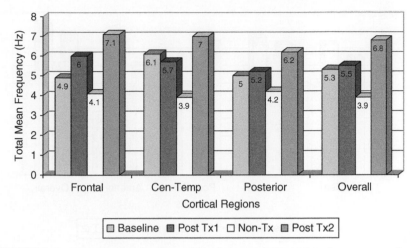

FIGURE 3.7   Graph showing the effects of AVE therapy at 10 Hz. Multivariate measures collapsed across regions for delta + theta are shown.

with various therapists was facilitated and communication skills were increased with the patient beginning to use "yes/no" answers by eye blinks (for example once for yes, twice for no). Within about 6 weeks following initiation of this procedure, the patient transitioned from a Rancho Level I/II to a Rancho Level III, and emerged to Level IV. Next, the total mean frequency was derived over these same cortical regions and, noting that the background activity was significantly low for an "awake" state, AVE entrainment was begun using 10 Hz visual and auditory stimulation for 40 minutes of every hour, 6 hours/day for 4 weeks (the same A-B-A-B treatment designed for the brainstem stimulation). The graphs in Fig 3.7 and 3.8 show the changes in total mean frequency and consequential Z-scores changes in the Neurometric QEEG multivariate delta + theta measures.

The conclusions from this case study are that selective sensory stimulation can improve wakefulness and cortical function in coma patients. Cortical entrainment can be used to alter the brain responsiveness to stimulation and improve functionality sufficiently to utilize other therapies that can also be used to further improve recovery.

VIII.   QEEG AS A TOOL FOR MONITORING OTHER "EXPERIMENTAL" INTERVENTIONS

By now, it should be apparent to the reader that one of the benefits of using neurometric QEEG measurement is to not only clarify brain dysfunction that can be correlated with behavior feature sets, but also it can be used to identify and predict intervention strategies. QEEG provides a clinical means to validate intervention

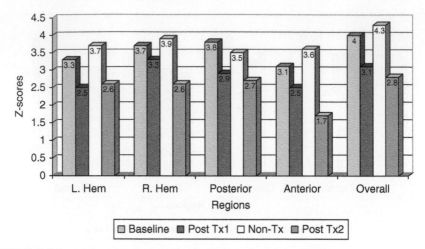

FIGURE 3.8   Graph showing the effects of AVE therapy at 10 Hz. Multivariate measures collapsed across regions for Delta + Theta are shown.

strategies that may be applied in otherwise refractory patients, in which, for example, traditional or the empirically based protocols do not yield the predicted positive outcomes. Such is the example provided above for AVE techniques.

Other paradigms may include implementing hormonal therapies for premenopausal depression (Morgan *et al.* 2007) or using combinatorial techniques where monotherapies have failed (Monastra *et al.*, 2002). The clinician may be called upon at times to consider "out-of-the-box" interventions when all standard or evidence-based methods may have failed. It is important to keep in mind that baseline measures that can objectively define deviations in function or behavior relative to age-expected values should be employed whenever possible, and to use such measures to demonstrate a normalizing of brain changes that can be correlated to such improved behavior changes validates the intervention methodology.

IX.   A COMMENT ABOUT THE FUTURE OF QEEG-BASED NEUROFEEDBACK

As the use of neurofeedback therapy has proliferated worldwide and has support of several professional societies (e.g., Society of Neuronal Regulation, EEG and Clinical Neuroscience, and American Association of Psychophysiology and Biofeedback), the validation of EEG neurofeedback has expanded across clinical populations. Historically, protocols for neurofeedback were first based on theories of mind and hypothesized correlates of EEG activity with states of consciousness and functioning. With the increased availability and understanding of QEEG analytic methods, deviations in brain measurement systems have guided clinicians using neurofeedback therapy to attempt to normalize QEEG measures with a concomitant change in behavior.

Newer techniques allowing the estimation of source localization from the surface recording used in QEEG are enabling a better understanding of the possible contribution of activity with subcortical structures and with hypothetical neurotransmitter systems associated with these structures. Emergent tools that help to understand the time dynamics of neural systems to be able to "share" information and to coordinate sensory-sensory interactions and sensory-response sets will eventually provide a window to understand the complexity of these unique networked systems. Ultimately, we will be able to better define the modes of intervention that can be used to "reset" the timing mechanisms that will facilitate the extent of elaborative information processing of information and optimize human intellectual performance. (John, 2005; Makeig *et al.*, 2004; Rizzuto *et al.*, 2003).

The emphasis in the field of neurotherapies in the manner we are discussing here is finding a way to reset or modulate functional brain activity which optimizes human performance without imposing the many risks that accompany the often forced and abrupt changes by psychopharmacotherapeutic interventions.

REFERENCES

Alberta, L., Ferréol, A., Cosandier-Rimélé, D., Merlet, I. and Wendling, F. (2008). Brain source localization using a fourth-order deflation scheme. *EEE Trans. Biomed. Eng*, **55(2)**, 490–501.

American Psychiatric Association, (2000). *Diagnostic and Statistical Manual of Mental Disorders* (4th edition).

Anderson, D. J. (1989). The Treatment of Migraine with Variable Frequency Photostimulation. *Headache*, **29**, 154–155.

Bares, M., Brunovsky, M., Kopecek, M., *et al.* (2007). Changes in QEEG prefrontal cordance as a predictor of response to antidepressants in patients with treatment resistant depressive disorder: a pilot study. *J. Psychiatr. Res.*, **41(3–4)**, 319–325.

Budzynski, T., Budzynski, H., Jordy, J., Tang, H. and Claypoole, K. (1999). Academic Performance with Photic Stimulation and EDR Feedback. *Journal of Neurotherapy*, **Fall/Winter**, 11–21.

Cantor, D. and Stevens, E. (unpublished manuscript). QEEG Evidence of Auditory-Visual Entrainment Treatment Efficacy of Refractory Depression. ECNS Conference, Munich, Germany, Sept 7, 2005.

Cantor, D. S., Pavlovich, M. and Brown-Lewis, R. (1994). *Electrical stimulation and classical conditioning of brain wave activity in a comatose TB1 patient.* Presented at annual conference of the National Academy of Neuropsychology.

Coburn, K., Lauterbach, E. C., Boutros, N., Black, K., Arciniegas, D. and Coffey, C. (2006). The Value of Quantitative Electroencephalography in Clinical Psychiatry: A Report by the Committee on Research of the American Neuropsychiatric Association. *The Journal of Neuropsychiatry and Clinical Neurosciences*, **18**, 460–500.

Clemens, B., Ménes, A., Piros, P., *et al.* (2006). Quantitative EEG effects of carbamazepine, oxcarbazepine, valproate, lamotrigine, and possible clinical relevance of the findings. *Epilepsy Res.*, **70(2-3)**, 190–199.

Duff, J. (2004). The usefulness of quantitative EEG (QEEG) and neurotherapy in the assessment and treatment of post-concussive syndrome. *Clinical EEG*, **35(4)**, 198–209.

Evans J., (ed.). (2006). *Forensics Applications of QEEG and Neurotherapy.* The Haworth Medical Press.

Fogelson, N., Kogan, E., Korczyn, A. D., Giladi, N., Shabtai, H. and Neufeld, M. Y. (2003). Effects of rivastigmine on the quantitative EEG in demented Parkinsonian patients. *Acta Neurol Scand.*, **107(4)**, 252–255.

Galderisi, S. (2002). Clinical applications of pharmaco-EEG in psychiatry: the prediction of response to treatment with antipsychotics. *Methods Find Exp. Clin. Pharmacol.*, **24(Suppl C)**, 85–89.

Goforth, H. W., Konopka, L., Primeau, M., *et al.* (2004). Quantitative electroencephalography in frontotemporal dementia with methylphenidate response: a case study. *Clin. EEG Neurosci. Apr,*, **35(2)**, 108–111.

Hallez, H., Vanrumste, B., Grech, R., *et al.* (2007). Review on solving the forward problem in EEG source analysis. *J. Neuroeng. Rehabil.*, **4**, 46. , Comment: Nov 30

Hansen, E. S., Prichep, L. S., Bolwig, T. G. and John, E. R. (2003). Quantitative electroencephalography in OCD patients treated with paroxetine. *Clin. Electroencephalogr., Apr,* **34(2)**, 70–74.

Hunter, A. M., Cook, I. A. and Leuchter, A. F. (2007). The promise of the quantitative electroencephalogram as a predictor of antidepressant treatment outcomes in major depressive disorder. *Psychiatr. Clin. North Am.*, **30(1)**, 105–124.

Hunter, A. M., Leuchter, A. F. and Morgan, M. L. (2005). Neurophysiologic correlates of side effects in normal subjects randomized to venlafaxine or placebo. *Neuropsychopharmacology*, **30(4)**, 792–799.

John, E. R. (2005). From synchronous neuronal discharges to subjective awareness?. *Progress in Brain Research*, **150**, 143–171.

John, E. R. and Prichep, L. S. (2006). The relevance of QEEG to the evaluation of behavioral disorders and pharmacological interventions. *Clin. EEG Neurosci.*, **37(2)**, 135–143.

John, E. R., Prichep, L. S., Friedman, J. and Easton, P. (1988). Neurometrics: Computer-assisted differential diagnosis of brain dysfunctions. *Science*, **293**, 162–169.

John, E. R., Prichep, L. S., Winterer, G., *et al.* (2007). Electrophysiological subtypes of Psychotic states. *Acta Psychiatr. Scand.*, **116**, 17–35.

Johnston, E., Cantor, D., Pavlovich, M., Brown-Lewis, R., and Hudson, D. (1992). *Quantitative Approaches for Designing Selective Sensory Stimulation Programs for Slow to Recover Head Injured Patients.* Presentation for the Georgia Speech and Hearing Association.

Kuano, H., Horie, H., Shidara, T., Kuboki, T., Suematsu, H. and Yasushi, M. (1996). Treatment of a depressive disorder patient with EEG-driven photic stimulation. *Biofeedback and Self-Regulation*, **21**, 323–334.

Makieg, S., Debener, S., Onton, J. and Delorme, A. (2004). Mining of event-related brain dynamics. *Trends in Cognitive Science*, **8(5)**, 204–210.

Manns, A., Miralles, R. and Adrian, H. (1981). The Application of Audiostimulation and Electromyographic Biofeedback to Bruxism and Myofascial Pain-Dysfunction Syndrome. *Oral Surgery*, **52**, 247–252.

Monastra, V. J., Monastra, D. M. and George, S. (2002). The effects of stimulant therapy, EEG biofeedback, and parenting style on the primary symptoms of attention-deficit/hyperactivity disorder. *Appl. Psychophysiol Biofeedback*, **27(4)**, 231–249.

Morgan, M. L., Cook, I. A., Rapkin, A. J. and Leuchter, A. F. (2007). Neurophysiologic changes during estrogen augmentation in perimenopausal depression. *Maturitas*, **56(1)**, 54–60.

Morse, D. and Chow, E. (1993). The Effect of the Relaxodont Brainwave Synchronizer on Endodontic Anxiety: Evaluation by Galvanic Skin Resistance, Pulse Rate, Physical Reactions and Questionnaire Responses. *International Journal of Psychosomatics*, **40**, 1–4.

Mucci, A., Volpe, U., Merlotti, E., Bucci, P. and Galderisi, S. (2006). Pharmaco-EEG in psychiatry. *Clin. EEG Neurosci.*, **37(2)**, 81–98.

Pascual-Marqui, R. D., Esslen, M., Kochi, K. and Lehmann, D. (2002). Functional imaging with low-resolution brain electromagnetic tomography (LORETA): a review. *Methods Find Exp Clin Pharmacol*, **24**, Suppl C: 91–5.

Prichep, L. S. and John, E. R. (1990). Neurometric studies of methylphendiate responders and non-responders. In *Dyslexia: A Neuropsychological and Learning Perspective* (G. Pavlidis, ed.), New York: John Wiley and Sons pp. 133–139.

Prichep, L. S. and John, E. R. (1992). QEEG Profiles in Psychiatric Disorders. *Brain Topography*, Vol. 4, No. 4, 249–257.

Rizzuto, D. S., Madsen, J. R., Bromfield, E. B., *et al.* (2003). Reset of human neocortical oscillations during a working memory task. *PNAS*, **100(13)**, 7931–7936.

Rodriguez, G., Vitali, P., De Leo, C., De Carli, F., Girtler, N. and Nobili, F. (2002). Quantitative EEG changes in Alzheimer patients during long-term donepezil therapy. *Neuropsychobiology*, **46(1)**, 49–56.

Russell, J. P. and Koles, Z. J. (2006). A comparison of adaptive and non-adaptive EEG source localization algorithms using a realistic head model. *Conf. Proc. IEEE Eng. Med. Biol. Soc.*, **1**, 972–975.

Saletu, B., Anderer, P. and Saletu-Zyhlarz, G. M. (2006). EEG topography and tomography (LORETA) in the classification and evaluation of the pharmacodynamics of psychotropic drugs. *Clin. EEG Neurosci.*, **37(2)**, 66–80.

Song, D. H., Shin, D. W., Jon, D. I. and Ha, E. H. (2005). Effects of methylphenidate on quantitative EEG of boys with attention-deficit hyperactivity disorder in continuous performance test. *Yonsei Med. J.*, **46(1)**, 34–41.

Sneddon, R., Shankle, W. R., Hara, J., Rodriquez, A., Hoffman, D. and Saha, U. (2006). QEEG monitoring of Alzheimer's disease treatment: a preliminary report of three case studies. *Clin. EEG Neurosci.*, **37(1)**, 54–59.

Suffin, S. and Emory, W. (1995). Neurometric subgroups in attentional and affective disorders and their association with pharmacotherapeutic outcomes. *Clin. Electroencephalog.*, **26(2)**, 76–83.

Thatcher, R. W., Walker, R. A., Gerson, I. and Geisler, F. H. (1989). EEG discriminant analyses of mild head trauma. *EEG Clin. Neurophysiol.*, **73**, 94–106.

Thatcher, R. W., Cantor, D. S., McAlaster, R., Geisler, G. and Krause, P. (1991). Comprehensive predictions of outcome in closed head-injured patients: The development of prognostic equations. In *Windows on the Brain: Neuropsychology's Technological Frontiers* (R. A. Zapulla, F. F. LeFever and J. Jaeger R. Bilder, eds), pp. 82–101. Ann. N.Y: Acad. Sri. 620.

Thatcher, R. W., Biver, C. J. and North, D. M. (2003). Quantitative EEG and the Frye and Daubert Standards of Admissibility. *Clinical EEG*, **34(2)**, 39–53.

Thomas, N. and Siever, D. (1989). *The effect of repetitive audio/visual stimulation on skeletometer and vasomotor activity*. Hypnosis: 4th European Congress at Oxford. London: Whurr Publishers.

CHAPTER 4

Diagnosing and treating brain function through the use of low resolution brain electromagnetic tomography (LORETA)

Leslie H. Sherlin, Ph.D.

Nova Tech EEG, Inc.; Southwest College of Naturopathic Medicine;
Q-Metrx, Inc.; University of Phoenix, USA

I. INTRODUCTION

As a brief introduction to this chapter I would like to say that it is not my intention to explain the technical details of any of the family of inverse solutions that were developed by Roberto Pascual-Marqui, Ph.D. and distributed as freeware from the KEY Institute for Mind-Brain Research. If your aim is to understand the technical principles of this inverse method you should refer to the writings of Pascual-Marqui and others that can be found in peer reviewed academic literature. Although there will be a very brief introduction to the method and its evolution, this will be inadequate for properly understanding the computational properties of the method. I will provide references and Internet addresses to find such details as citations within this chapter for your future reference and investigations.

Additionally, this chapter will describe some basic functions of various areas of the brain, and basic characteristics of the EEG, in order to illustrate the utility of the LORETA method as a tool for aiding in diagnostics and guiding intervention. In no way are these descriptions intended to be comprehensive in the ascertainment of brain structure and function. There are comprehensive textbooks, literature articles and even computer software that can be utilized as a resource for more in-depth understanding of the EEG characteristics and various structures of the brain and their functions.

With these factors in mind, it is my intention to provide you with a very straightforward and hopefully understandable way of using LORETA to understand your client or subject in language that is comprehensible. I hope to illustrate a method of integrating EEG characteristics, current source density localization, and brain structure's function to provide insight into your work.

Introduction to QEEG and Neurofeedback, Second Edition
ISBN: 978-0-12-374534-7

II. INTRODUCTION TO LORETA

Low resolution brain electromagnetic tomography (LORETA) is a specific solution to the inverse problem. The method was originally developed and described by Pascual-Marqui, Michel and Lehman in 1994 (Pascual-Marqui et al., 1994). This first paper presented the LORETA method as a new method for localizing the electric activity in the brain based on scalp potentials from multiple channel EEG recordings. This model was in contrast to previously described models because it did not require a limited number of point sources or a known surface distribution. Instead it computes the distribution of the current source density (CSD), measured in microamperes, through the full brain volume.

The LORETA analysis is unlike other quantitative EEG analysis techniques because it is capable of determining the relative activity of regions in the brain using surface electrodes (Pascual-Marqui et al. 1999). The EEG is a measure of electrical potential differences but the LORETA method estimates current densities at a deeper cortical level.

The LORETA method uses best estimate algorithms that localize the cortical generators of the observed summative neuronal firing. The LORETA-Key estimates the current source density for 2394 voxels which are $7 \times 7 \times 7$ mm. The solution is restricted to the gray matter. LORETA implements a three-shell spherical model of skin, skull, and cortex, which is co-registered to the MRI atlas of Talairach and Tournoux (Pascual-Marqui et al., 1994). By co-registering the solution space to a brain atlas it is possible to map electrical activity in all cortical structures (Congedo et al., 2004). An additional benefit of the LORETA method over scalp recordings is that the reconstruction is independent of the reference used in obtaining the EEG recordings (Pascual-Marqui et al., 1999).

In order for the LORETA to accurately solve the inverse solution there are some basic assumptions. As previously mentioned, the LORETA method is based upon a three-sphere head model which consists of a homogeneous medium within each sphere. Secondly, it is assumed that neurons that are side by side are synchronously and simultaneously firing. Finally, it is assumed that the solution is based upon maximal smoothness. This distribution concept is based on the solution in which the side by side neurons with least variability will be chosen. Finally, (Pascual-Marqui et al., 1994).

Since the original publication of LORETA methods in 1994, significant advancements have been made in the technique which now solves the inverse solution with zero localization error (Pascual Marqui, 2002). Standardized low resolution brain electromagnetic tomography (sLORETA) was demonstrated to localize test point sources with zero localization error more exactly. This is a characteristic that is unique among all other linear, distributed tomography techniques (Pascual Marqui, 2002).

Finally, the most recent release and development of this family of inverse solutions is exact low resolution brain electromagnetic tomography (eLORETA). eLORETA is not a linear imaging method but is a true inverse solution with exact and zero localization errors (Pascual Marqui, 2007a; Pascual Marqui *et al.*, 2006). The full details and technical specifications of each of the aforementioned methods can be found at the website of Roberto Pascual-Marqui and the KEY Institute for Mind-Brain Research (Pascual Marqui, 2007b), and in the cited publications. Despite there being several implementations of the LORETA method (sLORETA and eLORETA) I will refer to all of this family as LORETA for convenience.

A point that is made by Pascual-Marqui (Pascual Marqui, 2007b), which I wish to reiterate, is that the LORETA family of methods has very low spatial resolution. Spatial resolution will decrease as depth increases. In the words of its author, "sLORETA does not violate the law of conservation of garbage, i.e., 'garbage in, garbage out': if you feed sLORETA with noisy measurements, you will get noisy images" (Pascual Marqui, 2007b).

III. SOFTWARE REQUIRED TO PERFORM ANALYSES

The LORETA-KEY software package has always been a free academic software package independent of any profit-making ventures. Other third party software platforms have been developed which utilize the computational modules of the original LORETA software and have implemented reference sample databases with a variety of analysis features (Congedo, 2005). The sLORETA and eLORETA software packages were released also as free academic software from the KEY Institute, and are intended for use in a research setting only. Clinical or commercial use is strictly forbidden under the end user license agreement of the software (Pascual Marqui, 2007b). Despite the restrictions on the use of the sLORETA/eLORETA package from the KEY Institute, there has been one account of independent replication of the algorithms utilized in the sLORETA and eLORETA software packages that is also distributed as freeware and downloadable from the Internet (Congedo, 2005, 2008).

The third party software was developed to add additional features of analysis such as the ability to artifact continuous EEG (removal of selected transient events), computation of scalp topographies, customization of the spectral frequency bands, comparison to reference databases, and other analysis functions. The intention of the third party software was to increase the ease of LORETA computations by streamlining the processing procedures for the end user as well as adding the additional features.

IV. UTILITY OF SEGMENTATION OF EEG FREQUENCY BANDS BY FUNCTION

In order to establish the basic principles of using a LORETA method for interpretation of the EEG features, it is necessary to describe the most fundamental properties of the spectral EEG. As mentioned in the introduction to this chapter, it is not the intent to provide a detailed account of the EEG characteristics or the neuroanatomy involved, however it is essential that the reader realize that this is knowledge that must be obtained in order to utilize the LORETA methods as an aid to other diagnostic tools. In a very systematic way, the following frequency segments of band descriptions will attempt to provide you with the basic information to begin using LORETA analysis in a clinical setting.

When using the fast fourier transform (FFT) for computing the EEG it is common to group the individual frequencies into discrete defined bands based upon their function. There is variability in individuals' given frequency bands, but it is very common to utilize an average bandwidth. The most accurate approximation of the frequency bandwidths that can be used would be to evaluate each single Hz frequency band and define the appropriate lower and upper limits according to distribution. The segments would then be based upon generators of the EEG using factor analysis (Herrmann et al., 1978, Kubicki et al., 1979) and hierarchical clustering (Finelli et al., 2001). This concept is not new and has been suggested for use in defining LORETA bandwidths in a keynote lecture and an article by Pascual Marqui (Pascual Marqui et al., 2002). In this lecture a method for frequency band segmentation was presented which is based on neuronal generators. It is from this particular implementation that the following descriptions of frequency bands will be derived.

However the segmentation method, has been demonstrated in the writings cited in this chapter that the frequency bands segmentation may be very close in their lower and upper limits whatever the method utilized to create the limits. In this chapter, since the emphasis will be placed more on localization of generators rather than on specific limits that define the band, the Greek names will be used and the specific limits omitted when describing the localization of the neuronal generators. Again, it is important for the individual using the technique in this way to understand what they are doing when using frequency bands that are not determined based upon the individual. For the remainder of this chapter I will refer to the basic and most common frequency bands descriptors for ease in data presentation, however I strongly encourage the reader to understand the inherit limitations of arbitrarily defining the frequency bands, or the potential hazards in blindly accepting the classic frequency band definitions. As a reminder of the basic EEG frequency bands, and the state that is most commonly associated with the predominance of this frequency band, Fig. 4.1 can be utilized.

V. LOCALIZATION OF THE CORTICAL REFLECTION OF VOLTAGE

What has not been readily described is where the cortical representation or reflection of voltage is in the cortex. LORETA studies have provided us with such information (Pascual Marqui et al., 2002), and I have personally found this technique to be extremely valuable in understanding the presentation of symptom patterns of individuals. This information can be used to help determine if

Frequency Band Name	Frequency Bandwidth	State Associated with Bandwidth	Example of Filtered Bandwidth
Raw EEG	0–45 Hz	Awake	
Delta	0.5–3.5 Hz	Deep Sleep	
Theta	4–7.5 Hz	Drowsy	
Alpha	8–12 Hz	Relaxed	
Beta	13–35 Hz	Engaged	

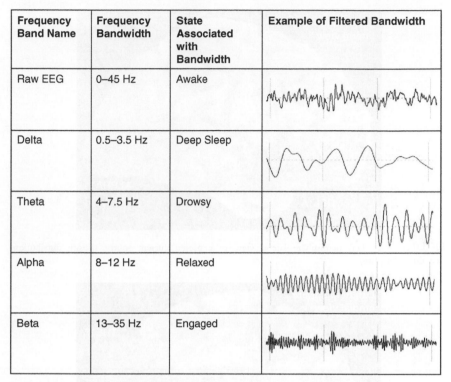

FIGURE 4.1   Common frequency band chart.

the brain is operating in an electrically optimal way or if there is the presence of *dysregulation*. The investigator, whether a clinician or researcher, will attempt to use the properties of the LORETA to determine if the individual has an *expected* or *atypical* frequency maxima localization. If an individual's scalp potentials are recorded and are artifact free, and the LORETA inverse solution computed, there is an expected distribution of the frequency band maxima. It is when the frequency band maxima is atypical that the skilled investigator must try to connect the symptoms of the individual with the characteristics of the EEG frequency band and the cortical area of localization.

The steps in the interpretation method I propose seem rather simplistic in structure but require a vast knowledge of:

1. EEG generators (sub-cortical and cortical structures that produce electrical activity).
2. The states associated with the presence of given electrical activity.
3. The function of the cortical structures where the representation of the voltage occurs.
4. If this localization is expected or atypical.

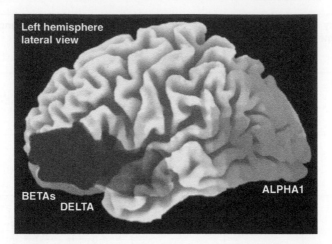

FIGURE 4.2   Left hemisphere lateral view of expected current source density distribution (see also color plate).

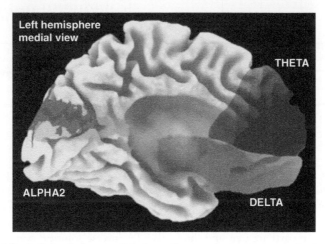

FIGURE 4.3   Left hemisphere medial view of expected current source density distribution (see also color plate).

In order to lay the foundation for LORETA interpretation I will systematically go through each common frequency band and describe these four fundamentals in the most basic way. Figs. 4.2 and 4.3 should be used as a reference point (Pascual Marqui *et al.*, 2002).

A.   The location of frequency generators

Surprisingly, there are still some unknown certainties about exactly where various frequencies may be generated. The theories that have the most evidence fall into

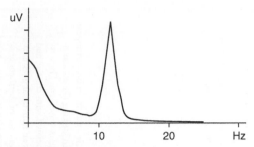

FIGURE 4.4   Expected frequency spectral distribution.

three categories. The first is the pacemaker theory that explains that the rhythmic frequencies are generated thalamically and drive the cortical activity. The second is that the cortex produces the frequency characteristics and imposes those upon the thalamus and, finally, the third is a combinatory theory that there is a dynamic process occurring between the thalamus and the cortex (Nunez, 1995). Nunez (1995) asserts that if the coupling is strong enough in this third model that the frequencies may not be able to be identified with a single structure. It has been thought for some time that it is known which structures of the brain are responsible for the generation of various electrical potentials and frequency bands (Steriade, 2005). However, these experiments may only localize the properties of a tested structure, and it is my assertion that it is important to consider all of the possible structures involved when interpreting the LORETA. For now I'll just remind the reader that we are seeing the voltage reflection in the cortex via LORETA that is the summation of the contribution of many structures to the electrical occurrence.

During the awake resting state the brain is producing electricity within all frequency bands. There is however an expected distribution of magnitude, which is illustrated in Fig. 4.4. It can be seen that alpha has the maximum magnitude values followed by delta, theta and the beta band has the lowest. Within the beta band, as the frequency increases the magnitude decreases. This basic spectral distribution is consistent although there are slight variations depending upon electrode site. There would be considerable variation across activation states of the individual. For this chapter I will only describe the awake resting condition unless otherwise stated. Of course in the awake resting state it is very common for the investigator to record and analyze both the eyes-closed and eyes-open conditions. The previously mentioned spectral properties continue to hold true with the apparent difference being that in the eyes-closed condition the alpha frequency band should have much higher amplitudes than in the eyes-open condition in the occipital (and immediately surrounding) electrode sites.

As previously indicated I am proposing a very systematic and straightforward method for using LORETA as a tool to aid in diagnosis and understanding of the individual client or subject in three steps. The first step of any EEG derived evaluation method is to carefully examine the raw unfiltered EEG data. This most

TABLE 4.1

Frequency Band Name	Frequency Range	Localization	Descriptors
Delta	Delta is the slowest, typically evaluated in the quantitative analysis including LORETA, and has the Greek letter designation of delta. Differing analysis systems and investigators are not consistent on the definitive bottom end of the frequency band ranging from 0.32 Hz up to 1.5 Hz. This is primarily due to differences of opinion in theory, thoughts on artifact vs. content, and technological capabilities (e.g. amplifier specifications). It is more agreeable that the delta band will go up to 3.5 Hz or 4 Hz.	Delta has been described as being generated from different structures. Delta activity can be found in two types. One type can be found to be generated in the cortex but its substrates are not well established (Steriade, 2005). The other is originating from the thalamus. Delta should be localized to the orbital frontal cortex, and may extend into the medial prefrontal region of the frontal lobe in the LORETA image. Please see the red color indicated as Delta in Figs 4.2 and 4.3.	Delta is primarily associated with sleep due to its predominance during sleep. It is additionally prominent in infants. Delta prominence in non-infants has been reported to be correlative with slowed cognitive processing, learning difficulties/disabilities, and even attention deficits.
Theta	Theta is defined as the frequency from 4 Hz up to 7.5 Hz or 8 Hz.	Theta waves may be described in the classic EEG literature as rhythmic slow activity. At the most basic level the theta is likely to be controlled by the septohippocampal cholinergic system (Steriade, 2005). Theta was first observed in the hippocampus of the rabbit, and later in humans as well (Buzsaki, 2006). Theta should be localized to the anterior cingulate gyrus and may extend superior into the frontal cortex in the LORETA image. The activity is represented by the blue color and labeled as Theta in Fig. 4.3.	Theta can be rhythmic or arrhythmic, and appear as square shaped often looking like a cursive r (t) in the raw complex waveform. Theta is most commonly associated with creative and spontaneous state. As an individual goes into a drowsy state the prevalence of the theta wave increases. Theta in excess has been contributed to the presence of attention deficits and other complaints that are consistent with an individual not being engaged but rather dissociated.

TABLE 4.1 *(Continued)*

Alpha	The alpha band is represented by the frequencies from 8 Hz to 12 Hz or 13 Hz. This frequency band is theorized to be primarily cortically generated, but it has been argued and assumed that there may be both corticothalamic as well as corticocortical systems involved (Niedermeyer, 2005). Niedermeyer (2005) says that : "No neurophysiological or psychophysiological alpha rhythm theory has yet found general acceptance, and there are still uncertainties about the origin and psychophysiological significance of this remarkable phenomenon. And yet, our insights into the nature of the alpha rhythm have been deepening".	See Alpha 1 and Alpha 2	Increased amplitudes of alpha have been found to be correlative with a variety of complaints. The best established is with depressed mood (major affective disorder). It has been shown that both elevated central alpha (Prichep and John, 1992), as well as frontal asymmetry of alpha (F3 > F4) (Davidson *et al.*, 2002, Davidson, 1998), may be an indication of emotional regulation deficits. Decreased amplitudes of alpha have conversely been indicated in the presence of anxiety spectrum disorders, and have been incorporated into several models of addiction (Prichep and John, 1992). Additionally, it has been reported and is theoretically sound that other complaints may be present with alpha aberrations. These complaints are varied and have been reported to range from attention deficits to pain regulation. Due to the complexity of the alpha rhythm it is likely to have an influence in a wide variety of clinical presentations.

(Continued)

TABLE 4.1 *(Continued)*

Frequency Band Name	Frequency Range	Localization	Descriptors
Alpha 1	Alpha 1 is defined as the frequency from 8 Hz up to 10 Hz. This low-frequency range of alpha is observed as the alpha below the posterior dominant rhythm.	The lower frequency of alpha (8–10 Hz) should be localized to the occipital lobe and the visual cortex in the LORETA image. Please see the green color indicated as Alpha 1 in Figs 4.2 and 4.3.	The low alpha or alpha 1 band are reflective of an unaware state of relaxation. They are present in a state of awake, predominant in eyes-closed condition, and perhaps meditative with no attention or awareness of the surroundings. This frequency band is more diffusely distributed in the eyes-closed condition as a result of the withholding of stimuli to the visual cortex. From this model we can associate the alpha 1 frequency as an "idle" rhythm, or one of decreased cortical activation.
Alpha 2	Alpha 2 is the faster component of the alpha band, and is defined as the frequency from 10 Hz up to 12 Hz or 13 Hz.	Alpha 2 should be localized to the precuneus areas of the medial parieto-occipital cortex in the LORETA image. Please see the pink color indicated as Alpha 2 in Fig 4.3.	Alpha 2 is most commonly associated with a state of awake and alert, but alpha 2 differs from alpha 1 as it has a generalized awareness of the surroundings with a focus on nothing specific. I refer to this state as "gaping cognizance of stimuli." The individual in this state has a wide and deep recognition of all sensory input, and holds focus on no specific thought or stimuli.
Beta	Beta activity is simply defined as any rhythmical activity that is above 13 Hz. This would of course exclude the posterior alpha rhythm if the individual's alpha was increased above 13 Hz. The beta frequency is generally accepted to be generated primarily by the corticocortical systems.	See Low Beta and High Beta.	When beta is elevated it has been associated with anxiety spectrum complaints. It may be associated with irritability or agitation as well as sleep disturbance and addictions (Prichep and John, 1992).

TABLE 4.1 (*Continued*)

Low Beta	Low beta is defined as the frequency from 13 Hz up to 21 Hz.	Low beta should be localized to the frontal cortex bilaterally, and may extend slightly posterior into the temporal cortex in lesser CSD values in the LORETA image. Please see the blue color indicated as betas in Fig. 4.2.	The low beta is primarily a reflection of activation of the cortex. Beta will increase under cognitive challenge as a result of increased cortical requirements of the task, and this will also change the location of maximal low beta activity in the LORETA image.
High Beta	High beta is defined as the frequency from 22 Hz up to 35 Hz.	High beta should be localized to the frontal cortex bilaterally, and may extend slightly posterior into the temporal cortex in lesser CSD values in the LORETA image. Please see the blue color indicated as betas in Fig. 4.2.	The high beta is most associated with higher levels of concentration. Beta will increase under cognitive challenge as a result of increased cortical requirements of the task and, just as with low beta, this will also change the location of maximal high beta activity in the LORETA image.

basic and essential step cannot be skipped—just because it is not discussed here, do not believe that LORETA is exempt from this step. A skilled investigator will begin to formulate hypotheses about the individual, and will begin to correlate complaints with findings in the EEG. Once the EEG has been examined, and carefully artifacted to remove any noise contribution to the signal that is not to be considered, the spectral LORETA analysis can be computed and the resultant images produced.

The second step in the interpretation method is to consider the frequency maxima distribution. Simply, does the localization within each frequency band match that described above? After making this consideration for each frequency band we can move to the third step of interpretation. If any frequency band were not localized as expected we would then derive some meaning from the atypical distribution. Examples of this will be following in the next section of this chapter.

The third step is to consider the amount of CSD of the given frequencies. From this I specifically mean to consider if the frequency spectral distribution follows what was expected (refer to Fig. 4.4). If it does not, then we have another data point for interpretation. This step is to evaluate the circumstance where the maximum CSD of a given frequency band is determined to have the expected localization but may be aberrant in the amount or ratio.

A final step can be added, which is to consider a reference database comparison. I have found that this final step is often unnecessary and, when the investigator has sufficient understanding of the EEG, the spectral properties and localization of the database will confirm their already determined findings. While this does have a certain utility for conveying exactly how far outside expected limits the individual might be, it is not necessary for understanding the presentation of the individual.

Often a database can be misleading if the first three steps are not followed with understanding. Simply finding a statistical anomaly in the individual's data does not necessarily imply a clinical relevance, and may cause the investigator to improperly determine a structure or frequency to be a contributor to the presentation when there are no other indications of such. If steps 1–3 do not indicate that the finding is correlative to the problem, certainly the finding of a database aberration should not be considered. It may be nothing more than a statistical "red herring." Even if it is a legitimate finding in the absence of clinical correlation and the finding's presence in steps 1–3, it should not be considered. The goal is to understand this individual and not to simply point out ways in which they are different from a reference population, which may be attributable to individual characteristics and not clinical relevance.

VI.   INTERPRETIVE EXAMPLES

In order to demonstrate the principles I propose, let's follow a few examples. Again, I will remind the reader that this assumes that the EEG has already been carefully examined and artifacted in each of the following examples.

Figure 4.5 illustrates the delta frequency band localized to Brodmann area 19, which is in the sensory cortical area in the medial and lateral aspect of the occipital lobe. This area is part of the extrastriate visual cortex that surrounds the primary visual cortex, and which processes visual information (Williams *et al.*, 2005). Recalling that delta is a frequency which is most predominant in the sleep state, it is no surprise that this individual has presented to the clinician with complaints of a visual processing learning disability.

The individual presents with complaints of mood regulation difficulties, and the clinician is trying to differentiate between bi-polar disorder and a combination of ADHD and possible depression. After performing an EEG and eLORETA analysis, Fig. 4.6 demonstrates the theta frequency maximum atypically distributed to Brodmann area 13, located in the associational cortical area in the insula. Being part of the associational cortex, it is involved in visceral sensory and emotional processing (Williams *et al.*, 2005).

Figure 4.7 identifies a diffuse distribution of beta 1 (low beta) across the occipital and parietal cortex. The frequency maximum is localized to the Brodmann area 40 which is part of the associational cortical area in the inferior parietal lobe, including

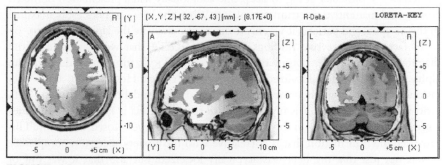

FIGURE 4.5   Displayed are the horizontal (left), sagittal (middle), and coronal (right) sections through the voxel with maximal current source density localized to Brodmann area 19; Precuneus in visual processing learning disability case (see color plate).

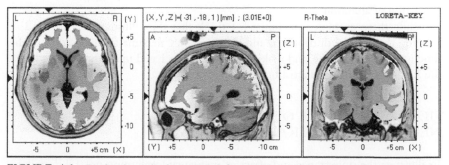

FIGURE 4.6   Displayed are the horizontal (left), sagittal (middle), and coronal (right) sections through the voxel with maximal current source density localized to Brodmann area 13; Insula in bi-polar disorder case (see color plate).

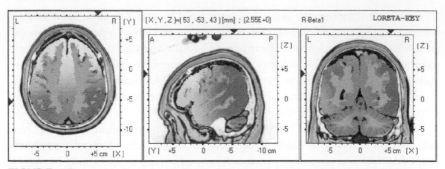

FIGURE 4.7   Displayed are the horizontal (left), sagittal (middle), and coronal (right) sections through the voxel with maximal current source density localized to Brodmann area 40; Inferior Parietal Lobule in anxiety and inattention case (see color plate).

the supramarginal gyrus. It is primarily involved in spatial orientation and semantic representation. This particular example was chosen to illustrate the point of correlating complaints with findings. This individual did not complain of difficulties around spatial orientation or semantic representation. She complained of sleep irregularities, particularly of difficulty going to sleep. She additionally had a presentation of mixed anxiety and inattentive spectrum complaints. When the beta was noticeably maximal in the occipital and parietal, it was necessary to also evaluate the alpha/beta ratio.

In fact there were two findings in the eLORETA that were valuable to the diagnostician. Firstly, the consideration of the alpha localization was indicated. The alpha was appropriately localized to the occipital cortex. However the alpha/beta ratio was 3.0. Although there are no well-defined ratio guidelines for the alpha/beta ratio in the eLORETA, it is my experience that the alpha is typically 8–10 times larger than the beta CSD in the occipital cortex of the eyes-closed condition. This provided the information that is correlative with the anxiety spectrum complaints. It was not just that the beta was atypically localized, but also that it was out of proportion in the spectral distribution. Secondly, the beta is absent frontally. This absence of beta frontally is correlative with the complaints of inattention. The lack of cortical activation frontally has been well established as playing a role in the regulation of attention.

While these examples are limited, I think that they illustrate the method of aligning the spectral distribution and the frequency maxima localization with the function of the structure, and making interpretation based upon the knowledge of the EEG frequency band attributes.

VII.   CASE EXAMPLE OF PRE-POST NEUROFEEDBACK TRAINING

To illustrate the importance and effect of frequency localization use, I'll describe a case from our teaching clinic. The 22-year-old client presented with complaints of general cognitive deficits with specific problems around attention and academic performance. The client also had secondary complaints processing social cues, and his family indicated that he would often not get jokes or understand sarcasm. It was unclear if the client had the diagnostic criteria for ADHD or if the presentation resulted more from a learning disability. After performing sLORETA analysis on the acquired EEG, I found that the client had an atypical localization of theta frequency to the occipital cortex.

Immediately, it was determined that the finding was in fact a slowed posterior dominant rhythm, or slowed alpha. The slowed alpha, or theta band, was maximally localized to Brodmann area 40, Parahippocampal Gyrus. Brodmann area 40 is the cortical component of the limbic system, and is involved in limbic associational

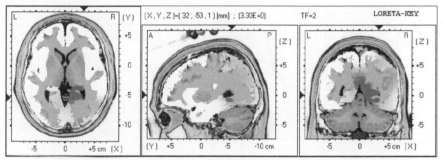

FIGURE 4.8   Displayed are the horizontal (left), sagittal (middle), and coronal (right) sections through the voxel with maximal current source density in the theta (4–7.5 Hz) band localized to Brodmann area 30; Parahippocampal Gyrus illustrating slowed alpha generator (see color plate).

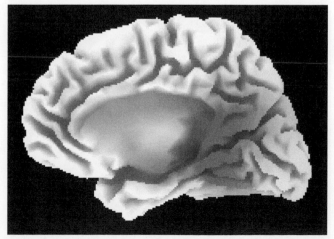

FIGURE 4.9   3-D surface sagittal image of theta (4–7.5 Hz) of the left hemisphere with maximal current source density localized to Brodmann area 30; Parahippocampal Gyrus illustrating slowed alpha generator (see color plate).

integration (Williams *et al.*, 2005). Not only does the slowed alpha correlate with the complaints of decreased cognitive processing, but additionally the localization is correlative to the client's secondary complaints of processing and integrating social cues. Based upon these findings, a scalp neurofeedback protocol was developed to decrease theta (4–7.5 Hz) and to increase alpha (9–12 Hz) at site POZ. The goal of the training was to "speed up" the alpha, and to normalize the localization of both alpha and theta.

Following 30 neurofeedback sessions the client reported complete symptom relief. He had began to experience improvements after six sessions, and this continued until session 24 when he indicated that he was noticing a plateau of effect from the neurofeedback training. He and his family indicated that his symptoms

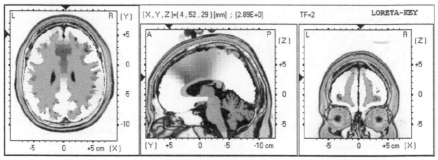

FIGURE 4.10   Displayed are the horizontal (left), sagittal (middle), and coronal (right) sections through the voxel with maximal current source density in the theta (4–7.5 Hz) band localized to the Anterior Cingulate post neurofeedback (see color plate).

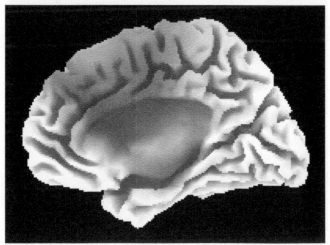

FIGURE 4.11   3-D surface sagittal image of theta (4–7.5 Hz) of the left hemisphere with maximal current source density localized to the Anterior Cingulate post neurofeedback (see color plate).

were no longer present. At that time it was suggested that he continue to session 30 to reinforce the positive learning that had occurred. He was discharged from the treatment plan at that time. Post sLORETA analysis indicated that the atypical distribution of theta had been normalized, and his posterior alpha was in the 8–12 Hz range.

VIII.   ADVANCED INTERVENTION—LORETA FEEDBACK

It wasn't long after myself and colleagues from the University of Tennessee, Brain Research and Neuropsychology laboratory, under the direction of Dr. Joel Lubar, began to utilize the LORETA technique for analysis that we began to consider whether we could use the method as a tool for intervention. We specifically had in mind LORETA feedback, a method for operant conditioning of deeper cortical structures. In a matter of a few years the first project to perform such analysis was being defined. It was in 2001 at an annual meeting of the International Society of Neurofeedback and Research (Society for Neuronal Regulation at that time) that we demonstrated in a workshop a participant's LORETA in real time (Lubar et al., 2001). As technology has advanced, the LORETA neurofeedback method has been refined and developed further, and validated for the first time as a technique that was able to be implemented (Congedo et al., 2004). Since that time several projects have followed which continue to demonstrate the utility of the method, and which are now expanding to explore the specific populations and techniques that might be able to be implemented (Canon et al., 2007).

Currently there are new studies being developed and carried out in the area of LORETA feedback. Additionally, there is some very exciting work taking place at the University of Alberta in Canada by the principle author, Douglas Ozier, in the area of chronic pain utilizing the updated algorithm of sLORETA for feedback with exact localization. So far these studies are replicating others findings in the areas of fMRI feedback with clinical populations, and they look to be a more cost-effective than fMRI feedback for treating deep cortical structures, and simultaneously are more specific than traditional scalp neurofeedback.

Ozier hypothesizes that regions of the cortex will show increased activation in the condition of pain catastrophize versus the condition of regulate pain (Ozier et al., 2008). During a trial investigation, a pilot subject participated in sLORETA feedback. The subject performed a baseline recording, and then was asked to "upregulate pain." In fact, as Ozier had predicted there was a cortical activation. One of the areas that showed a significant difference in Brodmann area 9 and 24. Brodmann area 9 participates in prefrontal associational integration. Brodmann area 24 is the associational cortical area in the anterior part of the cingulate gyrus; this area is part of the cortical components of the limbic system which is involved in the affective dimensions of pain (Williams et al., 2005).

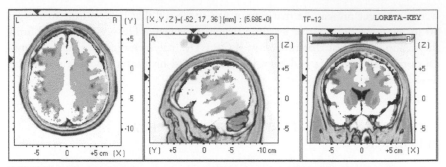

FIGURE 4.12   Displayed are the horizontal (left), sagittal (middle), and coronal (right) sections through the voxel with maximal current source density in the beta 4 (24–28 Hz) band localized to Brodmann areas 9 and 24 (see color plate).

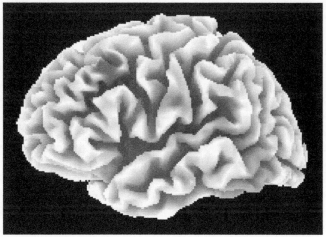

FIGURE 4.13   3-D surface sagittal image of beta (24–28 Hz) of the left hemisphere with maximal current source density localized to Brodmann areas 9 and 24 (see also color plate).

IX.   CONCLUSIONS

The field of neurofeedback and quantitative electroencephalography is constantly evolving. As technology advances and our understanding of the complex mechanisms of the brain systems increases, we will always be updating our windows to inquire and our reasoning for interpretation. At the present time, LORETA inverse solutions give us a reliable and cost-effective measure to use in a clinical and research setting. When the combination of frequency aberration in localization and value is paired with knowledge of brain structure and function, the investigator can draw conclusions and interpretations based on objective data that is consistent with the presentation of clinical complaints. Of course this is not completely objective, and is greatly dependent upon the knowledge and ability of the investigator.

There are many different approaches to interpretation of EEG, QEEG and even LORETA methods. The fundamentals and understanding of the underpinnings of the EEG are required, but standardization of the interpretation to a large part is not even desirable. "Because there is an element of science and an element of art in a good EEG interpretation; it is the latter that defies standardization" (Niedermeyer, 2005).

REFERENCES

Canon, R., Lubar, J. F., Congedo, M., Thornton, K., Towler, K. and Hutchens, T. (2007). The Effect of Neurofeedback Training in the Cognitive Division of the Anterior Cingulate Gyrus. *Internation Journal of Neuroscience*, **117**, 337–357.

Congedo, M. (2003). Tomographic Neurofeedback; a New Technique for the Self-Regulation of Brain Electrical Activity. *Department of Psychology*. Knoxville: University of Tennessee.

Congedo, M. (2005). *EureKa! 3.0 ed.* Mesa, AZ: Nova Tech EEG, Inc.

Congedo, M. (2008). Recent Advances in Minimum Norm Inverse Solutions: Model-Driven and Data-Driven sLORETA and eLORETA. *First trimestral advancement meeting of the Open-ViBE project*. France.

Congedo, M., Lubar, J. F. and Joffe, D. (2004). Low-resolution electromagnetic tomography neurofeedback. *IEEE Trans. Neural Syst. Rehabil. Eng.*, **12**, 387–397.

Finelli, L. A., Borbely, A. A. and Achermann, P. (2001). Functional topography of the human nonREM sleep electroencephalogram. *European Journal of Neuroscience*, **13**, 2282–2290.

Herrmann, W. M., Fichte, K. and Kubicki, S. (1978). The mathematical rationale for the clinical EEG-frequency-bads. 1. Factor analysis with EEG-power estimations for determining frequency bands. *EEG-EMG Zeitschrift fur Electroenzephalographie Electromyographie und Verwandte Gebiete*, **9**, 146–154.

Kubicki, S., Herrmann, W. M., Fichte, K. and Freund, G. (1979). Reflections on the topics: EEG frequency bands and regulation of vigilance. *Pharmakopsychiatrie Neuro-Psychopharmakologie*, **12**, 237–245.

Lubar, J. F., Congedo, M., Joffe, D. and Sherlin, L. (2001). LORETA 3-D Neurofeedback, Normative Database and New Findings. *Society for Neuronal Regulation*. CA: Monterey.

Niedermeyer, E. (2005). The Normal EEG of the Waking Adult. In *Electroencephalography: Basic Principles, Clinical Applications, and Related Fields* (E. Niedermeyer and F. L. Da Silva, eds). Philadelphia, PA: Lippincott Williams & Wilkins. pp.

Nunez, P. L. (1995). *Neocortical Dynamics and Human EEG Rhythms*. New York: Oxford University Press.

Ozier, D., Whelton, W., Mueller, H., Lampman, D. and Sherlin, L. (2008). Comparing the efficacy of thermal biofeedback and sLORETA neurotherapy as interventions for chronic pain. *Psychology*. Edmonton: University of Alberta.

Pascual Marqui, R. D. (2002). Standardized low-resolution brain electromagnetic tomography (sLORETA): technical details, Methods Find. *Experimental Clinical Pharmacology*, **24**, 5–12.

Pascual Marqui, R. D. (2007a) Discrete 3D distributed, linear imaging methods of electric neuronal activity. Part 1: exact, zero error localization. arXiv:0710.3341 [math-ph].

Pascual Marqui, R. D. (2007b). LORETA: low resolution brain electromagnetic tomography. Zurich, Switzerland: The KEY Institute for Brain-Mind Research.

Pascual-Marqui, R. D., Michel, C. M. and Lehmann, D. (1994). Low resolution electromagnetic tomography: a new method for localizing electrical activity in the brain. *Int. J. Psychophysiol.*, **18**, 49–65.

Pascual-Marqui, R. D., Lehmann, D., Koenig, T., *et al.* (1999). Low resolution brain electromagnetic tomography (LORETA) functional imaging in acute, neuroleptic-naive, first-episode, productive schizophrenia. *Psychiatry Res.*, **90**, 169–179.

Pascual Marqui, R. D., Esslen, M. and Lehmann, D. (2002) Frequency structure and neuronal generators of eyes-closed EEG. *International Society of Neurofeedback and Research 12th Annual Conference.* Scottsdale, AZ.

Pascual Marqui, R. D., Pascual-Montano, A., Lehmann, D., *et al.* (2006). Exact low resolution brain electromagnetic tomography (eLORETA). *Neuroimage*, **31**, S86.

Steriade, M. (2005). Cellular Substrates of Brain Rhythms. In *Electroencephalography: Basic Principles, Clinical Applications, and Related Fields* (E. Niedermeyer and F. L. Da Silva, eds), 5th edition. Philadelphia, PA: Lippincott Williams & Wilkins. pp.

Williams, S. M., White, L. E. and Mace, A. C. (2005). *Sylvius VG: Visual Glossary of Human Neuroanatomy.* Sunderland, MA: Puramis Studios, Inc.

CHAPTER 5

EEG biofeedback training using live Z-scores and a normative database

Thomas F. Collura, Ph.D.[1], Robert W. Thatcher, Ph.D.[2], Mark Llewellyn Smith L.C.S.W.[3], William A. Lambos, Ph.D., BCIA-EEG[4], and Charles R. Stark, M.D., BCIA-EEG[5]

[1] *BrainMaster Technologies, Inc., Oakwood, Ohio, USA*
[2] *EEG and NeuroImaging Laboratory, Applied Neuroscience, Inc., St. Petersburg, and Professor, Department of Neurology, University of South Florida, Florida, USA*
[3] *Private Practice, New York, USA*
[4] *Cognitive Neuro Sciences, Inc. and University of South Florida, Florida, USA*
[5] *Cognitive Neuro Sciences, Inc., Melbourne, Florida, USA*

I. INTRODUCTION

This chapter discusses the technical background, and initial clinical results obtained in an implementation of live Z-score-based training (LZT) in an EEG biofeedback system. This approach makes it possible to compute, view, and process normative Z-scores in real-time as a fundamental element of EEG biofeedback. While employing the same type of database as conventional QEEG post-processing software, LZT software is configured to produce results in real-time, suiting it to live assessment and training, rather than solely for analysis and review.

The Z-scores described here are based upon a published database, and computed using the same software code that exists in the analysis software, when used in "dynamic JTFA" mode. The database includes over 600 people, age 2 to 82. The system computes real-time Z-scores using JTFA (joint time frequency analysis) rather than using the FFT (fast fourier transform), which is more commonly used for obtaining post-processed results. As a result, Z-scores are available instantaneously, without windowing delays, and can be used to provide real-time information.

Live Z-scores can be used either for live assessment or for feedback training, depending on how the system is configured and used. When used for assessment, live Z-scores can be viewed during data acquisition, and can also be recorded and reviewed, as a simple, fast assessment. When used for training, the Z-scores must be integrated in some fashion into the feedback design, so that they are used to control displays, sounds, or other information, for purposes of operant conditioning and related learning paradigms.

Introduction to QEEG and Neurofeedback, Second Edition
ISBN: 978-0-12-374534-7

When used for training, the targeting method is important. There is a considerable range of possible approaches, ranging from the obvious use of a single Z-score as a training target, to more complex approaches that combine Z-scores in various ways, to produce more comprehensive training information. Upon first consideration, Z-scores can be used simply as an alternative means to produce a single target, for example to train a particular amplitude, amplitude ratio, or coherence value. While the core Z-score software in different systems may be uniform, there are further refinements regarding the incorporation into useful feedback including visual, auditory, or vibrotactile information. It is in this level of integration and system design that much of the "art" of Z-score biofeedback resides.

When combining Z-scores, one might initially consider presenting multiple targets to the trainee, and instructing them to train using several bar graphs, or similar displays. This may lead to complexity, and difficulty in presenting a simple and intuitive display. However, it is also possible to combine Z-scores internally to the software, and to present a simple feedback display to the trainee, such as a single graph or animation, that reflects the combined results. When doing so, we may have concern that the individual needs to "sort it out" or somehow "figure out" what is expected. However, this tendency to complicate both the system and the trainee's task may be unnecessary.

In the case studies shown here, Z-score training was accomplished with two or four channels of EEG. This provides an enormous amount of potential information in the form of Z-scores, and begs for a way to manage it. Protocols and entire approaches were innovated on-the-fly, as clinical changes and EEG observations motivated increasingly integrated yet simple-to-use protocol designs. We have found that it is possible to use combined Z-scores for training, and that up to 248 such scores can be used simultaneously with four channels, and with a simple and intuitive user interface. Even though the feedback may be controlled by an exceedingly complex internal design, when simple and intuitive feedback displays are presented, the trainee's brain does indeed appear capable of "sorting out" the targeted brain state, quickly, and efficiently. Key issues here relate to the methods for selection and decision-making relative to a plethora of Z-scores, and the reporting of meaningful results and statistics.

When inspecting individual live Z-scores, it is observed that their typical values are not the same as those observed when using post-processed QEEG results, as is explained in technical detail below. Initially, this was a cause for confusion and concern, until the underlying reasons are understood. To pursue this, let us use height as an example, rather than an EEG metric. To view a live Z-score in this case is analogous to watching an individual in action, for example playing a game, or working, in contrast to standing still. Post-processed Z-scores may be compared to taking single height measurements of individuals standing still, and using the data to produce a population statistic. The population statistics of static height might typically produce, for adult males, for example, a mean of 5 feet 10 inches, and a standard deviation of 2–3 inches. Thus, if an individual has a standing height of 6 feet 3 inches, that would be considered tall, perhaps more than 3 standard deviations out, and hence produce a Z-score of 3 or more.

However, if individuals are working or playing, for example jumping up and down, then the range is considerably larger. For anyone playing basketball to be 6 feet 3 inches above the ground is not so unusual, and may produce a Z-score of 2 or even less. Based upon this consideration, it can be understood that, if an individual has a conventional QEEG Z-score of 3 for a particular parameter (say absolute power), then when they are evaluated using live Z-scores, their score may be more like 2, or even less. This is not a problem or defect in the system, it is a natural consequence of watching a live statistic, versus a static statistic.

Despite this difference in the quantitative characteristics of live versus static Z-scores, LZT can be used as a valid and effective training paradigm, and is consistent with established QEEG-based practice. Live Z-scores can be used to train a combination of variables including absolute and relative power, power ratios, coherence, phase, and asymmetry. When used in this manner, the system is no longer targeting just a single variable or attribute. Rather, the possibility arises of training the brain in a complex multidimensional manner, so that it learns a comprehensive brain state. For example, if an individual learns to self-regulate along the concentration/relaxation dimension, but also learns to regulate the amplitude relationship between different frequency component bands, or between different sites, or the connectivity between sites, then a more complex target is produced. This may be thought of as moving the biofeedback training in the direction of a complex task such as riding a bicycle or reading a book, rather than simply "bench pressing" a single parameter, such as theta amplitude, up or down.

When viewed in this way, live Z-score training is not simply a convenience or a method for establishing training targets. It is a way to comprehensively define a brain state, and to train the individual to find and sustain it. More significantly, it provides an entirely new conceptual framework for designing protocols. It amplifies the value of the QEEG, and the QEEG significantly informs the use of Z-score training. LZT can be used as a combination GPS and navigator for the brain. It guides the trainee in a set of complex relationships including absolute and relative neuronal activation, as well as neuronal connectivity and interoperation. Rather than simply instructing the trainee to "make this larger" or "do more of that," it provides a comprehensive feedback reflecting a balanced, coordinated set of neuronal activities and relationships.

Nor is LZT limited to a strategy or "training to the norm." With LZT, we can also choose to up-train or down-train any components we like, including combinations of components, or relationships between components; so we can train to a Z-score of −2 or −3, or +2 or +3, or even +6 if we choose. The use of Z-score training does not dictate the targets used to create contingent feedback; rather, it casts targets in a new dimension. It is also important to emphasize that using Z-scores does not automatically relegate us to the domain of normalizing the EEG, although that is certainly an obvious and valuable option. For example, simultaneously normalizing multiple coherences in a single band between F3 and P3 is a promising direction for those with language challenges. At the same time, we can tweak any metrics we like up or down, based on judicious choices and stated goals. The use of Z-scores really provides an alternative to the concept of thresholding, and provides us with "portals" through which we can shoot the metrics, based on our own needs and persuasions.

LZT can also be combined with other protocol approaches, if the system and software will allow it. For example, the situation may arise in which conventional alpha or SMR enhancement training is desired, but it is also desired to maintain a normal connectivity metric. In other words, it may be desirable to train an individual to produce 12–15 Hz in a particular area, but to get rewards only insofar as the connectivity between certain areas is normal. As another example, one may wish to encourage synchronous alpha across the head, while at the same time ensuring that a collection of Z-scores is in the normal range.

When employing LZT, the conceptual and quantitative framework underlying the EEG training may differ from that commonly encountered, while at the same time, certain familiar elements may remain. For example, the size of the Z-score targets, expressed in "standard deviations," may replace the concept of threshold in conventional training. When multiple Z-scores are used, then the number of Z-scores that are within a certain target range may become a training goal, replacing the traditional "how big" or "how much" of some metric such as amplitude or coherence.

Despite this shift in thinking, the ultimate performance of feedback and training can be achieved without any change in the trainee's task or conceptual load. For example, it is possible to convert the results of multiple Z-scores into a single metric, and to train on that metric using a conventional trend line, bar graph, animation, or sound. In the clinical studies described here, one such approach has been to use a large number of Z-scores, possibly all that are available, to set a particular target size, and to use the number of achieved targets as the training variable, by watching that quantity on a graph, and using the current score as a parameter to control sound and visual feedback. Despite this rather radical shift in thinking, it is still possible to use a familiar feedback mechanism so that the trainee is not aware of any change in the underpinnings, and experiences only a change in the exact brain state(s) that are accompanied by reward feedback.

Some comments are in order regarding the overall role of LZT in the EEG biofeedback arsenal. One regards the idea that LZT training somehow obviates the need for the QEEG. The thinking is that, since LZT incorporates normative scores into its operation, there is less (or no) need to perform a full-head assessment. We do not agree with this point of view. The conventional QEEG remains an essential tool for assessing the overall condition of the trainee, and to plan interventions. There may be situations in which simply training to the norm may not be indicated. In any case, it is essential that the therapist understands the anticipated changes, and is prepared to deal with them. For example, a client may be expected to change as a result of feedback training, and it is the clinical training and experience of the clinician that will be needed to deal with these changes.

The second consideration is how LZT impacts the need for the clinician. We do not see LZT in any way reducing the role of the clinician, any more than an autopilot in a commercial airliner obviates the need for a trained, experienced pilot, or a laser-guided laparoscopic surgery obviates the need for a good surgeon. LZT ultimately provides a new targeting method, and a new way to teach the brain to achieve desired states. However, the core goal remains to treat an individual, which is the role of the clinician. Someone is needed to determine optimal placement, protocols, and clinical actions, and to oversee the process.

Two additional comments are in order. One has to do with what LZT can do in regard to peak performance and mental fitness, and the other has to do with how it relates to "normal" individuals.

There has been concern expressed regarding the possible effects of LZT on otherwise "normal" people. It has been posited that LZT training may "dumb down" individuals, by training them to a normal, hence mediocre, population. Ultimately, this is something that only experience can reveal. We have seen various reactions in this situation.

We have seen cases in which a normal or high-performing individual actually finds LZT training beneficial, pleasant, relaxing, and stimulating. In one situation, we observed an individual (a workshop attendee) who showed a slightly high C4 SMR signal, as well as mild hypo-coherence between C3 and C4. This may be interpreted as a "high-performance" EEG, since C4 SMR training is well recognized as a beneficial treatment, and also a mild amount of inter-hemispheric independence is not necessarily a bad trait. When given a comprehensive Z-score training, this individual reported benefits including being more relaxed, yet feeling energized. These are consistent with the fact that she received two components of training via LZT. The first was a mild "squash" training on the motor strip in the 12–15 Hz range (energizing), as well as some coherence up-training on the motor strip (relaxing).

In another situation, however, we observed another workshop attendee who showed more markedly pronounced motor strip SMR, and further informed us that he had developed the habit of sitting very still, and attending to his clients. When presented with LZT training, he simply reported that he did not like it. This is consistent with findings that individuals who have their alpha or SMR "where they like it" do not respond well to training that attempts to alter it. In summary, LZT training may be fine for certain individual from the normal spectrum, and may be undesirable for others.

With regard to peak performance and related issues, it should be noted that LZT does not automatically target the attributes typically used in this realm. For example, one common training approach is to encourage global alpha synchrony. While LZT could be used to target this type of EEG change, if one wants to increase alpha synchrony there are more direct methods to do so. LZT might be of value in monitoring such training, but is not specifically beneficial when the goal is simply to "make more alpha." Another peak-performance paradigm, the "squash" protocol, is also not specifically targeted using LZT. In this case, the goal is to acquaint the trainee with a "low voltage fast" (activated) state of EEG, in contrast to "high voltage slow" (relaxed) state. Again, we do not see LZT in any way replacing this approach, although it can provide a valuable adjunct. A third form of training that is not addressed by LZT is alpha/theta training, in which the goal is to achieve an altered, hypnogogic state of consciousness, useful for therapeutic purposes.

When put in context, LZT is a significant advance, and may prove revolutionary. At the core, it remains a form of operant conditioning, which teaches the brain to exercise the cycle of concentration and relaxation, in a systematic and defined manner. What has changed is the source of information informing the feedback, providing a biofeedback version of the "$1000 golf lesson." The following technical details and clinical case studies provide insight into its clinical utility, and possible ultimate effectiveness.

II.   DESIGN OF THE INSTANTANEOUS Z-SCORE NORMATIVE DATABASE

The number of subjects (N = 625), selection criteria, age range (2 months to 82 years), cross-validation tests, demographics, and other details of the Z-score normative database have been published, and are recommended reading for those interested in more detail than is briefly reviewed in this chapter (see Thatcher *et al.*, 1983, 1986, 1987; Wolf and Thatcher, 1990; Thatcher, 1998, 1999; Thatcher *et al.*, 2003). There are four basic concepts used in the design of Z-score biofeedback as described below:

A.   Use of Gaussian probabilities to identify "de-regulation" in the brain

The fundamental design concepts of Z-score biofeedback were first introduced by Thatcher (1998, 1999, 2000a, 2000b, 2000c). The central idea of the instantaneous Z-score is the application of the mathematical Gaussian curve or 'bell shaped' curve by which probabilities can be estimated using the auto and cross-spectrum of the electroencephalogram (EEG) in order to identify brain regions that are deregulated and depart from expected values. Linkage of symptoms and complaints to functional localization in the brain is best achieved by the use of a minimum of 19-channel EEG evaluation so that current source density and LORETA source localization can be computed. Once the linkage is made, then an individualized Z-score protocol can be devised. However, in order to make a linkage to symptoms, an accurate statistical inference must be made using the Gaussian distribution.

The Gaussian distribution is a fundamental distribution that is used throughout science, for example the Schrodinger wave equation in Quantum mechanics uses the Gaussian distribution as basis functions (Robinett, 1997). The application of the EEG to the concept of the Gaussian distribution requires the use of standard mathematical transforms by which all statistical distributions can be transformed to a Gaussian distribution (Box and Cox, 1964). In the case of the EEG, transforms such as the square root, cube root; $\log_{10}$, Box–Cox, etc. are applied to the power spectrum of the digital time series in order to approximate a normal distribution (Gasser *et al.* 1988; John *et al.* 1987, 1988; Duffy *et al.* 1994; Thatcher *et al.* 2003, 2005a, 2005b). The choice of the exact transform depends on the accuracy of the approximate match to a Gaussian distribution. The fact that accuracies of 95–99% match to a Gaussian are commonly published in the EEG literature encouraged Thatcher and colleagues to develop and test the Z-score biofeedback program.

B. Application of Gaussian probability distributions to instantaneous Z-score biofeedback, and why JTFA Z-scores are smaller than FFT Z-scores

The second design concept is the application of the Gaussian distribution to averaged "instantaneous" time domain spectral measures from groups of normal subjects, and then to cross-validate the means and standard deviations for each subject for each instant of time (Thatcher, 1998, 1999, 2000a, 2000b). The cross-validation is directly related to the variance of the distribution (Thatcher *et al.*, 2003, 2005a, 2005b). However, in order to achieve a representative Gaussian distribution it is necessary to include two major categories of statistical variance:

1. The moment-to-moment variance or within session variance.
2. Between subject variance across an age group.

In the case of the Fast Fourier Transform (FFT) there is a single "integral" of the power spectrum for each subject and each frequency and, therefore, there is only between subject variance in normative databases that use non-instantaneous analyses such as the FFT. Thus, there is a fundamental and important difference between an instantaneous Z-score and an integrated FFT Z-score, with the former having two sources of variance while the latter has only one source of variance. Figure 5.1 illustrates the relationship between an FFT-based normative database versus an "instantaneous" or joint time frequency analysis (JTFA) database, such as used for the computation of instantaneous Z-scores.

C. Simplification and standardization

The third design concept is simplification and standardization of EEG biofeedback by the application of basic science. Simplification is achieved by the use of a single

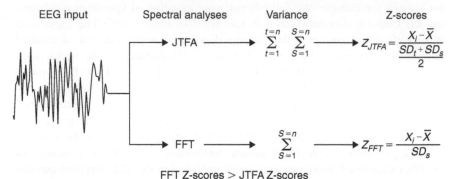

FIGURE 5.1   JTFA normative databases are instantaneous and include within session variance plus between subject variance. In contrast, FFT normative data only contains between subject variance. t = time, s = subjects and SD_t = standard deviation for the within session and SD_s = standard deviation between subjects. Thus FFT Z-scores are larger than JTFA Z-scores, and a ratio of 2:1 is not uncommon. (From Thatcher *et al.*, www.appliedneuroscience.com)

metric, namely, the metric of the "Z-score" for widely diverse measures such as power, coherence, and phase delays. Standardization is also achieved by EEG amplifier matching of the frequency response of the normative database amplifiers to the frequency characteristics of the EEG amplifiers used to acquire a comparison subject's EEG time series.

D.   Individualized EEG biofeedback protocols

A fourth and intertwined clinical concept in the design of Z-score biofeedback is "individualized" EEG biofeedback, and non-protocol drive EEG biofeedback. The idea of linking patient symptoms and complaints to functional localization in the brain as evidenced by "deregulation" of neural populations is fundamental to individualized biofeedback. For example, deregulation is recognized by significantly elevated or reduced power or network measures such as coherence and phase within regions of the brain that sub-serve particular functions that can be linked to the patient's symptoms and complaints. The use of Z-scores for biofeedback is designed to "re-regulate" or "optimize" the homeostasis, neural excitability, and network connectivity in particular regions of the brain. The functional localization and linkage to symptoms is based on modern knowledge of brain function as measured by fMRI, PET, penetrating head wounds, strokes and other neurological evidence acquired over the last two centuries (see Heilman and Valenstein, 1993; Braxis *et al.*, 2007; the Human Brain Mapping database of functional localization at: http://hendrix.imm.dtu.dk/services/jerne/brede/index_ext_roots.html).

Thus, the false concern that Z-score biofeedback will make exceptional people dull and an average individual a genius is misplaced. The concept is to link symptoms and complaints, and then monitor improvement or symptom reduction during the course of treatment. For peak-performance applications, a careful inventory of the client's personality style, self-assessment of weaknesses and strengths, and identification of the client's specific areas that they wish to improve must be obtained before application of Z-score biofeedback. Then, the practitioner attempts to link the client's identification of areas of weakness that they want improved to functional localization as expressed by "deregulation" of deviant neural activity that may be subject to change.

As mentioned previously, the instantaneous Z-scores are much smaller than the FFT Z-scores in NeuroGuide™ which uses the same subjects for the normative database. Smaller Z-scores when using the instantaneous Z-scores is expected. One should not be surprised by a 50% reduction in JTFA Z-scores in comparison to FFT Z-scores, and this is why it is best to first use 19-channel EEG measures and the highly stable FFT Z-scores to link symptoms to functional localization in the brain to the extent possible. Then use the Z-score program inside of NeuroGuide™ to evaluate the patient's instantaneous Z-scores in preparation before the biofeedback procedure begins. This will allow one to obtain a unique picture of the EEG instantaneous Z-scores of each unique patient prior to beginning Z-score biofeedback.

The clinician must be trained to select which Z-scores best match the patient's symptoms and complaints. A general rule is that the choice of Z-scores to use for biofeedback depends on two factors obtained using a full 19-channel EEG analysis: 1) scalp location(s) and, 2) magnitude of the Z-scores. Deregulation by hyperpolarization produces slowing in the EEG, and deregulation due to reduced inhibition produces deviations at higher frequencies. The direction of the Z-score is much less important than the location(s) of the deviant Z-scores, and the linkage to the patient's symptoms and complaints.

It is possible to review a patient's EEG prior to designing a Z-score biofeedback protocol. The Z-score biofeedback program inside of NeuroGuide™ is the same program as used by BrainMaster and other EEG system providers.

III.   INSTANTANEOUS Z-SCORES ACCESSED FROM INSIDE OF NEUROGUIDE™

Figure 5.2 is an example of the instantaneous Z-score screen inside of NeuroGuide™ while the instantaneous Z-scores are being reviewed.

A P4 and C4 theta and delta deviation from normal is evident as well as bilateral occipital delta deviations from normal. There is diminished alpha and theta in the instantaneous Z-scores, but on the average the dynamic FFT provides a much clearer picture of the right parietal and right central Z-scores. For illustration

Click View > Dynamic JTFA > Color Maps to view instantaneous power, coherence, phase, amplitude asymmetry, derivatives and phase reset

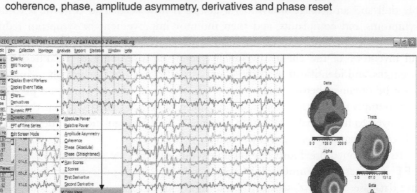

FIGURE 5.2   Screen capture from NeuroGuide™ in the Demo mode from a patient with right parietal and right central injury. Instantaneous Z-scores are on the right; EEG traces are on the left. Depress the left mouse button and move the mouse over the traces. Move the mouse to the right border and watch a movie of the dynamic Z-scores. Download the free NeuroGuide™ Demo at www.appliedneuroscience.com (see color plate)

purposes only, a biofeedback protocol would be to reward Z-score values less than and greater than 2 standard deviations in the theta frequency band in P4 and C4; most of the feedback rewards will automatically occur in the delta and theta frequency band. As mentioned previously, Fig. 5.2 is an example of an individualized Z-score biofeedback procedure after reviewing the patent's EEG using the same instantaneous Z-score program that is employed in the live Z-score DLL and incorporated into EEG biofeedback systems.

IV.   IMPLEMENTATION OF THE Z-SCORE BIOFEEDBACK

Step one is to compute means and standard deviations of instantaneous absolute power, relative power, power ratios, coherence, phase differences, and amplitude asymmetries on selected age groups of normal subjects from the 19-channel 10/20 electrode locations using the within session and between session variance as described previously. The inclusion/exclusion criteria, number of subjects, number of subjects per age group, cross-validation procedures, and other details of the means and standard deviation computations are published (Thatcher *et al*, 1987; 2003).

Step two is to develop a dynamic link library (DLL) that can be distributed to EEG biofeedback system manufacturers, which allows the manufacturers to integrate the instantaneous Z-scores inside of their already existing software environments. The DLL involves only four command lines of code, and is designed for software developments to easily implement the instantaneous Z-scores by passing raw digital data to the DLL and then organizing the Z-scores that are returned in less than one microsecond. This rapid analysis and return of Z-scores is essential for timely feedback when specific EEG features are measured by the complex demodulation JTFA operating inside of the DLL.

V. JTFA COMPLEX DEMODULATION COMPUTATIONS

The mathematical details of complex demodulation used to compute the instantaneous Z-scores as contained in the Applied Neuroscience, Inc. "DLL" are published in Otnes and Enochson (1977), Granger and Hatanaka (1964), Bloomfield (2000), and Thatcher *et al.* (2008). Complex demodulation is a time domain digital method of spectral analysis whereas the fast fourier transform (FFT) is a frequency domain method. These two methods are related by the fact they both involve sines and cosines; both operate in the complex domain, and in this way represent the same mathematical descriptions of the power spectrum.

The advantage of complex demodulation is that it is a time domain method and less sensitive to artifact, and it does not require windowing nor even integers of the power of 2 as does the FFT. The FFT integrates power in a frequency band over the entire epoch length and requires windowing functions, which can dramatically affect the power values, whereas, as mentioned previously, complex demodulation does not require windowing (Otnes and Enochson, 1972). Complex demodulation was computed for the linked ears and eyes-open and eyes-closed conditions for all 625 subjects in the normative database.

Figure 5.3 is an illustration of the method of complex demodulation for the computation of power, coherence and phase. The mathematical details are in Thatcher *et al.*, 2007.

VI. Z-SCORES AND QEEG NORMATIVE DATABASES

Matousek and Petersen (1973) computed means and standard deviations in one-year age groups, and were the first to use Z-scores to compare an individual to

TABLE 5.1 Center frequencies and bandwidths of the Z-score biofeedback DLL and NeuroGuide

	Center Frequency	Band Width
Delta	2.5 Hz	1–4 Hz
Theta	6.0 Hz	4–8 Hz
Alpha	10.0 Hz	8–12 Hz
Beta	18.5 Hz	12–25 Hz
Hi-Beta	27.5 Hz	25–30 Hz
Beta 1	13.5 Hz	12–15 Hz
Beta 2	16.5 Hz	15–18 Hz
Beta 3	21.5 Hz	18–25 Hz
Alpha 1	9.0 Hz	8–10 Hz
Alpha 2	11.0 Hz	10–12 Hz
Gamma 1*	FFT only	30–35 Hz
Gamma 2*	FFT only	35–40 Hz
Gamma 3*	FFT only	40–50 Hz

* = NeuroGuide only

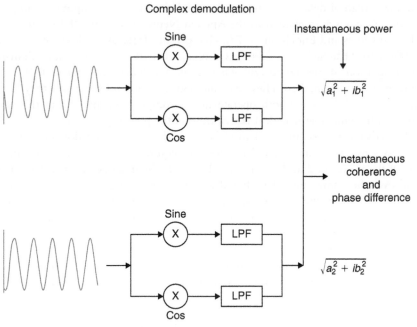

FIGURE 5.3 Diagram of complex demodulation. Left is a sine wave as input, which is multiplied by the sine and cosine waves at the center frequency of a given frequency band as described in Table 5.1, which transforms the digital time series to the complex plane. A 6th order Butterworth low-pass filter is used to shift the frequency to zero where power at the center frequency is then calculated using the Pythagorean theorem. Complex numbers are then used to compute coherence and phase as described in Appendix, section 4.0. (From Thatcher *et al.*, 2007, www.appliedneuroscience.com)

the normative database means and standard deviations. The Z-score is an excellent statistic defined as the difference between the value from an individual and the mean of the population divided by the standard deviation of the population or

$$Z = \frac{x_i - \bar{X}}{SD}$$

John and collegues (John *et al.*, 1987) expanded on the use of the Z-score for clinical evaluation, including the use of multivariate measures such as the Mahalanobis distance metric. A direct normalization of the Gaussian distribution using Z-scores is useful in comparing individuals to a QEEG normative database. That is, the standard score form of the Gaussian is where the mean $= 0$ and standard deviation $= 1$ or, by substitution into the Gaussian equation for a bell shaped curve, then

$$Y = \frac{1}{\sqrt{2\pi}} e^{-z2/2}$$

where Y $=$ Gaussian distribution and the Z-score is a deviation in standard deviation units measured along the baseline of the Gaussian curve from a mean of 0 and a standard deviation $= 1$, with deviations to the right of the mean being positive and those to the left negative. By substituting different values of Z then different values of Y can be calculated. For example, when $Z = 0, Y = 0.3989$ or, in other words, the height of the curve at the mean of the normal distribution in standard-score form is given by the number 0.3989. For purposes of assessing deviation from normal, the values of Z above and below the mean, which include 95% of the area of the Gaussian, are often used as a level of confidence necessary to minimize Type I and Type II errors. The standard-score equation is also used to cross-validate a normative database, which again emphasizes the importance of approximation to a Gaussian for any normative QEEG database.

A.   Standardization by amplifier matching and QEEG normative databases

Surprisingly, matching of amplifier frequency characteristics as a standard was largely neglected during much of the history of QEEG normative databases. In 1982 to 1987 E. Roy John and colleagues formed a consortium of universities and medical schools that were using QEEG who met several times over a few years; the consortium was one of the supporters of the edited volume by John titled "Machinery of the Mind" (John, 1990). One of the important issues consistently raised at the consortium meetings was the need for "standardization." In the 1980s it was technically difficult to match different EEG systems because of the infantile development of analysis software. This forced most QEEG users to use relative power, because absolute power was not comparable between different EEG machines. There was no frequency response standardization between different EEG machines, and thus there was no cross-platform standardization of QEEG.

It was not until the mid 1990s that computer speed and software development made amplifier matching and normative database amplifier equilibration a possibility. The first use of standardized matching of amplifiers was to the University of Maryland (UM) database (Thatcher *et al.*, 2003). The procedure involved injecting microvolt calibration sine waves into the input of amplifiers of different EEG machines, and then injecting the same microvolt signals into the normative database amplifiers, thus obtaining two frequency response curves. Equilibration of a normative QEEG database to different EEG machines is the ratio of the frequency response curves of the two amplifiers that are then used as coefficients in the power spectral analysis. This was an important step because suddenly absolute power Z-scores and normative database comparisons became possible.

The frequencies in absolute power are independent of each other, and are not distorted. It is always best to use absolute values whenever possible and not relative values, or even ratios. A ratio can change due to the denominator, or the numerator, and one cannot determine which has changed without evaluating the absolute values used to compute the ratios.

A simple method to exactly match the frequency characteristics of different amplifiers, by amplifier equilibration, is to calibrate the amplifiers using microvolt sine waves at discrete frequencies from 1–40 Hz, and inject the sine waves into the inputs of the EEG amplifiers (see Fig. 5.4). Then take the ratio of the microvolt values at each frequency, and use the ratios to exactly equate the spectral output values at different frequencies for different amplifiers. This method creates a universal equilibration process so that microvolts in a given amplifier are equal to microvolts in all other amplifiers, including the normative database amplifiers. By equilibrating amplifiers, direct comparisons between a given patient's EEG and the normative database means and standard deviations are valid and meaningful.

B. General method to produce a valid instantaneous Z-score EEG database

Figure 5.5 illustrates a step-by-step procedure by which the Z-instantaneous-score normative EEG database was validated, and sensitivities calculated. The left side of the figure is the edited, artifact clean, and reliable digital EEG time series, which may be re-referenced or re-montaged, and is then analyzed in either the time domain or the frequency domain.

Normative database amplifier matching—microvolt sine waves 0–40 Hz
Equilibration ratios to match frequency responses

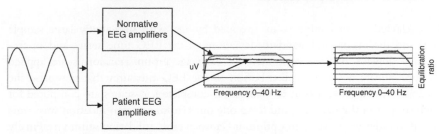

FIGURE 5.4 Flow chart of the amplifier standardization procedure. Microvolt sine waves are injected into the input of amplifiers, and the frequency responses are calculated. The frequency response of the normative database amplifiers and the frequency response of other EEG amplifier systems are then equated, and the spectral analysis is adjusted so that there is a standardized import and matching of amplifier systems with the common unit being microvolts (uV). (Adapted from Thatcher and Lubar, 2008, in press.)

Normative database validation steps

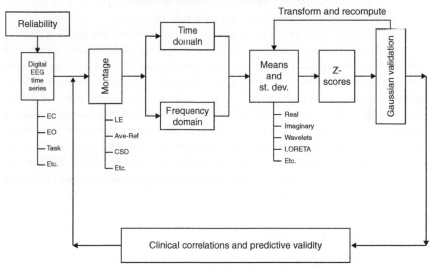

FIGURE 5.5 Illustration of the step-by-step procedure to Gaussian cross-validate, and then validate by correlations with clinical measures in order to estimate the predictive and content validity of any EEG normative database. The feedback connections between Gaussian cross-validation and the means and standard deviations refer to transforms to approximate Gaussian if the non-transformed data is less Gaussian. The clinical correlation and validation arrow to the montage stage represents repetition of clinical validation to a different montage, or reference, or condition such as eyes-open, active tasks, eyes-closed, etc. to the adjustments and understanding of the experimental design(s). (From Thatcher *et al.*, 2003.)

C. Age groupings of the instantaneous Z-score normative population

The selected normal subjects are grouped by age, with sufficiently large sample size, and the means and standard deviations of the EEG time series and/or frequency domain analyses computed for each age group. Transforms are applied to approximate a Gaussian distribution of the EEG measures that comprise the means. Once approximation to Gaussian is completed, Z-scores are computed for each subject in the database, and leave one out Gaussian cross-validation was computed in order to arrive at an optimum Gaussian cross-validation sensitivity. Finally, the Gaussian validated norms are subjected to content and predictive validation procedures such as correlation with neuropsychological test scores and intelligence, etc., and also discriminant analyses, neural networks, and outcome statistics, etc.

The content validations are with respect to clinical measures such as intelligence, neuropsychological test scores, school achievement, clinical outcomes, etc. The predictive validations are with respect to the discriminative, statistical, or neural network clinical classification accuracy. Both parametric and non-parametric statistics are used to determine the content and predictive validity of a normative EEG database.

Thatcher and Lubar (2008) show the number of subjects per year in the normative EEG lifespan database. It can be seen that the largest number of subjects are in the younger ages (e.g., 1–14 years, N = 470) when the EEG is changing most rapidly. As mentioned previously, a proportionally smaller number of subjects represent the adult age range from 14–82 years (N = 155). The Z-score normative database includes a total of 625 carefully screened individual subjects ranging in age from 2 months to 82 years. In order to increase the time resolution of age, sliding averages were used for the stratification in NeuroGuide™, and for instantaneous Z-scores (Thatcher *et al.*, 2003). Two-year means were computed using a sliding average with 6-month overlap of subjects. This produced a more stable and higher age resolution normative database, and a total of 21 different age groups. For the 21 age groups, age ranges, and number of subjects per age group see Thatcher and Lubar (2008).

VII.   CASE STUDY 1: JACK

In recent years, several neurofeedback approaches have been used to treat human epilepsy but only two have received extensive research and publication. The first, and original approach, as determined by Sterman and Friar (1972) enhances SMR activity while inhibiting the lower frequencies. The second, as illustrated by Kotchoubey *et al.* (2001), trains patients to control slow cortical potentials. Both techniques are effective in reducing seizure activity.

Recent advancements in the reliability of QEEG databases, most notably single-HZ bins and broadly-based coherence determinations, have led to the development of a third approach to the normalization of EEG in patients with epilepsy. These innovations have made it possible to more precisely characterize the power and coherence abnormalities of drug-resistant epilepsy. As demonstrated by Walker (2005), the general methodology is to identify the most significant abnormalities and train those areas with neurofeedback. Abnormal magnitude (power) indices are addressed first followed by deviant coherence values. This treatment method, combined with Z-score training, eventually proved successful with a client with medication-resistant, focal epilepsy.

Jack was a three-year-old male. The client's epilepsy was expressed as atonic, absence, and myoclonic seizures. After approximately one year of symptom-based neurofeedback treatment that produced brief periods of seizure control, Jack suffered a mild concussive head injury in the right orbital region. His seizure activity increased significantly. Three to four hundred microvolt inter-ictal epileptiform discharges were observed in the raw EEG trace. His paroxysmal activity began to generalize with a multi-spike focus. These new clinical developments proved resistant to symptom-based neurofeedback training. A new treatment strategy was developed that consisted of 2-channel inhibit protocols followed by coherence training based on the abnormalities revealed in a QEEG analysis.

These protocols were focused on the slower frequencies that tend to propagate seizure activity. The inhibit training had an immediate positive effect on seizure frequency, as well as the frequency and voltage of the patient's spike and wave complexes. The patient gained seizure control during this phase of treatment. Coherence training was begun with a focus on hypo-coherence in the lower frequencies. Seizure activity reappeared during the coherence phase of training.

This pattern was repeated during a subsequent trial of inhibit- and coherence-based training. The client gained seizure control during the inhibit phase of training only to relinquish it while undergoing coherence work. It appeared that the patient was responding negatively to traditional coherence training as evidenced by the second QEEG (Fig. 5.7). A slight variant in this round—the paroxysmal activity reappeared during the end of power training—suggested power training alone was not enough. Since standard coherence training seemed to make the patient worse, another form of coherence training was needed.

Traditional coherence training attempts to move coherence in a linear fashion from greater to lesser, or vice versa. Coherence is rewarded only when it moves in one direction. Z-score range training reinforces coherence when it remains inside a range of positive and negative Z-scores—a ceiling and a floor. Coherence is allowed to fluctuate between hyper-coherence and hypo-coherence. Z-score training exercises coherence within a range that can be altered as the trainee improves performance. The band of Z-scores trained can be narrowed, shaping the coherence toward less deviance.

This form of coherence training may be superior to traditional methods. Initial clinical results suggest that unlike conventional coherence approaches, Z-score coherence range training is less likely to produce the iatrogenic effects common to

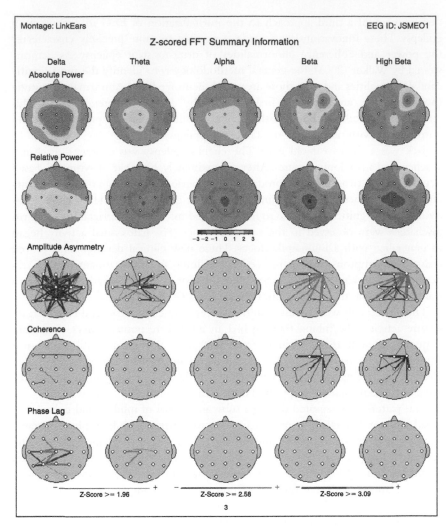

FIGURE 5.6   Jack's first QEEG revealing abnormal slow wave activity in central and parietal regions combined with delta and beta coherence abnormalities (see color plate).

overtraining. Two rounds of standard coherence training had not produced positive clinical results with Jack. After several weeks of Z-score coherence range training, he gained lasting seizure control. The post-treatment brain maps reveal a largely resolved set of coherence values (Fig. 5.8). As of the time of writing, the patient has maintained seizure control with a brief lapse for over one and one half years.

That lapse occurred when the patient was removed from medication, and a 24-hour video EEG was performed in an attempt to eliminate medication. In addition to the seizure activity, the test revealed continuous spike and wave

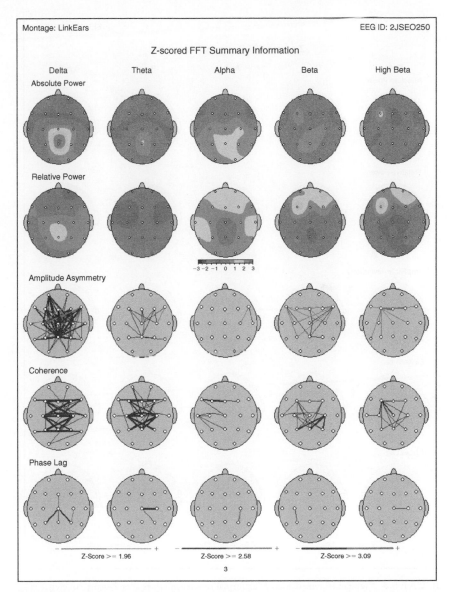

FIGURE 5.7 Significant increase in hypo-coherence in all bands after traditional coherence training (see color plate).

complexes during slow wave sleep. This prompted the review of a previous overnight EEG which had determined that, at that time, the patient had reached the diagnostic criteria for electrical status epilepticus during slow wave sleep (ESES). ESES is a rare disorder that causes neuropsyhological impairment in almost all cases according to Tassinari and colleagues (Tassinari et al., 2000). Despite a positive

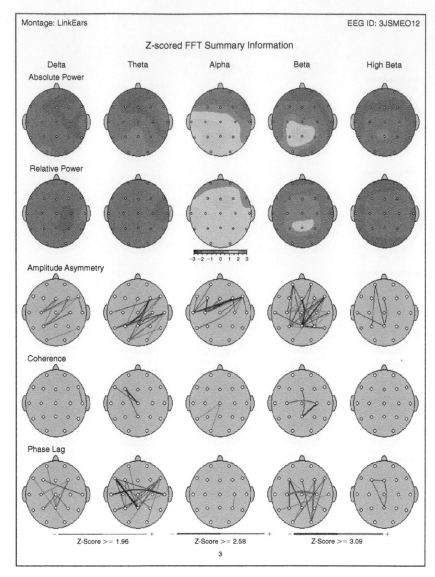

FIGURE 5.8   Substantial remediation of abnormal coherence values after Z-score coherence range training (see color plate).

seizure prognosis, ESES leaves 50% of children diagnosed with the syndrome with profound cognitive deficits (Tassinari and Galanopoulou, 1992, 2000). The most recent overnight EEG revealed a significant reduction in the frequency and magnitude of inter-ictal epileptiform discharges. While he no longer met the criteria for ESES, the continued presence of spike and wave activity created a significant vulnerability to the development of cognitive dysfunction. Additionally, Jack could not be without medication for his seizure disorder. For those reasons, it was determined that another round of neurofeedback was indicated.

The client sat for an additional course of 2-channel inhibit and coherence training. This time Z-score monitoring and training were employed from the beginning of treatment with two positive clinical effects. Because of the software's ability to reveal instantaneous coherence and magnitude values compared to Neuroguide's normative database, it was possible to alter clinical decisions that were initially based on the QEEG. Three coherence and four magnitude protocols were indicated by the QEEG. Traditionally, these protocols would be trained approximately five times each, totaling 35 sessions. The observation of absolute power values during inhibit training indicated resolution of those deviances in less than five sessions at several locations. Moreover, the Z-score software suggested far less deviance in slow wave activity at two locations than did the QEEG. After repeated monitoring of those sites, demonstrating flexibility within normal limits, they were eliminated from the training regimen.

At the end of power training, a Z-score assessment of coherence revealed significant differences from the results of the QEEG suggesting that the resolution of magnitude impacted coherence in a normative direction. Four 2-channel coherence Z-score range training sessions at three locations comprised the connectivity protocols in this round of treatment. At 20 total sessions, this treatment course was approximately one-third to one half the number of a traditional neurofeedback treatment course of 30–40 sessions. In this case the shortened treatment is the direct result of the combination of symptom resolution and the observation of less deviant magnitude and coherence values made possible by real-time Z-score monitoring.

The client has been seizure-free for one year since his brief lapse. He is currently prescribed a small fraction of his anticonvulsive medication with possible elimination in the near future. The patient tested into a gifted and talented program, and is thriving in the first grade with no indication of cognitive deficit.

VIII.   CASE STUDY 2: JOHN

John, a seventy-three-year-old Caucasian male, presented in treatment after suffering a brain tumor. A pre-treatment biopsy of the tumor caused hemorrhaging in the left temporal lobe just below T5. He submitted to several rounds of chemotherapy resulting in the complete elimination of all evidence of the cancer. At presentation the client could not read or drive due to right vision field neglect. He struggled to use the telephone, listen to the radio, watch television, or make sense of conversation. The patient suffered with Acoustico–agnostic Aphasia, an inability to recognize phenomes (Luria 1973). In addition, expressive speech was severely compromised. He had difficulty with articulation and word finding. He struggled to sustain attention and concentration. Moreover, the client had memory deficits such that he would forget the activity he was engaged in while performing it, and would often have trouble recalling the simplest instructions immediately after they had been given. He was frequently in a state of confusion and befuddlement.

The client's QEEG revealed increases in absolute and relative power of delta and theta in the area of his hemorrhage, and diffuse increases of absolute power of 6 and 7 Hz (Fig. 5.9). There were decreases in coherences of delta and theta—some greater than five standard deviations— involving the entire left hemisphere. The client completed approximately 66 sessions of traditional 2–channel inhibit and coherence training. All his symptoms improved. He was better able to drive, talk on the telephone, read, and watch television. There were several deficits that had not completely resolved. He experienced words "jumping around" on the page while he read. He was unhappy with his processing speed. Accustomed to reading several papers per day, he now struggled to read one. The patient continued to exhibit right vision field neglect. He often labored with word finding difficulty.

The client submitted to another QEEG. It revealed little change in left hemisphere coherence and power values from the first QEEG (Fig. 5.10). The left hemisphere remained almost completely disconnected from the right. However, the second QEEG discovered increased hyper–coherence in delta, theta and high beta in the right, undamaged hemisphere. Several studies suggest this shift as a possible compensatory mechanism in patients with traumatic brain injury (Just and Thornton, 2007, 2005). The Z–score software confirmed the findings of the second QEEG. Two–channel inhibit training based on a reading difference map was employed in the occipital and temporal lobes to immediate positive effect. The magnitude deviations were substantially improved with a rapid remediation in symptoms. The client reported that the words on the page no longer moved and he was reading more efficiently.

Right vision field neglect was still evident. Despite significant improvement in reading, the client reported that he often "missed" the last several words of a sentence. The patient reported that the right rear tail light of the car traveling in front of him was not perceptible. A four–channel Z–score protocol targeting 23 training parameters was employed. Included in that protocol were delta and theta absolute power, and delta, theta, and beta coherence. Simultaneously, 6–7 Hz was inhibited in all four channels. Visual, memory, and association areas were targeted. This protocol was based on a combination of the results of the QEEG and visual inspection of the real–time Z–score values (Fig. 5.11).

After three sessions, the trained Z–scores showed remarkable movement toward normative values. Absolute power and coherence indices improved, in some cases demonstrating flexibility of almost two standard deviations. All Z–scores revealed a shift toward more plasticity and less deviance (Fig. 5.12). The patient reported

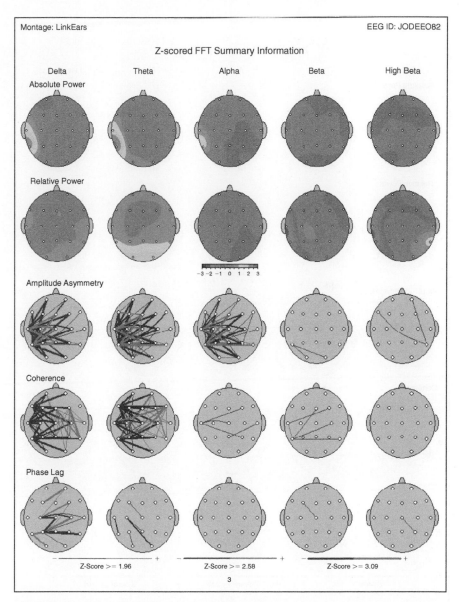

FIGURE 5.9 John's first QEEG demonstrating focal slow wave activity over the area of the hemorrhage, and theta abnormalities in occipital, parietal and temporal lobes with left hemisphere hypocoherence and right hemisphere hyper-coherence (see color plate).

that his right vision field neglect was greatly improved. He was consistently able to read the last several words of each sentence. He reliably observed the right rear tail light of cars preceding him. Several sessions later, he stated that he was able to perceive the cars stopped at intersections on his right.

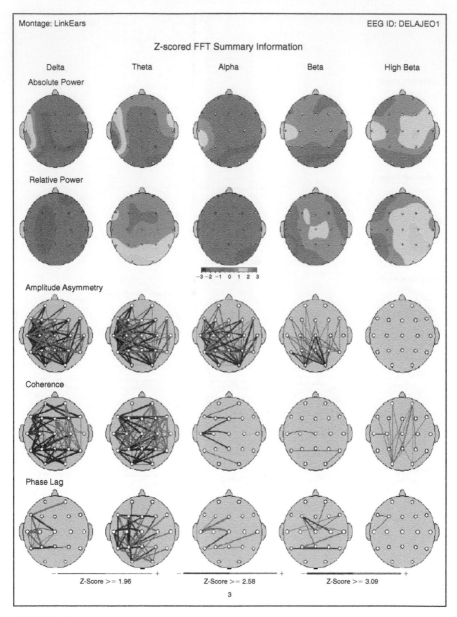

FIGURE 5.10   After 60 sessions of traditional inhibit and coherence training. Note the significant increase in hyper-coherence in the right hemisphere (see color plate).

SITES: O1 Pz (EO)	Abs	Rel	Rat/T	Rat/A	Rat/B	Rat/G	SITES: T4 P4 (EO)	Abs	Rel	Rat/T	Rat/A	Rat/B	Rat/G
Delta (1.0-4.0)	0.6	0.1	-0.4	0.4	0.3	0.5	Delta (1.0-4.0)	1.7	0.2	-0.2	0.5	0.2	0.4
Theta (4.0-8.0)	1.0	0.7		0.8	0.6	0.8	Theta (4.0-8.0)	1.8	0.5		0.8	0.4	0.6
Alpha (8.0-12.5)	-0.0	-0.6			-0.2	0.0	Alpha (8.0-12.5)	0.8	-0.6			-0.4	-0.1
Beta (12.5-25.5)	0.2	-0.3				0.0	Beta (12.5-25.5)	1.3	-0.1				0.3
Beta 1 (12.0-15.5)	-0.1	-0.5					Beta 1 (12.0-15.5)	0.9	-0.4				
Beta 2 (15.0-18.0)	0.3	-0.1					Beta 2 (15.0-18.0)	1.4	-0.1				
Beta 3 (18.0-25.5)	0.8	0.4					Beta 3 (18.0-25.5)	1.7	0.3				
Gamma (25.5-30.5)	0.2	-0.2					Gamma (25.5-30.5)	1.1	-0.2				
Delta (1.0-4.0)	1.0	0.3	-0.1	0.5	0.2	0.6	Delta (1.0-4.0)	1.3	0.4	0.0	0.7	0.4	0.8
Theta (4.0-8.0)	1.1	0.4		0.6	0.3	0.7	Theta (4.0-8.0)	1.3	0.4		0.8	0.4	0.8
Alpha (8.0-12.5)	0.2	-0.6			-0.3	0.0	Alpha (8.0-12.5)	0.2	-0.8			-0.4	-0.0
Beta (12.5-25.5)	0.7	-0.1				0.4	Beta (12.5-25.5)	0.8	-0.2				0.4
Beta 1 (12.0-15.5)	0.2	-0.5					Beta 1 (12.0-15.5)	0.2	-0.7				
Beta 2 (15.0-18.0)	0.8	-0.0					Beta 2 (15.0-18.0)	0.9	-0.1				
Beta 3 (18.0-25.5)	0.9	0.2					Beta 3 (18.0-25.5)	1.1	0.1				
Gamma (25.5-30.5)	0.5	-0.2					Gamma (25.5-30.5)	0.7	-0.3				

	O1-Pz ASY	COH	PHA	O1-T4 ASY	COH	PHA	O1-P4 ASY	COH	PHA	Pz-T4 ASY	COH	PHA	Pz-P4 ASY	COH	PHA	T4-P4 ASY	COH	PHA
Delta (1.0-4.0)	-0.4	-0.5	0.4	-0.9	0.4	-0.3	-0.8	-0.1	0.1	-0.6	-0.0	0.1	-0.4	-1.7	1.4	0.4	0.1	0.1
Theta (4.0-8.0)	-0.1	0.5	-0.2	-0.7	1.0	-0.5	-0.3	0.6	-0.3	-0.7	1.1	-0.5	-0.3	0.4	-0.1	0.7	1.1	-0.6
Alpha (8.0-12.5)	-0.3	0.3	-0.2	-0.8	-0.3	-0.1	-0.2	-0.0	-0.0	-0.6	-0.3	-0.0	-0.0	-0.1	0.1	0.7	0.2	-0.2
Beta (12.5-25.5)	-0.5	1.4	-0.4	-0.9	1.0	-0.4	-0.6	1.5	-0.4	-0.6	0.8	-0.3	-0.2	0.7	-0.2	0.5	0.5	-0.2
Beta 1 (12.0-15.5)	-0.3	0.2	-0.1	-0.8	-0.0	-0.0	-0.3	0.5	-0.3	-0.6	-0.3	0.0	-0.1	-0.0	-0.1	0.6	-0.3	0.1
Beta 2 (15.0-18.0)	-0.5	0.8	-0.4	-0.9	0.2	-0.4	-0.5	0.7	-0.4	-0.5	0.2	-0.3	-0.2	0.4	-0.2	0.4	0.2	-0.1
Beta 3 (18.0-25.5)	-0.2	1.0	-0.6	-0.8	0.6	-0.6	-0.3	1.1	-0.7	-0.7	0.5	-0.4	-0.2	0.5	-0.4	0.6	0.3	-0.2
Gamma (25.5-30.5)	-0.3	1.0	-0.4	-0.7	0.3	-0.3	-0.4	1.1	-0.5	-0.5	0.2	-0.2	-0.2	0.4	-0.2	0.5	0.2	-0.2

FIGURE 5.11   Four-channel Z-score protocol based on the QEEG and this Z-score assessment (see color plate).

SITES: O1 Pz (EO)	Abs	Rel	Rat/T	Rat/A	Rat/B	Rat/G	SITES: T4 P4 (EO)	Abs	Rel	Rat/T	Rat/A	Rat/B	Rat/G
Delta (1.0-4.0)	0.8	0.3	-0.0	0.4	0.4	0.6	Delta (1.0-4.0)	1.3	0.5	0.1	0.5	0.6	0.9
Theta (4.0-8.0)	0.8	0.4		0.4	0.4	0.7	Theta (4.0-8.0)	1.2	0.3		0.4	0.5	0.8
Alpha (8.0-12.5)	0.2	-0.3			-0.0	0.0	Alpha (8.0-12.5)	0.6	-0.3			0.1	0.4
Beta (12.5-25.5)	0.3	-0.2				0.0	Beta (12.5-25.5)	0.5	-0.5				0.3
Beta 1 (12.0-15.5)	-0.1	-0.6					Beta 1 (12.0-15.5)	0.1	-0.8				
Beta 2 (15.0-18.0)	0.2	-0.3					Beta 2 (15.0-18.0)	0.6	-0.3				
Beta 3 (18.0-25.5)	0.4	-0.1					Beta 3 (18.0-25.5)	0.6	-0.3				
Gamma (25.5-30.5)	0.2	-0.3					Gamma (25.5-30.5)	0.4	-0.5				
Delta (1.0-4.0)	0.7	0.2	0.1	0.2	0.0	0.4	Delta (1.0-4.0)	0.8	0.3	0.2	0.4	0.3	0.7
Theta (4.0-8.0)	0.5	0.0		0.1	-0.1	0.3	Theta (4.0-8.0)	0.6	0.1		0.3	0.1	0.6
Alpha (8.0-12.5)	0.3	-0.1			-0.2	0.2	Alpha (8.0-12.5)	0.2	-0.4			-0.2	0.2
Beta (12.5-25.5)	0.7	0.2				0.4	Beta (12.5-25.5)	0.5	-0.1				0.5
Beta 1 (12.0-15.5)	0.2	-0.3					Beta 1 (12.0-15.5)	0.1	-0.7				
Beta 2 (15.0-18.0)	0.5	-0.0					Beta 2 (15.0-18.0)	0.3	-0.3				
Beta 3 (18.0-25.5)	0.8	0.4					Beta 3 (18.0-25.5)	0.7	0.1				
Gamma (25.5-30.5)	0.7	0.2					Gamma (25.5-30.5)	0.5	-0.1				

	O1-Pz ASY	COH	PHA	O1-T4 ASY	COH	PHA	O1-P4 ASY	COH	PHA	Pz-T4 ASY	COH	PHA	Pz-P4 ASY	COH	PHA	T4-P4 ASY	COH	PHA
Delta (1.0-4.0)	0.0	0.4	-0.3	-0.5	0.6	-0.5	-0.1	0.3	-0.3	-0.5	0.4	-0.3	-0.2	0.1	-0.0	0.5	0.3	-0.3
Theta (4.0-8.0)	0.3	0.1	-0.1	-0.4	0.2	-0.1	0.2	-0.0	0.1	-0.6	0.6	-0.2	-0.1	0.2	0.1	0.6	0.9	-0.4
Alpha (8.0-12.5)	-0.2	0.1	-0.2	-0.4	-0.1	-0.0	0.0	-0.1	-0.1	-0.2	-0.1	-0.1	0.2	-0.6	0.2	0.4	0.1	-0.2
Beta (12.5-25.5)	-0.4	1.0	-0.4	-0.2	0.5	-0.3	-0.2	0.7	-0.2	0.1	0.5	-0.3	0.3	-0.7	0.1	0.1	0.7	-0.3
Beta 1 (12.0-15.5)	-0.2	0.4	-0.3	-0.2	-0.0	0.0	0.0	0.5	-0.3	0.0	-0.4	0.1	0.3	-0.5	0.2	0.2	-0.5	0.2
Beta 2 (15.0-18.0)	-0.3	0.5	-0.3	-0.3	0.1	-0.1	-0.1	0.4	-0.3	-0.1	-0.0	-0.1	0.2	-0.6	0.3	0.3	0.1	-0.0
Beta 3 (18.0-25.5)	-0.5	0.6	-0.4	-0.2	0.2	-0.4	-0.2	0.5	-0.4	0.2	0.1	-0.1	0.3	-0.8	0.4	-0.0	0.3	-0.3
Gamma (25.5-30.5)	-0.6	0.9	-0.4	-0.1	0.4	-0.5	-0.2	0.7	-0.4	0.3	0.5	-0.4	0.4	-0.5	0.1	-0.0	0.7	-0.5

FIGURE 5.12   After three sessions of training, Z-scores reveal substantial remediation (see color plate).

Birnbaumer (2007) has suggested that if the neuronal assemblies adjacent to the injury, rather than the homolog in the contra-lateral hemisphere, assume the function of damaged neurons more recovery is possible. Incorporating this strategy to address the client's expressive speech difficulties, a protocol targeting the left hemisphere was developed.

In addition to the damaged area of the supramarginal gyrus, Broca's area, the ventral frontal and posterior parietal lobes were trained (Illustration 10). Twenty-six training parameters including delta and theta absolute power and coherences of delta, beta and gamma were employed. After 11 sessions of Z-score training the measures had improved substantially. Coherence values were demonstrably more flexible, frequently moving within one standard deviation. Absolute power indices

SITES: F3 P3 (EO)	Abs	Rel	Rat/T	Rat/A	Rat/B	Rat/G	SITES: F7 T5 (EO)	Abs	Rel	Rat/T	Rat/A	Rat/B	Rat/G
Delta (1.0-4.0)	0.6	-0.1	-0.3	0.1	-0.2	0.7	Delta (1.0-4.0)	0.5	-0.2	-0.3	0.1	-0.3	0.7
Theta (4.0-8.0)	1.0	0.4		0.4		1.0	Theta (4.0-8.0)	1.0	0.4		0.5	0.0	1.0
Alpha (8.0-12.5)	0.4	-0.2			-0.3	0.6	Alpha (8.0-12.5)	0.3	-0.3			-0.4	0.6
Beta (12.5-25.5)	0.7	0.2				1.0	Beta (12.5-25.5)	0.9	0.4				1.1
Beta 1 (12.0-15.5)	-0.4	-1.0					Beta 1 (12.0-15.5)	-0.4	-1.0				
Beta 2 (15.0-18.0)	0.8	0.2					Beta 2 (15.0-18.0)	1.0	0.4				
Beta 3 (18.0-25.5)	1.3	0.8					Beta 3 (18.0-25.5)	1.5	0.9				
Gamma (25.5-30.5)	0.4	-0.1					Gamma (25.5-30.5)	0.6	-0.0				
Delta (1.0-4.0)	0.1	-0.6	-0.7	-0.3	-0.5	0.2	Delta (1.0-4.0)	1.0	-0.6	-1.0	-0.5	-0.0	0.7
Theta (4.0-8.0)	0.9	0.5		0.3	0.2	0.8	Theta (4.0-8.0)	2.2	0.8		0.4	0.9	1.5
Alpha (8.0-12.5)	0.4	-0.1			-0.2	0.5	Alpha (8.0-12.5)	1.4	0.2			0.4	1.1
Beta (12.5-25.5)	0.7	0.2				0.7	Beta (12.5-25.5)	1.0	-0.5				0.8
Beta 1 (12.0-15.5)	-0.2	-0.7					Beta 1 (12.0-15.5)	0.0	-1.4				
Beta 2 (15.0-18.0)	0.9	0.3					Beta 2 (15.0-18.0)	1.3	-0.1				
Beta 3 (18.0-25.5)	1.1	0.6					Beta 3 (18.0-25.5)	1.5	0.0				
Gamma (25.5-30.5)	0.6	0.1					Gamma (25.5-30.5)	0.8	-0.7				

	F3-P3:			F3-F7:			F3-T5:			P3-F7:			P3-T5:			F7-T5:		
	ASY	COH	PHA	ASY	COH	PHA	ASY	COH	PHA	ASY	COH	PHA	ASY	COH	PHA	ASY	COH	PHA
Delta (1.0-4.0)	0.4	0.0	0.4	-0.1	-0.3	0.6	-0.4	-0.2	0.9	-0.3	-0.3	0.4	-1.0	-1.6	1.1	-0.4	-0.0	0.4
Theta (4.0-8.0)	-0.0	-0.4	0.4	-0.0	-0.5	0.3	-1.1	0.1	0.7	0.0	-0.2	0.6	-1.5	-0.9	0.3	-1.0	0.3	0.5
Alpha (8.0-12.5)	-0.1	-0.4	0.3	0.1	0.1	-0.1	-1.1	0.2	0.4	0.1	-0.2	0.2	-1.3	-0.4	0.2	-1.0	0.1	0.3
Beta (12.5-25.5)	0.0	0.9	-0.3	-0.1	1.7	-0.7	-0.2	0.6	-0.3	-0.2	1.7	-0.5	-0.4	0.4	-0.1	-0.1	1.2	-0.5
Beta 1 (12.0-15.5)	-0.2	-0.1	0.0	-0.0	0.7	-0.5	-0.4	0.2	0.1	0.2	-0.2	-0.1	-0.2	-0.5	0.2	-0.4	0.1	-0.1
Beta 2 (15.0-18.0)	-0.1	0.2	-0.3	-0.2	0.9	-0.5	-0.5	0.0	-0.2	-0.1	0.5	-0.4	-0.6	0.2	-0.1	-0.3	0.5	-0.3
Beta 3 (18.0-25.5)	0.2	0.7	-0.5	-0.2	1.1	-0.8	-0.1	0.8	-0.4	-0.3	1.0	-0.7	-0.4	0.5	-0.3	-0.0	0.9	-0.5
Gamma (25.5-30.5)	-0.1	0.8	-0.5	-0.1	1.5	-0.7	-0.3	0.4	-0.3	-0.0	1.5	-0.7	-0.2	0.2	-0.1	-0.2	0.8	-0.5

FIGURE 5.13   First Z-score training of F3/P3/F7/T5. Note the damage in the temporal area at T5 reflected in abnormal absolute power Z-scores, and the significant deviation in connectivity measures (see color plate).

including the damaged area of the temporal lobe that had resisted traditional training, demonstrated similar remediation (Fig. 5.13). More importantly, the client was able to express himself with much more precision. More often appropriate and precise nouns such as "barn" took the place of the more general "animal house." Overall, the improvement in the production of coherence in conversation was marked, and confirmed by report of family and friends.

IX.   CASE STUDY 3: SL

This section will describe the experience of two of the chapter authors, Lambos and Stark, with Z-score training in SL, a seven-year-old right-handed male who was brought to us by his parents for help with discipline problems, both at home and in the classroom, and a possible diagnosis of ADHD. As per our usual procedures, we carefully interviewed the child and his parents, and conducted appropriate neuropsychological testing as well as a 19-channel QEEG.

S's history includes a normal vaginal delivery following an unremarkable gestation. He developed normally, and met developmental milestones within normal time periods. He was breast-fed, and has had few infectious disease problems. No head trauma, encephalitis or other common causes of insult to the brain were reported. With respect to his school experience, S has been a rapid learner but his teachers noted a tendency to become easily excited and aggressive with other children. Some teachers and professionals felt he could be classified as ADHD. The interview revealed that his home environment was somewhat chaotic. S is the oldest of four children age 2 to 7, all of whom we would describe as highly active. During his interview, S approached levels of activity that could be classified as hyperactive. His mother reported that she is constantly dividing her attention among the children and S's due to his hyperactive behavior.

We collected neuropsychological data from the Conner's parent and teacher rating scales, and administered the Connors CPT-II, and the NEPSY neuropsychological battery for children. His results on the neuropsychological tests showed both strengths and weaknesses in the standard scores, but none of the NEPSY domains were statistically significant. Both the Connor's scales and the CPT-II showed a mixture of normal responding, inattention and impulsivity. The only statistically significant measure on the CPT-II was perseverations. The test reported an equal probability of his belonging to the ADHD and non-clinical populations. Observation of his behavior during testing showed the majority of his difficulties were associated with excess activity rather than an inability to attend.

After analyzing his QEEG results (see below), we decided to train S with targeted EEG-biofeedback using the BrainMaster Z-score normalization protocol over four channels using the "Percent Z-OK" protocol. The threshold for percent Z in target was initially set at 85%, and the range of Z-scores was initially set at $+/- 2.0$. Sensors were placed at sites F3-F4/P3-P4 as per the QEEG results. Following 21 sessions of Z-score training with these parameters, we conducted a second QEEG, which is shown below compared to the pre-training results (QEEG #1). The results are described below for the eyes-closed and eyes–open recording conditions, respectively.

A. Eyes–closed condition

Raw tracings, amplitude frequency distributions and Z-score frequency distributions: See Figs 5.14A and 5.14B. Even in the raw wave and amplitude by frequency graphs, normalization of S's EEG pattern is obvious. The large aberrant wave forms seen in frontal sites (presumably caused by motor activity) during Q1 decreased significantly, and the overall distribution approached normality. More importantly, his Z-score distribution in the eyes-closed state following training was entirely within $+/- 1.5$ standard deviations of the reference population mean with the single exception of his dominant frequency, which we deemed not to be of clinical concern. S's brain function in the eyes-closed state has normalized as a result of EEG biofeedback.

Z-scored summary information (brain maps): See Figs 5.15A and 5.15B. The change in S's brain function is most apparent in the Z-scored summary maps. All of the measures with the exception of phase lag completely normalized in every frequency band except for the low 1–4 Hz delta range, and these significantly improved. Some coherence and amplitude asymmetry in the delta range remained, but these are difficult to interpret, and we view these as having less diagnostic relevance than the other bands (columns). The single area that remained in need of complete normalization was phase. Overall, the reduction in neural disregulation is exceptional. We have rarely seen improvements of this magnitude over the course of 20 sessions.

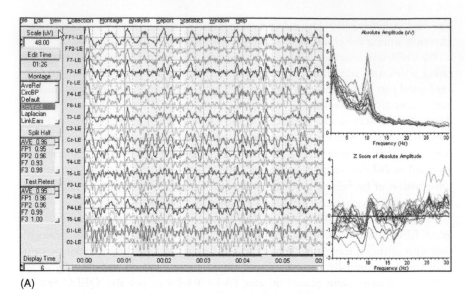

(A)

FIGURE 5.14A   Q1, FFT frequency distribution, eyes–closed (see color plate).

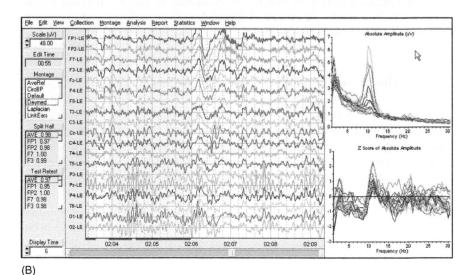

(B)

FIGURE 5.14B   Q2, FFT frequency distribution, eyes–closed (see color plate).

Source localization (LORETA): See Figs 5.16A and 5.16B (Pascqual Marqui *et al.*, 1994; Pascual-Marqui, 1999). These maps show a marked reduction in localized aberrations and network communication measures consistent with the previous maps. Visually, the changes are just as striking. The extreme disregulations in parietal lobe areas, which include the pre-motor cortex, have completely normalized. The

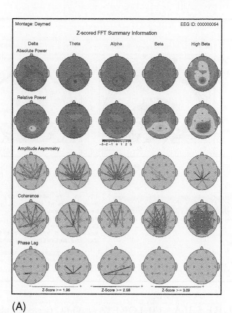

(A)

FIGURE 5.15A   Q1, FFT summary EC (see color plate).

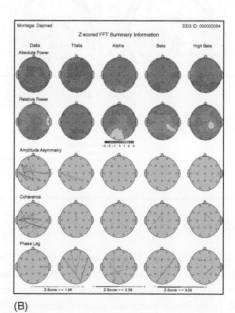

(B)

FIGURE 5.15B   Q2, FFT summary EC (see color plate).

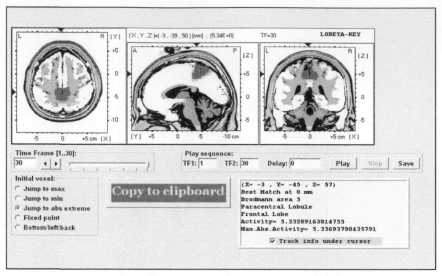

(A)

FIGURE 5.16A   Q1, LORETA @ 30 EC (see color plate).

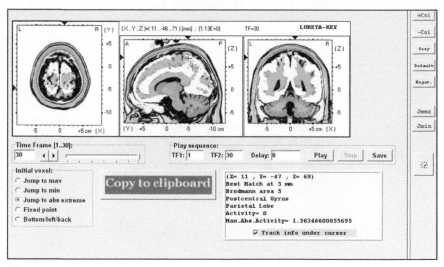

(B)

FIGURE 5.16B   Q2, LORETA @ 30 Hz EC (see color plate).

dorsolateral cortex is closely associated with executive function and response inhibition, and this finding predicts significant increases in S's ability to control disruptive behaviors. SKIL network maps also show significant improvements in coherence and co-modulation at all areas. Phase measures showed more modest improvement or less reduction of significant deviations than did power, coherence or co-modulation.

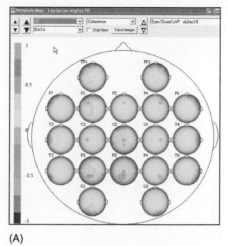

(A)

FIGURE 5.17A   Q1, coherence @ 30 EC (see color plate).

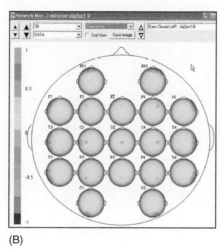

(B)

FIGURE 5.17B   Q2, coherence @ 30 EC (see color plate).

The conclusion for the eyes–closed analysis is that S's pattern of neural disregulation has improved dramatically. Clinical improvements are expected to correspond to the improvement in brain functioning.

B.   Eyes-open condition

Raw Tracings, Amplitude Frequency Distributions and Z-Score Frequency Distributions: See Figs 5.19A and 5.19B. Similar to the eyes–closed condition, normalization

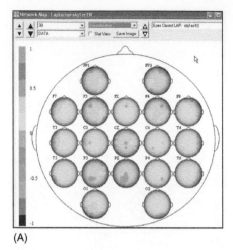

(A)

FIGURE 5.18A   Q1, comod @ 30 EC (see color plate).

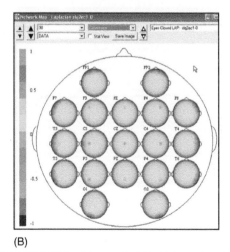

(B)

FIGURE 5.18B   Q2, comod @ 30 EC (see color plate).

of S's raw wave EEG pattern is obvious. Motor ticks causing large aberrant wave forms seen in frontal sites during Q1 have decrease in both frequency and amplitude, and the overall distribution is again approaching normality. Although at first glance the high Z-scores in the 23–30 Hz beta range seem to have increased in magnitude, the diminution in delta amplitudes in Q2 has caused the scale of the Z-score graph to change from Q1 to Q2, and the relative scores are close. Site F7 remains significantly elevated in Q2, but this site is close to the junction of the massiter and frontalis (jaw and forehead) muscles, and appears to be

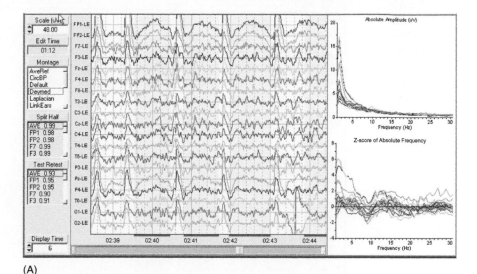

(A)

FIGURE 5.19A   Q1, FFT frequency distribution, eyes-open (see color plate).

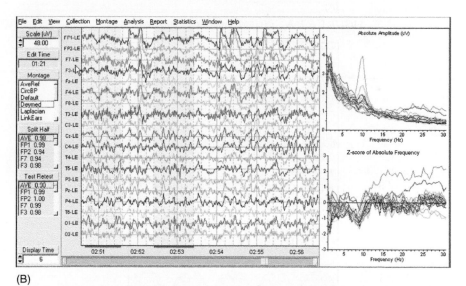

(B)

FIGURE 5.19B   Q2, FFT frequency distribution, eyes-open (see color plate).

muscle artifact. This is confirmed by examination of the raw wave patterns as well as by inspection of the summary maps in Figs 5.20A and 5.20B. All other sites are within the normal range of the reference population. Similar to the eyes-closed data, S's brain function in the eyes-open state has normalized as a direct result of EEG biofeedback.

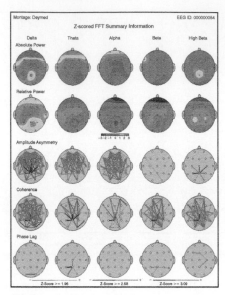

(A)

FIGURE 5.20A   Q1, FFT summary EO (see color plate).

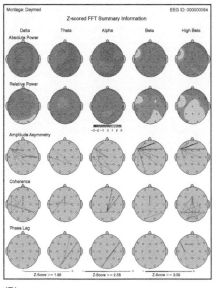

(B)

FIGURE 5.20B   Q2, FFT summary EO (see color plate).

Z-scored summary information (brain maps): See Figs 5.20A and 5.20B. The change is S's brain function is also significant, although some coherence aberrations remain in the beta frequency bands. Interestingly, phase measures are improved relative to the eyes-closed condition. The low 2–4 Hz delta range measures

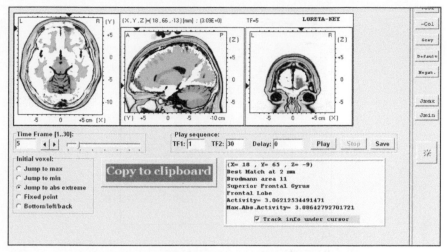

(A)

FIGURE 5.21A   Q1, LORETA @ 5 Hz EC (see color plate).

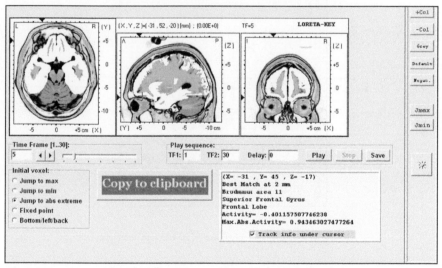

(B)

FIGURE 5.21B   Q2, LORETA @ 5 Hz EC (see color plate).

approach normalization in Q2 relative to Q1; these have significantly improved. Some coherence and amplitude asymmetry in the delta range remain, but these are difficult to interpret in any case, and have less diagnostic relevance than the other bands (columns). The reduction in neural disregulation remains striking. As with the eyes-closed condition, we are greatly encouraged by these results.

Source localization (LORETA): See Figs 5.21A and 5.21B. The LORETA analyses (Pascual Marqui *et al.*, 1994; Pascual-Marqui, 1999) once again showed

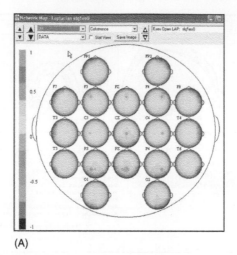

(A)

FIGURE 5.22A   Q1, coherence @ 20 EO (see color plate).

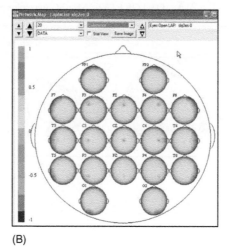

(B)

FIGURE 5.22B   Q2, coherence @ 20 EO (see color plate).

a marked reduction in localized disregulation. Visually, the changes are similarly striking. SKIL network maps in DATA mode, i.e., within subject comparisons that do not use the SKIL reference database, also show significant improvements in coherence and co-modulation at all areas. Once again, phase measures show the need for continued training. The conclusion for the eyes-open analysis is thus consistent with the eyes-closed condition: S's pattern of neural disregulation has improved dramatically. Clinical improvements were noticed in training sessions and recording in session notes, and conform to markedly improved behavior reported by his teachers in school, and at home as reported by S's parents.

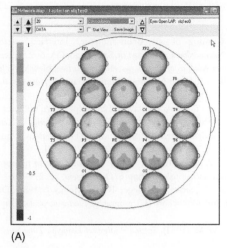

(A)

FIGURE 5.23A   Q1, comod @ 20 EO. (see color plate)

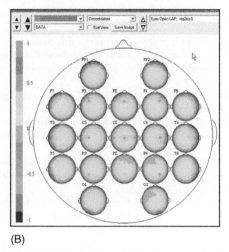

(B)

FIGURE 5.23B   Q2, comod @ 20 EO (see color plate).

X. CONCLUSIONS

Considering all of the data presented above, and the historical data at hand, 20 sessions of targeted EEG-biofeedback training using the Z-score normalization protocol resulted in significant normalization of S's neural functioning. Phase lag and related measures continue to show patterns outside the reference population norms, but all other measures normalized. His parents reported significant clinical and behavioral improvements in his presenting symptoms, which was also obvious to us in his training sessions.

REFERENCES

Birbaumer, N. (2007). Coming of age, brain-computer interface research. *Annual Conference, International Society of Neurofeedback and Research*, San Diego, CA, 6–9 September, pp.

Bloomfield, P. (2000). *Fourier Analysis of Time Series: An Introduction*. New York: John Wiley & Sons.

Box, G. E. P. and Cox, D. R. (1964). An Analysis of Transformations. *Journal of the Royal Statistical Society*, 211–243. discussion 244–252.

Brazis, et al. (2007). *Localization in Clinical Neurology*. Philadelphia, PA: Williams and Wilkins.

Byers, A. P. (1995). Neurofeedback therapy for a mild head injury. *Journal of Neurotherapy*, **1(1)**, 22–37.

Duffy, F., Hughes, J. R., Miranda, F., Bernad, P. and Cook, P. (1994). Status of quantitative EEG (QEEG) in clinical practice. *Clinical. Electroencephalography*, **25(4)**, VI–XXII.

Galanopoulou, A. S., Bojko, A., Lado, F., *et al.* (2000). The spectrum of neuropsychiatric abnormalities associated with electrical status of sleep. *Brain & Development*, **22**, 279–295.

Gasser, T., Jennen-Steinmetz, C., Sroka, L., Verleger, R. and Mocks, J. (1988). Development of the EEG of school-age children and adolescents. II: Topography. *Electroencephalography Clinical Neurophysiology*, **69(2)**, 100–109.

Granger, C. W. J. and Hatanka, M. (1964). *Spectral Analysis of Economic Time Series*. New Jersey: Princeton University Press.

Heilman, K. M. and Valenstein, E. (1993). *Clinical Neuropsychology*, 3rd edition. New York: Oxford University Press.

John, E. R. (1990). *Machinery of the Mind: Data, theory, and speculations about higher brain function*. Boston: Birkhauser.

John, E. R., Prichep, L. S. and Easton, P. (1987). Normative data banks and neurometrics: Basic concepts, methods and results of norm construction. In *Handbook of electroencephalography and clinical neurophysiology: Vol. III. Computer analysis of the EEG and other neurophysiological signals* (A. Remond, ed.), pp. 449–495. Amsterdam: Elsevier.

John, E. R., Prichep, L. S., Fridman, J. and Easton, P. (1988). Neurometrics: Computer assisted differential diagnosis of brain dysfunctions. *Science*, **293**, 162–169.

Just, A. M. and Shashank, V. (2007). The organization of thinking: What functional brain imaging reveals about the neuroarchitecture of complex cognition. *Cognitve, Affective and Behavioral Neuroscience*, **7(3)**, 153–191.

Kotchoubey, B., Strehl, U., Uhlmann, C., *et al.* (2001). Modification of slow cortical potentials in patients with refractory epilepsy: A controlled outcome study. *Epilepsia*, **42(3)**, 406–416.

Luria, A. R. (1973). *The Working Brain*. Basic Books.

Matousek, M. and Petersen, I. (1973). Frequency analysis of the EEG background activity by means of age dependent EEG quotients. In *Automation of clinical electroencephalography* (P. Kellaway and I. Petersen, eds), pp. 75–102. New York: Raven Press.

Otnes, R. K. and Enochson, L. (1978). *Applied Time Series Analysis*. New York: John Wiley & Sons.

Pascual-Marqui, R. D. (1999). Review of Methods for Solving the EEG Inverse Problem. *International Journal of Bioelectromagnetism*, **1**, 75–86.

Pascual-Marqui, R. D., Michel, C. M. and Lehmann, D. (1994). Low resolution electromagnetic tomography: a new method for localizing electrical activity in the brain. *International Journal of Psychophysiology*, **18**, 49–65.

Robinett, R. W. (1997). *Quantum Mechanics: Classical Results, Modern Systems and Visualized Examples*. New York: Oxford University Press.

Sterman, M. B. and Friar, L. (1972). Suppression of seizures in an epileptic following sensorimotor EEG feedback training. *Electroencephalography and Clinical Neurophysiology*, **33(1)**, 89–95.

Tassinari, C. A., Bureau, M., Dravet, C., *et al.*, (1992). Epilepsy with continuous spikes and waves during slow sleep otherwise described as ESES (epilepsy with electrical status epilepticus during slow sleep). In *Epileptic Syndromes in Infancy, Childhood and Adolescence* (J. Roger, M. Bureau, C. Dravet., *et al.*, eds) pp. John Libbey.

Thatcher, R. W., McAlaster, R., Lester, M. L., Horst, R. L. and Cantor, D. S. (1983). Hemispheric EEG Asymmetries Related to Cognitive Functioning in Children. In: *Cognitive Processing in the Right Hemisphere*, A. Perecuman (ed.), New York: Academic Press.

Thatcher, R. W., Krause, P. and Hrybyk, M. (1986). Corticocortical Association Fibers and EEG Coherence: A Two Compartmental Model. *Electroencephalog. Clinical Neurophysiol,* **64**, 123–143.

Thatcher, R. W. (1998). EEG normative databases and EEG biofeedback. *Journal of Neurotherapy,* **2(4)**, 8–39.

Thatcher, R. W. (1999). EEG database guided neurotherapy. In *Introduction to Quantitative EEG and Neurofeedback* (J. R. Evans and A. Abarbanel, eds), 1st edition. San Diego, CA: Academic Press pp. 72–93.

Thatcher, R. W. (2000a). EEG Operant Conditioning (Biofeedback) and Traumatic Brain Injury. *Clinical EEG,* **31(1)**, 38–44.

Thatcher, R. W. (2000b). An EEG Least Action Model of Biofeedback. *8th Annual ISNR conference,* St. Paul, MN, September.

Thatcher, R. W. (2000c). 3-Dimensional EEG Biofeedback using LORETA. Society for Neuronal Regulation, Minneapolis, MN, September 23.

Thatcher, R. W., Walker, R. A. and Guidice, S. (1987). Human cerebral hemispheres develop at different rates and ages. *Science,* **236**, 1110–1113.

Thatcher, R. W., Biver, C., McAlaster, R., *et al.* (1998). Biophysical linkage between MRI and EEG amplitude in closed head injury. *Neuroimage,* **7**, 352–367.

Thatcher, R. W., Walker, R. A., Biver, C., North, D. and Curtin, R. (2003). Quantitative EEG Normative databases: Validation and Clinical Correlation. *J. Neurotherapy,* **7(No. 3/4)**, 87–122.

Thatcher, R. W., North, D. and Biver, C. (2005a). EEG inverse solutions and parametric vs. non-parametric statistics of Low Resolution Electromagnetic Tomography (LORETA). *Clin. EEG and Neuroscience,* **36(1)**, 1–9.

Thatcher, R. W., North, D. and Biver, C. (2005b). Evaluation and Validity of a LORETA normative EEG database. *Clin. EEG and Neuroscience,* **36(2)**, 116–122.

Thatcher, R. W., North, D., and Biver, C. (2008). Self-organized criticality and the development of EEG phase reset. *Human Brain Mapping* Jan 24, (pub ahead of print).

Thatcher, R. W., & Lubar, J. F. (2008, in press). History of scientific standards of QEEG normative databases. In *Introduction to QEEG and Neurofeedback: Advanced theory and applications,* 2nd edition. (T. H. Budzynski, J. R. Evans and A. Abarbanel, eds) Ch 2, Elsevier Inc.

Thornton, K. E. and Carmody, D. P. (2005). Electoencephalogram biofeedback for reading disability and traumatic brain injury. *Child and Adolescent Psychiatric Clinics of North America,* **14**, 137–162.

Wolff, T. and Thatcher, R. W. (1990). Cortical reorganization in deaf children. *J. of Clinical and Experimental Neuropsychology,* **12**, 209–221.

CHAPTER 6

Alpha–theta neurotherapy and the neurobehavioral treatment of addictions, mood disorders and trauma

Nancy E. White, Ph.D. and Leonard M. Richards, Th.D.

The Enhancement Institute, Houston, Texas, USA

I. INTRODUCTION

The appearance of alpha–theta neurofeedback coincides with a major shift in the course of psychotherapy, one which appears to be leading us toward a much broader and more complex paradigm that might be described as *neurobehavioral therapy*. Neurobehavioral therapy approaches brain, mind, emotion, feeling and their behavioral expressions as a multilevel matrix, a complex functional system of many dimensions—physical and perceptual, local and non-local, quantum in nature—about which mechanisms of change are just beginning to be understood. Ongoing research into the structure, function and development of the brain/mind system and its interrelationship with the physical body is taking us there whether we want to go there or not.

Freud, trained as a neurologist, may have presaged this turn of events when, in 1914, he said, "All our provisional ideas in psychology will someday be based on organic substructure" (quoted in Schore, 1994). Freud also told us that the unconscious is the home of our emotions which, he said, were often dissociated from normal thought processes, and largely unavailable to us in waking consciousness (LeDoux, 1996). The late Eugene Peniston may have given us an elegant process, increasingly supported by emerging neurobehavioral research, to unlock the unconscious and alter perceptions, rewrite personal history, heal the self and enhance one's life.

In support of Peniston's work, the burgeoning field of neuroscience has provided groundbreaking studies in areas such as neuroplasticity (e.g., Buonomano and Merzenich, 1998), the malleability of memory (e.g., Cozolino, 1994), and the physics of neurological function (Cowan, 2008). These relatively recent concepts tend to merge with and extend the extensive research already published in the areas of learning and retrieval (e.g., Budzynski, 1971, 1997; Cowan, J., 1993;

Hartmann, 1997; Rossi, 1986), the mind–body connection (e.g., Manchester, 1995, 1997; Manchester *et al.*, 1998; Perry, 1992, 1997; Wolpe *et al.*, 1993; White, 1994, 1995, 1996; Wuttke, 1992), and neurochemistry (e.g., Blum, 1994; Bower, 1996; Pert, 1993, 1997). All of these concepts impact and lend credence to the workings of the alpha–theta deep-state approach to neurobehavioral healing, as we will discover.

The purpose of this chapter, then, is to introduce and describe the alpha–theta protocol, explain how and why it works to the extent current research supports such explanations, and discuss some implications for its use in clinical practice. The central thesis of the chapter is that alpha–theta neurotherapy, specifically the Peniston protocol of alpha–theta neurofeedback therapy and its modifications, provides a powerful therapeutic medium by which neurobehavioral healing can and does take place. In that connection, we propose to show that there is significant support for the effectiveness of this healing process, as well as provide some insight into the mechanisms by which it may work, in the literature of neuroscience, neurotherapy and related fields.

The chapter has four distinct parts. First, we reprise the original research of Peniston and Kulkosky (1989, 1991), and define the nature and function of the protocol itself. Next, we offer some explanations as to its broad range of effectiveness, both literature-based and theoretical. Then we discuss some of the ways in which the protocol opens a multilevel matrix of healing, effective on a wide range of seemingly disparate diagnoses. Finally, we describe how alpha–theta neurofeedback may be used effectively in a multi-modality approach to treating addictions, mood disorders and emotional trauma.

II. THE PENISTON PROTOCOL

With the publication of the research of Peniston and Kulkosky (1989), the field of neurotherapy began to come into its own, growing into and expressing Freud's original, almost forgotten, promise. Peniston's initial focus was a population of alcoholics, all of whom had been heavily addicted for more than 20 years and had been in rehabilitation unsuccessfully four to five times. Using his protocol of alpha–theta brain wave training combined with imagery of desired outcome, he was able to show reduction to elimination of craving for alcohol. The study showed an 85% success rate for the elimination of the alcoholic behavior of the men in the experimental group. Not fully trusting this level of success, Menninger did its own private follow-up study 36 months later (Walters, personal communication). They talked to each study subject, their wives and their family members, and found that the original outcomes were holding. The men were still free of alcohol dependence and, more importantly perhaps, their lives were more functional as confirmed by many family members' comments on how much the subjects' moods and behaviors had changed.

Intrigued by the significant changes in their original subjects' moods and affect, Peniston and Kulkosky (1991) subsequently extended their research to a population of Vietnam veterans who were hospitalized for post-traumatic stress disorder (PTSD). Peniston and Kulkosky randomly assigned 29 pre-screened Vietnam theater veterans with 12 to 15 year histories of chronic combat-related PTSD to one of two groups. The first (BWT) group received alpha–theta brainwave neurofeedback training while the second (CT) group received traditional medical treatment, i.e., psychotropic drugs, and combined individual and group therapy. The BWT group received a modified quantitative EEG, and both groups were administered the Minnesota Multiphasic Personality Inventory (MMPI) before and after completion of the study. The BWT group showed both a significant improvement in scores across testings, and significantly better scores than the TC group on the post tests. In follow-up studies, by 30 months after treatment all 14 subjects comprising the TC group had relapsed, while only three of the 15 BWT subjects had relapsed by then.

Perhaps the most remarkable outcome of both of these studies was the major personality shifts that were recorded in the scales of their pre- and post-Minnesota Multiphasic Personality Inventories (MMPI) and Millon Clinical Multiaxial Inventories (MCMI). According to these well-validated inventories most of the pathology of these personalities had normalized (Peniston and Kulkosky, 1990).

The protocol originally used by Dr. Peniston in his research began with several sessions of thermal biofeedback and autogenic training as a relaxation technique, and as pre-training for EEG feedback. In the original research the protocol involved fifteen 30-minute sessions, typically performed twice a day, 5 days a week, on Veterans Administration Hospital in-patients. In today's typically outpatient settings there are many versions of this original configuration, with the most common employing the original thermal and autogenic training followed by approximately 30 EEG feedback sessions conducted once daily four or five times a week, and including an imagined scene of the rejection of the undesired behavior and/or imagery of desired outcome. The agreed-upon scenario is introduced at the beginning of each EEG session, and repeated at the beginning of each session throughout the treatment.

This visualization of the desired state also includes images of being already healed as an explicit way of instructing the unconscious to make it so, thus avoiding ambiguities that may leave the door open to unintended interpretations. Moreover, inundating the unconscious with mental rehearsals of new conditions, and clear intentions of desired change, seems to effect healing and change both physiologically and psychologically (Green & Green, 1977; Achterberg, 1985; Simonton and Simonton, 1978).

Imagery is one of the earliest forms of healing. There is archaeological evidence suggesting that the techniques of the shaman using imagination for healing are at least 20,000 years old, with vivid evidence of their antiquity in the cave paintings in the south of France. Asclepius, Aristotle, Galen, and Hippocrates, often regarded as the fathers of medicine, used imagery for diagnosis and therapy (Achterberg, 1985).

Drs. Dean Ornish, Bernard Siegel, Norman Shealy, Larry Dossey, and Dr. Carl Simonton collectively emphasize the role of the imagination in healing. Imagination is now known to have a measurable effect on one's physical condition. That is, images may communicate with tissues and organs, even cells, to effect change (Simonton and Simonton, 1978; Achterberg, 1985; Rossi, 1986; Siegel, 1986).

Peniston's original electrode placement was O1, monopolar, referenced to linked ears and a forehead ground with feedback tones of the computer rewarding attainment of clinician-set thresholds of increasing alpha and theta brain wave amplitudes. Current placements might be CZ, PZ, or O2 with ear-based reference and ground. At our Institute we generally set the electrode at P4, near the area of the brain associated with boundaries of the self, and we set thresholds to assure at least 70% positive feedback with a warning signal for excessive delta (sleep wave) amplitudes. Each clinician seems to have his or her own variations on the theme, and today's more sophisticated software makes it easier to create the "dance" between alpha and theta frequency bands. Regardless of the differences in placement, and varying ideas on feedback, results seem to be consistently positive in treatment of addictions and other symptomology.

Hand warming with autogenic training and temperature biofeedback preceded the deep-state sessions of Peniston's original protocol. Hand warming has been used in the field of biofeedback for many years as an effective tool to correct hypertension and other symptoms of sympathetic overarousal, and many alpha–theta clinicians still begin with this practice. It can be helpful in teaching one to relax and be calm in any situation. Hand warming trains the circulatory aspect of the sympathetic branch of the autonomic nervous system involved in the "fight or flight" response. In the fight or flight response, the body is alerted and blood flow is increased to the major organs. This can become a chronic stress response. To counter this state, as the peripheral circulation is increased with training, the body relaxes. In addition, rhythmic diaphragmatic breathing may be taught to still body functions and focus attention.

Some clinicians believe that preparing the patient with a layman's explanation of the brain (e.g., the limbic area and neurochemistry), and some of the ways it effects change, gives the patient both a conscious and an unconscious understanding of the process which, along with the clarification of goals, helps create a clear intention for the desired outcome. This is expected to enhance the effect of imagery of the desired outcome.

III. THE EFFECTIVENESS OF ALPHA–THETA NEUROTHERAPY

Researchers and clinicians in the field of neurotherapy have proposed many theories for the apparently remarkable success of alpha–theta brain wave training. Is it practical to take this protocol apart in its different aspects to find its power, or would this be reductionist thinking akin to examining the vocal cords to see how one is a talented singer and another is not? The power of this protocol seems to lie in its non-linear interaction with many aspects of the brain/mind, and it may be of greater value to examine how these aspects contribute to an overall impact that creates a positive outcome for most patients treated.

Empirical science, as we know it, seeks to understand reality from the point of view of the five senses. However, alpha–theta neurofeedback, while it contains elements of the five senses, by its very nature takes one beyond the five senses to abilities that may lie latent within us all. This protocol seems to represent a technology designed for the induction of higher states of consciousness and insight, helping to alter one's relationship to self and the world as a result of what is seen and understood in those higher states. That is, alpha–theta is a transpersonal therapy.

Toward the end of his life, Abraham Maslow, one of the major pioneers in humanistic psychology, called attention to possibilities beyond self-actualization in which the individual transcended the customary limits of identity and experience. In 1968 he concluded, "I consider Humanistic, Third Force Psychology, to be transitional, a preparation for a still 'higher' Fourth psychology, transpersonal, transhuman, centered in the cosmos, rather than in human needs and interest, going beyond humanness, identity, self-actualization, and the like" (Maslow, 1968; Walsh and Vaughan, 1980). This protocol seems to express Maslow's vision, at least to some degree, even as his vision is progressively being fleshed out by research in neuroscience. In the paragraphs that follow we describe some of the more important aspects of brain/mind function that may contribute to the remarkable impact of the alpha–theta protocol.

A. Autopoiesis and the malleability of memory

Life is not a static condition but a process. Rose (2005) states: "Not only during development but throughout the lifespan, all living organisms are in a state of dynamic flux which insures both moment by moment stability (homeostasis) and steady change over time (homeodynamics)". It is the process of self-creation known as *autopoiesis*. Autopoiesis sees the brain in a constant state of non-linear development and redevelopment down to the dendrites themselves, which may extend into the synapse and retract with startling frequency, some extensions lasting only a few days (Trachtenberg *et al.*, 2002). Thus we are as humans both being and becoming at once, and at all levels of existence.

The earlier, linear view of the brain is based on the idea of specificity, which looks at the seeming invariants of the human brain as it develops. The emerging, dynamic (quantum) view of the brain focuses more on plasticity or the variations that develop as the brain adapts to environmental contingencies (Rose, 1994). We propose that neurofeedback in all its forms rides on the back of neural plasticity and may be described more by developmental systems theory, of which autopoiesis is a specific expression, than by anatomy alone. Systems are inherently non-linear and heuristic. Applied to the brain, systems theory recognizes that the brain is in a constant state of change along a continuum of probable shifts, and that its momentary stability, or homeostasis, is a point of pure potential along such a continuum. Neuroplasticity tells us that the brain can be directed in that process of change by appropriate interventions. This may be one of the reasons neurofeedback so confounds medicine's rigid view of science. It is not that the effectiveness of neurofeedback is not provable; rather, that medical science has yet to incorporate systems theory in its approach.

Consequently, the effectiveness of alpha–theta neurofeedback may be explained in large part by a psychological concept related to neuroplasticity known as the *malleability of memory*. The malleability of memory is a behavioral manifestation of the plasticity of neural systems (Cozolino, 2002). Conversely, the plasticity of memory opens an avenue to the alteration of neural systems. Cozolino (2002) illustrates how revisiting and re-evaluating early experiences from the adult perspective can allow the neurological rewriting of one's history. That is, the introduction of new information or new scenarios can modify affective reactions, and alter the nature of memories.

Alpha–theta neurotherapy facilitates this process by giving the patient and the empathetic therapist fairly direct access to unconscious processes that allow the reception and processing of memory-altering information. Alpha–theta software creates the dance between the alpha and theta amplitudes, called *crossovers*, which indicate that the brain is potentially in its most receptive state. In this state the patient not only has the opportunity to change the emotional content of the past, but can redirect his or her potential future from that new foundation. May this not be a form of Freud's organic sub-structure underlying the psychodynamic process?

B.   State-dependent memory and retrieval

Malleability of memory depends in part on states of consciousness and arousal, known to psychology as the concept of *state-dependent memory and retrieval,* or state-context dependent learning and retrieval as Jon Cowan (1993) has expressed it. Budzynski (1971, 1997) reported that a predominance of theta in the EEG was the ideal state for rescripting or reimprinting the brain, eliminating destructive behaviors or attitudes that are a result of scripts laid down in childhood (during a period when the child lives predominately in open focus) and replacing them with more suitable and more positive scripts for a mature adult. Rossi (1986) states that each time we access the state-dependent memory, learning, and behavior processes that encode a problem, we have an opportunity to reassociate and reorganize, or reframe, that problem in a manner that resolves it. This reliving, releasing, and rescripting may be one of the few ways in which an adult can modify old scripts, and store new information in the subconscious.

The surfacing of memories from early childhood during the alpha–theta brain wave training fits observations of state-dependent memory. Because information learned while in one state of consciousness may be more difficult to access when in another state of consciousness, the natural shift in dominant brain wave frequencies during maturation could result in dysfunctional childhood learning being preserved in the unconscious as an adult. To gain access to most of these state-bound memories, one may have to return to the state in which they were created, that is, a *theta state*, that state of consciousness just above sleep characterized by a dynamic balance between the alpha and theta frequency bands.

In utilizing the Peniston protocol of alpha–theta neurotherapy there is often a profound alteration in the state of consciousness of the patient. As subconscious (emotional) memories become more available to conscious (episodic) process in this deeply altered state, traumatic memories are often released and appear as flashbacks from the past. As these flashbacks are relived in the context of current adult resources and perceptions, the subconscious memories may become more readily available for healing and alteration.

C.   Causative properties of consciousness and arousal states

The reader may recall at this point that brain wave frequencies are correlated with various states of consciousness or arousal. To recapitulate briefly, a predominance of beta waves (approximately 13 Hz and higher) signals a state encompassing the thinking process with its accompanying ego reactions. In this state one is focused on the external world, while at the opposite end of the arousal spectrum one is basically disassociated from the external world and exhibits a predominance of delta, or sleep waves (0–4 Hz). With a predominance of theta waves (4–8 Hz) one's focus is on the internal world. This is the theta state described earlier, a world of hypnogogic imagery where a number of alpha–theta patients have encountered an "inner healer" who represents their shift out of victim consciousness into empowerment. Alpha brain waves (8–13 Hz) may be considered a bridge from the external world to the internal world, and vice versa.

In everyday existence, the ideal state of the ego may well be a state of poise between the inner world of self and the outer world of objects. With some addicts, and patients previously exposed to major trauma, alpha amplitudes can be low, creating an inflexibility that keeps one from shifting readily between inward and outward states (M. Sams, personal communication, May 1996). Patients exhibiting low alpha amplitudes may tend to avoid those internal states where one does the work to find awareness of self. As one increases alpha amplitudes via neurotherapy, such patients can gain the ability to shift with greater ease and appropriateness. Any overly intense concern with the outer world is tempered, and the individual may gain detachment with a sense of humor and loss of ego-centeredness. As one turns inward and attains deeper states, sensorimotor awareness tends to decrease, and consciousness centers on questions concerning the meaning of life. Patients exposed to these states usually describe the latter experience as serene and peaceful, providing them with new abilities and possibilities. They seem to develop a powerful coping skill, and may have access to such inner calm no matter what is occurring in their environment (Wuttke, 1992).

A related notion is suggested by the work of Thom Hartmann (1997), who states: "Everybody is familiar with the edge between normal waking consciousness and sleep: it's often a time of extraordinary feelings, sensations, and insights, particularly as we move from sleep into wakefulness. When the brain is brought to the edge of the world of God, the place of 'true' consciousness, a fractal intersection occurs. An unstable and dynamic system is created, and, like the rainbow colors of water and oil, new energies and visions are created". The Peniston alpha–theta protocol seems to enhance this ability to shift states, to move to this edge. In such states many aspects of the self involving wisdom and insight may be encountered and awareness of earlier traumas occurs, making them more accessible for healing.

D.   Neural function in the effectiveness of alpha–theta neurotherapy

Robert Boustany (personal communication, 1998), a biophysicist involved in neu-rofeedback research, suggests that, since NMDA (N-methyl D-aspartate) receptors act as a double lock and key to encoded patterns of behavior in the individual (LaMantia and Katz, 2001), activation of NMDA receptors in the region of the hippocampus may be essential to personal transformation. As proposed, this acti-vation may occur in the amygdala and a few other areas.

The use of the term *encoded patterns* indicates that individuals learn certain sur-vival response patterns while they are very young and the brain is still forming. These patterns are reflected in the subtle structure of the brain and are correlated with behavior. They may be considered as electro-chemical circuits that respond in specified ways. The response patterns encoded in the brain of the young child lead to unconscious responses later in life, some of which may be maladaptive. As an older child or as an adult, a cognitive awareness that a certain behavior causes problems will not change the behavior until the person develops enough emotional pliability to handle that insight. Alpha–theta neurofeedback may be one means of creating more adaptive behavior by encouraging the development of sufficient emotional pliability to facilitate change in these encoded patterns.

The hypothesis relating to NMDA receptors seems particularly well demon-strated in the treatment of alcoholism. The excitatory neurotransmitter glutamate has a protective effect against alcohol, and is expended in the process of reducing the effects of inebriation. It also relates to the functioning of NMDA receptors. Glutamate is required at the first stage of the two-stage process of reaching long-term potentiation (LTP) in NMDA receptors. Long-term potentiation refers to patterns of synaptic activity in the central nervous system that produce a long-lasting increase in synaptic plasticity (laMantia and Katz, 2001). Without LTP in certain brain regions, individuals show rigid aversion to change. Although ade-quate levels of glutamate normally are required for LTP, certain types of repeated stimulation and theta wave production also are reported to facilitate LTP, effects of which may persist for hours or even days. In the absence of sufficient glutamate, training to enhance theta amplitudes (relative to other frequencies) using neurofeedback is believed to facilitate LTP in certain cells of the hippocampus, with resulting decreases in rigidity and an increased ability to access and change encoded patterns of maladaptive behaviors.

In the alcoholic, glutamate is present in reduced quantities; consequently, the process of LTP is reduced. When LTP is reduced, individuals tend to be tense and rigid, and have great difficulty spontaneously producing high-amplitude theta waves. Nevertheless, with a sufficient number of alpha–theta neurofeedback sessions, these persons' brains often become capable of producing such waves. In treating alcoholism, the capability of producing high-amplitude theta waves developed during the alpha–theta protocol can result in a more adaptive individual, as indicated by pre–post MMPI 2 testing. This may explain how individuals who have undergone the alpha–theta protocol tend to recognize both cognitively and emotionally the nature of their behavior, and seem generally more able to walk away from addictive behaviors.

Moreover, the individual who has undergone the alpha–theta neurofeedback protocol is likely to have remarkable insights into the underlying reasons for his or her addiction, which is a strong indication that learning, flexibility, and adaptability have increased. Expressed in another way, a process known as *phase transition* occurs in which a new neural pattern begins to take the place of the old encoded patterns (Cowan, 2008). This neural process is explained in more detail below.

In summary, Boustany's explanation asserts that in addiction, as in other conditions, NMDA receptors act as a double lock and key on encoded patterns of behavior. When LTP occurs in the appropriate NMDA receptors, the individual can gain conscious access to these patterns, change them using both inner resources and those offered in the therapeutic environment, becoming in the process more adaptable, more physically predisposed to stop alcohol use, and emotionally more able to embrace the need for change

E.   Phase transition and alpha–theta's effectiveness with trauma

In trauma the brain suffers a conflict shock that induces a state of involuntary homeostasis engendered by survival terror. This is expressed via a neural network already sensitized to stimuli seen as a potential threat to one's existence (Iverson *et al.*, 2008). The result is the separate generation of both unconscious (emotional) memory and conscious (episodic) memory (Stein and Kendall, 2004), which may generalize, distorting the individual's pattern of noticing of what is in the environment (hypervigilance), and can result in inappropriate, even aberrant responses (abreactions, repetition compulsion). Survival terror shuts down aspects of autopoiesis, the process of becoming, with both behavioral and, in chronic cases especially, measurable physiological consequences (Bower, 1996).

The alpha–theta protocol works to neutralize the cause of the stuck pattern by introducing a much desired new condition or pattern while the brain is residing predominantly in the frequency band (theta), at which such change is most likely to be activated. Alpha–theta software rewards the brain for remaining largely in a theta state, described earlier as a dynamic balance, or dance, between the theta and alpha frequencies, even as the brain overall tends to be at rest. The brain at rest tends to produce random frequency patterns, opening the door to a potential *phase transition* into a new pattern (Cowan, 2008), in this case one suggested by the scenario of desired outcome recited to the person during the induction phase of each session. Support in the form of adjunctive treatments and individual or group psychotherapy amplifies the new state while participation in related community or religious activities can provide external verification of the new state.

With addiction the process appears similar to that described in the previous section. The brain in its way is convinced that it cannot survive without the exogenous substance of choice or a reasonable substitute. It will cause the organism to manipulate, rationalize, avoid, lie, cheat, steal and worse to maintain the existing chemical homeostasis. Certain aspects of addictive behavior, then, may be described as affects of survival terror. The alpha–theta protocol can introduce the possibility of a more desirable state (i.e., escape from annihilation), while adjunctive procedures such as cranial electrical stimulation (CES) and cognitive behavioral therapy, along with detoxification, dietary management and appropriate supplement therapies, support the opportunity for a phase transition to a recovery process.

F. Importance of the patient–therapist relationship

In most forms of therapy the relationship between the patient and his or her therapist is a key ingredient of the neurobehavioral healing process. Brugental (1987) states, "The art of psychotherapy . . . insists that what goes on inside the therapist, the artist, is crucial to the whole enterprise". Others such as Dr. Edgar Wilson have reported brain wave synchrony between healer and patient at the time of peak effectiveness (Cowan, 1993). Similarly, Fahrion *et al.* (1993) found that this interpersonal EEG synchrony was highest during times of apparent healing, especially in the alpha frequencies between left occipital areas of the practitioner and the patient. Clinicians have reported a number of instances in which the thoughts of the therapist in another room simultaneously seemed to influence the subject matter of a patient's spontaneous imagery. In short, within the arena of therapy, and in deep-state, open focus therapy especially, there is no objective observer.

Neurotherapy clinicians generally agree that trust of the therapist and rapport between therapist and client are crucial to successful treatment. White and Martin (1998) state that the quality of the patient–therapist relationship appears to be a significant component in the healing process, especially during any period of abreaction/catharsis. The therapist's empathy with, and sensitivity to, the patient's experience during the highly charged, vulnerable theta state supports the atmosphere of trust required for the patient to let go. The seasoning of the therapist, not so much by years lived as by the degree to which he or she has resolved their own traumas, may have awakened an "inner healer" that connects with the patient's own latent inner healer and offers hope. While the exact nature of any such connection may be difficult to measure, the idea finds support in Bell's theorem (Herbert, 1988), which states that two entities, once in connection, remain in connection and continue to affect each other. The therapist and patient can no longer be considered as separate and independent units, because both are affected in the process of healing.

G. Summary of the effectiveness of alpha–theta neurofeedback

The alpha–theta protocol taps into aspects of neural functioning only partly describable by traditional views of the brain, and only recently begun to be more fully defined by scientific research. The brain is in a lifelong autodynamic process, so change is its nature. Autodynamic change is also the ally of alpha–theta, making neural networks malleable and responsive to new information, however introduced. Neuroplasticity and its behavioral corollary, the malleability of memory, allow the alpha–theta patient to alter the impact of the past and effectively rewrite his or her history.

These concepts allow us to theorize that, by rewarding the patient for remaining predominantly in the theta state, state-dependent memories are retrieved and their emotional charges integrated and neutralized in a process of long-term potentiation induced by emotional identification with the desired outcome. By this same process new, more functional perceptions are implanted, effective for emotionally healthier living in the waking state. This process may also be viewed, in Jack Cowan's (2008) terms, as a *phase transition*, in which neural networks in a resting state may be benignly perturbed with new information, embodied in emotional identification with desired outcome, to shift to a more functional pattern. A critical factor in this process is the empathic therapist who, as an involuntary participant, provides support and the sense of safety that encourages the patient to go into the slow wave resting state where neurological shifts, which we call healing, can occur.

As the field of neurotherapy comes of age we are finding that many seemingly disparate diagnoses are being treated successfully using the Peniston protocol. In addition to Peniston and Kulkosky's (1989, 1990, 1991) published research on populations presenting with alcohol addiction and post-traumatic stress disorder, Dr. Carol Manchester (1995, 1997; Manchester *et al,* 1998) reported achieving integration of dissociative identity disorder in 30–60 alpha–theta sessions, a disorder usually requiring years of therapy, and even then with inconsistent results.

Brownback and Mason (1998) have reported similar results. Psychological disorders, including affective disorders, personality disorders, "rage-aholism," eating disorders, substance abuse, and relational dysfunctions (including marital conflict and codependency) presumably are being successfully treated (White, 1994). Somatic complaints, hypertension, cardiovascular problems, chronic fatigue, and immune dysfunction (Schummer, 1995) were reported to be improved using the alpha–theta protocol.

Several clinicians have been offering peak performance training, and there is now a certification in this specialty. Several have worked successfully with Olympic athletes (R. Patton, personal communication, April 1991) and international sports teams such as the Italian World Cup soccer team, whose neurofeedback training program was covered by *The Wall Street Journal*. Similarly, at the Institute we have achieved favorable outcomes with a number of amateur, college and professional athletes.

Further, addictions and dissociative identity disorder (DID) frequently present with multiple diagnoses. It is not unusual for a DID patient to meet the diagnostic criteria for several currently described psychiatric disorders, including depression, borderline personality disorder, somatization disorder, substance abuse, bulimia, anorexia nervosa, and panic disorder. Addicts frequently present with multiple diagnoses and the literature is clear on the negative effect of these conditions on recidivism (Wolpe *et al.*, 1993; Continuum, 1993), and yet these patients are reported to be good candidates for this protocol of an altered state therapy.

In our work at the Enhancement Institute in Houston, multiple diagnoses are being addressed with a high degree of favorable outcomes as measured by the MMPI and the MCMI administered both pre- and post-treatment. For example, the Institute had two post-doctoral fellows conduct an outcome analysis focusing on the five scales of depression found in these two personality tests. The population was 44 heterogeneous patients taken in order of presentation, all but six of whom had primary diagnoses other than depression. In four of the five scales they found a statistically significant reduction ($p > 0.001$) in depression (White, 1995, 1996).

The appearance of additional research and clinical reports describing the multiplicity of disorders being addressed, most of them quite successfully, has aroused quite a few skeptics. Speaking for many such skeptics Dr. Russell Barkley, one of the most vocal early critics of neurofeedback, publicly stated during an interview by Russ Mitchell for the *Eye to Eye with Connie Chung* television show (Mitchell, 1994): "We have a rule of thumb in this business. The more things you claim you can cure, the less effective your treatment is likely to be. It's a good rule of thumb to keep in mind".

It may indeed be a good rule to keep in mind; yet, we see consistently favorable shifts in individuals presenting with multiple diagnoses after undergoing the Peniston protocol. What accounts for the far-reaching effects of this protocol on so many disorders? Since we are working with brain and central nervous system regulation with all its manifestations, perhaps alpha–theta helps access the source of the problem. With the feedback tones of a computer set to reward the production of alpha and theta frequencies, the slowed cortical activity may simply set the stage for generalized healing in the form of retrieval, resolution and phase shifts to higher states of consciousness (Wuttke, 1992, Cowan, 2008).

Perhaps it may be that trauma is simply trauma after all, despite its many apparent causes and the many guises it takes in presenting symptomology. Perhaps the alpha–theta protocol has helped pull back the curtain, not only on a largely singular way of encouraging the brain to let go of trauma, but on trauma itself as a largely singular condition with many manifestations.

In support of this idea, Colin Ross (1989), an authority on dissociative identity disorder (DID), writes that the Diagnostic and Statistical Manual (DSM-IV) (American Psychiatric Association, 1994) should have a category for chronic trauma disorder, of childhood or adult onset, with or without DID. Ross sees chronic trauma disorder as a single field with distinct regions. The various regions could be called *affective disorder, eating disorder, substance abuse disorder,* and so on. More than one region of the field may be activated simultaneously in a given patient, and can occur in different combinations in different patients.

This would be a hierarchical diagnosis of which currently disparate diagnoses were a part, forming a sort of decision tree with chronic trauma disorder as the overarching diagnosis, and with modifiers for periods of onset (childhood/adult), nature of onset (acute/chronic), and whether or not DID were present. The various regions (e.g., affective disorder) and sub-regions (e.g., depression) then become branches. For instance, chronic trauma, childhood onset, would become the source out of which currently defined disorders and their multiple symptoms flow. From this point of view, the stress effects of trauma, from whatever source, may be seen as a single diagnosable condition modified by its specific expressions.

This view of trauma, and the apparent facility with which alpha–theta neurofeedback deals with its myriad symptoms, may give more than an answer to skeptics; it may offer significant clues to its effective treatment as well.

IV. ALPHA–THETA NEUROFEEDBACK IN THE NEUROBEHAVIORAL TREATMENT OF TRAUMA DISORDER

A. A closer look at trauma disorder

Earlier in this chapter we described the onset of trauma as an overwhelming situation inducing survival terror (Iverson *et al.*, 2008) which creates an implicit (unconscious) memory imprint and an explicit (conscious) memory imprint. These memories reside in different structures of the brain, i.e., the amygdala and the hippocampus, respectively, which are usually mediated by the orbital frontal cortex (Stein and Kendall, 2004). According to a number of researchers these structures, and especially the hippocampus, once overwhelmed by the onslaught of stress chemicals, produce fractured memories. For instance, the hippocampus may store conscious memory of a traumatic event as sights, sounds, smells, tastes and bodily sensations, but lacking a clear narrative. This leads to post-traumatic expression in ways described by the various emotional and behavioral fields we currently see as disparate diagnoses, e.g., affective disorders (anxiety, depression), behavioral disorders, and the like.

The literature is clear as well that susceptibility to trauma depends in large part on the person's perception of the event, and that something as intangible as one's perception of an event alters the chemistry of the body (Pert, 1997). For instance, Iverson and his colleagues (2008) found in their recent study involving British armed forces personnel that "personal appraisal of threat to life during the trauma emerged as the most important predictor of post-traumatic stress symptoms".

Predictors of susceptibility to the effects of survival terror, as well as resilience in the face of it, also are well documented in the literature, but the most important single predictor appears to be adverse childhood events. For example, in one recent study from the US Army Medical Research Unit in Heidelberg 4,529 male soldiers who had not been deployed to the conflict in Iraq were surveyed in 2003. Then, in 2004, a separate group of 2,392 male soldiers were surveyed three months after returning from duty in Iraq. The results of this study confirmed a close relationship between adverse childhood experiences and "key mental health outcomes" (Cabrera *et al.*, 2007). Other studies suggest that one-third of individuals who suffered physical or sexual abuse or neglect in childhood developed trauma disorder (*New York Times, Health Guide* 3/29/2008).

The neurological process of childhood sensitization arising from abuse or neglect is well documented (e.g., Schore, 1994; Siegel, 1999; Cozolino, 2002; Stein and Kendall, 2004). Bruce Perry (1992, 1997), a specialist in childhood trauma and attachment disorder, states that prolonged alarm reactions induced by traumatic events during infancy and childhood can result in altered development of the central nervous system (CNS).

He hypothesizes that with this altered development one would predict a host of abnormalities related to catecholamine regulation of affect including anxiety, arousal/concentration, impulse control, sleep, startle, and autonomic nervous system regulation. That is, a child who is reared in an unpredictable, abusive, or neglectful environment may have evoked, in his or her developing CNS, a milieu that will result in a poorly organized, dysregulated CNS catecholamine system. Schneider (1998) states that a child who lives in a constant state of fear from abuse, particularly in the first year, frequently shows an overdevelopment of the sympathetic pathways. Then, when the child encounters a traumatic episode later in life, the now-vulnerable system from childhood may elicit symptoms of trauma disorder emerging from a heightened excitation of both the sympathetic and parasympathetic systems. Even if the brain itself is not injured, the old symptom-eliciting circuits apparently remain.

On the other hand, if the infant's or young child's caregiver engages in frequent face-to-face attunement, using mirroring and mediating techniques, he or she facilitates the development of the right orbito-frontal cortex, which mediates functions of the amygdala and hippocampus, promoting autonomic regulation and resiliency to subsequent stress or trauma (Schore, 1994).

Blum (Miller and Blum, 1996) offers further information on the brain's ability to mediate stress. His research proposes a reward deficiency syndrome (RDS), caused by a variant of the Al allele of the dopamine receptor gene (DRD2), which reduces one's ability to autonomously achieve pleasure states. To feel pleasure or relief from pain, the brain's receptors must be stimulated with large amounts of dopamine, particularly in times of high stress. Pert (1993, 1997) has shown how stress elicits neuropeptides, and that the whole body undergoes physical changes when it is under stress. It follows that a person with a shortage of dopamine and other pleasure-related chemicals, genetically induced or otherwise, may be predisposed to manage stress poorly. Blum cites one report indicating that 59% of Vietnam veterans diagnosed with PTSD showed this DR2 gene variant (Miller and Blum, 1996).

Other predictors of susceptibility to trauma disorder that researchers generally consider important are pre-existing psychological disorders, genetic predispositions, and inadequate support systems. There are additional predictors of susceptibility which may have been discussed elsewhere in this book. They tend to join those we've mentioned to define a single perceptual framework toward which they all seem to lead: the perception of helplessness, powerlessness and inefficacy that erodes resilience and causes the individual to crumble—and his or her neural systems to become overwhelmed—in the face of traumatic events.

Without effective intervention these individuals tend to lead a fear-based life in which they evaluate as life-threatening many events or situations others may consider simply bothersome. The already sensitized systems of such individuals are incapable of mediating substantial stress, yet such levels of stress may be instigated in many instances by their own way of looking at things, which in turn reinforces the activation of their sensitized neural systems. Standard treatment regimens tend to focus on resolution of the trauma itself rather than on redirecting this systemic loop. These approaches may help the person to integrate implicit emotional memories into the explicit (conscious) memory system, and then reframe those memories in a way that defuses the trauma (Stein and Kendall, 2004), but the underlying perceptual set that fuels the belief systems of the ego tends to remain unaltered for the most part. Consequently, the person remains susceptible to new trauma.

Alpha–theta neurofeedback, on the other hand, bypasses the ego's belief systems by encouraging the person to remain in a theta state, a frequency band below those at which the ego is operative. The alpha–theta protocol then can break the sensitization loop at the source of the negative perceptual set itself. In the theta state, painful unconscious memories of adverse childhood circumstances or events, even those of very early childhood, may be reframed by having an empathetic therapist give the person, repetitively over a significant number of sessions, a scenario of desired outcome that depicts the person as already healed, empowered and efficacious. The presenting symptomology usually is resolved in the process.

Other supportive therapies can reinforce the phase shift to a new perceptual framework in which the person is much more resilient to major stressors, and to stress overall. The following section shows the clinician how this may be accomplished with a high proportion of favorable outcomes based on a multi-modal model we have developed and used successfully for some time.

B.   Resolving trauma with alpha–theta neurofeedback: A multi-modality model

Alpha–theta neurofeedback often is used as a stand-alone therapy, and as such it has been shown to work effectively to resolve symptoms of many disorders. Many therapists have done excellent work using the alpha–theta protocol by itself. On the other hand, a review of Peniston's original research shows that it was conducted in the context of support provided by an in-patient environment with an ongoing twelve-step program in place. In our experience we have found that the resolution of trauma disorder symptoms frequently benefits from more than alpha–theta alone, that the use of additional primary therapy modalities may be required, and that treatment often can be enhanced by selectively including one or more adjunctive modalities.

Moreover, as research and clinical practice have progressed it seems increasingly clear that many factors previously not considered can impinge on the alpha–theta treatment domain, affecting the quality and nature of the outcome. One major function of a multi-modality model is to identify the most impactful contributing factors, and deal with them in the treatment plan. Here are some examples compiled from case files of the Enhancement Institute.

- A number of trauma patients have presented with excessive cortical slowing attributable to an attention deficit condition (ADHD) or a mild head injury (TBI). The specific patterns become evident from a quantitative EEG (qEEG) administered to incoming neurofeedback patients. From its results one can prescribe a number of appropriate neurofeedback training sessions for the person prior to undergoing the alpha–theta protocol in order to increase the brain's resilience during the time of slow-wave feedback.
- Patients presenting with high stress, substance abuse, and insomnia or other conditions indicating a potentially significant neurotransmitter imbalance, can be given a neurotransmitter panel and receive targeted amino acid therapy (TAAT) to bring their neurochemistry into better balance, thus facilitating treatment outcomes.
- When a person presents with numerous medications, chronic health problems, dietary deficiencies or physical impairments, they undergo a medical evaluation prior to treatment and its results are expected to impact the overall treatment program (e.g., benchmarks for reducing medication).

The Institute retains a medical director for this purpose; other practices may refer the person to a physician in their referral network or to the person's own medical provider.

- In order to gain a picture of the patient's mental and emotional state prior to the onset of treatment, it helps to administer one or more psychological profiles. The profile(s) helps the practitioner see pathologies that might otherwise remain undetected, and also provides a pretreatment baseline. One would be well advised to administer these profiles again at the conclusion of treatment as a means of assessing overall improvement.

- A number of persons present with acute conditions (e.g., suicidal ideation) or major life problems (e.g., impending divorce), indicating the need for one-on-one intervention. These persons receive immediate psychotherapeutic attention and ongoing therapy sessions as part of their treatment plan.

- If substance abuse disorder presents, the person is required (1) to find, attend and undergo the program of an appropriate 12-step or faith-based support group during the treatment period, and (2) to break contact with enablers. The therapist has to monitor these requirements, and might also have the person undergo periodic unannounced drug testing during the period of treatment.

- Families and other caregivers frequently have an impact on the person's perception of treatment. With the person's consent we find it helpful to engage family and/or regular caregivers in the treatment process with periodic updates and opportunities for them to get their questions answered.

Another major function of a multi-modality model is to augment and amplify the impact of the alpha–theta protocol. Supportive treatments such as support groups, ocular light therapy (OLT), cranial electrical stimulation (CES), low energy neurofeedback (LENS) (Larsen, 2005), cognitive behavioral therapy, life skills coaching or family therapy, as well as acupuncture and other forms of body work (e.g., Rolfing, Reiki, cranio-sacral therapy and deep-tissue massage) can have a significant impact on the alpha–theta healing process when administered before, after or during the alpha–theta treatment protocol, as indicated by the initial evaluation and testing process.

The interactive modalities such as psychotherapy, beta training, and cognitive behavioral therapy are best administered in-house because they directly impinge on the alpha–theta process of healing. In addition, therapies such as CES and LENS can be easily and relatively inexpensively administered in-house with proper training. These two modalities also may have a broader use in the practice. Specialized modalities, such as the various forms of body work, can be referred out to the practitioner's referral network. The Institute maintains a room with a massage table for body workers to come in on a contract basis to work on specified patients.

From this matrix of treatment options the overall framework of a treatment program begins to emerge, one that can be tailored to each patient's specific needs. It begins with (a) an evaluation phase in two parts: (1) testing, including personality inventories and a qEEG, and (2) consultation and agreement on a treatment plan. It continues through (b) a treatment phase with up to three elements: (1) the alpha–theta protocol, (2) supportive treatment modalities (e.g., beta neurofeedback and/or individual psychotherapy), and (3) adjunctive modalities such as cranial electrical stimulation (CES) or body work. Other primary therapies generally are conducted either before (e.g., beta training), during (e.g., psychotherapy) or after the alpha–theta protocol proper (e.g., LENS sequences). The program concludes with (c) a post-testing and final evaluation phase. The effectiveness of this format may be illustrated best by using an actual situation; consequently, we present in the following paragraphs a case study using alpha–theta in the multi-modality context.

C. Resolving trauma using alpha–theta in a multi-modality context: A case study

CS, a sixty-year-old male, came to our office for his first appointment March 29, 2006. At this first meeting he presented with severe anxiety, depression, insomnia, and excessive worry. He reported that he had no suicidal tendencies, and said that in the past he had been upbeat even though haunted by chronic anxiety. His medications at intake were Xanax, Zoloft, Diovan and Armour Thyroid, plus periodic use of Ambien or Seroquel.

By way of history, CS had entered the hospital the previous September with an anxiety attack. He stated that he had three anxiety attacks in college. He also stated that his mother, who was periodically abusive, had an alcohol problem and may have been addicted to prescription drugs, was subject to anxiety attacks as well. He mentioned in that connection that his father was demanding and sometimes verbally abusive, yelling at him and demeaning him for perceived shortcomings. In 1993, at his employment, CS was feeling pressure to complete a major project when his past anxiety reasserted itself and he began to feel depressed. He then saw several physicians, and took the medications they prescribed to help his depression and anxiety. The next year his mother died leaving him an estate so that he could retire and avoid the anxiety of work pressure. He played golf frequently and enjoyed playing duplicate bridge three times a week as a Silver Life Master, stabilized with successive medications.

In early 2006 CS underwent a thorough physical examination which showed he had developed a stenosis, or degenerative constriction, of the aorta. He was prescribed Biovan for this condition. After this news, however, he began having panic attacks, a strong conscious fear of death, an emergent fear of heights, melancholy, hypertension, and intensified insomnia largely unmitigated by sleep medications. Generally upbeat despite his underlying anxiety, he became despondent and increasingly passive with diminished affect. CS experienced panic attacks during hurricanes Katrina and Rita, even after it became clear that they would largely bypass Houston, where he lived. These developments drove CS to seek treatment at the Institute.

His initial testing and evaluation consisted of an intake interview, a quantitative EEG (qEEG), the MMPI-2 and MCM-II personality profiles, an integrated visual/auditory test of attention (IVA), a medical evaluation, a neurotransmitter panel, and extensive personal history and health questionnaires.

Prior to testing, however, the physician at the Institute became concerned about the effect of CS' high dosage of thyroid medication (Armour Thyroid 60 mg/d) on his symptoms, and referred him to an endocrinologist for further evaluation. During this appointment CS made a statement the endocrinologist construed as being suicidal and, startled, she sent him directly to a nearby psychiatrist who immediately hospitalized him in the mental lock-up. After four days he returned to us, on a completely different complement of medication, for his testing and evaluation.

The results of CS' qEEG, adjusting for the effects of medication, showed insufficient alpha and significant overall disorganization. The IVA indicated no significant deficits in visual and auditory attention. Neurotransmitter testing revealed extremely low catecholamine levels and sub-optimal serotonin. The results of CS' personality profiles substantiated high levels of anxiety and dysthymia in a person appearing needy of approval, highly dependent and relatively self-absorbed, with possible addictive tendencies. A medical evaluation revealed that CS had not slept for the previous four nights and that he reflected the symptoms of high stress, but was otherwise in good physical condition.

In diagnostic terms we can see that the primary presenting conditions are anxiety and dysthymia. However, a closer look at CS' history reveals a person with adverse childhood experiences, a previous history of emotional problems, and a possible genetic susceptibility to trauma. Further, his reactions to the discovery of his stenosis indicated that CS *perceived* the condition to be potentially fatal, bringing fear of death (annihilation in ego's terms) to consciousness, much like the immediacy of death may strike the soldier in battle (Cabrera *et al.*, 2007, Iverson *et al.*, 2008). This perception by CS was generally confirmed in personal interviews. Such a perception would have been sufficiently potent to decisively pierce the armor of upbeat amiability CS had built up against the fears of a child traumatized by abusive parents and, perhaps, the demands of life. At this point CS faced in full force the feelings that had lingered below the surface for decades, venting from time to time in the form of anxiety and depression. This interpretation of the situation, pieced together from reviews of testing and evaluation, history and personal interviews, justified a diagnosis of trauma disorder of which anxiety and dysthymia were symptoms.

In an attempt to get at cause, we developed an intensive outpatient treatment program for CS with alpha–theta neurofeedback at its core supported by two types of waking-sate neurofeedback as well as several adjunctive therapies. This was the sequence:

- CS began treatment with up to 20 sessions of standard neurofeedback training for general reorganization and brain resilience. Concurrently with this initial protocol CS did 20 half-hour sessions of ocular light therapy (OLT) in the green (calming) spectrum and 20 half-hour sessions of cranial electrical stimulation (CES) while resting in our energy enhancement system (www.eesystem.com). Both adjunctive modalities were designed to mitigate anxiety by helping to stimulate and normalize the command centers of the brain: the pituitary, pineal and hypothalamus. CS also began a targeted amino acid therapy (TAAT), consisting of oral administration of medical grade amino acid formulas twice daily, to normalize neurotransmitter levels. He also began a program of progressive, moderate reduction of drug dosages in cooperation with his psychiatrist.
- This phase of treatment was followed by 30-plus sessions of alpha–theta. CS met with his alpha–theta therapist, discussed his desired outcomes, and together they developed a healing and empowering scenario especially languaged for the subconscious to take on in place of its encoded patterns of early trauma. CS began sessions at the rate of four times a week, tapering at the end of the protocol to twice weekly for two weeks, then once weekly for two weeks. CS was encouraged to refrain from alcohol consumption while he was undergoing alpha–theta, which he did.
- At the conclusion of alpha–theta CS was administered a LENS map and underwent two sequences of LENS neurofeedback, helping to consolidate the gains made during the foregoing program. Following this modality CS again took the MMPI and MCMI inventories for comparison with pretreatment levels.

CS responded well to this program from the beginning. The metrics of his neu-rofeedback sessions indicated a significant reduction both in mean amplitudes and in the variability of amplitudes throughout the observed spectrum, implying better organization. He began to feel somewhat better, partly because his brain was functioning better and partly because his condition was getting considerable attention. During the alpha–theta protocol CS' affect progressively improved. He undertook on his own to progressively change his diet, reducing his consumption of red meat and starches and increasing his consumption of vegetables and whole grains. By the time he completed his LENS training he seemed to be in a con-sistently brighter mood. He reported that his brain seemed sharper than ever. His family reported that CS had returned to his positive and upbeat self.

The results of CS' immediate post-treatment testing showed him to be symptom-free. On the MCMI-II only the desirability and histrionic scales remained elevated: CS still liked to be liked and still felt free to express his feelings. A third adminis-tration of the MMPI and the MCMI at approximately 18 months post-treatment showed that the results of treatment were holding well (Tables 6.1 and 6.2).

TABLE 6.1   CS—Millon Clinical Multiaxial Inventory-III (MCMI-III)

	Pre 5–2006	Post 9–2006	Follow-up 3–2008
Disclosure	51	38	48
Desirability	80	94	94
Debasement	52	0	0
Schizoid	48	24	12
Avoidant	47	0	0
Depressive	67	20	20
Dependent	87	30	60
Histrionic	87	87	92
Narcissistic	73	73	75
Antisocial	60	22	52
Sadistic	34	0	9
Compulsive	51	58	58
Negativistic	22	0	0
Masochistic	67	0	20
Schizotypal	39	0	0
Borderline	69	20	20
Paranoid	0	0	0
Anxiety	78	0	0
Somatoform	62	0	0
Bipolar: Manic	48	12	12
Dysthymia	71	0	0
Alcohol Dependence	60	15	30
Drug Dependence	45	30	45
Post-Traumatic Stress	45	15	15
Thought Disorder	60	0	0
Major Depression	60	20	20
Delusional Disorder	60	25	25

TABLE 6.2   CS—The Minnesota Report (MMPI-2)

T Score Pre 5–2006		Post 10–2006	Follow Up 3–2008
Hs—Hypochrondriasis	51	48	48
D—Depression	70	45	40
Hy—Hysteria	59	52	47
Pd—Psychopathic Deviance	57	40	42
Mf—Male/Female	44	44	42
Pa—Paranoia	42	46	49
Pt—Psychasthenia	77	49	47
Sc—Schizophrenia	56	49	45
Ma—Mania	53	47	43
Si—Social Introversion	49	38	40
MAC-R	53	48	46
APS	65	38	44
AAS	41	41	41
PK	50	38	38
MDS	46	37	42

V. CONCLUSION

The Peniston protocol of alpha–theta neurofeedback therapy has shown itself to be a powerful healing modality. Emerging research, especially in the areas of neuroplasticity and related concepts, combines with well-supported psychological concepts to explain its efficacy, while developments in the area of brain function are now beginning to explain the mechanisms by which may work. Combined with appropriate supportive therapies and adjunctive treatments, alpha–theta's effectiveness can be amplified to provide a powerful multi-modality means of dealing with causal factors of trauma disorder.

REFERENCES

Achterberg, J. (1985). *Imagery in Healing*. Boston: New Science Library.

American Psychiatric Association (1994). *Diagnostic and Statistical Manual of Mental Disorders*, 4th edition. Washington, DC: American Psychiatric Association.

Bohm, D. (1983). *Wholeness and the Implicate Order*. London: Routledge & Kegan Paul.

Bower, B. (1996). Child sex abuse leaves mark on brain. *Science News*, **147**, 340.

Brownback, T. and Mason, L. (1998). Brownback–Mason protocol utilizing neurotherapy with dissociation/addiction. Presented at the *Futurehealth Conference*, Palm Springs, CA.

Brugental, J. F. T. (1987). *The Art of Psychotherapy*. New York: W. W. Norton.

Budzynski, T. (1971). Some applications of biofeedback-produced twilight states. Presented at the *Annual Meeting of the American Psychological Association*, Washington, DC.

Budzynski, T. (1997). The case for alpha–theta: a dynamic hemispheric asymmetry model. Presented at the *Annual Conference of the International Society for Neurotherapy and Research,* Aspen, CO.

Buonomano, D. V. and Merzenoch, M. M. (1998a). A neural network model of temporal codegeneration and position – invariant pattern recognition. *Neural Comput.*, **11**, 103–116.

Buounomano, D. V. and Merzenich, M. M. (1998b). Cortical plasticity from synapses to maps. *Ann Rev. Neuroscience*, **21**, 149–186.

Cabrera, Hoge, Bliese, *et al.* (2007). Childhood adversity and combat as predictors of depression and post-traumatic stress in deployed troops. *Am. J. Prev. Med.*, **33(2)**, 77–82.

Campbell, J. (1988). *The Power of Myth with Bill Moyers*. New York: Doubleday.

Capra, F. (1975). *The Tao of Physics*. Boulder, CO: Shambhala.

Capra, F. (1996). *The Web of Life*. New York: Doubleday.

Chopra, D. (1989). *Quantum Healing*. New York: Bantam Books.

Chopra, D. (1993). *Ageless Body, Timeless Mind*. New York: Harmony Books.

Continuum (1993). Dual disorders: High recidivism presents challenge to professionals. *Hazelton Educational Materials*, October–November.

Cowan, J. (1993). Alpha–theta brain wave biofeedback: The many possible theoretical reasons for its success. *Biofeedback*, **21(2)**, 11–16.

Cowan, J. D. (2008). *Brain waves pattern themselves after rhythms of nature*. University of Chicago news office, February 15, 2008

Cozolino, L. (2002). *The Neuroscience of Psychotherapy*. New York: W. W. Norton.

Fahrion, S. (1995). Observations of the psychophysiology of personality transformation. Presented at the *Futurehealth Conference*, Key West, FL.

Fahrion, S., Wirkus, M. and Pooley, P. (1993). EEG amplitude, brain mapping, and synchrony in and between a bioenergy practitioner and client during healing. *Subtle Energies*, **3(1)**, 19–51.

Goswami, A. (1993). *The Self Aware Universe. New Instincts, Archetypes and Symbols*. Los Angeles: J. P. Tarcher.

Green, F. and Green, A. (1977). *Beyond Biofeedback*. New York: Knoll Publishing.

Grof, S. (1976). *Realms of Human Unconscious*. New York: B. P. Dutton.

Grof, S. (1980). *LSD Psychotherapy*. Pomona, CA: Hunter House.

Grof, S. (1985). *Beyond the Brain*. New York: State University of New York Press.

Grof, S. (1993). *The Holotropic Mind*. San Francisco: HarperCollins.

Hartmann, T. (1997). *The Prophet's Way*. Northfield, VT: Mythical Books.

Henry, J. P. (1992). *Instincts, Archetypes and Symbols: An Approach to the Physiology of Religious Experience*. Dayton, OH: College Press.

Herbert, N. (1985). *Quantum Reality*. New York: Doubleday.

Herbert, N. (1988). How Bell proved reality cannot be local. *Psycholog. Perspect.*, **20(2)**, 313–319.

Iverson, Fear, Ehlers, *et al.* (2008). Risk factors for post-traumatic stress disorder among UK armed forces personnel. *Psychol. Med.*, **38(4)**, 511–522.

LaMantia, A. S. and Katz, L. C., (eds) (2001). Plasticity of mature synapses and circuits. Neuroscience, 2nd edition. Sunderland, MA: Sinauer Associates, Inc., 535–62.

Larsen, S. (2006). *The Healing Power of Neurofeedback*. Rochester, Vermont: Healing Arts Press.

Manchester, C. (1995). Application of neurofeedback in the treatment of dissociative disorders. Presented at the *Mid-Atlantic Regional Biofeedback Conference*, Atlantic City, NJ.

Manchester, C. (1997). Treating high risk patients with neurofeedback under managed care. Presented at the *Futurehealth Conference*, Palm Springs, CA.

Manchester, C., Allen, T. and Tachiki, K. (1998). Treatment of dissociative identity disorder with neurotherapy and group self-exploration. *J. Neurother.*, 40–53.

Maslow, A. (1968). *Toward a Psychology of Being*, 2nd edition. New York: Van Nostrand Reinhold.

Miller, D. and Blum, K. (1996). *Overload: Attention Deficit Disorder and the Addictive Brain*. Kansas City: Andrews and McMeel.

Mitchell, R. (1994). *Eye to Eye with Connie Chung*. CBS Television Show, June 30, 1994.

Peniston, E. G. and Kulkosky, P. J. (1989). Alpha–theta brain wave training and beta-endorphin levels in alcoholics. *Alcohol. Clin. Exp. Res.*, **13**, 271–279.

Peniston, B. G. and Kulkosky, P. J. (1990). Alcoholic personality and alpha–theta brain wave training. *Med. Psychother.*, **3**, 37–55.

Peniston, E. G. and Kulkosky, P. J. (1991). Alpha–theta brain wave neurofeedback for Vietnam veterans with combat-related post-traumatic stress disorder. *Med. Psychother.*, **4**, 47–60.

Perry, B. (1992). Neurobiological sequelae of childhood trauma. In *Catecholamine Function in Post-traumatic Stress Disorder: Emerging Concepts* (M. Murberg, ed.), Washington, DC: American Psychiatric Press.

Perry, B. (1997). Incubated in terror. In *Children in a Violent Society*, (xxxxx, ed.), pp. New York: Guilford Press.

Pert, C. (1993). In Healing and the Mind (Moyers, B., ed.) pp. New York: Doubleday.

Pert, C. (1997). *Molecules of Emotion*. New York: Scribner.

Rose, S. (2005). *The Future of the Brain*. New York: Oxford University Press.

Ross, C. (1989). *Multiple Personality Disorder*. New York: John Wiley & Sons.

Rossi, E. (1986). *The Psychobiology of Mind–Body Healing*. New York: W. W. Norton.

Schneider, C. (1998). Considerations of right frontal lobe damage and the Phineas Gage phenomenon. Presented at the *Futurehealth Conference*, Palm Springs, CA.

Schurnmer, G. (1995). Self-regulation of the immune system. *J. Mind Technol. Optimal Performance. Megabrain Report*, **111(l)**, 30–39.

Siegel, B. (1986). *Love, Medicine & Miracles*. New York: Harper & Row.

Siegel, D. J. (1999). *The Developing Mind*. New York: Guilford Press.

Simonton, C. and Simonton, S. (1978). *Getting Well Again*. Los Angeles: J. P. Tarcher.

Sterman, M. B. (1995). How does the brain make waves, what do they mean and where should I place my electrodes? Presented at the *Futurehealth Conference*, Key West, FL.

Stein, P. T. and Kendall, J. (2004). *Psychological Trauma and the Developing Brain*. Binghamton, NY: Haworth Press.

Trachtenberg, J. T., Chen, B. E., Knott, G. W., *et al.* (2002). Long-term in vivo imaging of experience-dependent synaptic plasticity in adult cortex. *Nature*, **420**, 788–794.

Walsh, R. and Vaughan, F. (1980). The emergence of the transpersonal perspective. In *Beyond Ego* (R. Walsh and F. Vaughan, eds.) pp. xxx, Los Angeles: J. P. Tarcher.

Walsh, R., Elgin, D., Vaughn, F. and Wilber, K. (1980). Paradigms in collision. In *Beyond Ego* (R. Walsh and F. Vaughan, eds.) pp. xxx, Los Angeles: J. P. Tarcher.

White, N. (1994). Alpha–theta brain wave biofeedback: The multiple explanations for its clinical effectiveness. Presented at the *Annual Meeting of the Association for Applied Psychophysiology and Biofeedback*, Atlanta, GA.

White, N. (1995). Alpha–theta training for chronic trauma disorder. *J. Mind Technol. Optimal Performance. Megabrain Report*, **11(4)**, 44–50.

White, N. (1996). Alpha/theta feedback in the treatment of alcoholism. Presented at the *Annual Meeting of the Association for Applied Psychophysiology and Biofeedback*, Albuquerque, NM.

White, N. and Martin, K. (1998). Alpha–theta neurotherapy as a multi-level matrix of intervention. In *Applied Neurophysiology & Brainwave Biofeedback* (R. Kall, J. Kamiya and G. Schwartz, eds.) pp. xx, Bensalem, PA: Futurehealth.

Winson, J. (1990). The meaning of dreams. *Sci. Am.*, November, 86–96.

Wolpe, P. R., Gorton, G., Serota, R. and Stanford, B. (1993). Prediction compliance of dual diagnosis inpatients with aftercare treatment. *Hosp. Community Psychiat.*, **44(1)**, 45–49.

Wuttke, M. (1992). Addiction, awakening, and EEG biofeedback. *Biofeedback*, **20(2)**, 18–22.

[name of author of article] (2006). [title of article]. *Wall Street Journal*, 29 July, p. 1.

PART 3

Alternative Treatment Approaches to Neurofeedback

Hemoencephalography: Photon-based blood flow neurofeedback

Hershel Toomim[1], Ph.D. and Jeffrey Carmen[2], Ph.D.

[1]*Biocomp Research Institute, Los Angeles, California, USA*

[2]*Clinical psychology practice, Manlius, New York, USA*

This chapter provides information about the voluntary control of cerebral blood flow as a form of neurofeedback. The formal name of the process is hemoencephalography, but we have shortened the term to HEG for ease of pronunciation. A list of FAQs (frequently asked questions) can be found at the end of this chapter. For those who are unfamiliar with the concepts involved with HEG, reading the FAQs first may make the rest of the chapter easier to understand.

Natasha had been blind for three years as a result of toxic encephalopathy. Her SPECT study showed severe hypoperfusion in the right medioposterior temporal lobe. This is exactly where face and object recognition begins. Her visual processing functions were destroyed by exposure to toxic hydrocarbon emissions from freshly laid asphalt paving in the atrium next to her art studio. Although her brain continued to receive visual input, she was no longer able to make sense out of this data. She had become functionally blind. Differential diagnosis ruled out a conversion disorder. She was certified legally blind by the Braille Institute.

Hemoencephalography (HEG) and Hyperbaric Oxygen (HBO) helped her recover her sight after three years. She now proudly drives her own car. She has 20/20 vision—better than before the toxic exposure.

I. HEG AS A FORM OF NEUROFEEDBACK

The training of body functions to achieve restoration to health is now broadly accessible through complex instrumentation which is capable of capturing a variety of body responses. The term *biofeedback* refers to the process of "feeding back" physiological signals non-invasively from externally reached areas of the body. The feedback has the intent of teaching control over these signals. It has a long and respected history of assisting people in the management of troublesome physiological and emotional conditions. The term *neurofeedback* is a distinctive subset of biofeedback. It makes use of physiological signals that originate within the brain, as opposed to signals that originate from other sites such as cardiac or skeletal muscle activity. Neurofeedback includes both electroencephalography (EEG) and hemoencephalography (HEG) feedback.

Hemoencephalography (nirHEG) is the system developed by Hershel Toomim. The term, introduced by Marjory and Hershel Toomim at the AAPB annual meeting in 1995 (Toomin, 1995), implements near infrared spectroscopy (NIRS) to voluntarily control cerebral blood flow changes through increasing blood oxygen levels. The process involves the use of light in red and near infrared wavelengths (blood color) instead of magnetic fields as in functional magnetic resonance imaging (fMRI).

Passive infrared hemoencephalography (pirHEG) is the system developed by Jeffrey Carmen. This system increases voluntary cerebral blood flow changes through exerting changes in brain thermal activity. The process involves the use of light in far infrared wavelengths.

A.   Details of nirHEG development

Near infrared spectroscopy (NIRS) emerged from the work of F. F. Jobsis in 1977 (Proctor *et al.*, 1982). Jobsis invented non-invasive infrared monitoring of the oxygen content of brain tissue and blood flow. Britton Chance, Department of Biochemistry and Biophysics at the University of Pennsylvania School of Medicine, with his students, developed significant progress in the measurement of intercellular oxidation through his systematic efforts (Chance, 1962; Chance *et al.*, 1988).

Hershel Toomim, while concurrently investigating a new field of training brain waves using an electroencephalograph, sought to understand the physical principle of how brain wave training succeeded. Toomim's study was to investigate if there was a lasting blood flow change in the brain area being trained, in line with studies by Ingvar and Anders (1976). Alas, the history of development of a line of research is frequently replete with events that block its progress. Toomim's experiment used what was at the time the gold standard of brain blood flow measurement: single photon emission computed tomography (SPECT). In this test a bolus of radioactive material is injected into a vein. As the material circulates in the blood stream some of it lodges in brain tissues where it can be detected with a radiation scanner.

The experiment was planned as follows. The experiment was to train an individual to achieve a lasting change in brain waves that could be detected by SPECT blood flow activity. The experiment required SPECT studies before and after brain wave training. Arrangements were made with Dr. Russ Hibler of the Union Memorial Hospital in Baltimore, Maryland to do the SPECT studies with two Ph.D. psychology students (Julie Weiner of N.Y. University and Jean Scammon of the University of Maryland) to conduct the experiment. As politics would have it, a new doctor was appointed to be in charge of the Nuclear Medicine Service at Union Memorial Hospital who withdrew his support. In the meantime a Britton Chance study (Chance *et al.*, 1988), measuring brain blood oxygenation with near infrared spectroscopy (NIRS), provided an alternative method for conducting the experiment.

The spectroscope idea presented by Britton Chance's paper was a simple model for Toomim to build. Even without a stimulus, simply through self regulatory control, it was possible to easily control the readings. Testing began with volunteers who had various brain disorders such as ADHD, toxic encephalopathy, stroke, aging memory loss, depression, and even schizophrenia. Every test result turned to gold. All these people improved. One person who regained his memory wrote a testimonial saying "He has a gold mind." HEG was born! This instrument provided the makings of a new way to exercise the brain.

Toomim describes the use of the instrument experience thus: nirHEG shines a light on your brain. "A light on my brain? How can you do that?" Have you ever shone a flashlight on your palm and noticed that the dark side glows? Light travels through your tissue. Your skull is like that. It's not dark in there! It glows like a lampshade lighted from the outside. Light that gets in can also get out. Light coming out is the color of your brain.

Your brain changes color and warms when you use any part of it. Metabolism makes it warmer and bright red when you are using it, cooler and purple when you aren't. If you have seen the blood being drawn from your arm for a blood test you have seen the dark purple blood collect in the evacuated vial. On the other hand, when you cut yourself you see bright red blood. Blood turns red when it collects oxygen from your lungs or the air.

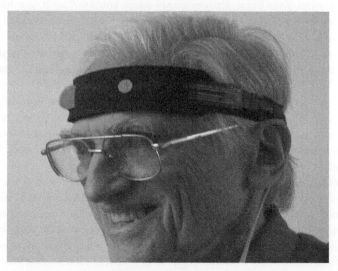

FIGURE 7.1   Present nirHEG sensor. Training area is marked by the white disc. Cerebral blood flow dynamics from the nir perspective.

Blood arrives in your lungs as used blood, a deep purple color. It absorbs oxygen and leaves your lungs bright red to begin its journey to your brain. It may come as a surprise that your brain is the most voracious user of fresh red blood in your body. Your brain weighs about three pounds, about one fiftieth of your body weight, yet at rest it uses about one fifth of all the fresh blood leaving your heart. It uses about 10 times as much blood per pound as the rest of your body.

When you use your brain it uses more blood. To keep your brain alive it has to be very careful in the way it uses blood. It keeps the blood supply to a minimum when it is at rest, and calls for more blood only in the nuclei being used at any time. When you use a nucleus it turns red. This feature has led to the important advance in the brain science we are seeing today a powerful scientific tool, the functional magnetic resonance imager (fMRI). With this instrument we can see the red areas being used at any time. We can see what parts of your brain are red when you talk, sing, or even think. Great instrument—too bad it costs so much. These are voluntary functions, right? So you can voluntarily change the color of your brain!

Now what is hemoencephalography? It is the poor man's fMRI. Hemoencephalography (HEG), literally brain blood graphics, is a form of neurofeedback whereby voluntary increases in cerebral blood flow form the basis of cerebral exercise.

Cerebral exercise has been shown to increase synaptogenesis (more synapses) and angiogenesis (more capillaries and arterioles) in rats (Diamond *et al.*, 1977). Further work with humans has reinforced this concept (Taub *et al.*, 1993; Maguire *et al.*, 2000). We now know that physical exercise improves brain function via angiogenesis, and mental exercise improves brain function by both synaptogenesis and angiogenesis. Your brain actually grows when you exercise it, just like a muscle does. It gets larger. And, like a muscle, your brain gets tired when you exercise it. Also, like a muscle, it wastes away when you don't use it. As Marion Diamond said "Use it or lose it." (Diamond, 1964). This suggests it is continually shrugging off old cells and building new ones. When the rate of loss equals the rate of cell gain, your brain is stable.

You might ask where it finds the room to grow. The brain has fluid filled spaces called *ventricles*. These spaces are filled with cerebral spinal fluid (CSF) that is continually being secreted and absorbed to maintain a constant pressure in your brain and spinal cord. New tissue displaces CSF. The growth is very small; Einstein's brain was hardly larger than the normal variation in brain sizes.

We harness HEG in the service of brain exercise. nirHEG shines a light through the skull onto the brain. Reflected light is the color of the brain. pirHEG monitors the radiation of excess thermal energy. Brain color and temperature is our clue to brain use. You can change the color and temperature at will. When you choose a brain action, like solving a problem, your brain requests more oxygen and glucose from the blood stream. As fresh oxygenated blood infuses the requesting tissue it becomes redder. As it uses the new blood-borne nutrients it warms. The increased blood flow then helps maintain thermal homeostasis in these cells.

The NIR probe light, reflected from the redder tissue, informs a computer of the change in color, it warms as the new energy is used. We can harness the computer to control a display of sound and video as a lure toward more energy use. We find we can control the computer display. We get tired when we overdo it. We have a brain gymnasium!

The brain is built of many compartments, each for a basic function. Vision, for example, resides in the back of the brain. So it is with functions like speech, muscle control, face recognition, etc. Each has its own nucleus. Our brain gymnasium can work with most of these. We merely have to exercise the chosen nucleus.

A simple experiment shows the loss of efficiency due to training at a distance from the module of primary interest. Two nirHEG headbands were simultaneously activated. One was at the top of the head at Cz, and the other was just above where the eyebrows meet at Fpz. Sound feedback, the only feedback, derived from the top site, Cz, was supplied to the subject for the first 5 minutes. A high level of action at the Cz headband was measured. The sound was then switched for control by Fpz, the frontal site, without the testee's knowledge. Choice of the headband controlling the sound required the operator only to press a different computer key. The testee unknowingly, by following the feedback, activated the headband that was the source of the sound. He began with the sound from the Cz headband then, after 5 minutes, sound was switched to the Fpz headband. Activation position on the head, by brain activation, followed the sound feedback as well.

As you can see in Fig. 7.2 there was a subsequent switch in the elicited activity from the top of head site to the frontal site. During the first 5 minutes the frontal

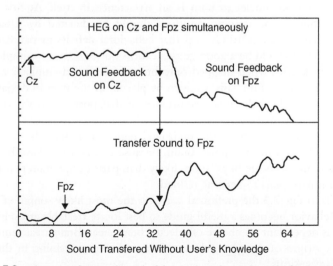

FIGURE 7.2   The ratio of Fpz at the end of the graph to that at the end of 5 minutes is approximately 3 to 1. Treating at the prefrontal cortex for prefrontal disorders is three times more effective than training at Cz for this disorder.

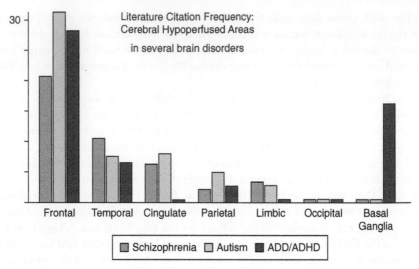

FIGURE 7.3   Number of references using brain imaging for locating specified brain disorders. Note the predominance of the prefrontal cortex.

activity at Fpz increased to a value approximately one third as large as the action at the top site, Cz. After the switch this activity at Fpz rapidly increased to about the level achieved earlier at the top site, Cz. Action at the sound source, now at Fpz, is shown in the lower panel to be about three times higher than when the controlling source was at Cz.

Selection of brain nuclei to train is an art/science in itself. At first thought it seems as though the training positions should be dictated by Quantitative Electroencephalography (QEEG), and that behavioral deficits in standard deviations from normal would be a good guide. It turns out to be not so simple.

Behavioral deficits, when mapped onto brain nuclei, need emphasis not given by standard deviations. Emphasis needs to be placed on the map in deviation values that represent the behavioral importance of that position to the behavioral deficit being investigated.

The frontal lobes, especially the prefrontal region, represent the most recent evolutionary changes in the human brain. Because of this, there have been fewer iterations making "software bugs" more likely than parts of the brain that have had more evolutionary years to become refined.

As shown in Fig. 7.3 the prefrontal cortex is the most likely source of aberrant behavior. Behavior becomes a useful guide to best locate treatable areas. Efficiency of training is dependent on choice of selected brain areas. Brain areas remote from the primary origin of disorder reduce training efficiency; training in these areas requires more sessions.

However, Fig. 7.4 nevertheless illustrates that a remote effect exists. In this SPECT study, a measure of abnormal blood flow, one can see the posterior cingulate

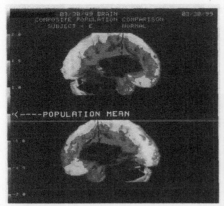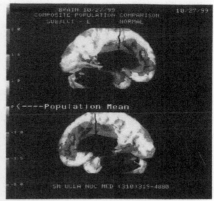

Before HEG   After HEG

FIGURE 7.4   Hypoperfused (blue) area shrinks after 23 sessions of HEG training at Fp1 and Fp2. Illustrated here is the remote effect. In this SPECT study, a measure of abnormal blood flow, one can see the posterior cingulate gyrus becomes more normal even though the training was at the prefrontal cortex (see also color plate).

gyrus becomes more normal (the yellow area) even though the training was at the prefrontal cortex.

Given that behavioral deficits are the presenting symptoms, behavioral tests were applied before and after each 10 sessions as a guiding record of progress. Selected tests were MicroCog, Beck Depression Inventory, Beck Anxiety Inventory, TOVA, SCL90, and Elaine Aron's Sensitivity Test.

MicroCog, a computer administered and scored test, was selected because its subtests are readily mapped to well-known behavioral traits and point to involved brain nuclei. The advantage is that poor response on a behavioral subtest points to the brain position involved that needs improvement (Fig. 7.5).

To partially satisfy the need for a method of finding an appropriate brain training location, and also because of dissatisfaction with a single reference for training positions, Toomim developed a questionnaire in order to establish important behavioral/cognitive areas for training. He used the categories as named in the MicroCog Test, including: Mental Control, Reasoning and Calculation, Memory, Spatial Processing, Response Time, Processing Speed, Processing Accuracy, and Cognitive Proficiency to categorize behavioral/cognitive activities. Responses to the questionnaire established the behaviorally important areas reported by the patient, and helped to measure improvement in behavioral categories in relation to a scale set to 100 for changes in hemoencephalography. Details of the questionnaire can be found on the web site www.Biocompresearch.org.

The TOVA (test of variables of attention) is also useful as a measurement of behavioral/cognitive change. It was originally designed to optimize medication dosage for attention deficit disorder. The test constructs a race between two brain pathways to reach the motor strip, activation areas C3 and C4. One route,

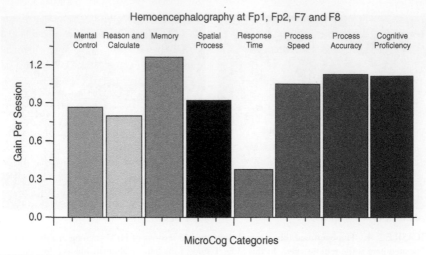

FIGURE 7.5   Effectiveness of nirHEG brain exercise is shown in improved cognitive characteristics. MicroCog relates cognitive changes in points per session on a 100 point scale for various trained behavioral functions.

the impulsive one, has primitive evolutionary advantages in activating life-saving action with a minimum of thought. Another cognitive pathway, a later, slower development, takes time for thought. A fast brain can afford that time. If an early, timely non–response decision reaches the muscle activation area in the brain, a correct non–response can be made. Otherwise, in error, it seems the thumb on the button has a mind of its own, and an incorrect button press occurs. The number of incorrect button presses becomes the basis for a score where 100 is the score for the average number of errors made by a population of normal subjects distributed by age and education level.

B.   Details of pirHEG development

In 1997, while Hershel Toomim was developing the concept of near infrared spectroscopy as a way to monitor cerebral blood flow, Jeffrey Carmen had been exploring the use of infrared detection without direct contact with the skin as a way to monitor body thermal behavior. Initially he had applied this concept to the task of training fingers and hands to increase blood flow. Training for increased blood flow using contact thermometry had already been well established in the biofeedback field as a training procedure for relaxation in general, and migraine treatment in particular. Training without the need for skin contact was a new concept.

The infrared detector used had a round field of view approximately 32 mm in diameter. It responded to infrared wavelengths in the 7–14 micron range, responding to signal changes with a very fast settling time of 80 milliseconds.

The results of this experimentation with infrared thermal monitoring yielded outcomes that were at least equivalent to contact thermometry and, in some cases, appeared to be more effective. There were three advantages for using a non-contact infrared system for monitoring human body thermal behavior. Firstly, the infrared sensor had a larger area of skin to which it responded. Secondly, since it was non-contact in nature it did not influence the thermal behavior of the surface being measured. Thirdly, the response time was very fast, taking about 80 milliseconds to reach 67% of the ultimate detected level.

Having validated the use of non-contact infrared technology as at least equivalent in efficacy to contact thermal training, the technology was applied to a disorder that was known at the time as reflex sympathetic dystrophy (RSD). The term has subsequently been renamed as Complex Regional Pain Disorder (CRPD) to reflect more current understanding of the mechanism. This is a condition involving extreme pain of unknown etiology. Typically a relatively minor injury produces extreme pain in part or all of a limb. Typically also, there is a resting pain level that never drops to zero, and an episodic pain level that is almost intolerable, stimulated by minimal sensory stimuli to the affected area. The extreme pain resulting from even slight skin contact precludes the use of contact thermal training, although on a theoretical basis this type of training made sense as a physiologically-based behavioral treatment for RSD.

It was hypothesized that if a person with RSD were trained to increase blood flow to the symptomatic area, pain might be reduced, and possibly the disorder itself would become less severe. The use of non-contact infrared temperature training seemed like a natural fit. It worked quite well, more or less. The technique was very effective in training the RSD sufferer to increase blood flow to the affected area. The negative side to this observation was that the increase in blood flow was accompanied by an extreme increase in pain. In essence, the treatment backfired but also validated the use of non-contact infrared technology for training control over thermal activity.

A second focus for application of pirHEG was in migraine headache events. The generally accepted theory of migraine pathophysiology involved excessive dilation of extra-cranial and intra-cranial blood vessels (Diamond, 1994). If the migraine sufferer could learn to voluntarily constrict these excessively dilated blood vessels, control over migraine activity might be achieved. However, attempts to teach people to reduce cerebral blood flow proved to be a complete failure. Physiologically this type of control may be a very difficult thing to achieve. Although cerebral blood flow responds to brain demand by increasing supply to the demand areas, the mechanism to create a local reduction in demand for blood is much less clear. To reduce localized cerebral blood flow would require reduction of brain activity in that area. It is very difficult to will a particular brain module to work less intensively, since attention to that function generally causes an increase in activity. It is the physiological equivalent to "not thinking about a pink elephant."

Concurrently with the observation that training people to reduce cerebral blood flow was very difficult, the theories of migraine pathophysiology began to change (Goadsby, 2001). The newly evolving theories centered around excessive brain excitability and irritability. Blood vessel behavior was hypothesized to be a correlate rather than a cause of migraine pain. Also, at about this same time, Carmen became aware of Toomim's work using NIR technology to train increases in brain activity in the prefrontal cortex.

Toomim observed that when individuals learned to increase brain activity in the prefrontal cortex, using the NIR technology, global brain control improved. Carmen hypothesized that it might be possible to achieve a similar training effect using non-contact infrared technology, and that the improved brain function might in some way be helpful with migraine management. This hypothesis was consistent with the newer theories regarding migraine pathophysiology. The effects turned out to be even stronger than anticipated. Toomim had been correct on two points. Firstly, it became clear that it was very easy to learn to increase brain activity using blood flow as a dependent variable. Secondly, increases in brain activity in the region of the prefrontal cortex resulted in a brain that functioned under better self-regulation.

This somewhat convoluted but serendipitous series of events led to a convergence between the ideas being explored independently by the two authors. They met for the first time at the Society for Neuronal Regulation conference in 1999, at which time they began to share ideas and plan cooperative research.

Carmen continued to develop this process with a major emphasis on the treatment of migraine headaches. In 2004 Carmen reported on the treatment of 100 migraine patients, using the passive infrared process. The reported effect for the more than 90% of migraine sufferers who continued for six sessions was a significant improvement in their migraines (Carmen, 2004).

Carmen reports the following as treatment guidelines: "I have established the following treatment guideline for session frequency and number of sessions. Once symptoms stabilize, I start to spread out the number of days between sessions. This process continues until or if the symptoms start to return. The effect of this process is that some people will end up needing to have practice sessions indefinitely, while others spread appointments out quickly, stabilize and never need another session."

C. Cerebral blood flow dynamics from the PIR perspective

The electromagnetic spectrum represents a continuum. Although all the wavelength bands have some characteristics that they share with all the other bands, there are also characteristics unique to each band. For example, X-rays can penetrate living tissue and can be recorded when they exit. Microwaves do not pass

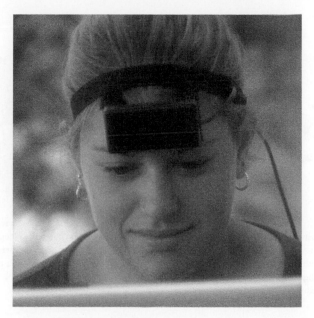

FIGURE 7.6   This is the current pirHEG sensor mounted on the forehead at Fpz, effectively covering a field of view 32 mm high by 46 mm wide.

through living tissue, but produce a heating effect as they transfer energy to the tissue. Within the infrared range of wavelengths (wavelengths longer than visible red light), NIR is close in frequency to visible light, but carries very little information regarding thermal activity. The wavelengths used by PIR are longer, and respond to changes in thermal activity, especially in the range of human body temperature.

The signal acquisition in the PIR system represents a conversion of excess brain thermal activity into a temperature equivalent. It is a very sensitive system for measuring and feeding back changes in regional thermal output of the brain. Its main usefulness is in "exercising" brain function. The underlying physiological mechanism is cellular metabolism. The dependent variable that is being measured to reflect these metabolic changes is cerebral blood flow. It is the change in regional cerebral blood flow that accounts for most of the transfer of thermal energy from metabolizing cells to the external environment.

The mechanism of infrared radiation and detection of this metabolic thermal waste product has been intensively studied in the rat brain by Shevelev (1992), and the human brain (Shevelev, 1998). He found a high degree of correlation between localization of thermal activity and localization of conditioned neural responses. He determined the relative contribution of increased thermal output to be predominantly a function of local cerebral blood flow increases with a smaller but significant contribution coming directly from local metabolic activity.

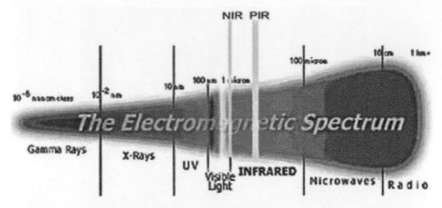

FIGURE 7.7   The wavelengths used in the NIR system are shorter than those used in the PIR system. The primary difference between short wavelength infrared and long wavelength infrared is that the longer wavelengths are sensitive to heat in the range of human body temperature whereas short wavelength infrared is insensitive to heat in that range. Both systems are based on photon detection, making them immune to electrical signal artifacts. By contrast, EEG neurofeedback is based on electron detection (see color plate).

There are parallels between the infrared detection system used with pirHEG and those infrared detection systems that already exist in nature. The PIR infrared sensor functions in a very similar manner to the infrared detection system of the pit viper. The pit viper monitors environmental thermal changes through the use of an infrared sensing organ. With this detection system, the pit viper monitors changes in the thermal environment produced by the motion of prey animals. In a similar manner, the PIR detector monitors changes in the environment. However the environment of interest is inside the skull, and the changes are the result of brain activity variations rather than physical motion.

For training purposes, the PIR headset detects changes in infrared radiation from the forehead. This radiation rises and falls with changes in regional cerebral blood flow, which in turn rises and falls in response to changes in regional cellular metabolism. The training signal is converted into analog and digital information that the individual can easily interpret. However it is not very useful as diagnostic data. The useful diagnostic data gets lost in the process of averaging across a large field of view for the purpose of feedback. Useful diagnostic data can be obtained from an infrared camera that presents pictures of the patterns of prefrontal cortical blood flow as the excess heat exits the forehead.

In terms of the specific signal components, some of the IR signal originating from brain tissue passes directly through the skull and surface tissues, and radiates directly into the environment in much the same way the beam from a flashlight would pass through a piece of translucent plastic. Secondly, some of the signal is absorbed by the skull and surface tissue as heat, which then gets reradiated as infrared. The pirHEG system measures a complex composite of these two signals.

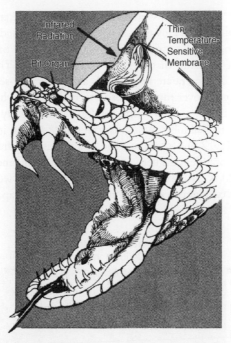

FIGURE 7.8   The wavelengths used in the PIR system are between 7 and 14 microns. The Pit Viper uses this portion of the electromagnetic spectrum for hunting. Image reproduced with permission from Exergen Corporation (Pompei and Pompei, 1996).

Since it measures only wavelengths longer than visible light, the visible intensity of light in the room has no effect on the signal.

Carmen's original work with the PIR system involved focal sensor placements that were consistent with the symptoms of the patient. He abandoned this focal approach in favor of a single Fpz placement for all interventions. Others using the PIR system have continued to use a variety of placements. Both approaches produce positive effects. The probable reason for the positive effects of the Fpz placement is that it picks up a large portion of the prefrontal cortex, and has the effect of gently increasing smooth arousal regulation. Toomim has followed a different path. He began his work mostly targeting brain areas directly under the forehead, but in recent years has begun to target a wide variety of brain locations.

D.   Infrared thermography

Using the Infrared Camera to Monitor Localized Changes in Brain Function

A very useful technique for monitoring cerebral blood flow in the prefrontal cortex is the use of infrared thermography. By definition, long wave infrared signals have no perceptible color when viewed by the human eye and, in fact, are not detectable by the human eye. However, some specially designed cameras are sensitive to those wavelengths. The use of such a camera can help monitor brain activity in those parts of the skull that are not covered by hair. The pattern changes viewed by this type of camera are meaningful as a pre-/post-session measure, and also as a change measure over multiple sessions. For people who are not bald, the area that is most easily monitored is the forehead. Fortunately the forehead is in the very front of the frontal lobes, which is a region of special interest.

This first image (Fig. 7.9) is the first stage of a precision infrared image capture. The camera captures wavelengths between 7 and 14 microns, and registers them on a grayscale with a 320 × 240 pixel resolution. The two image sequence is presented as an example of the type of precision the infrared camera is capable of providing.

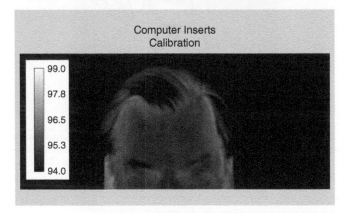

FIGURE 7.9   Calibration gives all images a common thermal reference (see color plate).

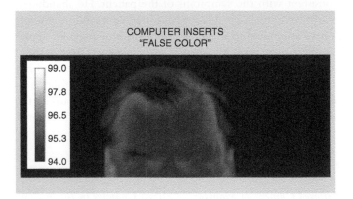

FIGURE 7.10   The final step in the sequence is the introduction of *false color*. This is called *false color* because wavelengths in this frequency have no color. The computer injects the color to make it easier for human interpretation of the image. This is an image of a "normal forehead." (see color plate)

Although the use of an infrared camera is not an essential part of the pir HEG system, its use can provide real time monitoring of cerebral blood flow changes. Both Hershel and Carmen have been using infrared imaging technology to monitor brain activity changes.

Using the Infrared Camera to Record Pre-/Post-Treatment Effects

One of the unanticipated benefits of developing the two separate HEG systems independently has been the evolution of different diagnostic and treatment styles. While Toomim emphasized cognitive testing and SPECT imaging to monitor treatment effects, Carmen developed a method of imaging brain activity in the prefrontal cortex by using an infrared camera. This is performed before and after each session. One of the fascinating aspects of this imaging is that it is very easy for a person to attribute meaning to the image. After a few sessions, people tend to be able to report what the image will look like prior to capturing the image. Typically, productive sessions produce a reduction of thermal variability in the image. Typically also, the baseline image taken before each session shows similar reductions in variation over time, paralleling symptom improvement.

Typically, for individuals who are left lateralized for language, dark areas on the forehead represent areas of relatively low brain activity. Dark areas in the center of the forehead are seen in individuals with attentional and emotional control difficulties. The dark region over the left eye is often seen in individuals with depression, however in this instance it is indicative of his language function difficulties rather than depression. Images must be captured without the person talking; otherwise the language side of the forehead produces too much thermal energy to

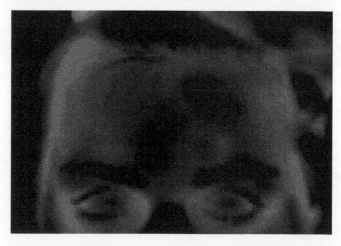

FIGURE 7.11   This is an example of a pre-session image captured with infrared camera. This image is of a 16-year-old male with severe concentration problems and severe word finding problems (see color plate).

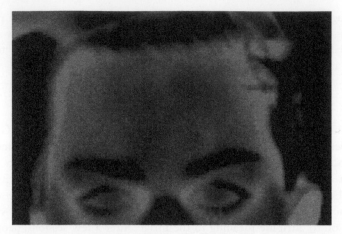

FIGURE 7.12   Post-session image. Previously dark areas on the forehead are lighter. Previously light areas on the forehead are less intense. There is less variability across the forehead. In this post-session image, the pinna of the left ear has a large increase in thermal output. Sometimes it is seen on the non-language side instead. Research on temperature changes of the pinna has not confirmed its meaning, although the general consensus is that it is probably related to language activity (Schiffer, 1998) (see color plate).

capture subtle patterns. Talking during image capture can represent artifact since it hides the baseline image, but because of that effect infrared imaging can also be a useful tool for helping to determine language lateralization.

Of equal importance to the reduction of thermal variability is the change in symptoms, even in such a short period of time. After a 25-minute pirHEG session, this young man's word-finding problems cleared up completely, and attentional patterns normalized. It is important to realize that the improvement initially does not last more than a day or two. That was the case here. In some situations, the symptoms eventually subside and don't reappear. However in other situations such as this one, the symptoms remain under control for a limited length of time. He can manage excellent symptom control for three to four weeks, after which the control fades.

With continued practice there are permanent improvements in brain function causing behavior patterns to permanently change. However, under intense stress people tend to revert to older stable behavior patterns. In other situations, the older stable behavior patterns are so strong that even without intense stress these patterns tend to re-emerge. This last response pattern describes the young man in these images. In his case he obtained his own HEG system, and practices with it when he feels the need.

II. A NEW PARADIGM

HEG represents a new paradigm. The two described techniques use light to access brain changes. They differ in the colors of light they use. Both depend on recording changes in characteristics of blood when changed during the course of brain metabolism. Carmen's PIR instrument measures the thermal waste product of cellular metabolism that is emitted through the forehead. This system uses long wavelength infrared light in the range of 7–14 microns (wavelengths sensitive to body temperature). Toomim's NIR instrument uses relatively short wavelengths, 680 and 850 nanometers (wavelengths sensitive to color). Blood warms and changes color as it is used as a result of oxygen and glucose metabolism. The generation of heat is also the result of oxygen and glucose metabolism.

The process of passive infrared hemoencephalography (pirHEG) seems similar in response characteristics and effects to the near infrared hemoencephalography (nirHEG) system. Reports from clinicians who have used both suggest similarities; especially similar responses to cognitive focus. As cognitive focus increases so does the signal. Experience with both systems suggests that the cognitive and affective state that produces a signal increase in the PIR system will also produce a signal increase in the NIR system.

One of the differences between the two systems is the size of the area of brain activity being monitored. Toomim's work has evolved in the direction of specificity of site monitoring, with a sensor that can target specific areas. Carmen's work has evolved in the direction of generalized monitoring, creating a sensor that has a very large field of view. Consequently, some of the differences in function between the two systems can be attributed to sensor specificity.

HEG has been used successfully in the treatment of attention deficit hyperactivity disorder of the inattentive and also hyperactive type, autistic spectrum disorders, bipolar disorder, traumatic brain injury, age-related memory loss, stroke, migraine headaches, epilepsy, Tourette's disorder, obsessive compulsive disorder, depression, schizophrenia, and toxic encephalopathy. We should point out that we are not typically talking about curing these disorders. We are talking about an intervention that reduces their severity, albeit sometimes dramatically so.

All these disorders (and many others) share a common element. Along with other symptoms, they represent a response by the brain to relatively minor stimuli that is excessive in terms of both rate and magnitude. This suggests that increasing the level of control the brain exerts over its own activities may be useful across a wide variety of disorders or dysfunctions.

We have learned that brain exercise via HEG has beneficial results. We have also learned that an approach that is too aggressive has the potential to produce side effects. The number of sessions, selection of brain nuclei, duration of sessions, and client sensitivity must all be considered in any treatment plan. Side effects will be discussed separately in this chapter. Typically they represent over-training or exhaustion of the area being targeted.

To avoid confusion in describing the concept of hemoencephalography, we decided to give suitable names to these two instruments. Toomim's system uses near infrared light and thus became known as *nirHEG*. Carmen's system required no light source and was passive, so in this regard it became known as passive, pirHEG.

pirHEG differs a bit from nirHEG in the nature of the cognitive and affective approach to increasing the signal output. For a person to increase the output of the PIR signal requires a simultaneously high level of "mental effort" (Pribram and McGuinness, 1975), combined with a relaxed, non-frustrated emotional state. Of particular interest is the effect of frustration. Even a very small level of frustration blocks the signal from increasing or may even produce a signal decrease. However, relaxation in the absence of mental effort has the same effect. The process requires a simultaneous combination of mental effort and a relaxed affective state. nirHEG is similar but is a little more tolerant of emotional discomfort. This may be due to the difference in technology or the difference in the volume of brain tissue monitored. At this point it is unclear which difference is responsible.

A. Human frontal lobes and behavioral pathology

The frontal lobes are the most recent evolutionary development of the human brain. The frontal lobes probably began to take their present form around 50,000 years ago (Jerison, 2007). In terms of evolutionary development, human frontal lobes have not had much time to be refined. Using a software analogy, the frontal lobes are still in "beta" format.

One of the major functions of the prefrontal region of the frontal lobes is smooth regulation of other brain modules so that they all work together. Damage or dysfunction of this region allows other modules to operate in an unregulated manner. In reviewing the DSM IV (American Psychiatric Association, 1994), it can be seen that many if not most of the diagnostic categories represent excesses of rate and magnitude in response to stimuli that are not very significant.

The latest hypotheses accounting for the aberrant action noted by the QEEG is that the prefrontal cortex determines the linkages between modules. Failure of this executive control system to adequately control the applicable modules results in improper operation of these modules. Unregulated brain modules operate in a manner inconsistent with a smoothly functioning organism.

For daily activities that are not emergency response activities, the brain works best when excitation and inhibition are smoothly regulated. This has often been named the "executive" system (Goldberg, 2001). It permits and favors careful thinking and analysis of life's challenges. This regulation is initiated in and regulated by the prefrontal portion of the frontal lobes. When the prefrontal cortex is functioning in a sub-optimal manner, the relationship between excitation and inhibition is compromised, resulting in other brain modules operating in an independent, unregulated manner.

A literature search for prefrontal cortex executive yielded 137,000 responses. A typical response: Tomita and Hyoe (1999) "The prefrontal cortex in intimately involved in emotion, memory, judgment, and error detection." Also it is noted that: "Interactions between the thalamus and the cortex mediate shifts in our states of consciousness, the sleep-wake cycle, quiet rest, or attention. Imbalances in the communication between thalamus and cortex is at the core of a host of psychiatric and neurological conditions. Yet, most of our ideas about thalamo-cortrical communication are based on sensory systems, but little is known about high-order association areas of the cortex that govern our thoughts, emotions, and actions" (Zikopoulos and Baras, 2007).

The frontal lobes, especially the prefrontal lobes, manage the balance between activation and inhibition for the rest of the brain (Chow and Cummings, 2007). As HEG science and clinical efficacy advance more and more, selection of training areas must follow the advancing understanding of brain functional connections. A recent advance has taken the thalamus and basal ganglia into consideration. The thalamus is controlled via the basal ganglia. We all know how we can focus attention at will on whatever we want. There must be some brain nucleus that makes focus possible. Now, evidence is available that the basal ganglia are involved in focus. It connects prefrontal areas to the thalamus. The thalamus is an information distributing nucleus. Except for the sense of smell all sensory organs send their information to the thalamus. From the thalamus information is distributed to function specialized nuclei.

We are all familiar with the highly variable intensity we perceive from our senses. The perceived intensity is controlled by the thalamus. We are also well aware that we can change the perception intensity at will by merely focusing on what we want to investigate. Two primary prefrontal areas have been found to activate separate individual basal ganglia focusing connections to the thalamus. One frontal position intensifies our responses while the other quiets these responses. These prefrontal areas are Brodmann's area 9, AFz, for quieting instructions to the thalamus, via the basal ganglia and the subthalamic nucleus, and the orbitofrontal areas between the eyebrows, Brodmann's areas 11 and 12, AFpz, then to the basal ganglia and thence to the subthalamic nucleus of the thalamus.

The thalamus, on receiving appropriate stimulation, then distributes intensity-controlled activation to function-specific nuclei in the cortex. With these two functions we have an accelerator between the eyebrows to intensity activity, and a brake at the middle hairline to quiet cerebral activity. These two areas serve in a balancing act to maintain an appropriate equilibrium between excitement and passivity. From the standpoint of neurotherapy we can arrange an appropriate balance by using nirHEG to appropriately adjust the tipping point between these levels (Viamontes and Beitman, 2007).

If the prefrontal cortex is functioning in a sub-optimal manner, improving its function will improve self-regulation. Even if the prefrontal cortex is functioning adequately, increasing the level of inhibition may also compensate for malfunctioning brain modules far removed from the front of the brain as illustrated in Fig. 7.2 (Toomim and Carmen, 1999).

III. BASIC HEG CONCEPTS

A summary of the basic concepts which can be gleaned from this chapter is as follows:

1. The brain is very plastic and has been shown to change as required to enhance its ability to deal with a challenge.
2. Brain exercise is a basic brain repair and growth promoting technique. Education level increases age of AD onset. Physical exercise increases brain angiogenesis. Brain exercise increases synaptogenesis and angiogenesis. Memory increases correlate with synaptic number increase. Brain nuclei volume has been shown to increase with brain use.
3. Brain activity can be measured non-invasively by cerebral tissue oxygenation and by brain blood temperature. fMRI measures the magnetic moment of deoxygenated hemoglobin and is an accepted scientific standard of brain activity. Blood temperature has been shown to correlate highly with brain metabolism. The Fick method of measuring energy use of the brain, the gold standard, depends on oxygen depletion in exiting venous blood vs. newly entering arterial oxygenated blood.
4. Brain activity is controlled voluntarily. Every voluntary body action or thought is consciously controlled. Body action/thought can be initiated by intent. Blood flow increases in affected brain nuclei to supply the energy that fuels the brain for life support, actions and thought.
5. Brain tissue oxygenation is easily measured by an external light operated spectrophotometer. Brain blood temperature, affected by brain metabolism, can also be used to train brain improvement. It is measurable with an infrared radiation sensitive thermometer.
6. With guidance from the blood flow or temperature mediated measurements, brain blood flow can be increased at will to levels beyond those reached in normal living. This is easily demonstrated with use of oxygen or temperature measuring instruments. We hypothesize that this higher than normal activity in the prefrontal cortex allows the brain to manage other brain modules that may otherwise malfunction.
7. Oxygen increase measurements with an external infrared spectrometer, voluntarily raised to maximum, routinely exceed 10% and have been shown to increase 100%.
8. Published studies have shown clinical improvements in brain function resulting from repeated brain exercise guided by temperature or oxygenation measurements.

A. Cautions, precautions, side effects

Although both authors are very enthusiastic about the use of this new technology, any system capable of having a powerful effect on the human brain has also, by definition, the ability to cause problems. Both forms of HEG have similar side effect profiles. Although the exact mechanism of these side effects remains unknown, most are consistent with the symptoms that would be expected from fatigue of the prefrontal cortex.

Headache: This is an interesting phenomenon because although it is described as a "headache," people often report that there is no real pain. The sensation is that of frontal throbbing rather than actual pain. It is likely that this represents a perception of a sensation with which the person is unfamiliar, and is due to increased cerebral blood flow to the prefrontal cortex. The sensation usually dissipates within one minute of stopping the session. This may not be due to frontal fatigue as much as the presence of an unfamiliar sensation.

Fatigue of the prefrontal cortex: If someone is trained for too long or too intensively, especially during the first session, that person may experience a general loss of self-regulation for the balance of that day. The symptoms are usually an exaggeration of the person's typical symptoms. Support for the hypothesis of frontal fatigue comes from the fact that the following day, after a night's sleep, the symptoms are dramatically reduced.

Difficulty initiating and maintaining sleep: It is unclear if this represents excessive arousal or failure of inhibition. Typically the person leaves with a high level of mental alertness but has difficulty sleeping that evening. This is especially true if the first session takes place late in the day. The effect is dimished after the first few sessions. The solution is to conduct the first few sessions in the morning if at all possible.

B. Overall training guidelines for both HEG systems

Applications: Both forms of HEG have been applied to a wide variety of conditions and disorders. It is becoming apparent to both of us that people who have focal brain modules that are malfunctioning, and people with arousal and inhibition difficulties, are likely to benefit from a trial with HEG technology.

Sensor location: Training locations should be carefully selected, based on current scientific knowledge of brain function. This is likely to change as knowledge of brain mechanisms becomes more precise. Both PIR and NIR systems can be used to target localized brain functions. The NIR system design is more efficient at targeting small areas while the PIR system is more efficient at targeting large areas. Hershel has primarily emphasized targeted placements while Jeff has primarily emphasized a frontal central training location.

Intensity and duration: The intensity and duration of training during each session should be guided by sensitivity and gentleness. Aggressive training is more likely to produce temporary side effects with no increase in training effectiveness.

Session frequency: Acceptable gains, possibly even maximum gains can be obtained with a frequency of once per week. HEG effectiveness is based on brain growth. Sessions that are too close to each other may not allow sufficient time to recover from brain exercise. The exact recovery and growth time varies with each individual, but sessions that are more frequent than twice a week are probably not a good idea.

Because some readers may be more familiar with EEG technology and dynamics than HEG, we decided to end this chapter with FAQs (Frequently Asked Questions). The answers will be provided by each of us, which will serve to demonstrate similarities and differences in personal perspectives as well as instrumentation.

IV.   FREQUENTLY ASKED QUESTIONS

Q: I have heard that PIR measures brain temperature. Is that true?

Jeff: No, at least not in the strictest sense. Having the display look like temperature was in retrospect a mistake, but it is too late to undo it. What is being measured is a thermal waste product from increased levels of cellular metabolism. This process of getting rid of extra heat is what keeps brain cells from overheating. The bare human forehead makes a nice exiting location for excess heat, as well as a convenient location for PIR and NIR sensors.

Q: If PIR measures thermal waste, what does NIR measure?

Hershel: nirHEG measures the color of brain blood flow. Higher demand placed on a brain requires energy to maintain life. The brain lives on glucose (sugar) and oxygen. Increased demand speeds the flow of capillary blood. Fresh blood enters the capillaries and brings oxygenated blood to the neural network. Fresh oxygen colors the brain red. In nirHEG we strive to make the brain as red as possible. With this effort we voluntarily speed blood flow and thereby exercise the targeted brain module. This is a natural activity. We do it all the time. We breathe life into our brains to solve problems, experience love, even to move.

Q: Can a person really be trained to directly control cerebral blood flow?

Hershel: No. This is a common misunderstanding of HEG. Both forms of HEG monitor changes of blood flow. However it is cellular activity, not blood flow, that is being trained. Using other means of inducing increases in cerebral blood flow does not alter focal symptoms.

Jeff: We agree on this. It is even possible that a person cannot be trained to directly control either cerebral blood flow or brain waves. Both blood flow and brain waves represent dependent variables. They are responses to brain cellular demand. However they are reliable in their response, and make convenient data to measure. In both cases, what is being trained is brain cellular activity rather than the dependent variables being monitored.

Q: Why does the brain demand localized increases in blood flow?

Hershel: Blood supply is determined by the load put upon localized areas. Often, in distant brain modules, poor operation can be traced to poor prefrontal control (see Fig. 7.7). Locating the most efficient training position is a science in itself largely dependent on existing prefrontal cortex nerve trunks and brain physiology.

Jeff: It is well known that the increase in blood supply is a response to increased cellular requirements for oxygen and glucose. What is less well known is that an equally important function is thermoregulation. A brain that overheats is at risk of self-destruction. Increased blood flow is one way to help maintain thermal stability. Humans have a forehead that is free from body hair, making the forehead a useful location from which excess brain heat can be transferred from within the skull to the external environment.

Q: Where on the head are the HEG sensors placed?

Hershel: NIR training is very targeted, based on symptoms and localized brain mechanisms. The forehead has widely varying effective areas. Each has a clearly defined function. There are areas for increasing and others for decreasing activity, areas for right brain emotional and others for left brain logical enhancements. The choice of training areas is determined by the needs of the client.

Jeff: This is an area in which Hershel and I have moved in opposite directions. Initially, I tried to apply PIR technology over a wide variety of skull placements based on neuropsychological assessment. This made intuitive sense. However, the strongest effects I found were always from frontal placements. For reasons partially related to differences in language lateralization, I have standardized on sensor placement at Fpz. It is possible to run into trouble by training the wrong side of the brain if the person has language lateralization on the right side of the brain rather than the left. Depression is one serious example in which training on the "wrong" side of the brain may worsen symptoms. Maintaining the sensor at Fpz avoids that problem. Another possible reason for my observations regarding differential placement effectiveness is the difference between PIR and NIR technology. PIR lends itself to monitoring larger more generalized changes whereas NIR lends itself to very focal measurement.

Q: What do you mean by generalized versus focal sensor placement?

Hershel: nirHEG lends itself beautifully to targeted placements. Because of the relatively small volume of brain tissue activity monitored, it can selectively monitor brain activity in a specific area while ignoring brain activity in adjacent areas. This can be very valuable in treatment of stroke where there is a penumbra of viable tissue surrounding the scar tissue damaged by the stroke.

Brain modules normally talk to each other. In autism, viable brain modules are often isolated from other brain modules by inadequate nerve connections. Activating viable brain modules wherever they exist, that often have never been used, exercises the connecting nerves and aids in development of supporting brain areas.

Jeff: pirHEG has a relatively large field of view. The original sensor monitored a circular area with a diameter of about 32 mm. The new sensor developed in 2007 monitors the same vertical response but expands the horizontal response to a 46 mm wide oval. It may be that the large volume of brain activity monitored lends itself more to a single central placement.

Q: So, if these two systems are so different, which one is better to use in a clinical setting?

Hershel and Jeff: This is an area in which we both completely agree. We feel there is a place for each type of technology, and that ideally a clinician should have access to both. Now, if you are new to HEG, reading these FAQs may help make the details of this chapter make more sense.

REFERENCES

Albert, T., Painted, C., Wienbruch, C., Rockstroh, B. and Taub, E. (1995). Increased cortical representation of the fingers of the left hand in string players. *Science*, **270**, 305–307.

Amen, D. G. (1994). New Directions in the Theory, Diagnosis, and Treatment of Mental Disorders: The Use of SPECT Imaging in Everyday Clinical Practice. In *The Neuropsychology of Mental Disorders* (L. F. Koziol and C. E. Stout, eds), pp. 286–311. Springfield, IL: Charles C. Thomas.

American Psychiatric Association (1994). *Diagnostic and Statistical Manual IV*. Washington, DC.

Bednarczyk, E., Remier, B., Weikert, C., Nelson, A. and Reed, R. (1998). Global blood flow, blood volume, and oxygen metabolism in patients with migraine headache. *Neurology*, **50(6)**, 1736–1740.

Berger, H. (1929). Das Electroenkephalogramm des Menchen. *Archive fur Psychiatrie und Nervenkrankheiten*, **87(40)**, 160–179.

Buchsbaum, M. S., Kessler, R., King, A., Johnson, J. and Capeletti, (1984). Simultaneous cerebral glucography with positron emission tomography and topographic electroencephalograph: Brain ischemia: quantitative EEG and imaging techniques. *Progress in Brain Research*, **62**, 263–370.

Carmen, J. A. (2002). Passive Infrared Hemoencephalography: Four years and 100 migraines later. Paper presented at *Society for Neuronal Regulation* annual conference, September, Scottsdale Arizona.

Carmen, J. A. (2004). Infrared Hemoencephalography: Four Years and 100 Migraines. *Journal of Neurotherapy*, **8(3)**, 23–51.

Chance, B., Cohen, P., Jobsis, F. and Schoener, B. (1962). Intracellular oxidation and reduction in vivo. *Science*, **137**, 499–508.

Chance, B., Leigh, J. S., Miyake, H., *et al.* (1988). Comparison of Time-Resolved and -Unresolved Measurements of Deoxyhemoglobin in Brain. *Proc. Natl Acad. Sci.*, July, **85(14)**, 4971–4975.

Chow, T. W. and Cummings, J. L. (2007). Frontal-Subcortical Circuits, 25–43, in Miller, B. L. and Cummings, J. L. (eds.) The Human Frontal Lobes, second edition. The Guilford Press, New York.

Diamond, M. C., Kretch, D. and Rosenzweig, M. R. (1964). The effects of an enriched environment on the histology of the rat cerebral cortex. *J. Comp. Neurol.*, **123**, 111–120.

Diamond, S. (1994). Head Pain: diagnosis and management. *Clinical Symposia*, **46(3)**, 2–34.

Goadsby, P. (2001). Pathophysiology of headache. In *Wolff's Headache and other Head Pain* (S. Silberstein, R. Lipton and D. Dalessio, eds), 7th edition, pp. 57–72. New York: Oxford University Press, Inc.

Goldberg, E. (2001). *The executive brain*. New York: Oxford University Press, Inc.

Gratton, G., Maier, J. S., Fabiani, M., Mantulin, and Gratton, E. (1994). Feasibility of intracranial near-infrared optical scanning. *Psychophysiology*, **31**, 211–215.

Gratton, G., Corballis, P. M., Cho, E., Fabiani, M. and Hood, D. C. (1995a). Shades of gray matter: Noninvasive optical images of human brain responses during visual stimulation. *Psychophysiology*, **32**, 505–509.

Gratton, G., Fabiani, M. and Corballis, P. M. (1995). Can we measure correlates of neuronal activity with non-invasive optical methods? Optical Imaging of Brain Function and Metabolism: Physiological Basis and Comparison to other Functional Neuroimaging Methods. In *Advances in Experimental Medicine and Biology* (A.Villinger and U. Dirnagel, eds). New York: N.Y. Plenum Press.

Gratton, G., Fabiani, M., Friedman, D., *et al.* (1995). Rapid changes of optical parameters in the human brain during a tapping task. *J. Cog. Neuro Sci.*, **7(4)**, 446–458.

Grey, and Walter, W. (1964). Contingent negative variation: An electrical sign of sensorimotor association and expectancy in the human brain. *Nature*, **203**, 380–384.

Hoshi, Y. and Tamura, M. (1993). Detection of dynamic changes in cerebral oxygenation coupled to neuronal function during mental work in man. *Neuroscience Letters*, **150**, 5–8.

Hoshi, Y. and Tamura, M. (1994). Multichannel near-infrared optical imaging of brain activity. *Neuro Science Protocols*, 94-070-04-02-15.

Ingvar, B. S. and Anders, A. (1976). Correlation between dominant EEG frequency, cerebral oxygen uptake and blood flow. *Enceph. Clin. Neurophysiol.*, **41**, 268–276.

Janzen, T., Graap, K., Stephanson, S., Marshall, W. and Fitzsimmons, G. (1995). Differences in baseline measures for ADD and normally achieving preadolescent males. *Biofeedback and Self Regulation*, **20(1)**.

Jerison, H. J. (2007). Evolution of the Frontal Lobes. In (B. L. Miller and J. L. Cummings, eds). The Human frontal lobes 2nd ed. pp. 107–118, New York: Guilford Press.

Kiyaikin, E. A. (2002). Brain temperature fluctuation: a reflection of functional neural activation. *European Journal of Neuroscience*, **16(1)**, 164–168.

Kurth, C. D., Steven, J. M., Benaron, D. and Chance, B. (1993). Near infra-red monitoring of the cerebral circulation. *J. Clin. Monitoring*, **9(3)**, July, 163–170.

Lassen, N. A. (1959). Cerebral blood flow and oxygen consumption in man. *Physiological Reviews*, **39(2)**, 183–238.

Lipton, R. B., Stewart, W. F., Diamond, S., Diamond, M. and Reed, M. L. (2001). Prevalence and burden of migraine in the United States: Results from American Migraine Study II. *Headache*, **41(7)**, 646–657.

Maguire, E. A., Gadian, D. G., Johnsrude, I. S., Good, C. D., Ashbrunner, J. and Frakowiack, R. S. (2000). Navigation-related structural change in the hippocampi of taxi drivers. *Proc. Natl Acad. Sci. U.S.A.*, **97**, 4398–4403.

Mann, C. A., Lubar, J., Zimmerman, A. W., Miller, C. A. and Muenchen, R. A. (1992). Quantitative analysis of EEG in boys with attention deficit disorder: Controlled study with clinical implications. *Pediatric Neurology*, **8(1)**, 30–36.

Meyer, J. S., Sakamoto, K., Akiyama, M., Yoshida, K. and Yoshitake, S. (1967). Monitoring cerebral blood flow, metabolism and EEG. *Electroenceph. Clin. Neuro.*, **23**, 97–508.

Moskowitz, M. (1998). Migraine and stroke – a review of cerebral blood flow. *Cephalalgia*, **18(22)**, 22–25.

Pinker, S. (1997). *How the mind works.* New York: W. W. Norton & Company, Inc.

Pompei, F. and Pompei, M. (1996). *Physicians Reference Handbook on Temperature; Vital Sign Assessment with Infrared Thermometry.* Watertown: Exergen Corporation.

Pribram, K. and McGuinness, D. (1975). Arousal, activation, and effort in control of attention. *Psychological Review*, **82(2)**, 116–149.

Proctor, H. J., Sylvia, A. L. and Jobsis, F. F. (1982). Failure of brain cytochrome alpha, alpha3 redox after hypoxic hypotension as determined by in vivo reflectance spectrophotometry. *Stroke*, **13(1)**, Jan–Feb, 89–92.

Raichle, M. E. (1987). Circulatory and metabolic correlates of brain function in normal humans. In *Handbook of Physiology* The Nervous System. (V. B. Mountcastle, F. Plum and S. R. Geiger, eds) **Vol. 5**. Bethesda Maryland: American Physiology Society.

Roland, P. E. (1993). *Brain Activation.* John A. Wiley & Sons. , Ch 18. 469–503

Roy, S. and Sherrington, C. J. (1890). On the regulation of the blood supply of the brain. *J. Physiol.*, **11**, 85–108.

Sacks, O. (1992). *Migraine.* England: University of California Press.

Shevelev, I. A. (1992). Temperature topography of the brain cortex: Thermoencephaloscopy. *Brain Topography*, **6(2)**, 77–85.

Shevelev, I. A. (1998). Functional imaging of the brain by infrared radiation (thermoencephaloscopy). *Progress in Neurobiology*, **56(3)**, 269–305.

Schiffer, F. (1998). *Of Two Minds*. New York: The Free Press.

Swerdlow, B. and Dieter, J. (1991). The value of medical thermography for the diagnosis of chronic headache. *Headache Quarterly*, **2(2)**, 96–104.

Taub, E., Miller, N. E., Novack, T. A., Cook, E. W., Fleming, W. C. and Nepomuceno, C. S. (1993). Technique to improve chronic motor deficit after stroke. *Archives of Physical Medicine*, **74**, 347–354.

Tinius T. ed. (2004). *New developments in blood flow hemoencephalogrqphy*. Binghamton, New York: Haworth Medical Press.

Tokarev, V. and Fleishman, A. (1998). Technical and engineering implementation of REG (Rheoencephalography) biofeedback training at the West Siberian Metallurgical Plant. *Russian Academy of Medical Science*, **20**, 432–435.

Tomita, M. and Hyoe, M. (1999). Top down signal from prefrontal cortex in executive control of memory retrieval. *Nature*, **461**, 10/14/99, 699–703.

Toomim, H. (1995). Brain blood flow and neurofeedback. Presented at annual meeting of the AAPB. Available from *Biocomp Research Institute*.

Toomim, H. (2002). Neurofeedback with hemoencephalography. *Explore for the Professional*, **11(2)**, 19–21.

Toomim, H. and Carmen, J. A. (1999). Hemoencephalography (HEG). *Biofeedback Society of California News letter*, **27(4)**, 10–14.

Toomim, H., Carmen, J.A., and Collura, T. F. (2007). Intelligent activation of stem cells. Paper presented at annual conference of *International Society for Neuronal Regulation*.

Toomim, H., Marsh, R., Kowalski, G. P., *et al.* (2004). Intentional Increase of Cerebral Blood Oxygenation Using Hemoencephalography (HEG): An Efficient Brain Exercise Therapy. *Journal of Neurotherapy*, **8(3)**, 5–21.

Toomim, H. and Marsh, R. (1999). *Biofeedback of Human Central Nervous System Activity Using Radiation Detection*. Washington D.C.: US Patent and Trademark Office. US Patent number 5,995,857.

van Prang, H., Christie, B. R., Terrence, J., Sejnowski, T. J. and Gage, F. H. (1999). Running enhances neurogenesis, learning, and long term potentiation in mice. *PNAS*, **96(23)**, 13427–13439.

Viamontes, G. I. and Beitman, B. D. (2007). Neural Substrates of Psychotherapeutic Change: Beyond Default Mode. *Psychiatric Annals*, . , 00:0 Month 200x 238–245. In Press.

Yamashita, Y., Maki, A. and Ito, Y. (1995). Noninvasive near-infrared topography of human brain activity. *J. Optical Society*, 212 650 5530;#7/16 8–7

Zametkin, A. J., Nordahl, T. E., Gross, *et al.* (1990). Cerebral glucose metabolism in adults with hyperactivity of childhood onset. *The New England Journal of Medicine*, **323(20)**, 1361–1366.

Zikopoulos, B. and Baras, H. (2007). Parallel driving and modulatory pathways link the prefrontal cortex and thalamus. *Public Library of Science*, **2(9)**, e848.doI10 1371/journal.pone 0000848.

CHAPTER 8

Audio-visual entrainment in relation to mental health and EEG

Thomas F. Collura, Ph.D.[1] and David Siever, CET[2]

[1]*BrainMaster Technologies, Inc., Oakwood, Ohio, USA*
[2]*Mind Alive Inc., Edmonton, Alberta, Canada*

I. OVERVIEW

If the language of the brain lies in its neuronal coding, then the expression of the brain lies in its rhythmicity and timing. The rhythmicity is due to the selective synchronization and desynchronization of the encoding within billions of pools of neurons which provide the sensory activity of everything that is sensed, thought, or done. Berger (1929) observed all four main rhythms—the alpha, beta, theta, and delta—in his very first EEG recording. It should come as no surprise, therefore, that since the earliest EEG studies, interest has turned toward rhythmic sensory stimulation, and its possible effects on brain function.

Auditory or visual stimulation (AVS) can take a wide variety of forms, generating different subjective and clinical effects. The simplest form of stimulation is to present a series of arbitrary light flashes or sound clicks to a subject, and investigate the resulting subjective or EEG effects, whereas audio-visual entrainment (AVE) would involve stimulation at a particular frequency. This "open loop" stimulation is not contingent on the EEG brainwave in any way. From this basic form, changes can be made in the type of stimulation, without dependence on the EEG waves.

Clinical reports of flicker stimulation appear as far back as the dawn of modern medicine. It was at the turn of the twentieth century when Pierre Janet, at the Salpêtrière Hospital in France, reported that by having his patients gaze into the flickering light produced from a spinning, spoked wheel in front of a kerosene lantern, there was a reduction in their depression, tension and hysteria (Pieron, 1982). With the development of the EEG, Adrian and Matthews published their results showing that the alpha rhythm could be "driven" above and below the natural frequency with photic stimulation (Adrian and Matthews, 1934). This discovery prompted several small physiological outcome studies on the "flicker following

Introduction to QEEG and Neurofeedback, Second Edition
ISBN: 978-0-12-374534-7

response," the brain's electrical response to stimulation (Bartley, 1934, 1937; Durup and Fessard, 1935; Jasper, 1936; Goldman *et al.*, 1938; Jung, 1939; Toman, 1941).

In 1956, W. Gray Walter published the first results on thousands of test subjects comparing flicker stimulation with the *subjective* emotional feelings it produced (Walter, 1956). Test subjects reported all types of visual illusions and in particular the "whirling spiral," which was significant with alpha production. Finally, in the late 1950s, as a result of Kroger's observations as to why US military radar operators often drifted into trance, Kroger teamed up with Sidney Schneider of the Schneider Instrument Company, and produced the world's first electronic clinical photic stimulator—the "Brainwave Synchronizer." It had powerful hypnotic qualities, and soon after studies on hypnotic induction began to be published (Kroger and Schneider, 1959; Lewerenz, 1963; Sadove, 1963; Margolis, 1966).

In the "open-loop" system of visual stimulation, flickering or flashing light can be replaced with sine wave and other types of modulated light. Generally, the more elaborate the photic stimulation, the greater the potential for the brain to interpret and respond. For example, sine-wave modulated light has a significantly greater effect on endogenous rhythms than a simple flickering light. In the case of auditory stimulation, simple clicks can be replaced with modulated or "warbling" sounds, or with binaurally presented "beats." In the case of binaural beats, two different signals are presented to each ear, and the reconstruction of the frequency difference or "beat" is performed within the brain itself.

It is also possible to introduce dependence of the stimulation on the EEG wave, so that it becomes EEG-driven, or "closed-loop," or "contingent." Contingent stimulation is produced when the parameters of the feedback are determined by the properties of the EEG. There is a variety of ways to achieve closed-loop control of feedback. These include both direct (phase-sensitive) and indirect (frequency or amplitude-sensitive) methods. Contingent stimulation greatly increases the possibility for learning to occur, and learning may even occur without conscious effort ("volition"). When the brain is presented with information (including stimulation that reflects EEG information), the possibilities for classical conditioning, operant conditioning, concurrent learning, and self-efficacy arise.

There is a variety of ways to make the stimulation contingent on the EEG, and these include approaches described by Carter *et al.* (2000), Davis (2005) and Collura (2005). These methods can be broken into two types: phase-sensitive and frequency-sensitive. In phase-sensitive feedback, the photic stimulation is determined by the exact details of the EEG wave, including the timing of peaks and valleys (Davis, 2005). The original Roshi I and Roshi II devices employed a proprietary algorithm that converted the complex EEG waveform into a pattern of flashes. The resulting stimulation was EEG-dependent, and reflected the details of the time behavior of the signal.

With frequency-sensitive methods, some EEG frequency parameters are first determined, such as peak or dominant frequency, and then the stimulation rate is set based upon this information (Russell, 1996; Ochs, 1994; Carter and Russell,

1993). It is further possible to control the onset and end of stimulation using EEG parameters. For an overview and bibliography of the technical and physiological issues see Collura (2002).

As EEG equipment improved, so did a renewed interest in the brain's evoked electrical response to photic and auditory entrainment, and soon a flurry of studies was completed (Barlow, 1960; Van der tweel and Lunel, 1965; Kinney, 1973; Townsend, 1973; Donker, 1978; Frederick et al., 1999; Chatrain et al., 1959).

II. EVIDENCE OF SENSORY EFFECTS OF AVE

Published work in AVE tends to fall into one of three categories: 1) Subjective experiential effects of AVE, 2) EEG changes associated with AVE with possible diagnostic value, and 3) clinical applications of AVE. The first type of work has been reported by Huxley (1954), Budzynski et al. (1999, 2007), and others. These have shown that rhythmic information can produce unique sensory experiences, associated with the properties of the stimulation. These can include sensations such as activation, relaxation, or discomfort, visual experiences, and "twilight" states.

Aldous Huxley (1954) was among the first to articulate the subjective correlates of what he described as the "stroboscopic lamp." In his view, "we descend from chemistry to the still more elementary realm of physics. Its rhythmically flashing light seems to act directly, through the optic nerves, on the electrical manifestations of the brain's activity." He described subjective experiences of incessantly changing patterns, whose color was a function of the rate of flashing. Between 10 and 15 flashes per second, he reported orange and red; above 15, green and blue; above18, white and gray. He also described enriched and intensified experiences when subjects were under the effects of mescaline or lysergic acid.

In his view, the rhythms of the lamp interacted with the rhythms of the brain's electrical activity to produce a complex interference pattern which is translated by the brain's apparatus into a conscious pattern of color and movement. He remained mystified, however, by one subject who reported seeing an abstract geometry described as a "Japanese landscape" of surpassing beauty, charged with preternatural light and color. Clearly, this simple procedure elicited brain responses far more complex than a simple interference pattern involving basic rhythmic interactions. It comprises the first report of the subjective responses to a simple, non-contingent stimulation.

The second type of work is reported by Gray Walter (1956), Regan (1989) , Collura (1996, 2001), Silberstein et al. (1990), and Frederick et al. (1999, 2004). These studies have shown that stimulation can produce both transient and lasting changes in the EEG. Collura (1978) articulated the relationship between the low-frequency and high-frequency components of the steady-state visual evoked potential as reflecting anatomically and physiologically distinct response mechanisms, and also demonstrated that the short-term waxing and waning in the steady-state visual evoked response reflects short-term changes in attention. It has been found that contingent stimulation has significantly greater effect in producing lasting changes, when compared to non-contingent stimulation.

The third type of work has been reported by Evans (1972), Hammond (2000), Carter and Russell (1993), Ochs (1994) and (Siever, 2007). This approach emphasizes clinical changes and applies the various forms of AVE, in an effort to delineate the visible effects which can be used therapeutically. When an empirical approach is used, benefits may be observed that would not be expected, based upon first principles. Clinical benefits have included improvements in attention and concentration, and reduction of depression.

Evans (1972) was particularly interested in the potential for simultaneous visual, auditory and tactile stimulation to assist with severely retarded children, and reported promising results. Davis (1999) developed a different type of EEG-controlled nonvolitional method that used parameters of the EEG signal to control light flashes. This approach incorporates particular aspects of the EEG signal in real-time. Hammond's (2000) report employs this system in a single case study that demonstrated efficacy in the case of depression. More recently, Davis has developed an open-loop method ("pRoshi") that provides similar stimulation dynamics, but does not utilize EEG control (Davis, 2005). Carter et al. (2000) described a method that extracts a determination of the dominant frequency in the EEG and uses this information to determine the frequency of stimulation. Both stimulation and entrainment are then non-contingent, consisting of a brief presentation of open-loop stimulation. They have reported clinical benefits, particularly in relation to learning and attention.

Additional clinical studies explored the use of photic entrainment to induce hypnotic trance (Kroger and Schneider, 1959; Lewerenz, 1963), to augment anesthesia during surgery (Sadove, 1963) and to reduce pain, control gagging and accelerate healing in dentistry (Margolis, 1966). More recently, the induction of dissociation was explored (Leonard et al., 1999; Leonard, et al., 2000), which aided the understanding of dissociative pathology and development of better techniques for relaxing people suffering from trauma and post-traumatic stress disorder (Siever, 2006).

III.   PHYSIOLOGICAL EFFECTS OF AVE SYSTEMS

Srinivarsan (1988) described a method to make the intensity of photic stimulation directly related to the instantaneous amplitude of the subject's EEG alpha wave. The stimulation was thus both phase-locked to, and proportional to, the size of the alpha signal. He reported enhanced alpha amplitude when subjects attended to the stimulator, with concomitant subjective reports consistent with enhanced alpha activity. Systems such as these do not appeal to any need for operant conditioning, or for instructions to the test subject. These methods are thus deemed "nonvolitional" in that they do not depend on the volition (intent) of the subject.

Collura (2005, 2007) has further described a nonvolitional method that employs selective photic entrainment at a predetermined flicker frequency, but which is presented contingent on the EEG meeting certain criteria. This approach can be used to inhibit particular EEG rhythms, and is also a nonvolitional method.

The following single-session example demonstrates the capability of EEG-controlled photic entrainment, when applied in an extinction learning model, to reduce excess theta activity. The trainee complained of not being able to control the level of their theta, and that it was known to be in excess in previous EEG analyses. The sensor was placed at Oz, and a single channel of EEG was used. The method was based on Collura (2005), as a means of reducing the theta activity by nonvolitional EEG-controlled training. The following results were obtained during a 60-minute test session with a 5-minute photic training period beginning at minute 30, with no additional instructions given to the trainee (see Fig. 8.1).

The chart shows theta (4.0–7.0 Hz) amplitude as a function of time, during a test session. Minutes 1–30: conventional neurofeedback. Minute 30: Contingent photic stimulation (14 Hz peripheral white LEDs flashed when theta > threshold) begins. Minute 35: Contingent photic stimulation is withdrawn. The continued effect of the learned extinction is evident. Minute 47: Trainee is talking, motion artifact is present.

The initial 30 minutes of monitoring showed the expected high levels of theta, averaging above 20 microvolts peak-to-peak. During this time, conventional feedback was presented in the form of bar graphs and sounds indicating when theta was below a threshold. At minute 31, photic stimulation was introduced, so that flashes at 14 per second were delivered, whenever the momentary theta value exceeded a second threshold value. For the next 5 minutes, the trainee experienced the intermittent

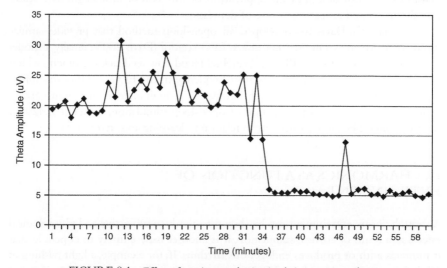

FIGURE 8.1   Effect of contingent photic stimulation on excess theta.

14 Hz photic stimulation in both eyes, using peripheral LED glasses, so that they could continue to watch the EEG biofeedback display. At minute 35, the stimulation was discontinued, and the trainee continued to watch the neurofeedback display, as before.

Figure 8.1 shows that the theta amplitude changed abruptly, from its standing level of over 20 microvolts to a level below 10 microvolts, within the 5-minute learning period. Moreover, the theta amplitude remains at the new level well after the removal of the stimulation, and does not show any tendency to recover or "creep up" for the remainder of the session. The "blip" at minute 47 occurs when the trainee is talking, basically remarking that "my theta level is staying down."

It appears from these results that the effect of the 5-minute learning interval was to produce a sustained change in theta activity that persisted well after the stimulation was withdrawn. Therefore, in contrast to "open-loop" stimulation, this method produces a robust and clear learning effect that is lasting. Furthermore, this learning did not depend on intention, as the trainee was given no instructions. Rather, the training was nonvolitional. The learning process was thus a result of intrinsic brain processes mediating the change directly, as a result of the effect of the stimulation on theta production.

A variety of modifications of audio-visual entrainment have been tested, with promising results. Rozelle and Budzynski (1995) used a prototype "EEG-Driven AVS" device developed by Ochs to augment neurofeedback in the successful treatment of a stroke client. This device sampled the client's EEG then automatically adjusted the AVE frequency to either lead or lag the dominant EEG frequency. Davis (1999) has developed a different type of EEG-controlled nonvolitional method that uses parameters of the EEG signal to control light flashes. This approach incorporates particular aspects of the EEG signal in real-time. Hammond (2000) describes the application of this system in a single case study that demonstrated efficacy in a case of depression.

More recently, Davis has developed an open-loop method that provides similar stimulation dynamics, but does not utilize EEG control (Davis 2005). Finally, a model of photic entrainment using EEG and cerebral blood flow feedback is eminent, which extracts a determination of the dominant frequency in the EEG, and uses this information to establish the frequency of stimulation. Entrainment is then non-contingent, consisting of a brief presentation of open-loop stimulation. Carter et al. (2000) reported clinical benefits, particularly in relation to learning and attention.

IV.   HARMONICS AS A FUNCTION OF ENTRAINMENT

Although photic entrainment can be shown to produce subjective and physiological effects as a result of cortical stimulation, it is another issue entirely to conclude that it interacts with or produces endogenous rhythms. If, for example, a light flashing at 10 flashes per second produces EEG responses at 10 cycles per second, this does not imply that the flashing is producing an "alpha" rhythm. Endogenous rhythms are associated with particular thalamocortical and corticocortical mechanisms, and are self-sustaining (Sterman, 1996). Responses to flickering light, on the other hand, are produced by the same mechanisms that produce simple evoked potentials, and thus involve sensory and perceptual mechanisms that are different from the innate cortical rhythmic generators. This is confirmed by the fact that photic "entrainment" effects in the EEG are invariably seen to vanish when the stimulation is withdrawn. In other words, the EEG is not "entrained" in the sense of "driving" an alpha rhythm. Rather, a repetitive evoked potential is produced, whose frequency content is simply related to the stimulating flashes, and the presence of these frequencies reflects an entirely different mechanism and functional anatomical basis when compared with endogenous rhythms.

Harmonics are also commonly seen in the EEG responses to photic stimulation. Again, these do not need to be interpreted as "beta" or "gamma" rhythms produced by the stimulation. Rather, the presence of higher harmonics is understood as a simple product of the complex waveform that is elicited. True beta, gamma, and similar high-frequency EEG rhythms are produced by particular cortico-cortical mechanisms, and are modulated as a function of cortical excitability. When a visual evoked response is produced, it has its own low-frequency and high-frequency components, regardless of the frequency of stimulation. The high-frequency components are the primary cortical responses, and low-frequency components reflect secondary cortical mechanisms. It so happens that when the stimulation occurs at certain rates, the overlapping of the separate evoked potential components reinforces a particular component, due to the linear superposition of the waveforms. Thus, the frequencies elicited by repetitive stimulation reflect different neuronal mechanisms than those producing endogenous rhythms.

As a result, the benefits of AVE are not simple or "automatic." That is, by stimulating at or near the alpha frequency, for example, we should not expect to elicit the same effects as the brain producing its endogenous alpha rhythm. There may be subjective correlates to the stimulation that resemble an alpha state, but this is not an intrinsic alpha state. In furthering the field, both the short-term and long-term EEG and clinical effects of the stimulation must be studied, in order to produce solid scientific and clinical rationale.

V.   EFFECTS OF AUDIO-VISUAL ENTRAINMENT

AVE is believed to achieve its effects through several mechanisms simultaneously. These include:

A. Altered EEG activity
B. Dissociation/hypnotic induction
C. Limbic stabilization

D. Improved neurotransmitter production

E. Altered cerebral blood flow.

It is important to delineate the difference between audio-visual stimulation (AVS) and audio-visual entrainment (AVE). Watching TV, a car driving by, or being at a noisy mall or theme park all constitute AVS, where there is a great deal of stimulation; all of it, however, is quite random and unorganized. This type of stimulation doesn't necessarily leave a significant imprint on one's psyche, cerebral blood flow or brain wave activity.

AVE is a subset of AVS where constant, repetitive stimuli of the proper frequency and sufficient strength to "excite" the thalamus, and neo-cortex, must be present. These stimuli do not transfer energy directly into the cortex as TV and radio waves do into a tuned circuit, nor in the same manner as placing a tuning fork near another tuning fork that is vibrating at the same frequency thus making the silent fork "hum" as well. The direct transmission of energy from AVE only goes so far as to excite retinal cells in the eyes, and pressure-sensitive cilia within the cochlea of the ears. The nerve pathways from the eyes and ears carry the elicited electrical potentials into the thalamus. From there, the entrained electrical activity within the thalamus is "amplified" and distributed throughout other limbic areas and the cerebral cortexes via the *cortical thalamic loop*. In essence, AVE involves the continuous electrical response of the brain in relation to the stimulus frequency, plus the mathematical representation (harmonics) of the stimulus wave shape. Figure 8.2 shows the visual pathways for visual entrainment. Figure 8.3 shows an occipital record of square wave visual entrainment at 2, 4, 8, 12 and 20 Hz (Kinney *et al.*, 1973).

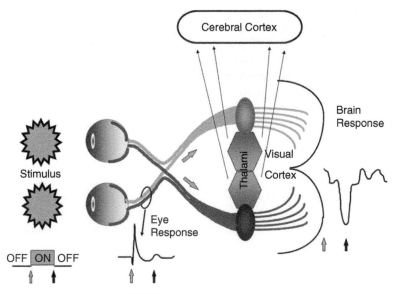

FIGURE 8.2   Visual pathways.

A. Altered EEG activity

The effects of AVE on the EEG are primarily found frontally, over the sensory-motor strip, and in parietal (somato-sensory) regions, and slightly less within the prefrontal cortex. It is within these areas where executive function, motor activation and somato-sensory (body) awareness are primarily mediated. It is believed this is why AVE lends itself well for the treatment of such a wide variety of disorders including PTSD, panic, anxiety, depression, cognitive decline, and attentional disorders. Eyes-closed AVE at 18.5 Hz has been shown to increase EEG brain wave activity by 49% at the vertex (CZ) (the only site examined in this study). Auditory entrainment (AE) is the same concept as visual entrainment with the exception that auditory signals are passed into the thalamus via the medial geniculate, whereas visual entrainment passes into the thalamus via the lateral geniculate (McClintic, 1978). At the vertex (with the eyes-closed) AE produced an increase in EEG brain wave activity by 21% (Frederick *et al.*, 1999). Successful entrainment leads to a meditative kind of dissociation, where the user experiences a loss of somatic and cognitive awareness.

Only a sine wave produces a single harmonic. Complex waves are made up of a multitude of harmonics; it is therefore reasonable to expect that a non-sine wave stimulus can generate harmonics in the brain. Figure 8.4 shows a combination sine-square stimulus with a second harmonic that shows up in the EEG record of this subject.

B. Dissociation/hypnotic induction

Dissociation occurs in varying degrees when we meditate, exercise, enter a hypnotic trance, read a good book, become involved in a movie or enjoy a sporting event.

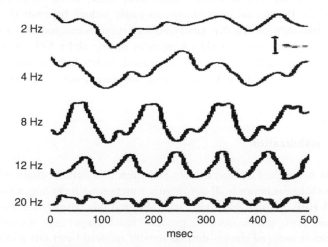

FIGURE 8.3   Visual entrainment effects on the occiput.

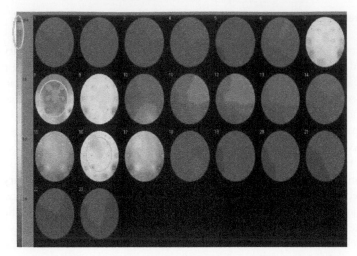

FIGURE 8.4   Brain map in 1 Hz bins during 8 Hz AVE ("SKIL" analysis—eyes-closed).

We get drawn into the present moment and let go of thoughts relating to our daily hassles, hectic schedules, paying rent, urban noise, worries, threats or anxieties and the resultant, often unhealthy, mental chatter. Dissociation involves a "disconnection" of self from thoughts and somatic awareness, as is experienced during deep meditation. As dissociation begins (after approximately 4–8 minutes) from properly applied AVE, a *restabilization* effect occurs where muscles relax, electrodermal activity decreases, peripheral blood flow stabilizes (hand temperature normalizes to 32–33° C), breathing becomes diaphragmatic and slow, and heart rate becomes uniform and smooth. Visual entrainment alone, in the lower alpha frequency range (7–10 Hz), has been shown to easily induce hypnosis (Lewerenz, 1963); and it has been shown that nearly 80% of subjects entered into a either a light or deep hypnotic trance within 6 minutes during alpha AVE (Kroger and Schneider, 1959), as shown in Fig. 8.5. Additional studies have shown that AVE provides an excellent medium for achieving an altered state of consciousness (Glickson, 1987).

C. Limbic stabilization

The amygdala is activated by fear, anxiety and stress (the fight-or-flight response), and the hypothalamus controls all autonomic functioning including muscle tension, electrodermal response, heart rate, arterial tone, body temperature, eating and satiety. Because AVE can be used to produce hand-temperature normalization, muscle relaxation, reduced electro-dermal activity, reduced heart rate and reduced hypertension, it is speculated that AVE may produce a calming effect on these

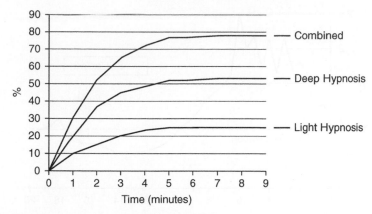

FIGURE 8.5   Photic stimulation induction of hypnotic trance (Kroger and Schneider, 1959).

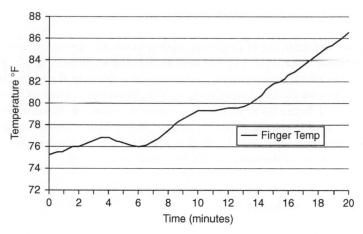

FIGURE 8.6   Finger temperature levels during AVE (n = 1).

limbic structures. AVE therefore lends itself very well to stabilizing panic and anxiety. When using white light as the stimulus, measures of finger temperature, electromyograph (EMG), electro-dermal response (EDR), and heart-rate variability (HRV) have been dramatically improved within 10 minutes.

Figure 8.6 shows increasing (normalizing) finger temperature in one subject. Figure 8.7 shows decreased electrodermal response using white-light AVE (DAVID system) at alpha frequencies. Notice that the normalization effect begins following roughly 6 minutes of AVE.

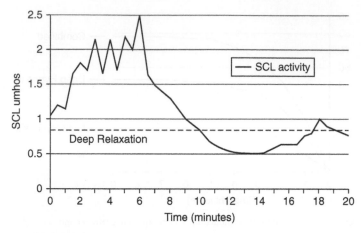

FIGURE 8.7   Reduced electrodermal activity during alpha AVE (n = 1).

D.   Improved neurotransmitter production

People under the influence of long-term anxiety eventually develop *adrenal fatigue* (hypo-adrenalis), characterized by exhaustion and fatigue (Wilson, 2001). And as both serotonin and norepinephrine production shuts down in the brain, depression sets in (Sapolsky, 2003). In one study of AVE, blood serum levels of serotonin, endorphine, and melatonin all increased considerably following 10 Hz, white-light photic stimulation (Shealy *et al.*, 1989). Several clinical studies showed declines in depression, anxiety and/or suicide ideation following a treatment program using AVE, e.g., Gagnon and Boersma, (1992); Berg and Siever, (2004).

E.   Altered cerebral blood flow

SPECT and FMRI imaging show that hypo-perfusion of cerebral blood flow (CBF) is associated with many forms of mental disorders (Rubin et al., 1994) including anxiety and depression (Wu *et al.*, 1992; Cohen, *et al.*, 1992), attentional problems (Teicher *et al.*, 2000), behavior disorders, and impaired cognitive function (Mortel *et al.*, 1994; Hirsch *et al.*, 1997).

AVE has been shown to increase brain glucose metabolism overall by 5%, and to increase CBF in the striate cortex, peaking at a 28% increase at 7.8 Hz.(Fox and Raichle, 1985). This, coincidentally, is the *Schumann Resonance*, the frequency that electro-magnetic radiation propagates around the earth (Schumann, 1952; Bliokh *et al.*, 1980; Sentam, 1987). In addition, AVE has been shown to increase CBF throughout various other brain regions including frontal areas (Mentis *et al.*, 1997; Sappey-Marinier *et al.*, 1992).

VI.   CLINICAL PROTOCOLS WITH FREE-RUNNING AUDIO-VISUAL ENTRAINMENT

Hundreds of thousands of people have successfully used audio-visual entrainment (AVE) to reduce or manage the symptoms of their disorders, syndromes, and ailments. To date, a number of AVE-related studies with clinical outcomes have been completed, and more are in progress. A number of the studies with clinical implications are listed below:

Attention deficit disorder	4 (n = 359, school children)
Academic performance in college students	2 (n = 22, college students)
Improved cognitive performance in seniors	4 (n = 86)
Reduced falling in seniors	1 (n = 80, seniors)
Dental—during dental procedures	2 (n = 36)
Temporo-mandibular joint dysfunction	2 (n = 43, middle-aged)
Seasonal affective disorder	1 (n = 74, middle-aged)
Pain and fibromyalgia	3 (n = 66, middle-aged)
Insomnia	1 (n = 10, middle-aged)
PTSD	~600 cases (public, police and military)
Migraine headache	1 (n = 7)
Hypertension	1 (n = 28)
Stroke	1 (n = 1)

A.   How AVE protocols (sessions) are designed

Since the inception of the original DAVID1 in 1984, designing sessions has been a multifaceted approach, and a lengthy process. Session designs are drawn from personal experience, results from clients and from practicing health professionals. The DAVID Session Editor (Fig. 8.8) is a valuable tool for allowing clinicians free reign over their customized session design. The Editor allows independent left and right frequency control from 0–25.5 Hz, including a steady-on state on either side. Intensity of light, type of auditory tone and heart beat pacer, plus its pitch and volume are also adjustable. Various waveforms (sine wave, triangle wave, sine-square combination, and square waves) of the light stimulation are also pre-settable.

Stimulation in the left visual field of both eyes and left ear evokes activity in the right hemisphere of the brain whereas stimulation in the right visual fields of both eyes and right ear evokes activity in the left hemisphere of the brain. Therefore, when this guide refers to left or right brain it is referring to the activity or side of the brain that is being activated. For example, "Left Brain Beta/Right Brain SMR" means that a beta frequency of auditory and visual stimulation is being presented to the right visual fields and right ear to produce a response in the left side of the brain, and SMR stimulation would come from the left side to produce a response in the right side of the brain.

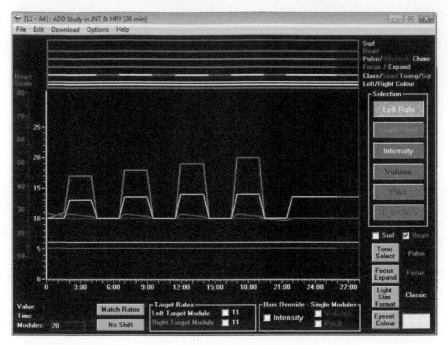

FIGURE 8.8   DAVID session editor.

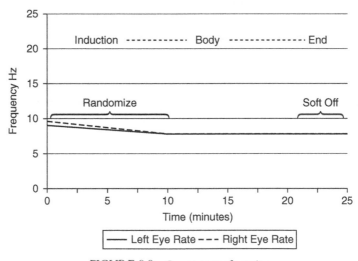

FIGURE 8.9   Components of a session.

B. Components of a session

As shown in Fig. 8.9, AVE sessions generally comprise three sections: an initial induction process, body, and ending. With eyes-closed AVE, the induction process is crucial in dissociating the user so that: a) the cortical-thalamic entrainable rhythm can maximize, and b) there can be calming of the autonomic nervous system as seen in Figs. 8.7 and 8.8 above. Most sessions in the DAVID systems begin with a 0.5 Hz difference between the left and right stimuli. This sets up a slow beat frequency, which is quite dissociating. A unique randomization process, which follows the frequency offset, also begins following the first minute of AVE. In the case of simple alpha, theta and delta sessions, this randomization continues until the target frequency is reached. Complex sessions do not generally require randomization as the complexity of the session provides its own dissociative induction. All DAVID sessions end with a "soft-off" process, where the session fades out gently, so as not to startle the user (Siever, 2000).

C. "Rules of thumb"

As with any intervention, there are guidelines as to when to receive treatment, and what the treatment should look like. In order to achieve the best results from AVE, we recommend the following as guidelines or "rules of thumb."

1. Drink a glass of water before every AVE session. Do this for at least the first six sessions and particularly with depression, ADD/ADHD, and cognitive decline in seniors where a condition of hypoperfusion of cerebral blood flow exists.
2. Close your eyes during the session for best effects, although keeping your eyes open is not harmful.
3. Use beta sessions in the morning, *not* at night.
4. Use the SMR session in the morning or early afternoon, and the longer "Dissociative SMR" at night for the anxious-mind/quiet-body type of insomnia.
5. Use 10 Hz alpha and theta sessions in the afternoon.
6. Use slower alpha sessions in the afternoon, evening or at bedtime, but not in the morning.
7. Use delta sessions at night only.

D. Session frequency ranges and types

By and large, the AVE frequency chosen is the same as is typically chosen for neurofeedback. About a dozen key session types can be identified. Session elements include a frequency, the time needed to induce a dissociative/meditative state of mind (the first crucial step toward deep induction), and a fading at the end. AVE sessions can span the entire brain wave range from sub-delta up to 25 Hz, and independently for each hemisphere. Beyond 25 Hz the effects of AVE diminish, and anxiety can be elicited. Marvin Sams (2007, personal communication) has also found that AVE up around gamma (40 Hz) can produce severe negative side effects. However, there are unique AVE sessions which are over and above traditional, straight-on entrainment. These are listed below.

1. *Beta 18–22 Hz*

Beta stimulation in the 18–22 Hz range has been shown to be the most effective for improving energy cognition (mental performance) and attention, and, to a lesser degree, for reducing depression. Beta has been proven useful for clearing mental "fog" in people with fibromyalgia (Berg *et al.*, 1999). However, AVE above 20 Hz may produce anxiety. Beta sessions increase arousal in non-ADHD users, whereas those with ADD-ADHD often fall asleep. A study treating seasonal affective disorder (SAD) using 20 Hz AVE showed large reductions in anxiety, depression, and carbohydrate cravings, while eliciting weight loss (Berg and Siever, 2004). Beta sessions are best used right after wakening, while the user is in bed, and run for 20 minutes.

Figures 8.10, 8.11 and 8.12 show results of the SAD study in 2004. Figure 8.10 shows reductions in depression (BDI or Beck Depression Inventory) while

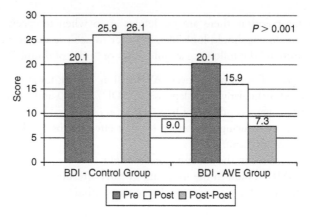

FIGURE 8.10   SAD study: change in depression, pre-, post- and post-post conditions (n = 74).

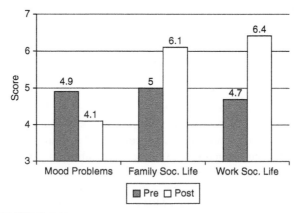

FIGURE 8.11   SAD study: social life, pre- and post- conditions (n = 74).

Fig. 8.11 shows improvement in mood and sociality. Figure 8.12 shows increased energy and reduced carbohydrate cravings. During the 2-week pre-test condition, the participants had an average weight loss of 3 pounds (1.36 Kg). They had further weight reductions of 6.5 pounds (4.3 Kg) during the two-week treatment condition.

2. Low beta/sensorimotor rhythm

The SMR (sensorimotor rhythm) is the idling rhythm for the motor strip—the long thin area located on top of the head between the ears (McClintic, 1978). As SMR increases, a person's body becomes more relaxed. Hyperactive (ADHD) children have very little SMR activity. In cortical regions outside of the motor strip, 12–15 Hz is considered to be low beta. Low beta relates to relaxed attention such as reading or engaging in a relaxing hobby such as knitting. SMR has also been used successfully with View-hole "Tru-Vu Omniscreen™" eyesets to improve reading speed and comprehension. Budzynski *et al.* (1999) used 14 Hz audio-visual stimulation to increase peak alpha frequency and A3/A1 ratios (11–13 Hz/7–9 Hz), which in turn enhanced mental clarity.

Use SMR for:

- Relaxed attention.
- Quieting the body down.
- Reading with the View-hole Omniscreen eyesets.
- Insomnia—"chattery" mind but relaxed body.

There are two variations of SMR. One variation is in keeping with Hauri's (1982) neurofeedback studies in which he found that uptraining in the 12–15 Hz frequency band helped reduce insomnia in people suffering from insomnia of the

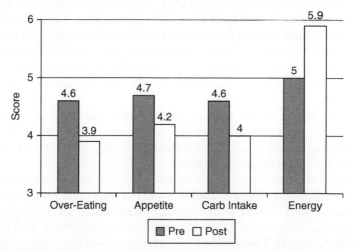

FIGURE 8.12   SAD study weight problems, pre- and post- conditions (n = 74).

"racy-head," relaxed-body type. The AVE session is typically 40 minutes with a long dissociated, randomized front end to help with sleep onset. The second variation involves ADD/ADHD children with whom this session is used with eyesets containing view-holes for reading. The session is then played while the person reads. No dissociation is added. Both left and right stimulation are locked in phase. Self-reports from these users indicate that visual tracking, attention, comprehension, and retention are improved.

3. Alpha sessions

The alpha AVE sessions in the range of 7–10 Hz are the most commonly used. They are used for meditating, going to sleep, calming anxiety and reducing post-traumatic stress syndrome (PTSD) symptoms. Clients have come into our office immediately following a panic attack, and they have been tense, pale and exhausted. Following a Schumann session these same clients have left feeling relaxed, calm, grounded, and stable for up to 2 days. Nothing settles down an irritated amygdala and hypothalamus as alpha AVE does. Most of the time people fall asleep during a slow alpha (7–9 Hz) session.

However, like meditation, deep relaxation and temperature biofeedback, alpha sessions can, in some cases, make the user unsettled and anxious if repressed memories begin to surface, although this is rare. People who are "controller" types and "guarded" don't generally like alpha sessions (or AVE sessions at all) because they feel like they are losing their control. People who have experienced trauma also often resist "giving in" to the session, not realizing that AVE may be the best thing for them.

Sometimes, continued daytime use of slowed alpha sessions can make a person feel sluggish, moody, and "foggy-headed." Brain maps we have done show that slowed alpha sessions often dramatically reduce depression but may increase depression as well. Presently, we don't know how to predict which way a person will go, so make mental body/mind checks when using these sessions during the daytime. Night-time use is okay, because our brainwaves slide through slow alpha and theta on the way to sleep. Afternoon use is also generally okay if the user falls asleep during the session.

All sessions have a natural element of dissociation just by the very nature of AVE. However, extra "chatter" reducing dissociation is achieved by using two slightly different frequencies, and randomization during the first portion of the session (see section on Dissociation above).

Jaw tension and degradation of the joint and its cartilage, more formally known as *temporo-mandibular dysfunction* (TMD), is often a direct physiological outcome in response to stress (Yemm, 1969). Auditory entrainment at 10 Hz, plus EMG biofeedback has been shown to directly reduce the symptoms of TMD (Manns et al., 1981). A study by Thomas and Siever, (1989) showed that many people with chronic TMD show *dysponesis* or bracing (tensing up) when asked to relax. AVE at 10 Hz produced deep masseter muscle relaxation and finger warming within 6 minutes. Cagnon and Boersma (1992) found that alpha AVE was effective in reducing chronic pain from back injury. Anderson (1989) found that alpha AVE effectively reduced migraine, and Siever (2003) found that alpha AVE normalized breathing and heart rhythms in minutes.

Alpha AVE at 10 Hz has also been shown to reduce jaw tension (Siever, 2003) during wide mouth opening. AVE has been used to reduce jaw pain, patient anxiety and heart rate during dental procedures (Morse and Chow, 1993). During this study, it was found that the most stressful part of a root canal procedure was during the injection (needle). With alpha AVE alone, heart rate was reduced significantly. With increased dissociation by listening to a relaxation tape, heart rate was further reduced.

A study by Williams, *et al.* (2006) found that as seniors approached 80 years of age, their ability to correctly identify real-language trigrams (three-letter words) versus fake words became impaired. They also found that seniors over 80 had difficulty remembering words they had heard previously in a test where they were required to identify random word-pairs. Based on the premise that healthy alpha near 10 Hz is associated with peak mental performance, a row of light-emitting diodes (LEDs) along the top of the computer testing monitor was flashed for just one second at a variety of frequencies (9 Hz, 9.5 Hz, 10 Hz, 10.2 Hz, 10.5 Hz, 11 Hz, 11.5 Hz, and 500 Hz, as a control) just before the task occurred. As expected, the seniors' performance was best following 10.2 Hz, in accordance with maximal healthy alpha production, as shown in Fig. 8.13.

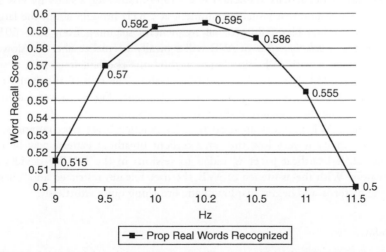

FIGURE 8.13   Results of declarative memory trials vs. photic stimulation frequency (Williams *et al.*, 2006) n = 30.

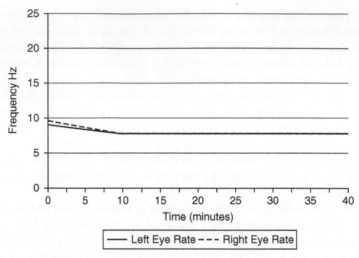

FIGURE 8.14   Schumann resonance session for sleep and meditation.

4. Alpha/theta and theta

Alpha/theta is a "twilight" state between awareness and sleep. It is associated with deep relaxation and creative insights (Budzynski, 1976). The alpha/theta range spans roughly from 7 to 8.5 Hz. The Schumann session (7.8 Hz) is likely the most popular of all AVE sessions (Fig. 8.14). Alpha/theta training is popular among neurofeedback practitioners for reducing the impact of stress. As has been shown in PET studies, a strong association exists between the perfusion of cerebral flow and slow wave EEG activity (Leuchter et al., 1999). However, a study by Fox and Raichle (1985), found that visual entrainment at 7.8 Hz brought about the largest increases in cerebral blood flow of all frequencies spanning from 1 to 60 Hz. Therefore, the *metabolism effect* of AVE will typically normalize aberrant slowed-alpha activity, even with AVE stimulation at the same aberrant frequency, as seen in this 22-year-old lady with ADD and fibromyalgia. Figure 8.15 shows the pre-AVE aberrant EEG activity. The post 7.8 Hz AVE results (Fig. 8.16) were taken 20 minutes following the cessation of the Schumann session.

Alpha/theta AVE provides an ideal time to practice heart rate training since autonomic activity is very low, thus an excellent breathing pattern may be easily achieved. A heartbeat pacer is added to sessions in the DAVID devices for these reasons. With the assistance of AVE, the user releases restricted and "chesty" breathing patterns, and begins diaphragmatic breathing quite effortlessly.

5. Delta

Sleep studies conducted within our office have shown that delta stimulation does not generally help with anxiety-based insomnia. Delta AVE does however reduce

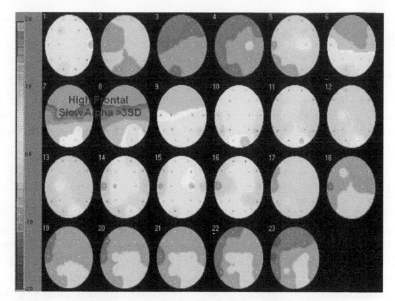

FIGURE 8.15   QEEG results on Skil Database—pre-AVE.

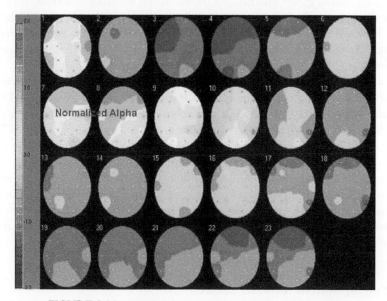

FIGURE 8.16   QEEG results on Skil Database—post 7.8 Hz AVE.

insomnia in those with fibromyalgia (Berg *et al.*, 1999). This coincides with Hauri's neurofeedback study with insomniacs.

6. Sub-delta

We believe that sub-delta (1–1.5 Hz) impacts the hypothalamus because of the way it has normalized both pain and hypertension in non-anxious, non-depressed clients. It also has been useful in re-establishing sleep in those with mid-night awakenings.

7. ADD/ADHD sessions

AVE sessions for treating ADD and ADHD generally comprise complex frequency stimulation. For instance, Carter and Russell (1993) developed a session to treat ADD/ADHD in school children. It provided entrainment at 10 Hz for 2 minutes, 18 Hz for another 2 minutes followed by one minute of silence, and repeated this pattern three times. They also noted that a second group using AVE and auditory entrainment with cassette tapes had greater improvement than those using AVE alone. A study by Budzynski *et al.* (1999) used an AVE device called *Biolight* for college students struggling with academic problems. Volunteers, at least one quarter of whom were university students, were randomly divided into a treatment (AVE) group and a waiting list control group. The Biolight produced one minute alternations of 14 and 22 Hz for 20 minutes. Following 30 sessions, mean alpha frequency and high/low alpha increased during memory tasks. Both groups' grade point average differences between the fall and spring quarters (they were trained during the winter quarter) showed that the AVE group had improved significantly over the controls.

A study of 99 children showed that treatment with AVE was more effective for inattention than using medications such as Ritalin and Adderall (Micheletti, 1998). Another study (n = 30) provided group treatment for 10 school children at a time who had attention deficits (Joyce and Siever, 2000). The session presented beta stimulation (19–21 Hz) to the left hemisphere and SMR (12–15 Hz) to the right hemisphere with a minute of alpha stimulation. Michael Joyce later conducted a follow-up ADD study involving 204 children from seven schools in Minnesota. Following 30 AVE sessions, there were reductions in anxiety, depression, inattention, and hyperactivity. On average, children from grades 1 to 11 showed average improvements in oral reading proficiency on the Slosson-R assessment of about one year (Joyce, 2001; Siever, 2003).

E. Special sessions for older adults

Cognitive decline in older adults is an ever-growing problem, not only because the numbers of older adults are increasing, but longer life increases the likelihood

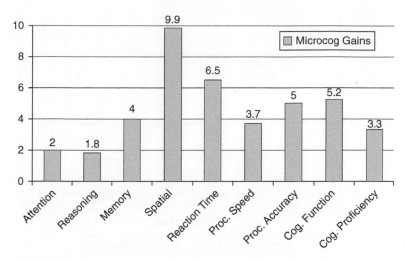

FIGURE 8.17   Microcog post–pre gains following AVE (Budzynski, 2007) n = 31.

of loss of memory and decline in cognitive performance. Cerebral blood flow has been shown to drop with age (Hagstadius and Risberg, 1989; Gur, *et al.*, 1987). It has also been shown that an increase in overall theta activity is the best and earliest indicator of cognitive decline (Prichep *et al.*, 1994).

Tom Budzynski developed the first "Brain Brightening" AVE session for seniors (Budzynski *et al.*, 2007). Participants were from two seniors' homes in Seattle. Ten seniors were simultaneously treated from a multiple DAVID system. Budzynski's session presented randomized light intensity, pulse-tone volume, and frequency from 9–22 Hz. The idea was to frequently initiate the orienting response while entraining with faster frequencies. Both of these effects helped to inhibit slow-wave alpha, and therefore improve cognition. Roughly 65–75% of the participants showed improvements for the measures of the Microcog computerized continuous performance test (CPT), shown in Fig. 8.17.

F. Depression session

Depression is the most common psychiatric disorder by far. About 14% of the population will experience clinical depression in their lifetime. Of these, an alarming 15% will unfortunately commit suicide (Rosenfeld, 1997). While acute (mild) stress seems to enhance mental function, chronic (severe) stress impairs hippocampal function which, in turn, may lead to multiple sclerosis, anxiety, depression, post-traumatic stress disorder, cognitive decline, and Alzheimer's disease (Esch *et al.*, 2002). As shown in Fig. 8.18, the Depression AVE session utilizes right-sided AVE at 19–20 Hz (left brain stimulation), and left-sided AVE at 10 Hz (right brain

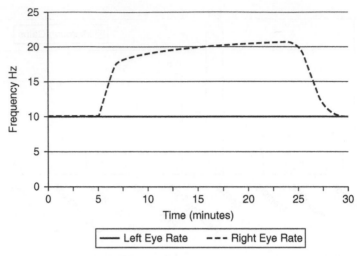

FIGURE 8.18   Depression reduction session.

stimulation). This approach normalizes the asymmetry in brain "alpha" activity that is typical of depression (Rosenfeld, 1997). Results have been seen 20 minutes later in QEEG records. Subjective case reports suggesting the effects may last up to 3 or 4 days.

Falls are the leading cause of injuries and injury-related deaths among persons aged 65 and older (Fife and Barancik, 1985; Hoyert, *et al.*, 1999). They are the cause of 95% of hip fractures in senior women (Stevens and Olsen, 1999). Hip fractures in turn are associated with decreased mobility, onset of depression (Scaf-Klomp *et al.*, 2003), diminished quality of life, and premature death (Zuckerman, 1996). A study by Berg and Siever (2004) showed that by treating with the depression AVE session, depression as recorded on the geriatric depression scale (GDS) was reduced significantly (Fig. 8.19), while balance and gait as measured with the Tinetti assessment tool (Tinetti, 1986) were improved (Fig. 8.20). As depression lifted, balance and gait improved.

VII.   APPLYING AVE WITH NEUROFEEDBACK

Neurofeedback (NF) and AVE complement each other. Many practitioners use photic entraining eyesets with view-holes during NF sessions. By manually adjusting the AVE frequency to be the same as the NF frequency, or by doubling the inhibition frequency, a patient can get a sense of what it "feels" like to make or inhibit that particular frequency. This speeds up the NF process considerably. In addition, an AVE device can be taken home to augment the session. Regardless of the approach, clinicians who combine the AVE with NF report that the typical 40-session NF process may often be reduced to 10 NF sessions. The use of AVE in the first couple of weeks of training can sharply decrease the patient's tension,

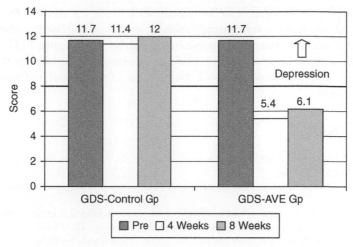

FIGURE 8.19   Reduction in geriatric depression (Berg and Siever, 2004) n = 80.

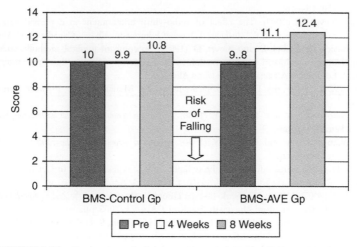

FIGURE 8.20   Improvement in balance mean scores (Berg and Siever, 2004) n = 80.

and reduce the frustration that many patients experience during the early sessions of NF.

VIII. CONCLUSION

A large and growing body of research and clinical experience demonstrates that AVE quickly and effectively modifies conditions of high autonomic (sympathetic and parasympathetic) activation and over- and under-aroused states of mind, bringing about a return to homeostasis. AVE exerts a powerful influence on brain/mind stabilization and normalization by means of increased cerebral flow, increased levels of certain neurotransmitters, and by normalizing EEG activity. AVE is proving to be a safe and cost-effective treatment, especially for the large numbers of disorders associated with dysfunctions of the central and autonomic nervous system.

REFERENCES

Adrian, E. and Matthews, B. (1934). The Berger rhythm: Potential changes from the occipital lobes in man. *Brain*, **57**, 355–384.

Anderson, D. (1989). The treatment of migraine with variable frequency photic stimulation. *Headache*, **29**, 154–155.

Barlow, J. (1960). Rhythmic activity induced by photic stimulation in relation to intrinsic alpha activity of the brain in man. *Electroencephalography and Clinical Neurophysiology*, **12**, 317–326.

Bartley, S. (1934). Relation of intensity and duration of brief retinal stimulation by light to the electrical response of the optic cortex of the rabbit. *American Journal of Physiology*, **108**, 397–408.

Bartley, S. (1937). Some observations on the organization of the retinal response. *American Journal of Physiology*, **120**, 184–189.

Berg, K. and Siever, D. (2004). The effect of audio-visual entrainment in depressed community-dwelling senior citizens who fall. *In-house manuscript*. Edmonton, Alberta, Canada: Mind Alive Inc.

Berg, K., Mueller, H., Seibel, D. and Siever, D. (1999). Outcome of medical methods, audio-visual entrainment, and nutritional supplementation in the treatment of fibromyalgia syndrome. *In-house manuscript*. Edmonton, Alberta, Canada: Mind Alive Inc.

Berger, H. (1929). Ueber das Elektroenkephalogramm des Menchen. *Arch Psychiatr Nervenkr*, **87**, 527–570.

Bliokh, P., Nikolaenko, A. and Filippov, Y. (1980). *Schumann resonances in the earth-ionosphere cavity*. London: Peter Perigrinus.

Bliokh, P., Nikolaenko, A. and Filippov, Y. (1980). *Schumann resonances in the earth-ionosphere cavity*. London: Peter Perigrinus.

Budzynski, T. H. (1976). Biofeedback and the twilight states of consciousness. In *Consciousness and Self Regulation* (G. E. Schwartz and D. Shapiro, eds), **1**. New York: Academic Press. pp.

Budzynski, T. H. (2007). AVS and Difficult-to-treat Disorders. *Proceedings of the 2nd Symposium on Music, Rhythm and the Brain*, Stanford University, Stanford, CA, 4/21/2008, pp.

Budzynski, T. H., Jordy, J., Budzynski, H. K., Tang, H.Y. and Claypoole, K. (1999). Academic Performance Enhancement with Photic Stimulation and EDR Feedback. *Journ. Of Neurotherapy*, **3**, 11–21.

Budzynski, T. H., Budzynski, H. K. and Tang, H. Y. (2007). Brain brightening: Restoring the aging mind. In *Handbook of Neurofeedback: Dynamics and Clinical Applications* (J. R. Evans, ed.), pp. 231–265. New York: Haworth Press.

Carter, J. and Russell, H. (1993). A pilot investigation of auditory and visual entrainment of brain wave activity in learning disabled boys. *Texas Researcher*, **4**, 65–72.

Carter, J., Russell, H., Vaughn, W. and Austin, R. (2000). Method and apparatus for treating an individual using electroencephalographic and cerebral flow feedback. US Patent 6,081,743.

Chatrian, G., Petersen, M. and Lazarte, J. (1959). Response to clicks from the human brain: Some depth electrographic observations. *Electroencephalography and Clinical Neurophysiology*, **12**, 479–489.

Cohen, R., Gross, M. and Lazarte, J. (1992). Preliminary data on the metabolic brain pattern of patients with winter seasonal affective disorder. *Archives of General Psychiatry*, **49**, 545–552.

Collura T. F. (1978). Synchronous Brain Evoked Potential Correlates of Directed Attention, Ph.D. Dissertation, Department of Biomedical Engineering, Case Western Reserve University.

Collura, T. F. (1996). Human Steady-State Visual and Auditory Evoked Potential Components During a Selective Discrimination Task. *Journal of Neurotherapy*, **3(1)**, 1–9.

Collura, T. F. (2001). Application of Repetitive Visual Stimulation to EEG Neurofeedback Protocols. *Journal of Neurotherapy*, **6(1)**, 47–70.

Collura, T. F. (2005). System for reduction of undesirable brain wave patterns using selective photic stimulation, U.S. Patent #6,931,275.

Collura, T. F. (2006). The Atlantis Visual/Auditory/Tactile system. AVS Journal, **5(2)**, 29–33.

Collura, T. F. (2007). Repetitive Visual Stimulation to EEG Neurofeedback Protocols, U.S. Patent #7,269,456.

Davis, C. (1999). Personal communication re "Roshi."

Davis, C. (2005). Personal communication re "pRoshi."

Donker, D., Njio, L., Storm Van Leewan, W. and Wieneke, G. (1978). Interhemispheric relationships of responses to sine wave modulated light in normal subjects and patients. *Encephalography and Clinical Neurophysiology*, **44**, 479–489.

Durup, G. and Fessard, A. (1935). L'electroencephalogramme de l'homme (The human electroencephalogram). *Annale Psychologie*, **36**, 1–32.

Esch, T., Stefano, G., Fricchione, G. and Benson, H. (2002). The role of stress in neurodegenerative diseases and mental disorders. *Neuroendocrinology Letters*, **23**, 199–208.

Evans, J. R. (1972). Multiple Simultaneous Sensory Stimulation of Severely Retarded Children: Results of a Pilot Study. Presented at the 1972 meeting of the Southeastern Psychological Association.

Fife, D. and Barancik, J. I. (1985). Northeastern Ohio Trauma Study, 3: incidence of fractures. *Annual Emergency Medicine*, **14**, 244–248.

Fox, P. and Raichle, M. (1985). Stimulus rate determines regional blood flow in striate cortex. *Annuls of Neurology*, **17(3)**, 303–305.

Frederick, J., Lubar, J., Rasey, H., Brim, S. and Blackburn, J. (1999). Effects of 18.5 Hz audiovisual stimulation on EEG amplitude at the vertex. *Journal of Neurotherapy*, **3(3)**, 23–27.

Frederick, J. A., Timmerman, D. L., Russell, H. L. and Lubr, J. F. (2004). EEG coherence effects of audio-visual stimulation (AVE) at dominant and twice dominant alpha frequency. *Journal of Neurotherapy*, **8(4)**, 25–42.

Gagnon, C. and Boersma, F. (1992). The use of repetitive audio-visual entrainment in the management of chronic pain. *Medical Hypnoanalysis Journal*, **7**, 462–468.

Glicksohn, J. (1987). Photic driving and altered states of consciousness: An exploratory study. *Imagination, Cognition and Personality*, **6(2)**.

Goldman, G., Segal, J. and Segalis, M. (1938). L'action d'une excitation inermittente sur le rythme de Berger. (The effects of intermittent excitation on the Berger rhythms (EEG rhythms). *C.R. Societe de Biologie Paris*, **127**, 1217–1220.

Gray Walter, W. (1956). Color illusions and aberrations during stimulation by flickering light. *Nature*, **177**, 710.

Gur, R. C., Gur, R. E., Obrist, W., Skolnick, B. and Reivich, M. (1987). Age and regional blood flow at rest and during cognitive activity. *Archives of General Psychiatry*, **44**, 617–621.

Hagstadius, S. and Risberg, J. (1989). Regional cerebral blood flow characteristics and variations with age in resting normal subjects. *Brain and Cognition*, **10**, 28–43.

Hauri, P. (1982). The treatment psychologic insomnia with feedback: a replication study. *Biofeedback & Self Regulation*, **7(2)**, 223–235.

Hammond, D. C. (2000). Use of the Roshi in a case of depression. *Journal of Neurotherapy*, **4(2)**, 45–56.

Hirsch, C., Bartenstein, P., Minoshima, S., *et al.* (1997). Reduction of regional cerebral blood flow and cognitive impairment in patients with Alzheimer's disease: Evaluation of an observer independent analytic approach. *Dementia and Geriatric Cognitive Disorders*, **8**, 98–104.

Hoyert, D. L., Kochanek, K. D. and Murphy, S. L. (1999). Deaths: Final data for 1997. *National Vital Statistics Report 1999*, **47**, 1–104.

Huxley, A. (1954). The Doors of Perception/Heaven and Hell, 1963 edition. New York: Harper & Row.

Jasper, H. H. (1936). Cortical excitatory state and synchronism in the control of bioelectric autonomous rhythms. *Cold Spring Harbor Symposia in Quantitative Biology*, **4**, 32–338.

Joyce, M. (2001). New Vision School. Report to the Minnesota Department of Education, unpublished.

Joyce, M. and Siever, D. (2000). Audio-visual entrainment program as a treatment for behavior disorders in a school setting. *Journal of Neurotherapy*, **4(2)**, 9–15.

Jung, R. (1939). *Das Elektroencephalogram und seine klinische Anwendung* (The electroencephalogram and its clinical application). *Nervenarzt*, **12**, 569–591.

Kinney, J. A., McKay, C., Mensch, A. and Luria, S. (1973). Visual evoked responses elicited by rapid stimulation. *Encephalography and Clinical Neurophysiology*, **34**, 7–13.

Kroger, W. S. and Schneider, S. A. (1959). An electronic aid for hypnotic induction: A preliminary report. *International Journal of Clinical and Experimental Hypnosis*, **7**, 93–98.

Leonard, K., Telch, M. and Harrington, P. (1999). Dissociation in the laboratory: A comparison of strategies. *Behaviour Research and Therapy*, **37**, 49–61.

Leonard, K., Telch, M. and Harrington, P. (2000). Fear response to dissociation challenge. *Anxiety, Stress and Coping*, **13**, 355–369.

Leuchter, A. F., Uijtdehaage, S. H., Cook, I. A., O'Hara, R. and Mandelkern, M. (1999). Relationship between brain electrical activity and cortical perfusion in normal subjects. *Psychiatry Res.*, **90(2)**, 125–140.

Lewerenz, C. (1963). A factual report on the brain wave synchronizer. *Hypnosis Quarterly*, **6(4)**, 23.

Manns, A., Miralles, R. and Adrian, H. (1981). The application of audiostimulation and electromyographic biofeedback to bruxism and myofascial pain-dysfunction syndrome. *Oral Surgery*, **52(3)**, 247–252.

Margolis, B. (1966). A technique for rapidly inducing hypnosis. *CAL (Certified Akers Laboratories)*, June, 21–24.

McClintic, J. (1978). *Physiology of the human body*. New York: John Wiley & Sons.

Mentis, M., Alexander, G., Grady, C., *et al.* (1997). Frequency variation of a pattern-flash visual stimulus during PET differentially activates brain from striate through frontal cortex. *Neuroimage*, **5**, 116–128.

Micheletti, L. (1998). Ph.D. dissertation, unpublished. Available through Mind Alive Inc.

Morse, D. and Chow, E. (1993). The effect of the Relaxodont™ brain wave synchronizer on endodontic anxiety: evaluation by galvanic skin resistance, pulse rate, physical reactions, and questionnaire responses. *International Journal of Psychosomatics*, **40(1–4)**, 68–76.

Mortel, K., Pavol, A., Wood. *et al.* (1994). Perspective studies of cerebral perfusion and cognitive testing among elderly normal volunteers and patients with ischemic vascular dementia and Alzheimer's disease. *Journal of Vascular Diseases*, **45**, 171–180.

Ochs, L. (1994). Method for evaluating and treating an individual with electroencephalographic disentrainment feedback, US Patent 5,365,939.

Pieron, H. (1982). Melanges dedicated to Monsieur Pierre Janet. *Acta Psychiatrica Belgica*, **1**, 7–112.

Prichep, L., John, E., Ferris, S., *et al.* (1994). Quantitative EEG correlates of cognitive deterioration in the elderly. *Neurobiology of Aging*, **15(1)**, 85–90.

Regan, D. (1989). Human Brain Electrophysiology. New York: Elsevier.

Rosenfeld, P. (1997). EEG biofeedback of frontal alpha asymmetry in affective disorders. *Biofeedback*, **25(1)**, 8–12.

Rozelle, G. R. and Budzynski, T. H. (1995). Neurotherapy for stroke rehabilitation: A single case study. *Biofeedback and Self Regulation*, **20**, 211–228.

Rubin, E., Sakiem, H., Nobler, M. and Moeller, J. (1994). Brain imaging studies of antidepressant treatments. *Psychiatric Annals*, **24(12)**, 653–658.

Russell, H. (1996). Entrainment combined with multimodal rehabilitation of a 43-year-old severely impaired postaneurysm patient. *Biofeedback and Self Regulation*, **21**, 4.

Sadove, M. S. (1963). Hypnosis in anaesthesiology. *Illinois Medical Journal*, 39–42.

Sams, M. (2007). Personal communication.

Sapolsky, R. (2003). Taming stress. *Scientific American*. September, 88–95.

Sappey-Marinier, D., Calabrese, G., Fein, G., Hugg, J., Biggins, C. and Weiner, M. (1992). Effect of photic stimulation on human visual cortex lactate and phosphates using 1H and 31P magnetic resonance spectroscopy. *Journal of Cerebral Blood Flow and Metabolism*, **12(4)**, 584–592.

Scaf-Klomp, W., Sanderman, R., Ormel, J. and Kempen, G. (2003). Depression in older person after fall-related injuries: a prospective study. *Age and Aging*, **32**, 88–94.

Schumann, W. O. (1952). Uber die strahlungslosen eigenschwingungen einer leitenden kugel, die von einer luftshicht und einer ionospharenhulle umbegen ist. *Zeitschrift fur Naturforsch*, **7a**, 149.

Sentam, D. (1987). Magnetic polarization of Schumann Resonances. *Radio Science*, **22**, 596–606.

Shealy, N., Cady, R., Cox, R., Liss, S., Clossen, W., and Veehoff, D. (1989). A comparison of depths of relaxation produced by various techniques and neurotransmitters produced by brainwave entrainment. Shealy and Forest Institute of Professional Psychology. *A study done for Comprehensive Health Care,* (unpublished).

Siever, D. (2000). *The rediscovery of audio-visual entrainment technology*. Unpublished manuscript. Available from Mind Alive Inc., Edmonton, Alberta, Canada.

Siever, D. (2003). Applying audio-visual entrainment technology for attention and learning: part III. *Biofeedback*, **31(4)**, 24–29.

Siever, D. (2003). *Techtalk: Matters of the heart*. Spring, 2003 Newsletter. Available from: www.mindalive. com/1_0/techtalkhrv.htm.

Siever, D. (2003). Audio-visual entrainment: II. Dental studies. *Biofeedback*, **31(3)**, 29–32.

Siever, D. (2004). The application of audio-visual entrainment for the treatment of seasonal affective disorder. *Biofeedback*, **32(3)**, 32–35.

Siever, D., (2006). Audio–visual entrainment: Finding a treatment for post-traumatic stress disorder. www.mindalive.com/1_0/article%207.pdf.

Siever, D. (2007). Audio-Visual Entrainment (AVE) in Overview. *Proceedings of the 2nd Symposium on Music, Rhythm and the Brain*, Stanford University, Stanford, CA May 11–13, 2007.

Silberstein, R.B, Schier, M.A, Pipingas, A., Ciorciari, J., Wood, S.R. and Simpson, D.G. (1990). Steady-state visually evoked potential topography associated with a visual vigilance task. *Brain Topography*, **3(2)**, 337–347.

Srinivarsan, T.M. (1988). Nonvolitional biofeed back as a therapy. In *Energy Medicine Around the World*. (T.M. Srinivarsan, ed.), pp. 157–166. Phoenix AZ: Gambel Press.

Sterman, M.B., (1996). Physiological origins and functional correlates of EEG rhythmic activities: implications for self-regulation. *Biofeedback of Self regulation*. 21(1), 3–33..

Stevens, J. and Olson, S. (1999). Reducing falls and resulting hip fractures among older women. *Home Care Provider*, **5**, 134–141.

Teicher, M., Anderson, C., Polcari, A., Glod, C., Maas, L. and Renshaw, P. (2000). Functional deficits in basal ganglia of children with attention-deficit/hyperactivity disorder shown with functional magnetic resonance imaging relaxometry. *Nature Medicine*, **6(4)**, 470–473.

Thomas, N. and Siever, D. (1989). The effect of repetitive audio/visual stimulation on skeletomotor and vasomotor activity. In *Hypnosis: 4th European Congress at Oxford* (D. Waxman, D. Pederson, I. Wilkie and P. Meller, eds), pp. 238–245. London: Whurr Publishers.

Tinetti, M. F. (1986). Performance-oriented assessment of mobility problems in elderly patients. *Journal of American Geriatric Society*, **34**, 119–126.

Toman, J. (1941). Flicker potentials and the alpha rhythm in man. *Journal of Neurophysiology*, **4**, 51–61.

Townsend, R. (1973). A device for generation and presentation of modulated light stimuli. *Electroencephalography and Clinical Neurophysiology*, **34**, 97–99.

Van der Tweel, L. and Lunel, H. (1965). Human visual responses to sinusoidally modulated light. *Encephalography and Clinical Neurophysiology*, **18**, 587–598.

Williams, J., Ramaswamy, D. and Oulhaj, A. (2006). 10Hz flicker improves recognition memory in older people. *BMC Neuroscience*, **7(21)**, 1–7.

Wilson, J. (2001). *Adrenal fatigue: The 21ˢᵗ century stress syndrome*. Petaluma, CA: Smart Publications.

Wu, J., Gillin, J., Buchsbaum, M., Hershey, T., Johnson, J. and Bunney, W. (1992). Effect of sleep deprivation on brain metabolism of depressed patients. *American Journal of Psychiatry*, **149**, 538–543.

Yemm, R. (1969). Variations in the electrical activity of the human masseter muscle occuring in association with emotional stress. *Archives of Oral Biology*, **14**, 873–878.

Zuckerman, J. D. (1996). Hip fracture. *New England Journal of Medicine*, **334**, 1519–1525.

CHAPTER 9

Brain music treatment:
A brain/music interface

Galina Mindlin, M.D., Ph.D.[1] **and James R. Evans, Ph.D.**[2]

[1]*Columbia, Univ. College of Physicians & Surgeons, New York, USA*
[2]*Professor Emeritus, Univ. of South Carolina, South Carolina, USA*

I. INTRODUCTION

Music's power to elicit or calm emotions, stimulate memories, energize, improve mental states, entertain, and heal has been recognized for centuries by civilizations around the world (Schullian and Schoen, 1948; Campbell, 1993; Sacks, 2007). Over the centuries armies have used the cadence of music to march to war, and babies all over the world fall to sleep with lullabies. Music is present in all cultures. In fact, the sub-title of a recent book refers to music as "a human obsession" (Levitin, 2006). A connection between healing and music is implied in the fact that Apollo was the Greek god of both music and medicine, and its links are supported by a long history of successful use of music therapy with many disorders. A recent report of a connection between learning and music stated that listening to Mozart music may enhance some learning abilities (Rauscher *et al.*, 1995).

Given these reports, it is not surprising that cognitive neuroscientists increasingly are joining with physiologists, musicians, music therapists and cognitive psychologists, and together are seeking to better understand the mechanisms through which music exerts it effects. With rapid developments in functional neuroimaging, a great deal is being learned about the neurology and neuropsychology of the musical experience.

The field of music therapy has a long history of using music in various ways to help restore, improve or maintain mental and physical health (Magee and Wheeler, 2006). Specific examples include: (1) brain injured clients playing musical instruments and/or listening to selected music to capitalize on the organizing properties of rhythm as an aid to synchronization of movements; (2) melodic intonation therapy being invoked where aphasic persons with intact ability to verbalize through singing are encouraged to sing (intone) selected words or sentences, with the melodic aspects gradually fading out with continued practice; and (3) behavior

Introduction to QEEG and Neurofeedback, Second Edition
ISBN: 978-0-12-374534-7

modification training incorporating music used as a powerful reinforcement (by providing a patient with the opportunity to listen to a favorite music piece) for engaging in desired behaviors.

A related and relatively new approach is brain music treatment (BMT) (Mindlin, 2006). It is a form of neurofeedback which involves converting aspects of a person's brain electrical activity (EEG) into two musical files recorded on a CD. The person then listens to these selections over a period of a few weeks. The specific underlying mechanisms have not been determined. Nonetheless, high rates of success in improving sleep patterns have been achieved through decreasing anxiety when using a relaxing file, and promoting focus and sustained attention when using an activating file. In this chapter we describe the clinical practice of BMT, review existing scientific literature on the topic, speculate on mechanisms for the therapeutic effectiveness of BMT (with special emphasis on entrainment/ disentrainment of brain electrical activity as a possible mechanism), and discuss the future promise of BMT as a therapeutic modality.

II.   BRAIN MUSIC TREATMENT AS A THERAPEUTIC MODALITY

BMT was developed in the early 1990s at the Moscow Medical Academy in Russia. Following long-term efforts of a group of neurophysiologists, clinicians and mathematicians led by Dr. Ya I. Levin, an algorithm was developed which effectively translates brain rhythms into music. The use of such "brain music" as a treatment modality was expanded in Europe, and then introduced into the United States a few years ago by the first author, Dr. Galina Mindlin. Prior to this, Dr. Mindlin had worked closely with Dr. Levin conducting research on neurological and other physiological variables in clients complaining of insomnia, anxiety and mood disorders. BMT proceeds as practiced by Dr. Mindlin are discussed in the following paragraphs.

After a brief diagnostic evaluation, each prospective patient completes two self-report type instruments: a subjective sleep scale and the Beck Depression Inventory. The former paper and pencil test includes the main contents of the Athen's Sleep Scale, allowing a quick assessment of one's insomnia, while the latter scale helps to determine depression and whether mood state is a factor in the sleep disorder.

If accepted for BMT, a client is evaluated by gathering 5–7 minutes of brain electrical activity (EEG), sampled from four scalp electrode sites (F3, F4, C3, C4 in the International 10–20 Electrode Placement System; monopolar, referenced to linked ears). The client is asked to sit with eyes closed, stay awake and try to maintain a state of relaxation. Data gathering commences when the EEG wave forms are relatively artifact-free, and appear to be reflecting such a state. The recorded EEG data then are translated into two musical files, and recorded on studio equipment. These files include a relaxing file which is derived from slower wave components of the person's EEG, and an activating file derived from the faster rhythms. Translation is accomplished using a "brain sound compiler" developed in the 1990s by D. G. Gavrilov (Levin, 1998).

A. Translation of EEG patterns to music

Tayloring the music into a personalized form is complex. Prior to translation, EEG wave patterns are edited and "cleaned" by removal of artifacts, transients and other abnormal features. Only edited epochs are translated into music. During translation, the EEG is registered and divided into 1-second intervals. By using harmonic Fourier expansion, each interval is transformed into frequency spectra, i.e., common frequency ranges (delta, theta, alpha, beta). Subsequently, K parameters are calculated using the ratios of frequency powers for each 1-second interval, i.e., $K = Ptheta/Pbeta$. The EEG patterns then are converted into a musical map consisting of 36 notes of three piano octaves (small, first and second), eight duration segments, and eight volume gradations to be used for conversion of K parameters into musical sounds.

The formulation of the music itself is composed of a number of steps programmed into the computer. Eighteen transformation algorithms in the compiler program allow for selection of one of 120 musical instruments for each EEG channel. Specific EEG parameters involved include percent power for five frequency ranges, and peak power frequency for each channel. Resulting musical compositions are derived from the compiler program's ability to vary volume and musical tempo from each channel, transpose the music of each channel to different octaves, make changes in musical parameters such as legato–staccato, add major and minor chords, and analyze the note patterns of each channel (Levin, 1998). It is believed that these procedures establish optimal rhythmic and tonal parameters for influencing brain neurophysiology to help create desired states of mind.

B. The brain music procedure

It is recommended that patients listen to their relaxing BMT recordings every night before falling asleep, and during the night anytime their sleep gets interrupted. Upon awakening patients listen to their activating file. During the day a person can listen to the BMT files as needed to help to promote a desired state. For example, to decrease feelings of being overwhelmed or anxious, or before going to a meditative state, a person would listen to his or her relaxing file. In order to increase focused attention, or more efficiently accomplish some mental or physical activity, a person would listen to his or her activating file. Positive results usually are reported within 3 to 4 weeks.

Since a patient's brain wave pattern is altered with BMT toward more adaptive functioning as his or her condition improves, it is recommended to repeat the recording and prepare new musical files after about 3 or 4 months to make an adjustment to any new brain wave pattern which may have developed. Some patients report a plateau or reduction of original positive effects after months of listening to their original files. In such cases one may have become desensitized to the therapy, and/or EEG patterns may have changed significantly. In such cases having a new EEG evaluation and obtaining modified music files is recommended in order to provide continuing improvement. In a few cases it may be necessary to have repeat EEG evaluations and new music files prepared a third or even fourth time in order to maintain optimal momentum of therapeutic effects.

There have been no reports of lasting negative side effects of BMT. However, about 5–7% of patients have reported a light headache or dizziness during the first days of BMT which would cease after about a week. Many people have been able, under their physician's supervision, to decrease or eliminate their psychotropic medications while maintaining the gains experienced after BMT. This suggests that this type of treatment either increases the efficiency of some medications, and/or stimulates one's "natural" production of deficient neurochemicals.

III. SUMMARY OF BMT RESEARCH AND CLINICAL FINDINGS

Existing research on use of BMT with anxious insomniacs is promising. In one double blind study (Levin, 1998) 58 patients ranging in age from 18 to 60 years (mean = 43 years) served as participants. All were assessed as free from "severe mental or somatic pathology." The majority were women (60.3%). Duration of illness ranged from one month to 20 years (mean = 30 months), and the mean frequency of insomnia was 5.4 times per week. Complaints of difficulty going to sleep were reported by 84.5% of participants, of frequent night waking by 75.9%, and of early morning awakening by 51.7%. Sixteen reported experiencing all three sleep difficulties. Eighty-five percent had used sleeping medications (primarily benzodiazepines), and 15% had been using various "plant-derived" sleeping medications. All stopped taking any psychotropic agent prior to BMT.

Forty-four participants (experimental group) were exposed to recordings of their own "brain music," and fourteen (control group) to that of other patients. The music was derived from an individual's EEG segments corresponding to different sleep phases. Four electrode sites (monopolar leads) were involved: right and left forehead, and right and left center. Each participant listened to the BMT tape before going to sleep over a 15-day period. Before and after measures were taken, including psychological testing with the MMPI and state-trait anxiety inventory (STAI), a questionnaire on which participants subjectively rated various sleep parameters on a five-point scale, and (for all but 12 participants) nocturnal sleep polyography including EEG and EMG. Before/after differences for each group were assessed using non-parametric statistics.

At the end of BMT the experimental group showed significant improvement on all subjective characteristics of sleep, with greatest changes in duration of sleep and evaluation of sleep quality. Significant decreases on anxiety measures and on the depression and hypochondriasis scales of the MMPI also were found for those in the BMT group. Polysomnographic EEG measures revealed increases in power in the alpha frequency range, and reductions in power of the beta range, as well as significant increase of total sleep time, decrease in sleep onset time, increase in duration of delta and REM sleep, decrease in nocturnal awakenings, and increase in number of completed sleep cycles.

The control group also showed significant improvement on all subjective sleep measures, as well as on the anxiety measures and the MMPI depression scale. However, other than an increase in alpha frequency power, the control group showed no significant improvements in the more objective physiological measures (even though 50% had increases in duration of sleep, reduction in time taken to go to sleep, and number of movements during sleep). These results suggest that, while BMT has a high placebo effect, the experimental group's greater gains on objective measures supports it as a highly effective non-pharmacological approach to treatment of insomnia which goes beyond any placebo value it may have.

In a smaller, double blind study by Kayumov *et al.* (2002), 18 participants with chronic insomnia of at least 2 years duration, and scores above 50 on the Zung self rating anxiety scale, were randomly assigned to listen to their own brain music recording or the recording of another patient for 4 weeks. The experimental group consisted of seven females and three males with a mean age 41.6 years, while the control (placebo) group contained five females and 3 males with a mean age of 42.8 years. Participants from both groups had slightly elevated scores on a depression inventory prior to beginning BMT. The Athens insomnia scale, Zung anxiety scale, and actigraphy (objective measures of movement) were used to assess subjective and objective quality of sleep before and after BMT. Statistical analysis involved independent samples T-tests with Bonferoni correction.

Both groups showed significant positive changes in sleep quality on the insomnia scale following BMT, with no significant difference between groups. However, while both experimental and control groups had reduced scores on the anxiety scale, the former group's improvement was significantly greater. Actigraphic measures showed significantly decreased intervening wakefulness and increased total sleep time following BMT, but only for the experimental group. Sleep onset latency did not change significantly. The authors concluded that BMT is a useful alternative to pharmaceutical therapy for treating insomnia and anxiety.

Levine *et al.* (1999) summarized findings from 250 patients suffering from insomnia, anxiety-related disorders and/or depression who were evaluated before and after 14 days of exposure either to brain music based on their own EEG or on the EEG of another. It was not clear whether this was one study involving patients with different diagnoses, or a compilation of results of several studies. Although they noted that the studies were of a double blind type, few details of research design were provided. They reported statistically significant decreases in levels of anxiety and depression based on before/after scores on a Spielberger anxiety scale and the Beck Depression Inventory.

Other significant changes for those receiving "authentic" BMT occurred on EEG measures, including "normalization of interhemispheric interrelations" and "recuperation of right hemisphere function", and on polysomnographic measures, including total sleep duration, increased delta sleep and REM duration, and decreased movement and wakefulness during periods of sleep. Subjective evaluation of improvement by participants and by their physicians indicated "excellent" or "good" ratings by 88.7% of participants, and by 84.1% of their physicians. Fifty percent of those who listened to brain music based on others' EEGs reported improvement but primarily only during the first days of "treatment," with diminishing effects in coming days.

To date, the first author and 18 BMT providers located in various locations in the United States have treated approximately 1,300 patients with insomnia, anxiety, mood disorders, ADHD, headaches and substance dependence. Patients with insomnia have demonstrated roughly the same effectiveness rate as shown in controlled research studies: 82–85% effectiveness. The sleep onset time generally decreases, by self-report, from about an hour to 10 minutes. Number of awakenings dropped from four or five to one or two on average. Patients, overall, report good nights' rests after BMT.

Patients with anxiety (generalized anxiety disorder) report significant decreases in anxiety symptoms and worry in about 80% of cases. The majority of patients with panic disorder report being panic attack-free after the treatment. Patients with social phobia who were instructed to listen to their relaxing BMT file 15–20 minutes before public speaking reported feeling much more relaxed and worry-free while "on stage." More than half the patients with insomnia and anxiety have been able to decrease the initial dosage of their medications, and about 30% of such patients were able to use BMT as their main treatment.

Patients with mood disorders (depression; bipolar disorder) reported that BMT helps bring them to more desired mood states. Depressed patients reported that listening to their activating file every morning, and during the times of day they feel withdrawn, unmotivated and otherwise depressed, was especially helpful in terms of their mood. Many bipolar patients were able to regulate their mood lability by listening to the relaxing file. The effectiveness rate (self-report) in patients with mood disorders was about 80%, and about 25% were able to reduce the dosage of their medications when using BMT as a complementary treatment.

Patients with ADHD listen to the activating files early in the morning, and around noon—the times they usually take their dosage of prescribed stimulants. Additionally, they are instructed to listen to their activating file 15–20 minutes before engaging in tasks which require sustained focus of attention. Most patients report increases in concentration and peak performance after a course of BMT. Some have been able to reduce the dosage of their medications under physician supervision, and some have used BMT as stand-alone treatment. Good results also have been observed with headache patients, both tension headache and migraine. After regularly listening to BMT files, patients commonly report overall decreases in frequency and intensity of headaches. During the aura phase when the parasympathetic system is activated and many patients feel dizzy, "heavy", "weak" or hypotensive, they are instructed to listen to the activating file to increase arousal and activate the sympathetic nervous system. If a migraine attack occurs, they may listen to the relaxing file to decrease arousal.

Certainly, there is need for data from controlled research to support the many clinical successes noted, and help clarify neurophysiological mechanisms of BMT. Currently, the main author is principal investigator for a study on effectiveness of BMT with insomnia at St. Lukes-Roosevelt Hospital. It is hoped that results of this research will facilitate multi-center studies in the United States needed to confirm the many clinically observed benefits.

While existing research supports the therapeutic value of BMT, there has been very little written regarding theories of its effectiveness. Various possibilities are discussed in the following section.

IV. THEORETICAL VIEWPOINTS

Undoubtedly, some health care professionals and prospective patients are skeptical when introduced to this new form of treatment. However, many people sense either intuitively, or through awareness of the power of music and the neurological basis of the musical experience, that the notion of translating brain activity into music is worth pursuing, even if a specific theoretical rationale is unclear. Persons working with EEG recordings who also are familiar with music have noted for some time the many apparent parallels between components of music and components of EEG wave forms, e.g., pitch/frequency, volume/wave amplitude, harmony/phase relationships and synchrony among wave forms. This connection was implied by the title of one of the first books published on neurofeedback, *A Symphony in the Brain: The Evolution of the New Brain Wave Biofeedback* (Robbins, 2000).

Some early attempts to translate brain waves into music occurred in 1965 when Alvin Lucier composed the first piece of music generated from human brain waves (Brouse, 2004). Subsequently, several others, perhaps most notably David Rosenboom at the Laboratory of Experimental Aesthetics at York University in Toronto (Rosenboom, 1990), have actively pursued the EEG/music connection. However, most of this study has been related to music as art. It has been only in very recent years that "brain wave music" has been used as a healing modality. Despite many apparent music–EEG parallels, some have disputed their practical relevance. Perhaps unaware of BMT and the work of Rosenboom and others, Kline *et al.* (2002) state that attempts to convert EEG to audible frequencies has resulted more in cacophony than symphony. They cite difficulty in removing artifacts and limited spatial resolution of the EEG as major impediments to accurate conversion.

Apart from any fascination with EEG and musical wave form similarities, some scientific research demonstrates that different types of music affect EEG measures (Levitin, 2006; Petsche and Etlinger, 1998). And, EEG-derived brain music seems to modify EEG activity, as evidenced by the occasionally slowed rate of progress following weeks of successful BMT training. The need for a new EEG evaluation and translation in order to enable continuing therapeutic progress further augments the understanding that the music has modified the initial EEG pattern. Below, we speculate on theoretical mechanisms by which music's therapeutic effects may occur, the possible mechanisms of EEG-music interactions, and BMT's unique potential for therapeutic value.

Dating back to at least the eighteenth century, it was speculated that the mechanical effects of sound vibrations on various body substances and organs accounted for many of music's effects (Roger, 1748, as cited in Schullian and Schoen, 1948). Related, updated support for the effect of sound vibrations on the body include findings that acoustic vibrations directly stimulate the autonomic nervous system by way of vagus nerve–ear connections (Rider, 1997).

Regarding BMT in particular, evidence from recent unpublished studies suggests that the mechanisms of its efficacy are a result of its effects on neurotransmitters, hormones and other neurochemicals. In one study at the University of Toronto (Kavumov *et al.*, 2003) levels of night melatonin in saliva increased ninefold after a course of BMT. This suggests that serotonin, which plays a significant role in sleep regulation, also is significantly increased after BMT. This finding is supported by clinical data indicating that many patients taking melatonin-enhancing medications prior to starting BMT were able to give it up when their "natural" melatonin production increased.

Changes in dosage and cessation of multiple symptom-alleviating drugs have been documented. Many patients with depressive disorders report decreases in symptoms after BMT, and are able to decrease their dosages of SSRIs and other medications commonly used for depression. And, many patients diagnosed with ADHD are able to quit using stimulant medications. These observations suggest that BMT influences seratonin, norepinephrine and dopamine levels. Research now in progress, or in planning stages, using self-report and objective measures such as fMRI, PET and QEEG to study BMT effects are expected to clarify the role of BMT-induced neurochemical changes in the positive effects of this treatment modality.

However, it is the central nervous system (CNS) which mediates perception of musical structures, and enables meaning and aesthetic value to be assigned to music. And, as noted earlier, the rhythms of the CNS (i.e., the EEG) are affected by music. Therefore, it seems logical that the CNS and, more specifically the EEG, should be a focus of attempts to understand the dynamics of music therapy in general, and of BMT in particular. This will be discussed in the following section.

A.   BMT: Is it operant feedback or entrainment?

BMT is a form of EEG biofeedback (neurotherapy) since a person's EEG is being "fed back," albeit in an edited and translated form. A main theory of EEG biofeedback's effectiveness is that it is a form of operant conditioning. That is, when a client is motivated to obtain feedback during neurotherapy (e.g., to see their score increase on a feedback screen, or successfully play a video game), the feedback serves as a reinforcement, thus increasing the likelihood that the EEG state eliciting the feedback will be more likely to occur in the future. Since neurotherapy training protocols usually are designed so that feedback is given only when certain poorly regulated or otherwise abnormal aspects of the client's EEG are moving in the direction of normalcy, this reinforcement presumably facilitates one's learning to develop and regulate mental states associated with normalization of the EEG. Neither music therapy nor BMT have such state-dependent requirements for feedback. Rather, both appear to involve entrainment of EEG as can occur with use of light/sound equipment or other sources of sensory stimulation which expose clients to rhythmic sensory stimulation of varying complexity. [1]

B.   The concept of entrainment

The effects of music may be due partially to its functioning as a means of entrainment. The concept of entrainment has a long history, dating back to 1665 when the Dutch physicist Huygens observed that pendulums of two clocks placed on a common support would become synchronized with each other. The concept has since been applied widely in mathematics, and in the physical, biological and social sciences. Although specifics of definitions vary at least slightly, entrainment basically is "a process whereby two rhythmic processes interact with each other in such a way that they adjust towards and eventually 'lock in' to a common phase or periodicity" (Clayton *et al.*, 2005).

Neurologists, neurotherapists and neuroscientists interested in neuronal regulation are well aware that simple, repetitive photic stimulation, e.g., a flashing light or a tone, can "drive"(entrain) one's EEG so that the dominant EEG frequency becomes or approximates that of the stimulus. This is the rationale for the photic driving component of medical EEG evaluations, as well as for the audio–visual stimulation or auditory–visual entrainment (AVS or AVE) sometimes used by neurotherapists and others to help clients modify abnormal EEG frequencies. The latter might be used, for example, to increase the power or duration of higher

---

[3]Traditional neurofeedback also may involve entrainment in that operantly trained rhythms may, in turn, entrain other internal rhythms. And, there may be an operant conditioning component to BMT in that positive internal changes may be sensed and serve to facilitate continuing listening to the musical files.

frequency activity in a client with abnormally excessive power at lower frequencies by exposing him or her to lights embedded in goggles flashing at a beta level frequency such as 25 Hz. It should be noted here, however, that this also could be conceived of as disentrainment, if it is assumed that the excessive lower frequency power had been dysfunctionally entrained in some manner at an earlier time.

Many positive effects of entrainment (or disentrainment) via auditory and/or visual stimulation have been reported (Sevier, 2007). These effects often are attributed to normalization and/or regulation of abnormal brain electrical activity. Some critics have claimed that effects are temporary, and advocate learned self-regulation of EEG activity with the aid of EEG biofeedback equipment rather than simply having EEG changes imposed via AVS type equipment. In regard to this, it may be that temporary effects of exposure to rhythmic sounds or other oscillating stimuli are due to the difference between resonance and entrainment. In the former, a vibratory pattern generates or amplifies the same pattern in another medium, but the vibratory pattern in the second medium ceases when that in the first is withdrawn. If no entrainment occurs, any effects are temporary.

While it remains for future research to determine the relative value of AVS and EEG biofeedback, both can be conceived of as means of bringing order to disordered brain activity—one through entrainment by ordered (consistent/rhythmic) external stimuli, and the other through operant conditioning and unconscious, semi-conscious or conscious self-regulation of the disordered brain activity using biofeedback equipment and an appropriate neurotherapy training protocol.

C.   BMT as entrainment

If, as suggested above, AVS, traditional music therapy, and other specific approaches, including BMT, involve use of external rhythms to influence internal rhythms via entrainment, are there any reasons why BMT should be an especially effective approach to healing? Listening to many different types of music or other organized sound, or being exposed to naturally rhythmic stimuli such as sounds of a waterfall, mountain stream or ocean waves very often is perceived as creating at least temporary improvements in our mental states. Do all of these rhythmic sounds entrain and, therefore, organize internal rhythms in an equally positive manner, or may BMT have greater healing potential?

One answer to these questions may lie in the statement sometimes made by BMT practitioners that "the brain 'recognizes' the translated musical selections," presumably because they are based on the individual's specific brain wave patterns. This may mean that features of the rhythms involved in the brain music, even though somewhat modified in the translation process, are close enough to those of one's ongoing brain electrical activity to facilitate entrainment more readily than if the features were more "foreign." Perhaps relevant to this, many music therapists use a related technique sometimes referred to as the "iso-moodic" principle in which they choose musical selections to "fit" the presumed mood of a client (e.g., depressed mood), then gradually incorporate other selections to move the person toward a more desirable mood.

While it may be true that a great variety of music and other rhythmic stimuli can entrain body rhythms, including the EEG, randomly chosen or even self-selected stimuli may not entrain as effectively, or may even entrain in a negative manner relative to one's psychological and physical health. It can be speculated that an individual's brain electrical activity and other physiological rhythms have developed over time in a highly idiosyncratic manner due to genetic and experiential influences, and entrainment by many external and internal rhythms, thus creating a one-of-a-kind "body symphony" which can be more or less chaotic or harmonious. By translating selected, edited components of a client's own EEG into music, BMT may function in a unique manner to more reliably produce beneficial entrainment or disentrainment of body rhythms.

As noted by Clayton *et al.* (2004), entrainment is not a simple process. For example, it can occur to varying degrees over varying time periods, with only a certain optimal degree being beneficial, and too little or too much being useless or even harmful. Optimal entrainment may occur more readily to a stronger, more intense signal than to a weaker oscillating signal, to a signal which is of a slightly different frequency than the one being entrained, or to one which is not consistent but, rather, is flexible and incorporates random variation. Furthermore, it may take time before any optimal degree of entrainment is achieved. Given these facts, the use of musical selections based on recorded individualized EEG signals (as involved in the translation algorithms in BMT) could be uniquely conducive to optimal entrainment for the following reasons:

1. The intensity of the music may give it especially strong entrainment potential.
2. The somewhat less than real-time processing involved in gathering EEG data, and the editing ("cleaning") of it prior to translating it to music, may necessarily change its characteristics to the degree that the entraining stimulus (the music) is slightly different from the frequency of the to-be-entrained oscillatory activity (the client's EEG).
3. EEG signals, or at least those as recorded and used in the BMT translation algorithms, may contain random variability which then is reflected in the music.
4. Listening daily to the BMT music over a period of several weeks allows ample time for an optimal degree of entrainment to occur.

Complex rhythmic stimuli such as brain electrical activity and music involve more components than frequency alone. Tempo and harmonic, melodic and intensity features, for example, are involved, and may all entrain to some degree during any process involving entrainment between two or more such complex rhythmic signals. This is in contrast to the relatively simple rhythmic signals involved in photic driving and most AVE equipment, and suggests that the more complex stimuli may enable "richer," more encompassing, and perhaps longer lasting healing effects. Given the above reasoning, it seems entirely possible that, through use of sophisticated technology, BMT effectively and uniquely enables optimal entrainment, and creates enduring improvement in mental state.

V. POSSIBILITIES FOR THE FUTURE OF BMT

Although the existing controlled research supports the efficacy of BMT as a treatment for insomnia and some anxiety disorders, its reported value for other disorders is based on clinical observations and anecdotal reports. Thus, there is a pressing need for well-designed research, especially for these other disorders. BMT lends itself well to controlled, double blind research. For example, it is a simple matter to provide "sham" music to control group participants, such as that based on another person's brain waves, or random, unknown musical selections. This is in contrast to traditional neurofeedback and some other auditory stimulation approaches where participants easily become aware of false feedback, and/or ethical concerns about potential harm may more readily be raised. Although there is great need for research on the frequently reported value of BMT for specific disorders such as ADHD, depression, autism, learning disabilities, headache and substance abuse, there also is a need for research on the relative effectiveness of BMT in comparison to other traditional and complementary/alternative approaches regarding such factors as speed and permanence of symptom removal, negative side effects and cost–benefit ratio.

While BMT in its present form is considered a very effective treatment modality, it likely will evolve, with applications to a wide variety of conditions. There have been clinical reports that combining BMT with more traditional neurofeedback has advantages with certain clients, and this may become more common in the future (Mindlin and Rozelle, 2006). As computer speeds increase and EEG hardware and software permit more accurate artifact rejection, localization of abnormalities and accurate measurement of more EEG parameters, it may prove possible, and therapeutically valuable, to incorporate data from more electrode sites and from other aspects of the EEG into the algorithms involved in creating individualized brain music. Parameters such as phase relationships, and other measures of neural connectivity are among such possibilities.

Brain music might be coordinated with color and/or tactual stimulation to provide a sort of "psychedelic brain music." And, if one accepts the concept of a "body symphony," music based on rhythmic body processes such as respiration and heart rhythms might be added to brain wave measures to have a more holistic impact. Of course, there is a possibility that too many measures could be incorporated. To do so would create an extremely complex "package" which could be extremely difficult to research. And, until perfected, it could invite many errors in translation, some of which might have adverse effects. Perhaps creating optimal entrainment in only one system (i.e., brain electrical activity) can enable that system to entrain other bodily systems in a therapeutic manner. Thus, "keep it simple" may be the best approach.

VI. SUMMARY

BMT is a new treatment technique which combines aspects of neurofeedback and music therapy. It involves sampling a client's EEG from four electrode sites, translating selected components of the EEG to individualized "brain music" recorded on a CD, and having the client listen to this music regularly over a period of several weeks. The CD contains two musical files—one to facilitate a relaxed state and one to induce activation. Controlled research supports the value of BMT in the treatment of insomnia and some anxiety disorders, while extensive clinical experience suggests its value for a wider range of disorders. It has proven to be a cost-effective treatment, with special advantages being lack of side effects, and the fact that clients listen to the CD when they wish in their own homes. Many clients have been able to reduce or completely eliminate medications.

Exact reasons for BMT's therapeutic effects are unknown. In this chapter we speculated on various reasons for its efficacy, including mechanical effects of sound vibrations, and influences upon neurochemicals. It was suggested that the ordered rhythms of the music may entrain, or disentrain, clients' EEG rhythms, creating greater order in formerly more or less chaotic brain electrical activity. It was speculated that BMT may have advantages over other healing approaches using rhythmic external stimulation because the brain music is based on each individual client's extremely unique EEG activity and, therefore, may be more readily "recognized" and "accepted" by the central nervous system as a source of entrainment. Also, it was suggested that, as compared to rhythmic stimulation by flashing lights or simple tones, the music may enable a "richer" entrainment involving features common to both EEG activity and music, such as harmonics and phase relationships among waveforms.

There is much need for further controlled research on BMT, including its value with regard to various mental disorders, and comparison of its cost–benefit ratio to that of traditional and other complementary/alternative treatment approaches. BMT of the future may be based on EEG from more sites, and may involve translation of other body rhythms to music. However, it also may be that increasing the complexity of BMT in this manner would interfere with optimal entrainment or otherwise prove to be counter-productive.

REFERENCES

Brouse, A. (2004). A young person's guide to brainwave music. *Horizonzero*, **(15)**. http://www. horizonzero.ca. Accessed 16 July, 2007.

Campbell, D. (1993). *Music: Physician for times to come.* Wheaton, IL: Theosophical Publishing House.

Clayton, M., Sager, R. and Will, U. (2005). In time with the music: The concept of entrainment and its significance for ethnomusicology. *EME* (European Meetings in Ethnomusicology), **11**.

Kayumov, L., Hawa, R., Lowe, A., Levin, Y., Golbin, A. and Shapiro, C. (2003). Increases in evening and night-time melatonin levels following brain music therapy for anxiety-associated insomnia. *Sleep*, **26**, abstract supplement, p. A99.

Kayumov, L., Soare, K., Serbine, O., *et al.* (2002). Brain music therapy for treatment of insomnia and anxiety. *Neuropsychiatry Review*, **3(8)**.

Kline, J., Brann, C. and Loney, B. (2002). A cacophony in the brainwaves: A critical appraisal of neurotherapy for attention deficit disorders. *The Scientific Review of Mental Health Practice*, **1(1)**, 46–55.

Levin, Y. (1998). "Brain music" in the treatment of patients with insomnia. *Neuroscience and Behavioral Physiology*, **28(3)**, 330–335.

Levine, I., Gavrilov, D., Goldstein, I., and Dallakian, I. (1999). Music of the brain – the new method of treatment of insomnia, anxiety and depression. *Proceedings of the 2nd Israel International Congress on Integrative Medicine* (Israel), **12**, 24–24.

Levitin, D. (2006). *This is your brain on music: The science of a human obsession*. New York: Hutton.

Magee, W. and Wheeler, B. (2006). Music therapy for patients with traumatic brain injury. In *Alternate therapies in the treatment of brain injury and neurobehavioral disorders* (G. J. Murrey, ed.), pp. 51–74. New York: The Haworth Press.

Mindlin, G. (2006). In step with Galina Mindlin, MD, PhD : Brain music therapy. *Psychiatry Weekly*. http://www.psychweekly.com. Accessed 14 September, 2006.

Mindlin, G. and Rozelle, G. (2006). Brain music therapy is take-home neurofeedback for insomnia, anxiety and stress-related conditions. Presented at the *14th Annual Conference of the International Society for Neurofeedback and Research*, Atlanta, GA.

Petsche, H. and Etlinger, S. (1998). *EEG and thinking*. Vienna: Austrian Academy of Sciences.

Rauscher, F., Shaw, G. and Ky, K. (1995). Listening to Mozart enhances spatial-temporal reasoning: Towards a neurophysiological basis. *Neuroscience Lett.*, **185**, 44–47.

Rider, M. (1997). *The rhythmic language of health and disease*. St. Louis: MMB Music Inc.

Robbins, J. (2000). *A symphony in the brain*. Boston: Atlantic Monthly Press.

Rosenboom, D. (1990). The performing brain. *Computer Music Journal*, **14(1)**, 48–65.

Sacks, O. (2007). *Musicophilia: Tales of music and the brain*. New York: Knopf.

Schullian, D. and Schoen, M. (1948). *Music and medicine*. New York: Henry Schuman, Inc.

Sevier, D. (2007). Audio-visual entrainment: History, physiology, and clinical studies. In *Handbook of neurotherapy: Dynamics and clinical applications* (J. R. Evans, ed.), pp. 155–183. New York: The Haworth Medical Press.

PART 4

Recent Clinical Applications of Neurofeedback

CHAPTER 10

Neurofeedback in alcohol and drug dependency

David L. Trudeau, M.D.[1], Tato M. Sokhadze, Ph.D.[2] and
Rex L. Cannon, M.A.[3]

[1]University of Minnesota, School of Health Sciences,
Department of Family Medicine and Community Health, Minneapolis, Minnesota, USA
[2]Department of Psychiatry and Behavioral Sciences,
University of Louisville School of Medicine, Louisville, Kentucky, USA
[3]The University of Tennessee, Knoxville, Tennessee, USA

I. INTRODUCTION

It is a privilege to contribute this chapter on neurofeedback and substance use disorder. While neurofeedback has been employed since the 1970s in the treatment of alcoholism and other addictions, it remains less than a mainstream treatment. This is not to imply that there are clearly successful and efficacious treatments for addictions that dominate the clinical mainstream. The treatment of addictive disorders remains based on short- and long-term strategies that employ and integrate various individual and group-based therapeutic interventions, case management, residential structure, values-based programs, cognitive behavioral therapies, pharmacological interventions, motivational techniques, and other methods. Addictive disorders are complex and associated with other comorbid conditions, and it seems unlikely that a simple and single approach will satisfy the needs of patients.

This chapter is addressed to the clinician that has limited experience with the techniques to be described, and is meant as an introduction to the topic. The information presented here can be found in greater detail in several recent reviews (Sokhadze et al., 2008; Sokhadze et al., 2007a; Trudeau 2000, 2005a, 2005b), which are a must read for anyone who wants to pursue the treatment of chemical dependencies using neurofeedback. These peer reviewed papers address the issues of validating the science of neurofeedback for addictive disorders, and offer comprehensive annotated reviews of the literature.

It is important to point out at the beginning of this chapter that neurofeedback is used as an add-on treatment to other therapies, namely 12-step programs, and/or cognitive behavioral therapies or other types of psychotherapies or residential programs. Neurotherapy is not validated as a stand-alone therapy for addictive disorders.

Introduction to QEEG and Neurofeedback, Second Edition
ISBN: 978-0-12-374534-7

241

Secondly, it is important to point out that many persons with substance use disorders have comorbid conditions that need to be considered in designing a treatment plan that incorporates neurotherapy. These include conditions such as MTBI or ADHD, which may require separate neurofeedback treatment for those specific conditions either preceding neurofeedback treatment for addiction, or incorporated into it. There are also conditions such as affective disorders and anxiety disorders that occur commonly in substance use disorders that may respond well to neurofeedback protocols for addictive disorders. These conditions may require separate assessments during the course of therapy to determine response and the need for changing protocols or adding other treatments, i.e., medication or psychotherapy to integrate into the treatment plan.

Substance use disorders (SUDs) include disorders related to the taking of a drug of abuse (including alcohol), and represent the most common psychiatric conditions that can result in serious impairments in cognition and behavior. Acute and chronic drug abuse results in significant alteration of the brain activity detectable with quantitative electroencephalography (QEEG) methods. The treatment of addictive disorders by electroencephalographic (EEG) biofeedback (or *neurofeedback*, as it is often called) was first popularized by the work of Eugene Peniston, and became popularly known as the Peniston protocol (Peniston and Kulkosky, 1989, 1990, 1991). This approach employed independent auditory feedback of two slow brain wave frequencies, alpha (8–13 Hz) and theta (4–8 Hz) in an eyes-closed condition to produce a hypnagogic state. The patient was taught prior to neurofeedback to use what amounts to success imagery (of sobriety, refusing offers of alcohol, living confident and happy) as they drifted down into an alpha–theta state. Repeated sessions resulted in long-term abstinence, and changes in personality testing.

Because the method worked well for alcoholics, it has been tried in subjects with mixed substance dependence and stimulant dependence—but with limited success until the work of Scott and Kaiser (Scott and Kaiser, 1998; Scott *et al.*, 2002, 2005). They described treating stimulant abusing subjects with attention-deficit type EEG biofeedback protocols, followed by the Peniston protocol, with substantial improvement in program retention and long-term abstinence rates. This approach has become known widely as the Scott–Kaiser modification (of the Peniston protocol). A third approach to neurofeedback in substance use disorders is to use QEEG-guided neurofeedback, although the efficacy of this method has not been studied as extensively.

This chapter will be divided into several sections: In the first section we will review SUD prevalence and describe QEEG changes typical for the most widespread drugs of abuse (alcohol, marijuana, heroin, cocaine, and methamphetamine). The second section will focus on treatment employing EEG biofeedback in SUD. First the Peniston protocol (alpha–theta training) will be described. In the second part of this section a description of the Scott–Kaiser modification (beta training followed by alpha–theta training) will be given, along with some discussion of a rationale for why this approach may be more successful with stimulant abusers. A third section will look at clinical implications of comorbidities in neurobiofeedback treatment of alcohol and drug abuse, with an eye towards integrating and individualizing treatment approaches. A rationale for the application of QEEG-guided neurofeedback intervention in SUD in conjunction with other therapies will also be given.

The fourth section will discuss how neurofeedback can be integrated with other therapies. This section includes discussion of some current research that looks beyond set protocol approaches to neurofeedback treatment of substance use disorder. These approaches focus on components of therapy such as retention enhancement and enhancement of cognitive behavioral and other therapies. A final section will discuss further directions for clinical research in this area, emphasizing that even though neurofeedback is probably an efficacious ancillary treatment for SUD, it is still a technique that is developing.

II. SUD PREVALENCE AND QEEG CHANGES

Drug addiction can be described as a mental disorder with idiosyncratic behavioral, cognitive and psychosocial features. The substance use disorder commonly referred to as "drug addiction" is characterized by physiological dependence accompanied by the withdrawal syndrome on discontinuance of the drug use, psychological dependence with craving, the pathological motivational state that leads to the active drug-seeking behavior, and tolerance, expressed in the escalation of the dose needed to achieve a desired euphoric state. Drug addiction is a chronic, relapsing mental disease that results from the prolonged effects of drugs on the brain (Volkow *et al.*, 2003). Drug addiction can take control of the brain and behavior by activating and reinforcing behavioral patterns that are directed to compulsive drug use (Di Chiara, 1999).

The incidence of SUD is staggering, leading to behavioral, cognitive and social adverse outcomes that incur substantial costs to society. For instance, in 2002, it was estimated from the Substance Abuse and Mental Health Service Administration that 22 million Americans have a substance abuse or dependence disorder, and 2 million of them were current cocaine users (SAMHSA, 2004). According to the 2004 revised *National Survey on Drug Use and Health*, nearly 12 million Americans have tried methamphetamine, and 583,000 of them are chronic methamphetamine users. The specific illicit drugs that had the highest levels of past year dependence or abuse in 2005 were marijuana, followed by cocaine and pain relievers. Marijuana was the most commonly used illicit drug (14.6 million past month users). In 2005, it was used by 74.2% of current illicit drug users. Among current illicit drug users, 54.5% used only marijuana, 19.6% used marijuana and another illicit drug, and the remaining 25.8% used only an illicit drug other than marijuana in the past month (SAMHSA, 2006).

Fatal poisoning, which include overdoses (ODs) on illicit drugs, alcohol, and medications, is the leading cause of injury death for individuals age 35–44, and the third leading cause of injury death overall, trailing motor vehicle accidents and firearm-related deaths (CDC, 2004). Heroin-related ODs have increased at an alarming rate in portions of the US and other countries (Darke and Hall, 2003; Landen *et al.*, 2003), and OD has surpassed HIV infection as the primary cause of death for heroin users. Not surprisingly, heroin is frequently associated with opioid-related ODs, both as a single drug and in combination with other substances (CDC, 2004).

Many patients seeking treatment for addiction have multiple drug dependencies and psychiatric comorbidities. Information from epidemiological surveys indicates that drug addiction is a common phenomenon, and is associated with significant effects on both morbidity and mortality. Large individual and societal costs of drug abuse make research and treatment of drug addiction an imperative problem (French *et al.*, 2000). Recently, through intensive clinical neurophysiological research and biological psychiatric studies, many specific components of cognitive, emotional, and behavioral deficits typical for substance use disorders have been identified and investigated. However, the practical values of these cognitive neuroscience and applied psychophysiology-based treatment (e.g., neurofeedback) findings depend on a further integration of these methodological approaches; this will be discussed later in this chapter in sections three and four.

The following paragraphs will summarize some of the important findings observed in EEG in SUD. From the 11 classes of substances listed in the DSM-IV (American Psychiatric Association, 2000), this chapter will discuss alcohol, cannabis (marijuana), heroin, and the psychostimulants cocaine and methamphetamine. For a more complete and annotated review of EEG in SUD please see the review paper by Sokhadze *et al.*, (2008).

A.   EEG in alcoholism

Electroencephalographic alterations have been described in alcoholic patients mainly in the beta and alpha bands (Bauer, 1997, 2001ab; Costa and Bauer, 1997; Finn and Justus, 1999; Franken *et al.*, 2004; Rangaswamy *et al.*, 2002, 2004; Winterer *et al.*, 2003a, 2003b). Decreased power in slow bands in alcoholic patients may be an indicator of chronic brain damage, while increase in beta band may be related to various factors suggesting cortical hyperexcitability (Saletu-Zyhlarz, 2004). Abnormalities in resting EEG are highly heritable traits, and are often associated with a predisposition to alcoholism development (Finn and Justus, 1999). The studies on the effects of alcohol dependence on EEG coherence can be summarized as lower frontal alpha and slow-beta coherence in alcohol-dependent patients with some topographical coherence abnormality differences between alcohol-dependent males and females.

B. EEG in marijuana abuse

Several lines of evidence suggest that cannabis may alter functionality of the pre-frontal cortex, and thereby elicit impairments across several domains of complex cognitive function. Several studies in both humans and animals have shown that cannabinoid exposure results in alterations in prefrontal cortical activity, provid-ing evidence that cannabinoid administration may affect the functionality of this brain area (Block *et al.*, 2002; Egerton *et al.*, 2006; O'Leary *et al.*, 2002; Whitlow *et al.*, 2002). QEEG studies on acute THC exposure reported a transient dose-dependent increase in relative power of alpha, decrease in alpha frequency, and decrease in relative power of beta at posterior EEG recording sites (Lukas *et al.*, 1995; Struve *et al.*, 1994; Trudeau *et al.*, 1999).

Chronic marijuana abuse is known to result in a number of physiological, percep-tual and cognitive effects, but persistent QEEG effects from continuing exposure to THC have been difficult to demonstrate (Wert and Raulin, 1986). However, recent studies by Struve and his colleagues (Struve *et al.*, 1998, 1999, 2003) have demonstrated a significant association between chronic marijuana use and topographic QEEG pat-terns of persistent elevations of alpha absolute power, relative power, and interhemi-spheric coherence over frontal cortex, as well as reductions of alpha mean frequency. Another important QEEG finding was the elevated voltage of all non-alpha bands in THC users. A third QEEG finding involved a widespread decrease in the relative power of delta and beta activity over the frontal cortical regions in marijuana users.

C. EEG in heroin addiction

Only few studies have investigated QEEG changes in heroin addicts. QEEG changes in heroin addicts in the acute withdrawal period have been described as low-voltage background activity with diminution of alpha rhythm, increase in beta activity, and large amounts of low-amplitude delta and theta waves in central regions (Fingelkurts *et al.*, 2006a, 2006b; Franken *et al.*, 2004; Polunina and Davydov, 2004). In general, pro-nounced desynchronization is characteristic for acute heroin withdrawal, but spectral power of EEG tends to normalize almost completely after several weeks of abstinence (Costa and Bauer, 1997; Papageorgiou *et al.*, 2001; Shufman *et al.*, 1996). The most con-sistent changes in EEG of heroin addicts were reported in alpha and beta frequencies, and included deficit in alpha activity and excess of fast beta activity in early heroin absti-nence. The excess of beta appears to reverse considerably when heroin intake is stopped for several months, and therefore it may be viewed as an acute withdrawal effect.

D. EEG in cocaine addiction

Qualitative and quantitative EEG measures are highly sensitive to the acute and chronic effects of neurointoxication produced by cocaine, as well as effects from withdrawal and long-term abstinence from cocaine use. Acute effects of smoked crack cocaine have been shown to produce a rapid increase in absolute theta, alpha, and beta power over the prefrontal cortex, lasting up to half an hour after administration of the drug (Alper *et al.*, 1990, 1998; Costa and Bauer, 1997; Herning *et al.*, 1985; Noldy *et al.*, 1994; Prichep *et al.*, 1996, 1999, 2002; Roemer *et al.*, 1995). The increase in theta power was reported to correlate with a positive subjective drug effect, while the increase in alpha power was reported to correlate with nervousness (Reid *et al.*, 2006).

QEEG measures are also sensitive to the acute and chronic effects of cocaine, as well as effects from withdrawal and long-term abstinence from cocaine use. Some EEG characteristics observed in cocaine addicts are considered to be due to the neurotoxic effects, whereas some EEG characteristics in cocaine addicts may also indicate a predisposition toward the development of cocaine addiction. During protracted abstinence from cocaine, long-lasting increases in alpha and beta bands together with reduced activity in delta and theta bands are seen (Alper *et al.*, 1990; Prichep *et al.*, 1996; Roemer *et al.*, 1995). Several recent studies employing QEEG techniques have demonstrated an association between the amount of beta activity in the spontaneous EEG and poor program retention and relapse in cocaine abuse.

E.   EEG in methamphetamine addiction

Only few studies have examined the QEEG consequences of methamphetamine dependence. They report that methamphetamine-dependent patients exhibited significant power increase in delta and theta bands as compared to non-drug-using control (Newton *et al.*, 2003, 2004). QEEG patterns associated with acute withdrawal and recent abstinence in methamphetamine dependence have not yet been sufficiently described. One study reported that abstinent methamphetamine-dependent patients had increased EEG power in the delta and theta but not alpha and beta bands (Newton *et al.*, 2003). In general, QEEG studies in methamphetamine addiction are in accordance with other neurocognitive studies (e.g., Kalechstein *et al.*, 2003), suggesting that methamphetamine abuse is associated with psychomotor slowing and frontal executive deficits.

F.   P300 abnormalities in cocaine, methamphetamine and heroin addiction, and alcoholism

The P300 is the most widely used EEG parameter in psychiatry and other clinical applications. The P300 is the component of the event-related potential (ERP) occurring 300–600 ms post-stimulus (Polich *et al.*, 1994; Pritchard, 1981). The amplitude of P300 reflects the allocation of attentional resources, while the latency is considered to reflect stimulus evaluation and classification time. The P300 is usually obtained in oddball paradigm, wherein two stimuli are presented in a random order—one of them frequent (standard) and another one rare (target) (Polich, 1990; Polich and Herbst, 2000).

Most ERP studies of P300 did not differentiate among patients character-ized by histories of either cocaine, or cocaine and alcohol, or heroin dependence (Cohen et al., 2002; Hada et al., 2000; Kouri et al., 1996; Porjesz et al., 2005; Porjesz and Begleiter, 1998). Across all the patient groups, P300 was significantly reduced in amplitude relative to P300 ERPs recorded from individuals with no history of alcohol or drug dependence. The latency of the frontal and parietal P300 was reported to be delayed, and amplitude reduced to novel non-targets in cocaine and alcohol-dependent subjects compared to controls in auditory and visual three-stimuli oddball tasks (Biggins et al., 1997; Fein, et al., 1996; Herning et al., 1994a; Kouiri et al., 1996; Patrick et al., 1997; Polich,1990). Continued absti-nence from heroin, and from cocaine and alcohol, was shown to be associated with a trend toward P300 normalization (Bauer, 2001a, 2001b).

Several studies have investigated ERP changes associated with methamphet-amine abuse and dependence (Iwanami et al., 1994, 1998). In general, chronic psychoactive substance abuse and drug dependence are associated with delayed and attenuated cognitive ERP in auditory and visual oddball tasks.

G.   QEEG and ERP abnormalities in addiction: Psychopharmacological effects or trait markers?

Whether QEEG alterations and P300 decrements found in most of SUD are only a coincident "marker" of vulnerability or make a direct etiologic contribution to risk for substance dependence is still unknown. The P300 reduction and abnormal QEEG patterns are seen in mental disorders that often are comorbid with substance abuse, such as conduct disorder, ADHD, bipolar or major affective disorder (Bauer, 1997; Bauer and Hesselbrock, 2001, 2002; O'Connor et al., 1994; Friedman and Squires-Wheeler, 1994). Reduced P300 amplitude related to prefrontal brain dys-function may suggest that a deficit in inhibitory control is an underlying mechanism shared by different psychopathologies (Clark et al., 1999; Tarter et al., 2003).

Taken together, the findings converge on the conclusion that there exists an inherited predisposition for an externalizing psychopathology that includes ADHD, conduct disorder, and substance abuse. PTSD seems to heighten the risk for addiction as well. Thus, the reviewed findings support the hypothesis that addicted subjects may manifest a P300 amplitude reduction and QEEG abnor-malities as a trait reflecting central nervous system (CNS) disinhibition, which may be a predisposing factor for addiction liability, resistance to drug habit extinc-tion, and relapse vulnerability.

II.   STUDIES OF EEG BIOFEEDBACK ON SUBSTANCE ABUSE TREATMENT

A.   The Peniston protocol (alpha–theta feedback)

The early studies on self-regulation of alpha rhythm elicited substantial interest in potential clinical applications of alpha biofeedback for SUD treatment (Nowlis and Kamiya, 1970). Several uncontrolled case studies and conceptual reviews on alpha EEG training for alcohol and drug abuse treatment were reported but the impact of alpha biofeedback training as an SUD therapy was not significant (Brinkman, 1978; DeGood and Valle, 1978; Denney et al., 1991; Goldberg et al., 1976, 1977; Jones and Holmes, 1976; Passini et al., 1977; Tarbox, 1983; Sim, 1976; Watson et al., 1978). The bulk of the literature to date regarding EEG biofeedback of addictive disorders is focused on simultaneous alpha and theta biofeedback.

The technique involves the simultaneous measurement of occipital alpha (8–13 Hz) and theta (4–8 Hz), and feedback by separate auditory tones for each frequency representing amplitudes greater than pre-set thresholds. The subject is encouraged to relax, and to increase the amount of time that signal is heard, that is to say, to increase the amount of time that amplitude of each defined bandwidth exceeds the threshold. A variety of equipment and software has been used to acquire, process and filter signal, and though there are differences in technique inherent with equipment and software, their impact on clinical outcome is unknown.

Alpha–theta feedback training was first employed and described by Elmer Green and colleagues (Green et al., 1974) at the Meninger Clinic. This method was based on Green's observations of single lead EEG during meditative states in practiced meditators, during which increased theta amplitude was observed following initial increased alpha amplitude, then drop-off of alpha amplitude (theta/alpha crossover). When the feedback of alpha and theta signal was applied to subjects, states of profound relaxation and reverie were reported to occur. The method was seen as useful in augmenting psychotherapy and individual insight. It could be seen as a use of brain wave signal feedback to enable a subject to maintain a particular state of consciousness similar to a meditative or hypnotic relaxed state over a 30- or 40-minute feedback session.

The first reported use of alpha–theta feedback in an SUD treatment program was in an integrated program started in 1973 at Topeka VA that included group and individual therapies. Daily 20-minute EEG biofeedback sessions (integrated with EMG biofeedback and temperature control biofeedback) were done over 6 weeks, resulting in free, loose associations, heightened sensitivity, and increased suggestibility. Patients discussed their insights and experiences associated with biofeedback in therapy groups several times a week, augmenting expressive psychotherapy (Goslinga, 1975; Twemlow and Bowen, 1976; 1977; Twemlow et al., 1977). These initial studies advanced the utility of biofeedback-induced theta states in promoting insight and attitude change in alcoholics, with the assumptions that biofeedback-induced theta states are associated with heightened awareness and suggestibility, and that this heightened awareness and suggestibility would enhance recovery. Outcome data regarding abstinence were not reported.

In the first reported randomized and controlled study of alcoholics treated with alpha–theta EEG biofeedback, Peniston and Kulkosky (1989) described positive outcome results. Their subjects were in-patients in a VA hospital treatment program—all males with established chronic alcoholism and multiple past failed treatments. Following a temperature biofeedback pre-training phase, Peniston's experimental subjects (n = 10) completed 15 30-minute sessions of eyes-closed occipital alpha–theta biofeedback. Compared to a traditionally treated alcoholic control group (n = 10), and nonalcoholic controls (n = 10), alcoholics receiving brainwave biofeedback showed significant increases in percentages of EEG record in alpha and theta rhythms, and increased alpha rhythm amplitudes (single lead measurements at international 10–20 system site O1).

The experimentally treated subjects showed reductions in Beck depression inventory scores compared to the control groups. Control subjects who received standard treatment alone showed increased levels of circulating beta-endorphin, an index of stress, whereas the EEG biofeedback group did not. Thirteen-month follow-up data indicated significantly more sustained prevention of relapse in alcoholics that completed alpha–theta brainwave training as compared to the control alcoholics, defining successful relapse prevention as "not using alcohol for more than six continuous days" during the follow-up period.

In a further report on the same control and experimental subjects, Peniston and Kulkosky (1990) described substantial changes in personality test results in the experimental group as compared to the controls. The experimental group showed improvement in psychological adjustment on 13 scales of the Millon clinical multiaxial inventory compared to the traditionally treated alcoholics who improved on only two scales, and became worse on one scale. On the 16-PF personality inventory, the neurofeedback training group demonstrated improvement on seven scales, compared to only one scale among the traditional treatment group. This small n study employed controls and blind outcome evaluation, with 80% positive outcome versus 20% in the traditional treatment control condition at 4-year follow up.

The protocol described by Peniston at Fort Lyons VA cited above is similar to that initially employed by Twemlow and colleagues at Topeka VA, and Elmer Green at the Menninger Clinic, with two additions: temperature training, and script. Peniston introduced temperature biofeedback training as a preconditioning relaxation exercise, and an induction script to be read at the start of each session. This protocol (described as follows) has become known as the "Peniston protocol," and has become the focus of research in subsequent studies. Subjects are first taught deep relaxation by skin temperature biofeedback employing autogenic phrases, and have at least five sessions of temperature feedback. Peniston also used the criteria of obtaining 94 degrees before moving on to EEG biofeedback.

Subjects then are instructed in EEG biofeedback and, in an eyes-closed and relaxed condition, receive auditory signals from EEG apparatus using an international site O1 single electrode. A standard induction script employing suggestions to relax and "sink down" into reverie is read. An example of such a script modified after Peniston that was used in the neurofeedback lab at Minneapolis VA by one of the authors (DLT) follows:

> "With your eyes closed—allow yourself to relax completely—as you listen to the tones—tell your brain to make more alpha waves—allow yourself to sink down into a mentally alert and relaxed state—imagine what your brain looks like—imagine the subconscious part of your brain—tell the subconscious part of your brain to guide you—see yourself in a drug/alcohol using situation with the people you have used with—see yourself being offered drugs/alcohol—see yourself rejecting drugs and alcohol by getting up and saying "no thanks" and leaving the situation and your using friends behind—ask your subconscious brain to mellow out your personality—sink down into a reverie state letting your thoughts flow—completely relaxed—do it".

When alpha (8–12 Hz) brainwaves exceed a pre-set threshold, a pleasant tone is heard and, by learning to voluntarily produce this tone, the subject becomes progressively relaxed. When theta brainwaves (4–8 Hz) are produced at sufficiently high amplitude a second tone is heard, and the subject becomes more relaxed and, according to Peniston, enters a hypnagogic state of free reverie and high suggestibility. Following the session, with the subject in a relaxed and suggestible state, a therapy session is conducted between subject and therapist where the contents of the imagery experienced are explored (Peniston and Kulkosky, 1989, 1990, 1991; Saxby and Peniston, 1995).

A number of case series studies have replicated the initial findings of Peniston in terms of personality, mood, and long-term abstinence with alcoholics; however, attempts to employ alpha–theta with mixed substance abuse, especially stimulants, has not met with the same success (Bodenhamer-Davis and Calloway, 2004; DeBeus et al., 2002; Fahrion et al., 1992; Finkelberg et al., 1996; Kelly, 1997). For a complete review of studies, and a critical discussion of efficacy and specificity of the Peniston protocol, please see Sokhadze et al., (2008).

The Scott–Kaiser modification of the Peniston protocol

Scott and Kaiser (1998) describe combining a protocol for attentional training (beta and/or SMR augmentation with theta suppression) with the Peniston protocol (alpha–theta training) in a population of subjects with mixed substance abuse, rich in stimulant abusers. The beta protocol is similar to that used in ADHD (Kaiser and Othmer, 2000) and was used until measures of attention normalized, and then the standard Peniston protocol without temperature training was applied (Scott et al., 2002, 2005). The study group is substantially different than that reported in either the Peniston or replication studies. The rationale is based in part on reports of substantial alteration of QEEG seen in stimulant abusers associated with early treatment failure likely associated with marked frontal neurotoxicity and alterations in dopamine receptor mechanisms. Additionally, pre-existing ADHD is associated with stimulant preference in adult substance abusers, and is independent of stimulant associated QEEG changes.

These findings of chronic EEG abnormality and high incidence of pre-existing ADHD in stimulant abusers suggest they may be less able to engage in the hypnagogic and auto-suggestive Peniston protocol. Furthermore, eyes-closed alpha feedback as a starting protocol may be deleterious in stimulant abusers because the most common EEG abnormality in crack cocaine addicts is excess frontal alpha (Herning et al., 1994b; Prichep et al., 2002).

Using their approach, Scott and Kaiser (Scott and Kaiser, 1998; Scott et al., 2002, 2005) described substantial improvement in measures of attention, and also of personality, similar to those reported by Peniston and Kulkosky. Their experimental subjects underwent an average of 13 SMR-beta (12–18 Hz) neurofeedback training sessions followed by 30 alpha–theta sessions during the first 45 days of treatment. Treatment retention was significantly better in the EEG biofeedback group, and was associated with the initial SMR-beta training. One-hundred-and-twenty-one in-patient drug program subjects randomized to condition, followed up at one year, were tested and controlled for the presence of attention and cognitive deficits, personality states and traits. The experimental group showed normalization of attention variables following the SMR-beta portion of the neurofeedback, while the control group showed no improvement. Experimental subjects demonstrated $p < 0.005$ level significant changes beyond the control subjects on five of the ten scales of the MMPI-2. Subjects in the experimental group were also more likely to stay in treatment longer, and more likely to complete treatment, as compared to the control group. Finally, the one-year sustained abstinence levels were significantly higher for the experimental group as compared to the control group (Scott et al., 2005).

The approach of beta training in conjunction with alpha–theta training has been applied successfully in a treatment program aimed at homeless crack cocaine abusers in Houston, Texas, with impressive results (Burkett et al., 2003). Two-hundred-and-seventy male addicts received 30 sessions of a protocol similar to the Scott–Kaiser modification. One-year follow-ups of 94 treatment completers indicate that 95.7% of subjects are maintaining a regular residence; 93.6 % are employed/in school or training, and 88.3 % have had no subsequent arrests. Self-report depression scores dropped by 50%, and self-report anxiety scores by 66%. Furthermore, 53.2% reported no alcohol or drug use 12 months after biofeedback, and 23.4% used drugs or alcohol one to three times after their stay, a substantial improvement from the expected 30% or less expected recovery in this group. The remaining 23.4% reported using drugs or alcohol greater than 20 times over the year. Urinalysis results corroborated self-reports of drug use.

The treatment program saw substantial changes in length of stay and completion. After the introduction of the neurofeedback to the mission regimen, length of stay tripled—beginning at 30 days on average, and culminating at 100 days after the addition of neurotherapy. In a later study the authors reported follow-up results on 87 subjects after completion of neurofeedback training (Burkett et al., 2005). The follow-up measures of drug screens, length of residence, and self-reported depression scores showed significant improvement. It should be noted that this study had limitations, since neurofeedback was positioned only as an adjunct therapy to all other faith-based treatments for crack cocaine abusing homeless persons enrolled in this residential shelter mission, and was an uncontrolled study. Yet the improvement in program retention is impressive, and may well be related to the improved outcome.

III.   COMORBIDITIES OF SUD AND IMPLICATIONS FOR INDIVIDUALIZED NEUROFEEDBACK

There are several conditions commonly associated with addictive disorders that have known neurophysiological aberrations. The co-occurrence of alcohol and other substance use disorders with other psychiatric disorders has been widely recognized. Co-occurrence of SUD and other psychiatric diagnosis (e.g., PTSD, antisocial personality disorder, ADHD, unipolar depression, etc.) is highly prevalent (Biederman et al., 1995; Drake and Walach, 2000; Evans and Sullivan, 1995; Grant et al., 2004; Jacobsen et al., 2001). Persons with co-occurring other mental disorders and SUD have a more persistent illness course, and are more refractive to treatment than those without dual diagnosis (Brown et al., 1995; O'Brien et al., 2004; Schubiner et al., 2000; Swartz and Lurigio 1999). In designing a treatment plan employing neurobio feedback it is important to consider comorbidities that may require either modification of protocol and/or ongoing assessment regarding response.

Depression occurs in approximately 30% of chronic alcoholics (Regier et al., 1990). In treatment settings, these depressed patients can be challenges to the clinician, as they may not respond as well to treatment as other patients, may have greater relapse, attrition, and readmission rates, and may manifest symptoms that are more severe, chronic, and refractory in nature (Sheehan, 1993). Several neurofeedback approaches have been described as efficacious for depression (Rosenfeld, 2000), and may be considered as part of a treatment plan. It should also be noted that alpha/theta training alone for alcoholics has been effective for associated depression.

Independent of other psychiatric comorbidity, ADHD alone significantly increases the risk for SUD. Associated social and behavioral problems may make individuals with comorbid SUD and ADHD treatment-resistant (Wilens et al., 1998). In males ages 16–23, the presence of childhood ADHD and conduct disorder is associated with non-alcohol SUD (Manuzza et al., 1989). Childhood ADHD associated with conduct disorder in males is an antecedent for adult non-alcohol SUD and antisocial personality disorder (Wender, 1995). The incidence of ADHD in clinical SUD populations has been studied, and may be as high as

50% for adults and adolescents (Downey *et al.*, 1997; Horner and Scheibe, 1997). Adult residual ADHD is especially associated with cocaine abuse, and other stimulant abuse. ADHD alone has positive treatment outcomes of just under 80% when treated by neurofeedback (Monastra *et al.*, 2005).

Rates of PTSD occurring in persons primarily identified with or in treatment for substance abuse vary from 43–59% (Breslau *et al.*, 1991; Triffleman *et al.*, 1999). Cocaine abusers are three times more likely to meet diagnostic criteria for PTSD compared to individuals without a SUD (Cottler *et al.*, 1992). Methamphetamine-dependent individuals are at greater risk to experience particular psychiatric symptoms, particularly PTSD in females (Kalechstein *et al.*, 2000). Alpha–theta training alone has been reported as an effective treatment of PTSD (Peniston and Kulkosky, 1991).

Finally, pharmacotherapies for comorbid conditions such as ADHD, PTSD, affective disorders, anxiety disorders, and other psychiatric conditions may work in concert with neurofeedback therapies for addictions. This is discussed more extensively in the following section IV.   INTEGRATING NEUROTHERAPY WITH OTHER THERAPIES. .

A.   QEEG-guided neurotherapy

A number of substance-specific QEEG abnormalities have been discussed in section II of this chapter. It may make good sense clinically to consider specific neurotherapy treatment of these QEEG aberrations either in place of or preceding alpha–theta therapy. Applicable neurotherapy approaches are attractive alternative therapies for coexisting or underlying conditions in SUD clients who have high-risk behaviors for medication treatment, such as overdosing, abuse, or poor compliance. While there are no published systematic studies of neurotherapy treatment of co-occurring depression, TBI, ADHD, PTSD, or drug neurotoxicity on the course and outcome of addictive disorders, several recent reports of neurotherapy for addictions based on QEEG findings, which in turn may be related to comorbidities, have been presented. Basically, this technique involves the use of QEEG to identify patterns of EEG that deviate from standardized norms, and individualized EEG biofeedback protocols to correct them.

DeBeus *et al.* (2002) are in the process of a randomized controlled study of neurotherapy for SUD that examines the difference between QEEG-based treatment, research-based (Scott–Kaiser) treatment, and wait-list control for alcohol- and drug-dependent outpatients. Preliminary results are promising. While historically alpha–theta training has been the accepted approach in treating alcohol and drug dependency, this study suggests QEEG-based training is a viable alternative, demonstrating similar outcomes for personality change and abstinence rates. Future directions include determination of those likely to benefit from one of the particular treatments or a combination of the two, and analysis of long-term abstinence rates.

Gurnee (2004) has presented data on a series of 100 sequential participants with SUD who were treated by QEEG-based neurotherapy, with marked heterogeneity of QEEG sub-types and corresponding symptom complexes. In this clinically derived scheme, QEEG's that deviate from normative databases, mainly with excess alpha amplitude, are associated more often with depression and ADD. Those with deficient alpha amplitude are associated with anxiety, insomnia, and alcohol/drug abuse. Beta excess amplitude is associated with anxiety, insomnia, and alcohol/drug abuse. Central abnormalities are interpreted as mesial frontal dysfunction, and are associated with anxiety, rumination, and obsessive compulsive symptoms. The therapeutic approach is to base neurotherapy on correcting QEEG abnormalities, i.e., train beta excess amplitude down when present, while monitoring symptoms.

B. QEEG-guided relapse prevention

There are tentative findings suggesting that QEEG variables may be used to predict those alcoholics and drug abusers most at risk for relapse. For instance, Winterer et al. (1998) were able to predict relapse among chronic alcoholics with 83–85% success, significantly outperforming prediction from clinical variables. Although they found more desynchronized (less alpha and theta, and more beta activity) over frontal areas in alcoholics in general, those individuals who relapsed displayed even more of this activity.

Bauer (2001a) obtained EEG data on alcohol-, cocaine- or opioid-dependent patients after 1–5 months sobriety. Those who had relapsed by 6 months later were also characterized by increased beta (19.5–39.8 Hz) activity relative to those maintaining abstinence. Relative beta power was superior to severity of the alcoholism, depression level, antisocial personality disorder, childhood conduct problems, family history, or age as predictors, and was unaffected by their substance of abuse. The EEG differences between relapse-prone and abstinence-prone groups was found to be related to the interaction of two premorbid factors: childhood conduct disorder and paternal alcoholism.

These findings receive further support from Bauer (2001a, 2001b, 2002) and from Prichep et al. (1996) who also found that beta activity was predictive of treatment failure. They found two clusters among cocaine addicts. One had more severe damage (alpha), and tended to remain in treatment. Those with less severe alpha excess, and more beta activity, tended to leave treatment. They also discovered that drop-outs could not be determined from anxiety, depression, or demographics.

IV. INTEGRATING NEUROTHERAPY WITH OTHER THERAPIES

A. Twelve-step programs

Historically, neurofeedback has been employed in 12-step programs, and has been compatible with developing key personal insights into concepts such as powerlessness, character defects, and rebuilding traumatic memories, as well as spiritual insights. Because of the transformational model of 12-step programs, alpha–theta training has been easily accepted as a potential component and, to date, there have been no reports of incompatibility.

B.   Pharmacotherapies

Pharmacological interventions for SUD have wide acceptance in certain situations. Aversive therapy for alcohol dependence, for example disulfuram or neuropeptide blocking therapy such as naltrexone, has been employed in alcoholics. Other new drugs designed to decrease alcohol consumption, binge drinking, or produce aversive reactions, regularly become available. There have been no studies on the combined effects of neurofeedback with these therapies but there is little reason to believe that there would be interactions. Peniston anecdotally described aversive effects on exposure to alcohol occurring in subjects who underwent alpha–theta training for alcoholism but who were on no aversive medication. There is a possibility that alpha–theta neurofeedback may potentiate aversive drug therapies for alcoholics.

Opioid substitution, i.e., methadone maintenance, or agonist antagonist therapies for opioid addiction are well accepted and widely acknowledged as efficacious. There is no study of neurofeedback per se in conjunction with these pharmacotherapies, but there is no reason to think that they could not be employed either in cases where there is a commorbidity such as ADHD, where stimulants might be a second choice, or anxiety where sedative type medication may be less than desirable because of abuse risk.

While effective agonist and antagonist pharmacotherapies as well as symptomatic treatments exist for opioid dependence, neither agonists nor antagonists have been approved as uniquely effective for treatment of stimulant abuse or dependence (Grabowski et al., 2004). There is no current evidence supporting the clinical use of carbamazepine (Tegretol) , antidepressants, dopamine agonists (drugs commonly used to treat Parkinson's and restless leg syndrome), disulfiram (Antabuse), mazindol (an experimental anorectic), phenytoin (Dilantin), nimodipine (Nimotop), lithium, and other pharmacological agents in the treatment of cocaine dependence (De Lima et al., 2002; Venneman et al., 2006). There is continued interest in developing pharmacotherapies that may be effective in stimulant abuse treatments.

C.   Cognitive behavioral therapies

Successful strategies for behavioral treatment in drug addiction may include:

1. Interventions aimed to decrease the reward value of the drug, and simultaneously increase values of natural reinforcement.

2. Approaches aimed to change stereotype conditioned drug-seeking behaviors.
3. Methods to train and strengthen frontal inhibitory control (Sokhadze et al., 2007a; Volkow et al., 2004).

Since stressful events can result in relapse to drug-taking behavior (Koob and Le Moal, 2001), an adjunct treatment strategy is to interfere with the neurobiological responses to stress. Current research with neurobiofeedback and addictive disorders is geared toward the use of EEG feedback to enhance one component of a cognitive behavioral therapy scheme. The research schemes described below also use more sophisticated electrophysiologic techniques such as brain electrical source localization and event-related potential (ERP) analytical approaches to temporally and spatially localize brain events.

Rex Cannon, Joel Lubar and Deborah Baldwin of the Brain Research and Neuropsychology Laboratory at University of Tennessee in Knoxville are studying "Self-Perception and Experimental Schemata in the Addicted Brain." They are performing this research with three goals in mind.

Firstly, to attempt to reconcile and integrate data from all disciplines involved in addiction research in order to develop a novel approach for neurophysiological study pertaining to SUD, and conceivably determine and describe EEG source generators that are instrumental in the processes of self-perception and experiential schemata utilizing a recently developed assessment instrument.

Secondly, to utilize this information to develop an integrative treatment model for addictive disorders based on this research, involving novel group processing methods and spatial specific neurophysiological operant learning (LORETA Neurofeedback).

Thirdly, to utilize both the assessment and neurophysiological data for development of statistical models for possible diagnostic and predictive purposes, and to provide a means for a neurophysiological treatment efficacy measure (Cannon et al., 2006, 2007; Congedo, 2003; Congedo et al., 2004).

To date, studies identifying neural source generators in self-perception schemata and their relationship with substance use disorders using QEEG and standardized low resolution electromagnetic tomography (sLORETA) are scant. This research is designed to assess the neural activation patterns relative to schemata regarding the self in recovering addicts, and identify possible generators in the cortex as compared to controls, with the hypothesis that there is dendritic pruning early in developmental phases that contributes to frequency-specific activity in neuronal populations in the ventromedial portions of the prefrontal cortex and limbic regions. Furthermore, it is proposed that these neural pathways hinder the integration of affect, cognition, reward and decision-making processes, and adversely influence the perception of self, and self in relation to experience and the development of adaptive schemata and personality characteristics.

In a current study at the University of Louisville, Tato Sokhadze and his colleagues (Sokhadze, 2005; Sokhadze et al., 2007a; Sokhadze et al., 2007b) utilize dense-array QEEG/ERP variables and measures of behavioral performance on mental tasks (reaction time, accuracy) to explore the cognitive functions in patients with cocaine abuse/dependence diagnosis. This research also studies recovery of these functions during bio-behavioral intervention based on an integrated neurofeedback (NFB, Scott–Kaiser protocol) and motivational enhancement therapy (MET) in an outpatient population. The purpose of this research is also to characterize changes in cognitive functioning associated with success rate of three arms for cocaine addiction treatment (MET, NFB, and combined MET + NFB). Prior, during, and subsequent to the above bio-behavioral therapies, individual differences in QEEG and dense-array ERP are assessed during cognitive tasks containing drug-related and generally affective cues, and during cognitive tasks aimed to test cortical inhibitory capacity, selective attention, response error processing, and cortical functional connectivity.

V.   FURTHER RESEARCH

While it is not the aim of this chapter to be an exhaustive treatise on the state of research in neurobiofeedback and addictive disorders (the appended references to recent review papers fill that function), it is still necessary to point out that neurotherapy is a new and developing field. Substantially more information is needed about many aspects of neurobiofeedback and SUD to validate clinical utility and efficacy.

More information is needed regarding QEEG-guided biofeedback and addictive disorder. Specific patterns of QEEG abnormality associated with specific substance use toxicity, such as those found in stimulant abuse or alcohol abuse or with comorbidities such as ADHD, PTSD or TBI, suggest underlying brain pathologies that might be amenable to individualized EEG biofeedback. These approaches would likely be individualized rather than protoco-based, and would be used independently or in conjunction with classic alpha–theta training. QEEG patterns and abnormalities depend significantly on whether the subject is still currently using, the chronicity of use, and the current stage withdrawal or protracted abstinence. A neurofeedback protocol selected for an individual client with SUD should be directly related to the level of current substance use or abstinence, especially in such classes of drugs as heroin, where withdrawal syndrome results in substantial physiological manifestations, including transient QEEG changes.

Even though there are no reported systematic studies of EEG biofeedback treatment of commonly occurring comorbidities of substance use disorders, it makes sense that clinical EEG biofeedback treatment study protocols consider the presence of ADHD, TBI, PTSD, depression and drug associated neurotoxicity. It is probable that this approach may improve outcome, especially in conventional treatment-resistant participants.

Unfortunately, only a few large-scale studies of neurofeedback in addictive disorders have been reported in the literature. Most, if not all, of the recommendations previously made regarding further research (Trudeau 2000, 2005a, 2005b) have yet to be implemented. These recommendations are summarized as follows:

1. Studies require external, systematic replicability of brain wave feedback methods and results in diverse populations with control condition treated, and traditionally treated matched control groups.
2. Details need to be given regarding equipment used and technical specifications, including details about amplification, filtering, spectral extraction, windowing, and other pertinent information needed by neurofeedback specialists for replication and comparison. Any attempt at drawing a common picture from QEEG data is difficult due to significant methodological differences, such as different definitions of frequency bands, different filtering methodology, number of channels, reference choice, etc.
3. The essential components and durations in brain wave feedback required for therapeutic advantage need to be stated, including double-blinded studies that control for all other possible therapeutic effects.
4. Open clinical trials that investigate efficacy of the types of protocols used for ADHD, PTSD, depression, and TBI remediation with SUD subjects comorbid for those conditions need to be reported.
5. Open clinical trials that assess the efficacy of EEG biofeedback in addressing the specific QEEG changes of chronic alcohol, heroin, cannabis, and stimulant abuse need to be reported.
6. The physiological and psychological processes of the therapeutic effects of EEG biofeedback, including studies of QEEG and ERP changes, need to be investigated and reported.
7. Studies need to adhere to clearly defined outcome measures of established validity.

Considering advances in ERPs, sampling rates and array density, other important recommendations for future development of the field should be listed:

- Increased number of channels in EEG and ERP recording (e.g., higher spatial sampling rate) have become available leading to important developments related to brain activity source localization.
- There are several specific functional diagnostic tools from the cognitive neuroscience arsenal that are very specific to test addictive disorders. Among those should be mentioned cue reactivity tests using QEEG and ERP measures. Cue reactivity is a very sensitive test of motivational relevance of drug-related items (Carter and Tiffany, 1999) that can be detected using electroencephalographic methods.

- Besides more traditional neurocognitive tests (TOVA, IVA + Plus, etc.) well recognized in neurofeedback research (e.g., in studies on effectiveness of neurotherapy in ADHD treatment) there might be used more relatively standardized tests with EEG/ERP recording to assess executive functions in addicts. Among those tests we may mention Continuous performance test (Go-NoGo task), Stroop test, Eriksen flanker test, etc. Some of these tests are sufficiently sensitive to assess recovery of cortical inhibition function commonly known to be impaired in patients with SUD.
- Testing emotional reactivity and responsiveness in addiction is another important domain where QEEG and ERP methods may help to obtain more effective evaluation of the affective state of recovering addicts.

Another important objective for future neurofeedback treatment for SUD should be attempts to integrate neurotherapy with other well-known behavioral interventions for drug abuse, such as cognitive behavioral therapy (CBT) (Crits-Christoph *et al.*, 1999), and motivation enhancement therapy (MET) (Miller and Rollnick, 2002), etc. As a population, drug addicts are very difficult to treat, characterized by a low motivation to change, and reluctance to enter treatment programs. CBT and MET are powerful psychotherapeutic interventions to bring about rapid commitment to change addictive behaviors. These behavioral therapies are especially useful to enhance compliance of the drug-dependent individuals, and facilitate their neurofeedback treatment engagement.

EEG biofeedback treatment of ADHD may be important in prevention for children and adolescents at risk for developing SUD. It may be possible that EEG biofeedback therapy of childhood ADHD may result in a decrease in later life SUD (Wilens *et al.*, 1998). There have been no reported studies of the effect of neurofeedback treatment on prevention of SUD in ADHD subjects to date.

There are several very important applications of the neurofeedback protocols for enhancement of cognitive performance in healthy subjects (reviewed in Vernon, 2005). This promising new line of neurofeedback-based cognitive neuroscience research has significant potential to elucidate neurobiological mechanisms explaining how neurofeedback training may alter and enhance cognition and behavioral performance in patients with SUD as well.

Drugs of abuse can impair cognitive, emotional and motivational processes. More QEEG and cognitive ERP research is needed to characterize the chronic and residual effects of drugs on attention, emotion, memory, and overall behavioral performance. More research is needed also to relate cognitive functionality measures to clinical outcome (e.g., relapse rate, drug screens, psychiatric status, etc.). Such QEEG/ERP studies may facilitate the translation of clinical neurophysiology research data into routine practical tools for assessment of functional recovery both in alcoholism and addiction treatment clinics.

We believe that some of the above described QEEG assessments at the pretreatment baseline might be useful as predictors of clinical outcome and relapse risk. Incorporation of cognitive tests with EEG and ERP (e.g., P300) measures into cognitive behavioral and neurofeedback-based interventions may have significant potential for identification of whether certain QEEG/ERP measures can be used as psychophysiological markers of treatment progress (and/or relapse vulnerability), and also may provide useful information in planning cognitive behavioral and neurotherapy treatment in substance abuse comorbid with mental disorder.

With the advances made in the last several years, it is hoped that continued interest will be generated to further study brain wave biofeedback treatment of addictive disorders. Effectiveness in certain hard to treat populations (conventional treatment-resistant alcoholics, crack cocaine addicts, cognitively-impaired substance abusers) is promising. The prospect of an effective medication-free, neurophysiologic, and self-actualizing treatment for a substance-based, brain impaired, and self-defeating disorder such as SUD is attractive.

REFERENCES

Alper, K. R. (1999). The EEG and cocaine sensitization. *Journal of Neuropsychiatry and Clinical Neuroscience*, **11**, 209–221.

Alper, K. R., Chabot, R. J., Kim, A. H., Prichep, L. S. and John, E. R. (1990). Quantitative EEG correlates of crack cocaine dependence. *Psychiatry Research*, **35**, 95–106.

Alper, K. R., Prichep, L. S., Kowalik, S., Rosenthal, M. S. and John, E. R. (1998). Persistent QEEG abnormality in crack cocaine users at 6 months of drug abstinence. *Neuropsychopharmacology*, **19**, 1–9.

American Psychiatric Association (2000). *Diagnostic and statistical manual of mental disorders*, Fourth edition [DSM-IV], Text revised, Washington, DC.

Bauer, L. O. (1997). Frontal P300 decrement, childhood conduct disorder, family history, and predisposition of relapse among abstinent cocaine abusers. *Drug & Alcohol Dependence*, **44**, 1–10.

Bauer, L. O. (2001a). Predicting relapse to alcohol and drug abuse via quantitative electroencephalography. *Neuropsychopharmacology*, **25**, 332–333.

Bauer, L. O. (2001b). CNS recovery from cocaine, cocaine and alcohol, or opioid dependence: a P300 study. *Clinical Neurophysiology*, **112(8)**, 1508–1515.

Bauer, L. O. (2002). Differential effects of alcohol, cocaine, and opiod abuse on event-related potentials recorded during a response competition task. *Drug and Alcohol Dependence*, **66**, 137–145.

Bauer, L. O. and Hesselbrock, V. (2001). CSD/BEM localization of P300 sources in adolescents "at risk": Evidence of frontal cortex dysfunction in conduct disorder. *Biological Psychiatry*, **50**, 600–608.

Bauer, L. O. and Hesselbrock, V. M. (2002). Lateral asymmetries in the frontal brain: effects of depression and a family history of alcoholism in female adolescents. *Alcoholism Clinical and Experimental Research*, **26**, 1662–1668.

Biederman, J., Wilens, T., Mick, E., Milberger, S., Spencer, T. J. and Farone, S. V. (1995). Psychoactive substance use disorders in adults with attention deficit hyperactivity disorder (ADHD): Effects of ADHD and psychiatric comorbidity. *American Journal of Psychiatry*, **152(11)**, 1652–1658.

Biggins., C. A., MacKay, S., Clark, W. and Fein, G. (1997). Event-related potential evidence for frontal cortex effects of chronic cocaine dependence. *Biological Psychiatry*, **42**, 472–485.

Block, R. I., O'Leary, D. S., Hichwa, R. D., *et al.* (2002). Effects of frequent marijuana use on memory-related regional cerebral blood flow. *Pharmacology, Biochemistry and Behavior*, **72**, 237–250.

Bodenhamer-Davis, E. and Callaway, T. (2004). Extended follow-up of Peniston Protocol results with chemical dependency. *Journal of Neurotherapy*, **8(2)**, 135.

Breslau, N., Davis, G. C., Andreski, P. and Peterson, E. (1991). Traumatic events and post traumatic stress disorder in an urban population of young adults. *Archives of General Psychiatry*, **48**, 216–222.

Brinkman, D. N. (1978). Biofeedback application to drug addiction in the University of Colorado drug rehabilitation program. *International Journal of Addiction*, **13(5)**, 817–830.

Brown, P. J., Recupero, P. R. and Stout, R. (1995). PTSD-substance abuse comorbidity and treatment utilization. *Addictive Behavior*, **20**, 251–254.

Burkett, S. V., Cummins, J. M., Dickson, R., and Skolnick, M. H. (2003). Neurofeedback in the treatment of addiction with a homeless population. Presented *at ISNR 11th annual conference*, Houston, TX, September 18–21.

Burkett, S. V., Cummins, J. M., Dickson, R. and Skolnick, M. H. (2005). An open clinical trial utilizing real-time EEG operant conditioning as an adjunctive therapy in the treatment of crack cocaine dependence. *Journal of Neurotherapy*, **9(2)**, 27–47.

Cannon, R., Lubar, J., Gerke, A. and Thornton, K. (2006). Topographical coherence and absolute power changes resulting from LORETA Neurofeedback in the anterior cingulate gyrus. *Journal of Neurotherapy*, **10(1)**, 5–31.

Cannon, R., Lubar, J., Congedo, M., Thornton, K., Hutchens, T. and Towler, K. (2007). The effects of Neurofeedback in the cognitive division of the anterior cingulate gyrus. *International Journal of Neuroscience*, **117(3)**, 337–357.

Carter, B. L. and Tiffany, S. T. (1999). Meta-analysis of cue-reactivity in addiction research. *Addiction*, **94**, 327–340.

CDC (Centers for Disease Control Prevention) (2004). Unintentional and undetermined poisoning deaths—11 states, 1990–2001. *Morbidity and Mortality Weekly Reports*, **53**, 233–238.

Clark, D., Parker, A. and Lynch, K. (1999). Psychopathology of substance related problems during early adolescence: a survival analysis. *Journal of Clinical Child Psychology*, **28**, 333–341.

Cohen, H. L., Ji, J., Chorlian, D. B., Begleiter, H. and Porjesz, B. (2002). Alcohol-related ERP changes recorded from different modalities: a topographic analysis. *Alcoholism: Clinical and Experimental Research*, **26**, 303–317.

Congedo, M. (2003). *Tomographic Neurofeedback: A new technique for the self-regulation of brain electrical activity*. An unpublished dissertation. University of Tennessee, Knoxville, 2003.

Congedo, M., Lubar, J. and Joffe, D. (2004). Low-resolution electromagnetic tomography neurofeedback. *IEEE Transactions On Neuronal Systems and Rehabilitation Engineering*, **12(4)**, 387–397.

Costa, L. and Bauer, L. (1997). Quantitative electroencephalographic differences associated with alcohol, cocaine, heroin and dual-substance dependence. *Drug & Alcohol Dependence*, **46**, 87–93.

Cottler, L. B., Compton, W., Mager, D., Spitznagel, E., and Janca, A. (1992). Post traumatic stress disorder among substance abusers from a general population. *American Journal of Psychiatry*, **149**, 664–670.

Crits-Christoph, P., Siqueland, L., Blaine, J., *et al*. (1999). Psychosocial treatments for cocaine dependence: National Institute On Drug Abuse Collaborative Cocaine Treatment Study. *Archives of General Psychiatry*, **56**, 450–493.

Darke, S. and Hall, W. (2003). Heroin overdose: research and evidence-based intervention. *Journal of Urban Health*, **80**, 189–200.

DeBeus, R., Prinzel, H., Ryder-Cook, A. and Allen, L. (2002). QEEG-based versus research-based EEG biofeedback treatment with chemically dependent outpatients: preliminary results. *Journal of Neurotherapy*, **6(1)**, 64–66.

De Bruin, E. A., Stam, C. J., Bijl, S., Verbaten, M. N. and Kenemans, J. L. (2006). Moderate-to-heavy alcohol intake is associated with differences in synchronization of brain activity during rest and mental rehearsal. *International Journal of Psychophysiology*, **60(3)**, 304–314.

DeGood, D. E. and Valle, R. S. (1978). Self-reported alcohol and nicotine use and the ability to control occipital EEG in a biofeedback situation. *Addictive Behaviors*, **(1)**, 13–18.

De Lima, M. S., de Oliveira Soares, B. G., Reisser, A. A. and Farrell, M. (2002). Pharmacological treatment of cocaine dependence: a systematic review. *Addiction*, **97**, 931–949.

Denney, M. R., Stelson, J. L. and Hardt, H. D. (1991). Sobriety outcome after alcoholism treatment with biofeedback participation: A pilot inpatient study. *International Journal of Addiction*, **26**, 335–341.

Di Chiara, G. (1999). Drug addiction as dopamine-dependent associative learning disorder. *European Journal of Pharmacology*, **375(1–3)**, 13–30.

Downey, K. K., Stelson, F. W., Pomerleau, O. F. and Giordani, B. (1997). Adult attention deficit hyperactivity disorder: psychological test profiles in a clinical population. *Journal of Nervous and Mental Diseases*, **185(1)**, 32–38.

Drake, R. E. and Wallach, M. A. (2000). Dual diagnosis 15 years of progress. *Psychiatry Services*, **51**, 1126–1129.

Egerton, A., Allison, C., Brett, R. R. and Pratt, J. A. (2006). Cannabinoids and prefrontal cortical function: Insights from preclinical studies. *Neuroscience and Biobehavioral Reviews*, **30**, 680–695.

Ehlers, C. L., Wall, T. L. and Schuckit, M. A. (1989). EEG spectral characteristics following ethanol administration in young men. *Electroencephalography and Clinical Neurophysiology*, **73**, 179–187.

Evans, K. and Sullivan, J. M. (1995). *Treating addicted survivors of trauma*. New York: Guilford Press.

Fahrion, S. L. (2002). Group biobehavioral treatment of addiction. Paper presented at *The 4th Meeting on the Neurobiology of Criminal and Violent Behavior. Research and Clinical Applications of Neurofeedback for Offender Populations with Substance Use Disorders.*

Fahrion, S. L., Walters, D., Coyne, L. and Allen, T. (1992). Alterations in EEG amplitude, personality factors and brain electrical mapping after alpha–theta brainwave training: a controlled case study of an alcoholic in recovery. *Alcoholism: Clinical Experimental Research*, **16**, 547–551.

Fein, G., Biggins, C. and Mackay, S. (1996). Cocaine abusers have reduced auditory PSO amplitude and suppression compared to both normal controls and alcoholics. *Biological Psychiatry*, **39**, 955–965.

Fingelkurts, A. A., Fingelkurts, A. A., Kivisaari, R., *et al.* (2006a). Reorganization of the composition of brain oscillations and their temporal characteristics in opioid dependent patients. *Progress in Neuro-Psychopharmacology and Biological Psychiatry*, **30(8)**, 1453–1465.

Fingelkurts, A. A., Fingelkurts, A. A., Kivisaari, R., *et al.* (2006b). Increased local and decreased remote functional connectivity at EEG alpha and beta frequency bands in opioid-dependent patients. *Psychopharmacology*, **188(1)**, 42–52.

Finkelberg, A., Sokhadze, E., Lopatin, A., *et al.* (1996). The application of alpha–theta EEG biofeedback training for psychological improvement in the process of rehabilitation of the patients with pathological addictions. *Biofeedback and Self-Regulation*, **21**, 364.

Finn, P. R. and Justus, A. (1999). Reduced EEG alpha power in the male and female offspring of alcoholics. *Alcoholism: Clinical and Experimental Research*, **23(2)**, 256–262.

Franken, I. H. A., Stam, C. J., Hendriks, V. M. and van den Brink, W. (2004). Electroencephalographic power and coherence analysis suggest altered brain function in abstinent male heroin-dependent patients. *Neuropsychobiology*, **49**, 105–110.

French, M. T., McGeary, K. A., Chitwood, D. D. and McCoy, C. B. (2000). Chronic illicit drug use, health services utilization and the cost of medical care. *Social Science and Medicine*, **50**, 1703–1713.

Friedman, D. and Squires-Wheeler, E. (1994). Event-related potentials (ERPs) as indicators of risk for schizophrenia. *Schizophrenia Bulletin*, **20(1)**, 63–74.

Goldberg, R. J., Greenwood, J. C. and Taintor, Z. (1976). Alpha conditioning as an adjunct treatment for drug dependence: part I. *International Journal of Addiction*, **11(6)**, 1085–1089.

Goldberg, R. J., Greenwood, J. C. and Taintor, Z. (1977). Alpha conditioning as an adjunct treatment for drug dependence: part II. *International Journal of Addiction*, **12(1)**, 195–204.

Goslinga, J. J. (1975). Biofeedback for chemical problem patients: a developmental process. *Journal of Biofeedback*, **2**, 17–27.

Grabowski, J., Shearer, J., Merrill, J. and Negus, S. S. (2004). Agonist-like, replacement pharmacotherapy for stimulant abuse and dependence. *Addictive Behaviors*, **29**, 1439–1464.

Grant, B. F., Stinson, F., Dawson, D. A., Chou, S. P., Ruan, W. J. and Pickering, R. P. (2004). Co-occurrence of 12-month alcohol and drug use disorders and personality disorders in the United States. *Archives of General Psychiatry*, **61**, 361–368.

Green, E. E., Green, A. M. and Walters, E. D. (1974). Alpha–theta biofeedback training. *Journal of Biofeedback*, **2**, 7–13.

Gurnee, R. (2004). Subtypes of alcoholism and CNS depressant abuse. Presented at The Winter Brain, Optimal Functioning, and Positive Psychology Meeting. Palm Springs, 2004 http://www.brain-meeting.com/2004_abstracts.htm

Hada, M., Porjesz, B., Begleiter, H. and Polich, J. (2000). Auditory P3a assessment of male alcoholics. *Biological Psychiatry*, **48**, 276–286.

Herning, R. I., Jones, R. T., Hooker, W. D., Mendelson, J. and Blackwell, L. (1985). Cocaine increases EEG beta: a replication and extension of Hans Berger's historic experiments. *Electroencephalography and Clinical Neurophysiology*, **60(6)**, 470–477.

Herning., R. I., Glover, B. J. and Guo, X. (1994a). Effects of cocaine on P3B in cocaine abusers. *Neuropsychobiology*, **30**, 132–142.

Herning, R. I., Glover, B. J., Koeppl, B., Phillips, R. L. and London, E. D. (1994b). Cocaine induced increases in EEG alpha and beta activity: evidence for reduced cortical processing. *Neuropsychopharmacology*, **11**, 1–9.

Horner, B. R. and Scheibe, K. E. (1997). Prevalence and implications of attention-deficit hyperactivity disorder among adolescents in treatment for substance abuse. *Journal of the American Academy of Child and Adolescent Psychiatry*, **36(1)**, 30–36.

Iwanami, A., Suga, I., Kaneko, T., Sugiyama, A. and Nakatani, Y. (1994). P300 component of event-related potentials in methamphetamine psychosis and schizophrenia. *Progress in Neuropsychopharmacology and Biological Psychiatry*, **18**, 465–475.

Iwanami, A., Kuroki, N., Iritani, S., Isono, H., Okajima, Y. and Kamijima, K. (1998). P3a of event-related potential in chronic methamphetamine dependence. *Journal of Nervous and Mental Diseases*, **186**, 746–751.

Jacobsen, L. K., Southwick, S. and Kosten, T. R. (2001). Substance use disorders in patients with post traumatic stress disorder. *American Journal of Psychiatry*, **158**, 1184–1190.

Jones, F. W. and Holmes, D. S. (1976). Alcoholism, alpha production, and biofeedback. *Journal of Consulting and Clinical Psychology*, **44(2)**, 224–228.

Kaiser, D. A. and Othmer, S. (2000). Effect of Neurofeedback on variables of attention in a large multi-center trial. *Journal of Neurotherapy*, **4(1)**, 5–15.

Kalechstein, A. D., Newton, T. F., Longshore, D., Anglin, M. D., van Gorp, W. G. and Gawin, F. H. (2000). Psychiatric comorbidity of methamphetamine dependence in a forensic sample. *Journal of Neuropsychiatry and Clinical Neurosciences*, **12**, 480–484.

Kalechstein, A. D., Newton, T. F. and Green, M. F. (2003). Methamphetamine dependence is associated with neurocognitive impairment in the initial phases of abstinence. *Journal of Neuropsychiatry and Clinical Neurosciences*, **15**, 215–220.

Katayama, J. and Polich, J. (1996). P300 from one-, two-, and three-stimulus auditory paradigms. *International Journal of Psychophysiology*, **23**, 33–40.

Katayama, J. and Polich, J. (1998). Stimulus context determines P3a and P3b. *Psychophysiology*, **35**, 23–33.

Kelly, M. J. (1997). Native Americans, neurofeedback, and substance abuse theory: three year outcome of alpha/theta neurofeedback training in the treatment of problem drinking among Dine' (Navajo) People. *Journal of Neurotherapy*, **2(3)**, 24–60.

Koob, G. F. and Le Moal, M. (2001). Drug addiction, dysregulation of reward, and allostasis. *Neuropsychopharmacology*, **24**, 97–129.

Kouri, E. M., Lukas, S. E. and Mendelson, J. H. (1996). P300 assessment of opiate and cocaine abusers: effects of detoxification and bupernorphine treatment. *Biological Psychiatry*, **40**, 617–628.

Landen, M. G., Castle, S. and Nolte, K. B. (2003). Methodological issues in the surveillance of poisoning, illicit drug overdose, and heroin overdose deaths in New Mexico. *American Journal of Epidemiology*, **157**, 273–278.

Lukas, S. E., Mendelson, J. H. and Benedikt, R. (1995). Electroencephalographic correlates of marihuana-induced euphoria. *Drug and Alcohol Dependence*, **37**, 131–140.

Manuzza, S., Klein, R. G., Konig, P. H. and Giampino, P. L. (1989). Hyperactive boys almost grown up, IV. Criminality and its relationship to psychiatric status. *Archives of General Psychiatry*, **46**, 1073–1079.

Miller, W. and Rollnick, S. (2002). *Motivational Interviewing*. New York: Guilford.

Monastra, V. J., Lynn, S., Linden, M., Lubar, J. F., Gruzelier, J. and LaVaque, T. J. (2005). Electroencephalographic biofeedback in the treatment of attention-deficit/hyperactivity disorder. *Applied Psychophysiology and Biofeedback*, **30**, 95–114.

Näätänen, R. (1990). The role of attention in auditory information processing as revealed by event-related potentials and other brain measures of cognitive functioning. *Behavioral and Brain Sciences*, **13**, 201–287.

Newton, T. F., Cook, I. A., Kalechstein, A. D., *et al.* (2003). Quantitative EEG abnormalities in recently abstinent methamphetamine-dependent individuals. *Clinical Neurophysiology*, **114**, 410–415.

Newton, T. F., Kalechstein, A. D., Hardy, D. J., *et al.* (2004). Association between quantitative EEG and neurocognition in methamphetamine-dependent volunteers. *Clinical Neurophysiology*, **115**, 194–198.

Noldy, N. E., Santos, C. V., Politzer, N., Blair, R. D. and Carlen, P. L. (1994). Quantitative EEG changes in cocaine withdrawal: evidence for long-term CNS effects. *Neuropsychobiology*, **30**, 189–196.

Nowlis, D. P. and Kamiya, J. (1970). The control of electroencephalograhic alpha rhythms through auditory feedback and the associated mental activity. *Psychophysiology*, **6**, 476–484.

O'Brien, C. P., Charney, D. S., *et al.* (2004). Priority actions to improve the care of persons with co-occurring substance abuse and other mental disorders: a call to action. *Biological Psychiatry*, **56**, 703–713.

O'Connor, S., Bauer, L. O., Tasman, A. and Hesselbrock, V. M. (1994). Reduced P3 amplitudes of ERPs are associated with both a family history of alcoholism and antisocial personality disorder. *Progress in Neuropsychopharmacology and Biological Psychiatry*, **18**, 1307–1321.

O'Leary, D. S., Block, R. I., Koeppel, J. A., *et al.* (2002). Effects of smoking marijuana on brain perfusion and cognition. *Neuropsychopharmacology*, **26**, 802–816.

Papageorgiou, C., Liappas, I., Asvestas, P., *et al.* (2001). Abnormal P600 in heroin addicts with prolonged abstinence elicited during a working memory test. *NeuroReport*, **12**, 1773–1778.

Papageorgiou, C., Liappas, I., Ventouras, E. M., *et al.* (2004). Long-term abstinence syndrome in heroin addicts: indices of P300 alterations associated with a short memory task. *Progress in Neuropsychopharmacology and Biological Psychiatry*, **28**, 1109–1115.

Passini, F. T., Watson, C. G., Dehnel, L., Herder, J. and Watkins, B. (1977). Alpha wave biofeedback training therapy in alcoholics. *Journal of Clinical Psychology*, **33(1)**, 292–299.

Patrick, G., Straumanis, J. J., Struve, F. A., Fitz-Gerald, M. J. and Manno, J. E. (1997). Early and middle latency evoked potentials in medically and psychiatrically normal daily marihuana users: a paucity of significant findings. *Clinical Electroencephalography*, **28(1)**, 26–31.

Peniston, E. G. and Kulkosky, P. J. (1989). Alpha–theta brainwave training and beta endorphin levels in alcoholics. *Alcoholism Clinical and Experimental Research*, **13**, 271–279.

Peniston, E. G. and Kulkosky, P. J. (1990). Alcoholic personality and alpha–theta brainwave training. *Medical Psychotherapy*, **2**, 37–55.

Peniston, E. G. and Kulkosky, P. G. (1991). Alpha–theta brain wave neurofeedback for Vietnam veterans with combat related post traumatic stress disorder. *Medical Psychotherapy*, **4**, 1–14.

Peniston, E. G., Marriman, D. A., Deming, W. A. and Kulkosky, P. G. (1993). EEG alpha–theta brain wave synchronization in Vietnam theater veterans with combat related post traumatic stress disorder and alcohol abuse. *Medical Advances in Medical Psychotherapy*, **6**, 37–50.

Polich, J. (1990). P300, probability, and interstimulus interval. *Psychophysiology*, **27**, 396–403.

Polich, J. and Herbst, K. L. (2000). P300 as a clinical assay: Rationale, evaluation and findings. *International Journal of Psychophysiology*, **38(1)**, 3–19.

Polich, J., Pollock, V. E. and Bloom, F. E. (1994). Meta-analysis of P300 from males at risk for alcoholism. *Psychological Bulletin*, **115(1)**, 55–73.

Polunina, A. G. and Davydov, D. M. (2004). EEG spectral power and mean frequencies in early heroin abstinence. *Progress in Neuropsychopharmacology and Biological Psychiatry*, **28(1)**, 73–82.

Porjesz, B. and Begleiter, H. (1998). Genetic basis of event-related potentials and their relationship to alcoholism and alcohol use. *Journal of Clinical Neurophysiology*, **15**, 44–57.

Porjesz, B., Rangaswamy, M., Kamarajan, C., Jones, K. A., Padmanabhapillai, A. and Begleiter, H. (2005). The utility of neurophysiological markers in the study of alcoholism. *Clinical Neurophysiology*, **116**, 993–1018.

Prichep, L. S., Alper, K. A., Kowalik, S. C. and Rosenthal, M. (1996). Neurometric QEEG studies of crack cocaine dependence and treatment outcome. *Journal of Addictive Disorders*, **15(4)**, 39–53.

Prichep, L. S., Alper, K. R., Kowalik, S. C., *et al.* (1999). Prediction of treatment outcome in cocaine dependent males using quantitative EEG. *Drug and Alcohol Dependence*, **54**, 35–43.

Prichep, L. S., Alper, K. A., Sverdlov, L., *et al.* (2002). Outcome related electrophysiological subtypes of cocaine dependence. *Clinical Electroencephalography*, **33(1)**, 8–20.

Pritchard, W. (1981). Psychophysiology of P300. *Psychological Bulletin*, **89**, 506–540.

Rangaswamy, M., Porjesz, B., Chorlian, D., *et al.* (2002). Beta power in the EEG of alcoholics. *Biological Psychiatry*, **52**, 831–842.

Rangaswamy, M., Porjesz, B., Chorlian, D., *et al.* (2004). Resting EEG in offspring of male alcoholics: beta frequencies. *International Journal of Psychophysiology*, **51**, 239–251.

Reid, M., Flammino, F., Howard, B., Nilsen, D. and Prichep, L. S. (2006). Topographic imaging of quantitative EEG in response to smoked cocaine self-administration in humans. *Neuropsychopharmacology*, **31**, 872–884.

Regier, D. A., Farmer, M. E., Rae, D. S., *et al.* (1990). Comorbidity of mental disorders with alcohol and other drug abuse: results from the Epidemiologic Catchment Area (ECA) Study. *Journal of the American Medical Association*, **264**, 2511–2518.

Roemer, R. A., Cornwell, A., Dewart, D., Jackson, P. and Ercegovac, D. V. (1995). Quantitative electro-encephalographic analysis in cocaine-preferring polysubstance abusers during abstinence. *Psychiatry Research*, **58**, 247–257.

Rosenfeld, J. P. (2000). An EEG biofeedback for affective disorders. *Clinical Electroencephalography*, **31(1)**, 7–12.

Saletu-Zyhlarz, G. M., Arnold, O., Anderer, P., *et al.* (2004). Differences in brain function between relapsing and abstaining alcohol-dependent patients, evaluated by EEG mapping. *Alcohol Alcoholism*, **39**, 233–240.

SAMHSA (Substance Abuse and Mental Health Services Administration) (2004). Results from the 2003 National Survey on Drug Use and Health (NSDUH Series H-25), Office of Applied Studies, Substance Abuse and Mental Health Services Administration, Rockville, MD.

SAMHSA (Substance Abuse and Mental Health Services Administration) (2006). Results from the 2005 National Survey on Drug Use and health: National Findings (Office of Applied Studies, NSDUH Series H-30, DHHS Publication No. SMA 06-4194). Rockville, MD.

Saxby, E. and Peniston, E. G. (1995). Alpha–theta brainwave neurofeedback training: an effective treatment for male and female alcoholics with depressive symptoms. *Journal of Clinical Psychology*, **51(5)**, 685–693.

Scott, W. and Kaiser, D. (1998). Augmenting chemical dependency treatment with neurofeedback training. *Journal of Neurotherapy*, **3(1)**, 66.

Scott, W. C., Brod, T. M., Sideroff, S., Kaiser, D., and Sagan, M. (2002). Type-specific EEG biofeedback improves residential substance abuse treatment. Paper presented at *American Psychiatric Association Annual Meeting 2002*.

Scott, W. C., Kaiser, D., Othmer, S. and Sideroff, S. I. (2005). Effects of an EEG biofeedback protocol on a mixed substance abusing population. *American Journal of Drug Alcohol Abuse*, **31(3)**, 455–469.

Schubiner, H., Tzelepis, A., Milberger, S., *et al.* (2000). Prevalence of attention-deficit/hyperactivity disorder and conduct disorder among substance abusers. *Journal of Clinical Psychiatry*, **61**, 244–251.

Sheehan, M. F. (1993). Dual diagnosis. *Psychiatry Quarterly*, **64**, 107–134.

Shufman, E., Perl, E., Cohen, M., *et al.* (1996). Electroencephalography spectral analysis of heroin addicts compared with abstainers and normal controls. *Israel Journal of Psychiatry Related Science*, **33**, 196–206.

Simon, S. L., Domier, C., Sim, T., Richardson, K., Rawson, R. and Ling, W. (2002). Cognitive performance of current methamphetamine and cocaine abusers. *Journal of Addictive Diseases*, **21**, 61–74.

Sokhadze, T. (2005). Neurofeedback and cognitive behavioral therapy based intervention in dual diagnosis: a neurobiological model. *Journal of Neurotherapy*, **9(4)**, 123–124.

Sokhadze, T., Stewart, C. M. and Hollifield, M. (2007a). Integrating cognitive neuroscience research and cognitive behavioral treatment with neurofeedback therapy in drug addiction comorbid with Post Traumatic Stress Disorder: A conceptual review. *Journal of Neurotherapy*, **11(2)**, 13–44.

Sokhadze, T., Tasman, A., Stewart, C. M., Singh, S., and Hollifield, M. (2007b). Dense-array QEEG/ ERP study of frontal deficits in patients with substance use disorder and PTSD. Presented at the *15th Annual Conference of ISNR*, San Diego, CA, September 6–9.

Sokhadze, E. M., Cannon, R. L. and Trudeau, D. L. (2008). EEG biofeedback as a treatment for Substance Use Disorders: review, rating of efficacy, and recommendations for further research. *Applied Psychophysiology and Biofeedback*. **33**(1) 1–28. *Journal of Neurotherapy*, **12**(1), 5–43.

Struve, F. A., Straumanis, J. J., Patrick, G. and Price, L. (1989). Topographic mapping of quantitative EEG variables in chronic heavy marihuana users: empirical findings with psychiatric patients. *Clinical Electroencephalography*, **20**(1), 6–23.

Struve, F. A., Straumanis, J. J. and Patrick, G. (1994). Persistent topographic quantitative EEG sequelae of chronic marihuana use: a replication study and initial discriminant function analysis. *Clinical Electroencephalography*, **25**, 63–75.

Struve, F. A., Patrick, G., Straumanis, J. J., Fitz-Gerald, M. J. and Manno, J. (1998). Possible EEG sequelae of very long duration marihuana use: pilot findings from topographic quantitative EEG analyses of subjects with 15 to 24 years of cumulative daily exposure to THC. *Clinical Electroencephalography*, **29**(1), 31–36.

Struve, F. A., Straumanis, J. J., Patrick, G., Leavitt, J., Manno, J. and Manno, B. R. (1999). Topographic quantitative EEG sequelae of chronic marihuana use: a replication using medically and psychiatrically screened normal subjects. *Drug and Alcohol Dependence*, **56**, 167–179.

Struve, F. A., Manno, B. R., Kemp, P., Patrick, G. and Manno, J. (2003). Acute marihuana (THC) exposure produces a "transient" topographic quantitative EEG profile identical to the "persistent" profile seen in chronic heavy users. *Clinical Electroencephalography*, **34**, 75–83.

Swartz, J. A. and Lurigio, A. J. (1999). Psychiatric illness and comorbidity among adult male jail detainees in drug treatment. *Psychiatry Service*, **50**, 1628–1630.

Tarbox, A. R. (1983). Alcoholism, biofeedback and internal scanning. *Journal Study of Alcohol*, **44**(2), 246–261.

Tarter, R. E., Kirisci, L., Mezzich, A., *et al.* (2003). Neurobehavior disinhibition in childhood predicts early age at onset of substance disorder. *American Journal of Psychiatry*, **160**, 1078–1085.

Triffleman, E., Carroll, K. and Kellogg, S. (1999). Substance dependence post traumatic stress therapy: an integrated cognitive-behavioral approach. *Journal of Substance Abuse Treatment*, **17**, 3–14.

Trudeau, D. L. (2000). A review of the treatment of Addictive Disorders by EEG biofeedback. *Clinical Electroencephalography*, **31**, 13–26.

Trudeau, D. L. (2005a). EEG Biofeedback for Addictive Disorders – The state of the Art in 2004. *Journal of Adult Development*, **12**, 139–146.

Trudeau, D. L. (2005b). Applicability of brain wave biofeedback to substance use disorder in adolescents. *Child and Adolescent Clinics of North America*, **14**, 125–136.

Trudeau, D. L., Thuras, P. and Stockley, H. (1999). Quantitative EEG findings associated with chronic stimulant and cannabis abuse and ADHD in an adult male substance use disorder population. *Clinical Electroencephalography*, **30**, 165–174.

Twemlow, S. W. and Bowen, W. T. (1976). EEG biofeedback induced self actualization in alcoholics. *Journal of Biofeedback*, **3**, 20–25.

Twemlow, S. W. and Bowen, W. T. (1977). Sociocultural predictors of self actualization in EEG biofeedback treated alcoholics. *Psychological Reports*, **40**, 591–598.

Twemlow, S. W., Sizemore, D. G. and Bowen, W. T. (1977). Biofeedback induced energy redistribution in the alcoholic EEG. *Journal of Biofeedback*, **3**, 14–19.

Venneman, S., Leuchter, A., Bartzokis, G., *et al.* (2006). Variation in neurophysiological function and evidence of quantitative electroencephalogram discordance: predicting cocaine-dependent treatment attrition. *Journal of Neuropsychiatry Clinical Neurosciences*, **18**(2), 208–216.

Vernon, D. J. (2005). Can neurofeedback training enhance performance? An evaluation of the evidence with implication for future research. *Applied Psychophysiology and Biofeedback*, **30**, 347–364.

Volkow, N. D., Fowler, J. S. and Wang, G. J. (2003). The addicted human brain: insights from imaging studies. *Journal of Clinical Investigations*, **111**, 1444–1451.

Volkow, N. D., Fowler, J. S. and Wang, G. J. (2004). The addicted human brain viewed in the light of imaging studies: brain circuits and treatment strategies. *Neuropharmacology*, **47**, 3–13.

Watson, C. G., Herder, J. and Passini, F. T. (1978). Alpha biofeedback therapy in alcoholics: an 18-month follow-up. *Journal of Clinical Psychology*, **34(3)**, 765–769.

Wender, P. H. (1995). *Attention-Deficit Hyperactivity Disorder in Adults*. New York: Oxford University Press.

Wert, R. C. and Raulin, M. L. (1986). The chronic cerebral effects of cannabis use. I. Methodological issues and neurological findings. *International Journal of Addiction*, **21**, 605–628.

Whitlow, C. T., Freedland, C. S. and Porrino, J. L. (2002). Metabolic mapping of the time-dependent effects of delta 9-tetrahydrocannabinol administration in the rat. *Psychopharmacology*, **161**, 129–136.

Wilens, T. E., Biederman, J. and Mick, E. (1998). Does ADHD affect the course of substance abuse? Findings from a sample of adults with and without ADHD. *American Journal of Addictions*, **7(2)**, 156–163.

Winterer, G., Kloeppel, B., Heinz, A., Ziller, M., Dufeu, P., Schmidt, L. G. and Herrmann, W. M. (1998). Quantitative EEG (QEEG) predicts relapse in patients with chronic alcoholism and points to a frontally pronounced cerebral disturbance. *Psychiatry Research*, **78**, 101–113.

Winterer, G., Enoch, M. A., White, K., Saylan, M., Coppola, R. and Goldman, D. (2003a). EEG phenotype in alcoholism: increased coherence in the depressive subtype. *Acta Psychiatrica Scandinavica*, **108**, 51–60.

Winterer, G., Smolka, M., Samochowiec, J., et al. (2003b). Association of EEG coherence and an exonic GABA$_B$R1 gene polymorphism. *American Journal of Medical Genetics*, **117B**, 51–56.

CHAPTER 11

EEG Evaluation of traumatic brain injury and EEG biofeedback treatment

Robert W. Thatcher Ph.D.

*EEG and NeuroImaging Laboratory, Applied Neuroscience, Inc.,
St. Petersburg, and Professor, Department of Neurology,
University of South Florida, Florida, USA*

I. INTRODUCTION

This chapter is a modification and update of a paper evaluating EEG and TBI in athletes (Thatcher, 2006). The update in this chapter includes a more general review and analysis of quantitative EEG (QEEG) for the evaluation of the locations and extent of injury to the brain following rapid acceleration/deceleration trauma, especially in mild traumatic brain injury (TBI). The earliest use of QEEG was by Hans Berger in 1932, and since this time over 2,000 peer reviewed journal articles have been published in which QEEG was used to evaluate traumatic brain injury. Quantitative EEG is a direct measure of the electrical energies of the brain and network dynamics which are disturbed following a traumatic brain injury. The most consistent findings are:

1. Reduced power in the higher frequency bands (8–40 Hz) which is linearly related to the magnitude of injury to cortical gray matter.
2. Increased slow waves in the delta frequency band (1–4 Hz) in the more severe cases of TBI, which is linearly related to the magnitude of cerebral white matter injury.
3. Changes in EEG coherence and EEG phase delays which are linearly related to the magnitude of injury to both the gray matter and the white matter, especially in frontal and temporal lobes.

A review of QEEG reliability and clinical validation studies showed high predictive and content validity as determined by correlations between QEEG and clinical measures, such as neuropsychological test performance, Glasgow coma scores, length of coma, and MRI biophysical measures. Inexpensive and high speed QEEG NeuroImaging methods were also discussed in which the locations of maximal deviations from normal in three-dimensions were revealed. Evaluation of the sensitivity and specificity of QEEG with a reduced number of EEG channels offers the feasibility of real-time monitoring of the EEG using Blue Tooth technology inside of a helmet, so that immediate evaluation of the severity and extent of brain injury can be accomplished. Finally, QEEG biofeedback treatment for the amelioration of complaints and symptoms following TBI is discussed.

An important fact to keep in mind when evaluating the clinical consequences of traumatic brain injury is that the brain, while only constituting about 2% of our body weight, consumes approximately 60% of blood glucose (Stryer, 1988). In other words, an approximately two and 1/2 pounds of soft tissue consumes approximately 60% of the total energy of the body, as much as muscles in active contraction at every moment of time (Stryer, 1988). A pertinent question is 'how is this disproportionate amount of energy utilized?' The answer is that most of the brain's metabolic energy is transformed into electricity by which the essential perceptual, cognitive, emotive, regulatory, and motor functions are carried out at each moment of time.

The human brain is vulnerable to traumatic injury by the fact that it sits on a hard bony vault. Rapid acceleration/deceleration forces often result in contusions or bruising of the frontal and temporal lobes, which are located at the interface between the soft tissues of the brain and the hard bone of the skull. For example, because of physics even blunt impacts to the occipital bone result in frontal and temporal brain injuries (Ommaya, 1986; 1994; Sano *et al.*, 1967). In addition to linear percussion forces, rapid acceleration/deceleration often produces shear forces in which different regions of the brain move at different rates, resulting in stretching of axons with effects on the myelin and on conduction velocities. Similarly, rotational forces can also be imparted to the brain, and both the shear and rotational forces can damage the cerebral white matter as well as brain stem structures even in whiplash injuries (McLean, 1995; Ommaya and Hirsch, 1971). The duration of reduced brain function following traumatic brain injury can be many years, even in the case of mild head injuries in which there is no loss of consciousness (Ommaya, 1995; Barth *et al.*, 1983; Rimel *et al.*, 1981).

II.   ELECTROCHEMISTRY AND THE ELECTROENCEPHALOGRAM

The electroencephalogram, or EEG, is typically recorded at the scalp surface with reference to the ear, and represents the moment-to-moment electrical activity of the brain. The electroencephalogram, or EEG, is produced by the summation of synaptic currents that arise on the dendrites and cell bodies of billions of cortical pyramidal cells that are primarily located a few centimeters below the scalp surface. The synaptic currents involve neurotransmitter storage and release which are dependent on the integrity of the sodium/potassium and calcium ionic pumps located in the membranes of each neuron. Metabolic activity is the link between EEG/MEG and PET, SPECT and fMRI which are measures of blood flow dynamics. Glucose regulation and restoration of ionic concentrations occurs many milliseconds, seconds, and minutes after electrical impulses and synaptic activity and, therefore, blood flow changes are secondary to the nearly instantaneous electrical activity and metabolic activities that give rise to the EEG at each moment of time (Thatcher and John, 1977).

The effects of traumatic injury on the electrical activity of the brain, due to injury to the number and integrity of ionic channels and electrical generators, and on the network dynamics involved in the distribution and coordination of the electrical energy, is easily measured with the EEG using high speed modern and inexpensive computers. As would be expected, EEG measurements are sensitive and accurate in the detection and evaluation of the effects of rapid acceleration/deceleration on brain electrical activity. This fact is supported in the sections that follow with citations to a vast scientific literature of EEG studies showing similar effects of traumatic brain injury, as would be expected when a small and energetic mass of tissue is suddenly accelerated and banged against a hard bony vault.

III. AMERICAN ACADEMY OF NEUROLOGY AND QUANTITATIVE EEG

In 1997 Marc Nuwer, as a spokesperson for the American Academy of Neurology (AAN), published a non-peer reviewed opinion paper that acknowledged the widespread use of "Digital EEG" in support of visual examination of EEG traces by a neurologist. In the same AAN opinion paper, QEEG was arbitrarily limited to the less worthy category "experimental" as distinct from "clinically acceptable" (Nuwer, 1997). This is important because the outdated, flawed and politically motivated 1997 ANN position opposing applications of QEEG still holds sway in 2008; it still influences insurance companies and it still restricts the availability of twenty-first century technology to people with serious clinical problems including brain injury in athletes.

One is struck by the fact that the less worthy categories of QEEG according to the Nuwer 1997 opinion involve a variety of serious neurological and psychological problems such as traumatic brain injury, learning disabilities, language disorders, schizophrenia, depression, addition disorders, obsessive compulsive disorders, and many others (Nuwer, 1997). One is also struck by the fact that the AAN has not revised its 1997 opinion given the prior and current scientific literature and scholarly rebuttals (Hughes and John, 1999; Hoffman *et al.*, 1999; Thatcher *et al.*, 1999).

Another remarkable fact is that the 1997 AAN assignment to the "unworthy" category occurred without a proper review of the scientific literature—without any citations that rebutted the prior 20 years of quantitative EEG studies. It is also remarkable that the AAN position paper supported visual examination of the EEG tracings as the "Gold Standard" for acceptance in courts and for third party reimbursement, when it is well known that subjective visual examination of EEG traces is unreliable and inferior to quantitative analyses (Cooper *et al.*, 1974; Woody, 1966, 1968; Niedermeyer and Lopez Da Silva, 1995).

The lack of objectivity, low reliability, and reliance on subjective opinion in the visual analysis of EEG tracings is well known by neurologists; for example, the primary textbook that neurologists are required to study before taking an EEG examination states:

> There is simply no firm rule concerning the manner in which the reader's eyes and brain have to operate in this process. Every experienced electroencephalographer has his or her personal approach to EEG interpretation. This is also true for the manner in which the EEG report is written. Although standardization is an important goal in many areas of EEG technology, experienced electroencephalographers should not abandon a certain individualistic spirit.... (Niedermeyer and Da Silva, 1995, p.185–86)

As mentioned previously, in response to the 1997 Nuwer opinion paper in opposition to quantitative EEG, Hughes and John (1999) wrote a rebuttal that included 258 publications, and systematically categorized and analyzed the consistency and high sensitivity of quantitative EEG studies in all of the areas that the AAN labeled as "experimental." They also showed that the sensitivity and specificity of the AAN's alleged "clinically valid" categories often had lower sensitivity and specificity than the category that the AAN labeled as "experimental," thus further proving that the opinion paper was biased and arbitrary. The Hughes and John (1999) rebuttal was the first paper to show that the Nuwer 1997 position paper was a sham, and it was followed by two additional rebuttals that cited the scientific literature and pointed out misrepresentations and omissions in the 1997 Nuwer AAN opinion paper (Hoffman et al., 1999; Thatcher et al., 1999).

The arbitrary and subjective opinion of the AAN is also contradicted by the fact that the National Library of Medicine database lists over 90,000 QEEG studies published since 1970 involving a wide variety of clinical conditions, thus proving that there is a very widespread use and acceptance of this technology. The disconnect between the 1997 Nuwer AAN opinion paper is further contradicted by a search of the National Library of Medicine database using the search words "EEG and traumatic brain injury" which resulted in 2,020 citations, with the majority of these articles involving quantitative EEG and not visual examination of EEG tracings drawn by ink pens or on a computer display. A similar search of the National Library of Medicine database for each of the restricted or alleged experimental uses of QEEG also yields a larger number of clinical publications.

Below is a partial list of organizations that, in contrast to the AAN, support or certify by examination trained and experienced Ph.D.s and M.D.s in EEG and QEEG including the use of QEEG for the evaluation of mild to severe traumatic brain injury. The list below helps demonstrate that the AAN does not constitute the relevant community using QEEG nor is the AAN a representative of the users of QEEG. The list of organizations below represents many more individuals than the membership of the AAN who do not use QEEG.

1. American Medical EEG Society
2. American Board of EEG and Clinical Neurophysiology

3. American Psychological Association
4. EEG and Clinical Neuroscience Society
5. International Society for NeuroImaging in Psychiatry
6. International Society for Brain Electrical Activity
7. American Board of Certification in Quantitative Electroencephalography
8. Biofeedback Certification Institute of America
9. Association for Applied Psychophysiology and Biofeedback
10. International Society for Neural Feedback and Research
11. Society for Applied Neuroscience

The large list of organizations and the large number of Ph.D.s and M.D.s that support the use of QEEG for the evaluation of TBI shows that the AAN "does not represent the relevant community" in a court of law. The definition of the "relevant community" is critical in medical-legal issues for the admission of evidence in a court of law under both Frye and Daubert criteria which are:

1. Acceptance by the relevant community of users of the methodology, and
2. Reliability.

Neurologists are in the minority of those using QEEG technology and, therefore, the first prong of Frye is not met by the ANN when it opposes admission of QEEG because neurologists do not represent the relevant community of users of QEEG. For example, in a July 2004 deposition[1] Dr. Nuwer admitted that he had never personally used QEEG for the evaluation of traumatic brain injury, and he was asked to guess the number of neurologists that use QEEG. Dr. Nuwer responded by estimating less than 100 neurologists use QEEG. This number is less than 1% of the total number of users of QEEG technology and, therefore, as a matter of mathematical fact Nuwer and the AAN do not represent the relevant community of users of the technology.

Under Frye and Daubert standards, if there are over 16,000 users of a technology that has produced over 70,000 peer reviewed scientific articles then how is it possible that Dr. Nuwer represents the opinion of a "relevant" or majority community when there are less than 1% of neurologists who even use the technology? The second prong of Frye is easily met by the facts because the reliability of QEEG is often 90–99% (Thatcher *et al.*, 1999; 2003).

IV. DEFINITIONS OF DIGITAL EEG AND QUANTITATIVE EEG (QEEG)

The AAN defined digital EEG as "… the paperless acquisition and recording of the EEG via computer-based instrumentation, with waveform storage in a digital format on electronic media, and waveform display on an electronic monitor or

---

[1]State of Florida vs. Samuel Harris case No. 05-2001-CF-041393-AXXX-XX.

other computer output device." The primary purposes of digital EEG is for efficiency of storage, the saving of paper, and for the purposes of visual examination
of the EEG tracings. The 1997 AAN position paper concluded that "Digital EEG
is an excellent technical advance and should be considered an established guideline for clinical EEG." (Nuwer, 1997, p. 278).

The American Academy of Neurology opinion paper (Nuwer, 1997) then
attempted to create a distinction between digital EEG and quantitative EEG by
defining quantitative EEG (qEEG or QEEG) as "the mathematical processing of digitally recorded EEG in order to highlight specific waveform components, transform
the EEG into a format or domain that elucidates relevant information, or associate
numerical results with the EEG data for subsequent review or comparison." (Nuwer,
1997, p. 278). However, the reality is that there is no clear distinction between digital
EEG and quantitative EEG because both involve mathematical transformations. For
example, the process of analog-to-digital conversion involves transforms by analog
and digital filtering, as well as amplification, sample and hold of the electrical scalp
potentials and remontaging and reformatting the EEG. Clearly, digital EEG involves
mathematical and transformational processing using a computer, and therefore the
distinction between quantitative EEG and digital EEG is weak and artificial.

It would appear that the AAN's artificial distinction between digital EEG and
quantitative EEG is aimed to support the practice of visual examination of EEG
tracings, which is highly unreliable and insensitive (Cooper *et al.*, 1974; Woody,
1966; 1968) while at the same time downplaying modern advances in quantitative
EEG, which is more reliable and more sensitive than visual examination alone.
Indeed, simultaneous QEEG with visual examination of EEG tracings can significantly aid a competent clinician in their assessment of a patient's problems.

V.   SIMULTANEOUS CONVENTIONAL EEG
TRACINGS AND QUANTITATIVE EEG

Figure 11.1 illustrates a common modern quantitative EEG analysis which can
be activated rapidly by a few mouse clicks on a small home computer using free
educational software or by using inexpensive FDA registered commercial QEEG
software. EEG traces are viewed and examined at the same time that quantitative
analyses are displayed so as to facilitate and extend analytical power.

Common sense dictates that the digital EEG and QEEG when simultaneously
available facilitate rapid, accurate and reliable evaluation of the electroencephalogram.
Clearly, the AAN's distinction between digital EEG and quantitative EEG needs to be
revisited, and a new and more clinically useful position should be adopted by the AAN.

Since 1929, when the human EEG was first measured (Berger, 1929), modern
science has learned an enormous amount about the current sources of the EEG
and the manner in which ensembles of synaptic generators are synchronously
organized. It is known that short distance local generators are connected by white

Examples of QEEG analyses

BESA
BioSemi
BrainMaster
Cadwell
CapScan
DeyMed
Lexicor
MindSet
Mitsar
NeuroNav
NeuroPrax
NeuroScan
Nicolet
NuAmps
ProComp
XLTEK
etc.

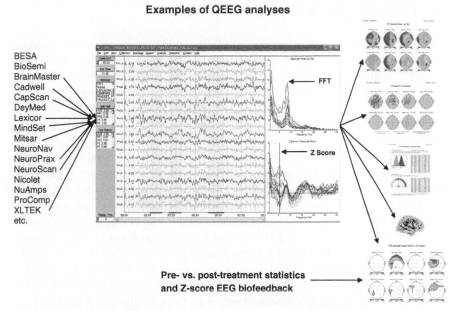

FFT

Z Score

**Pre- vs. post-treatment statistics
and Z-score EEG biofeedback**

FIGURE 11.1   Example of QEEG analyses in which calibrated EEG digital data are imported; test–retest and split half reliabilities are computed, spectral analyses are performed (FFT) and compared to a normative database (e.g., Z Scores); discriminant analyses and color topographic maps are produced; three-dimensional source localization is measured; and objective pre-treatment vs. post-treatment, or pre-mediation vs. post-medication, statistics within a few minutes using the same computer program (see color plate).

matter axons to other local generators that can be many centimeters distant. The interplay and coordination of short distance local generators with the longer distant white matter connections has been mathematically modeled and shown to be essential for our understanding of the genesis of the EEG (Nunez, 1981; 1995; Thatcher and John, 1977; Thatcher *et al.*, 1986).

The first QEEG study was by Hans Berger (1932, 1934) when, recognizing the importance of quantification and objectivity in the evaluation of the electro-encephalogram (EEG), he used the Fourier transform to spectrally analyze the EEG. The relevance of quantitative EEG (QEEG) to the diagnosis and prognosis of traumatic brain injury (TBI) stems directly from the quantitative EEG's ability to measure the consequences of rapid acceleration/deceleration to both the short distance and long distance compartments of the brain as well as to coup counter-coup patterns, focal contusions and neural membrane damage.

In this chapter I will first briefly review the present state of knowledge about the reliability, validity and diagnostic value of QEEG in TBI, with special emphasis on the integration of QEEG with MRI and other imaging technologies. I will also briefly discuss EEG biofeedback as a possible treatment to help ameliorate symptoms following traumatic brain injury.

VI.   TEST–RETEST RELIABILITY OF QEEG

The clinical sensitivity and specificity of QEEG is directly related to the stability and reliability of QEEG upon repeat testing. The scientific literature shows that QEEG is highly reliable and reproducible (Hughes and John, 1999; Aruda *et al.*, 1996; Burgess and Gruzelier, 1993; Corsi-Cabera *et al.*, 1997; Gasser *et al.*, 1985; Hamilton-Bruce *et al.*, 1991; Harmony *et al.*, 1993; Lund *et al.*, 1995; Duffy *et al.*, 1994; Salinsky *et al.*, 1991; Pollock *et al.*, 1991).

The inherent stability and reliability of QEEG can even be demonstrated with quite small sample sizes. For example, Salinsky *et al.* (1991) reported that repeated 20-second samples of EEG were about 82% reliable, at 40 seconds the samples were about 90% reliable, and at 60 seconds they were approximately 92% reliable. Gasser *et al.* (1985) concluded that: "20 sec. of activity are sufficient to reduce adequately the variability inherent in the EEG" and Hamilton-Bruce *et al.* (1991) found statistically high reliability when the same EEG was independently analyzed by three different individuals. Although the QEEG is highly reliable even with relatively short sample sizes, it is the recommendation of most QEEG experts that larger samples sizes be used, for example, at least 60 seconds of artifact-free EEG, and preferably 2–5 minutes should be used in a clinical evaluation (Duffy *et al.*, 1994; Hughes and John, 1999).

VII.   PRESENT USE OF QEEG FOR THE EVALUATION OF TBI

As mentioned previously, the National Library of Medicine lists 2,020 peer reviewed journal articles on the subject of EEG and traumatic brain injury. The vast majority of these studies involved quantitative analyses and, in general, the scientific literature presents a consistent and common quantitative EEG pattern correlated with TBI. Namely, reduced amplitude of the alpha, beta and gamma frequency bands of EEG (8–12 Hz, 13–25 Hz and 30–40 Hz) (Mas *et al.*, 1993; von Bierbrauer *et al.*, 1993; Ruijs *et al.*, 1994; Korn *et al.*, 2005; Hellstrom-Westas, 2005 Thompson *et al.*, 2005; Tebano *et al.*, 1988; Thatcher *et al.*, 1998a, 2001a; Roche *et al.*, 2004; Slewa-Younan, 2002; Slobounov *et al.*, 2002), changes in EEG coherence, and phase delays in frontal and temporal relations (Thatcher *et al.*, 1989, 1991, 1998b, 2001b; Hoffman *et al.*, 1995, 1996a; Trudeau *et al.*, 1998; Thornton, 1999, 2003[2]; Thornton and Cormody, 2005).

---

[2]Thornton (1999) incorrectly claimed that he used and tested the Thatcher *et al.* (1989) discriminant function. The facts are that Thornton did not use the Thatcher *et al.* (1989) discriminant function but instead used a modified and invalid version of the discriminant function, and the findings in his study regarding the Thatcher *et al.* (1989) discriminant function should be ignored. What is important, however, is that Thornton obtained high sensitivity and specificity using his own discriminant function which was developed independent of the Thatcher *et al.* (1989) discriminant function.

The reduced amplitude of EEG is believed to be due to a reduced number of synaptic generators, and/or reduced integrity of the protein/lipid membranes of neurons (Thatcher *et al.*, 1997, 1998a, 2001b). EEG coherence is a measure of the amount of shared electrical activity at a particular frequency, and is analogous to a cross-correlation coefficient. EEG coherence is amplitude independent, and reflects the amount of functional connectivity between distant EEG generators (Nunez, 1981, 1994; Thatcher *et al.*, 1986). EEG phase delays between distant regions of the cortex are mediated in part by the conduction velocity of the cerebral white matter, which is a likely reason why EEG phase delays are often distorted following a traumatic brain injury (Thatcher *et al.*, 1989, 2001a). In general, the more severe the traumatic brain injury then the more deviant the QEEG measures (Thatcher *et al.*, 2001a, 2001b).

Quantitative EEG studies of the diagnosis of TBI typically show quite high sensitivity and specificity, even for mild head injuries. For example, a study of 608 mild TBI patients and 103 age-matched control subjects demonstrated discriminant sensitivity = 96.59%, specificity = 89.15%, positive predictive value (PPV) = 93.6% (average of Tables II, III, V), and negative predictive value (NPV) = 97.4% (average of Tables III, IV, V) in four independent cross-validations. A similar sensitivity and specificity for QEEG diagnosis of TBI was published by Trudeau *et al.* (1998), Thornton (1999), and Thatcher *et al.* (2001b). All of these studies met most of the American Academy of Neurology's criteria for diagnostic medical tests of:

1. The "criteria for test abnormality was defined explicitly and clearly."
2. Control groups were "different from those originally used to derive the test's normal limits."
3. "Test–retest reliability was high."
4. The test was more sensitive than "routine EEG" or fMRI and PET "neuroimaging tests."
5. The study occurred in an essentially "blinded" design (i.e., objectively and without ability to influence or bias the results).

VIII.   DROWSINESS AND THE EFFECTS OF MEDICATION ON QEEG

Artifact removal is important in order to achieve high reliability and validity in the clinical assessment of EEG. Drowsiness is an artifact that is easy to detect, and is rarely a problem in EEG recording, especially when the first 30 seconds to 2 minutes of a recording session are utilized in the analysis as this is a time period in which it is difficult for patients to become drowsy. Eyes-open EEG analysis is another method used to avoid drowsiness. When the EEG recording is excessively long, then careful examination of the EEG to detect and remove drowsiness is necessary. Drowsiness is characterized by reduced amplitude of alpha activity in posterior regions, slow eye movements and, with deeper levels of drowsiness, theta rhythms in the frontal lobes. Focal deviations from normal cannot be explained by drowsiness; for example, drowsiness does not occur in only a single or a localized region of the brain.

Medications of various types can also affect the EEG. However, there is no evidence that a given medication only affects a localized and isolated region of the brain, or one hemisphere, and not the other hemisphere, as different receptor types that medication acts on are widely distributed and never exclusively present in only one region of the cortex (Wauguier, 2005). Consequently, the use of remontage procedures, such as the Laplacian montage, eliminates diffuse and global electrical fields produced by medication. For example, the Laplacian sets spatially common fields equal to zero and enhances focally present electrical activity, which can then be correlated with the point of impact on to the patient's skull in the case of traumatic brain injury, and by Low Resolution Electromagnetic Tomography (LORETA), in order to localize abnormal EEG activity. In addition, it appears that EEG coherence and phase delays are not very sensitive to effects of medications. This fact was illustrated in a QEEG study of 608 TBI patients in which no differences in an EEG discriminant function were observed when patients on medication were compared with patients with no medication, or when different types of medications were compared (Thatcher et al., 1989).

IX.   PREDICTIVE VALIDITY OF QEEG IN THE EVALUATION OF TBI—NEUROPSYCHOLOGICAL

Predictive (or criterion) validity has a close relationship to hypothesis testing by subjecting the measure to a discriminant or cluster analysis or to some statistical analysis in order to separate a clinical sub-type. Nunnally (1978) gives a useful definition of predictive validity as: "when the purpose is to use an instrument to estimate some important form of behavior that is external to the measuring instrument itself, the latter being referred to as criterion [predictive] validity." For example, science "validates" the clinical usefulness of a measure by its false positive and false negative rates, and by the extent to which there are statistically significant correlations to other clinical measures and, especially, to clinical outcomes (Cronback, 1971; Mas et al., 1993; Hughes and John, 1999).

Another example of predictive validity is the ability to discriminate traumatic brain injured patients from age-matched normal control subjects at classification accuracies greater than 95% (Thatcher et al., 1989, 2001b; Thornton, 1999). Another example of predictive validity is the ability of QEEG normative values to predict cognitive functioning in TBI patients (Thatcher et al., 1998a, 1998b, 2001a, 2001b). Table 11.1 shows correlations between QEEG and a variety of neuropsychological tests, and serves as another example of clinical predictive validity and content

TABLE 11.1   Correlations between neuropsychological test scores and QEEG discriminant scores in TBI patients (N = 108) (from Thatcher *et al.*, 2001a).

Pearson Product-Moment Correlation	Correlation	Probability
WAIS Test—scaled scores		
Vocabulary	−0.416	0.05
Similarities	−0.640	0.001
Picture arrangement	−0.576	0.01
Performance	−0.504	0.01
Digit symbol	−0.524	0.01
BOSTON Naming Test		
# of spontaneous correct responses	−0.482	0.05
WORD Fluency Test—total correct words		
COWA	−0.568	0.01
Animals	−0.630	0.001
Supermarket	−0.709	0.001
ATTENTION Test—raw scores		
Trail Making A—Response Time	0.627	0.001
Trail Making B—Response Time	0.627	0.001
Stroop—Word	−0.427	0.05
Stroop—Color	−0.618	0.001
Stroop—Color + Word	−0.385	ns
WISC Test—executive functioning—raw scores		
Perseverative responses	0.408	0.05
% Concept. level responses	−0.200	ns
Categories completed	−0.187	ns
Design fluency – # originals	−0.454	0.05
Design fluency – # rule violations	0.304	ns
WECHSLER Memory Test—raw scores		
Logical memory II	−0.382	ns
Visual production II	−0.509	0.01
Digit span (forward + backward)	−0.336	ns
Digit span (forward)	−0.225	ns
%-tile rank forward	−0.300	ns
Digit span (backward)	−0.213	ns
CVLT Test—raw scores		
Recall — List A	−0.509	0.01
Recall — List B	−0.554	0.01
List A — short-delay free	−0.518	0.01
Semantic Cluster ratio	−0.162	ns
Recall Errors — free intrusions	0.409	0.05
Recall Errors — cued intrusions	0.520	0.01
Recognition hits	−0.595	0.01
Recognition false positives	0.280	ns

validity. As seen in Table 11.1, relatively strong correlations exist between QEEG measures and performance on neuropsychological tests. Also, as the severity of TBI increases then there is a systematic increase in deviation from normal EEG values which correlates to a systematic decrease in neuropsychological test performance (Thatcher et al., 1998a, 1998b, 2001a, 2001b). Such relationships between clinical measures and the EEG demonstrate the predictive validity of EEG in the evaluation of TBI as well as normal brain functioning (Thatcher et al., 2003, 2005c).

The reliability and stability of the QEEG discriminant function was evaluated by comparing the discriminant scores at baseline to the discriminant scores obtained upon repeated EEG testing at 6 months and 12 months after the initial baseline EEG test. No statistically significant differences were found between any of the post-injury periods up to 4 years post-injury, thus demonstrating high reliability even several years after injury (Thatcher et al., 2001a).

The results of a cross-validation analysis of the QEEG and TBI are shown in Fig. 11.2. In this study, quantitative EEG analyses were conducted on 503 confirmed TBI patients located at four different Veterans Affairs hospitals (Palo Alto, CA; Minneapolis, MN; Richmond, VA; and Tampa, Fl), and three military hospitals (Balboa Naval Medical Center, Wilford Hall Air Force Medical Center, and Walter Reed Army Medical Center). Figure 11.2 shows histograms of the distribution of QEEG TBI discriminant scores in the 503 TBI subjects who were tested 15 days to 4 years post-injury. It can be seen that the distribution of the QEEG discriminant scores, and thus the severity of the injury, varied at the different hospitals. The VA patients exhibited more deviant QEEG scores than the active duty military personnel which was consistent with the clinical evaluations, including neuropsychological testing.

Table 11.2 shows the results of multivariate analyses of variance in which statistically significant differences in neuropsychological performance were predicted by the QEEG discriminant score groupings. The group which had lower EEG discriminant scores was associated with higher neuropsychological functioning when compared with the group which had higher EEG discriminant scores.

X. THE USE OF FEWER ELECTRODES TO EVALUATE THE EFFECTS OF TBI

As the number of recording channels decreases, then the ability of quantitative EEG measures to detect the consequences of rapid acceleration/deceleration forces should diminish. This is what is expected for a measure to be valid (predictive validation). A test of this assumption was carried out by systematically reducing the number of EEG recording channels from five to two, and then recomputing the best discriminant function to distinguish mild TBI patients from age-matched normal control subjects. The analyses still showed quite high sensitivity and specificity in discriminanting age normals from TBI patients. Figure 11.3 shows ROC curves (receiver operator curves) of discriminant accuracy for 2-, 3-, 4- and 5-channel EEG which range from 74–97.3% discriminant accuracy.

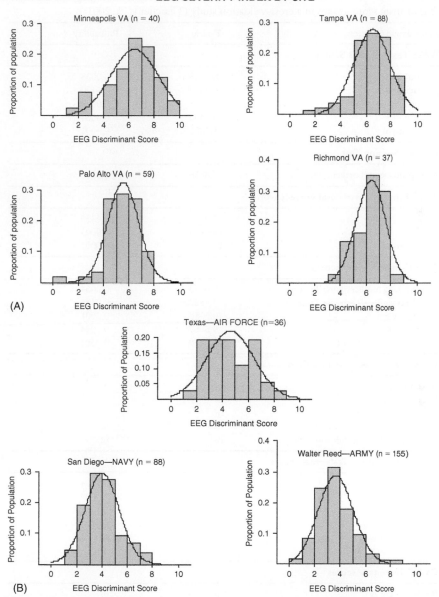

FIGURE 11.2   Histograms showing the QEEG discriminant score distribution from 503 TBI outpatients located at four different Veterans Affairs hospitals (A), and three military hospitals (B). Normal = 0 and most severe TBI = 10 (from Thatcher *et al.*, 2001a).

TABLE 11.2   Results of multivariate analyses of variance between low and high EEG discriminant score groups in a cross-validation study (Thatcher *et al.*, 2001a).

Multivariate Analyses:	F-ratio	Probability
WAIS Test—Scaled Scores		
Vocabulary	8.7448	0.0038
Similarities	6.3690	0.0130
Picture arrangement	8.2771	0.0048
Performance	13.2430	0.0004
Digit symbol	21.0620	0.0001
Boston Naming Test		
# of spontaneous correct responses	4.8616	0.0290
Word Fluency Test—total correct words		
COWA	5.2803	0.0230
Animals	14.0170	0.0003
Supermarket	18.8370	0.0001
Attention Test—raw scores		
Trail Making A—Response Time	7.6953	0.0064
Trail Making B—Response Time	4.6882	0.0324
Stroop—Word	16.5080	0.0001
Stroop—Color	9.6067	0.0024
Stroop—Color + Word	4.3879	0.0383
WISC Test—executive functioning-raw scores		
Perseverative responses	ns	ns
% Concept. level responses	ns	ns
Categories completed	ns	ns
Design fluency — # originals	ns	ns
Design fluency — # rule violations	ns	ns
Wechsler Memory Test—raw scores		
Logical memory II	3.9988	0.0484
Visual production II	7.1378	0.0089
Digit span (forward + backward)	ns	ns
Digit span (forward)	ns	ns
%-tile rank forward	ns	ns
Digit span (backward)	ns	ns
CVLT Test—raw scores		
Recall — List A	ns	ns
Recall — List B	ns	ns
List A — short—delay free	7.0358	0.0089
Semantic cluster ratio	ns	ns
Recall errors — free intrusions	ns	ns
Recall errors — cued intrusions	ns	ns
Recognition hits	ns	ns
Recognition false positives	ns	ns

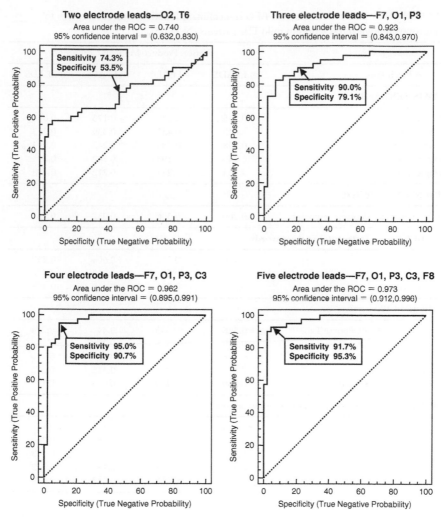

FIGURE 11.3   Receiver operating characteristics curves (ROC) of TBI discriminant functions using different numbers of electrode leads. As the number of leads increases from two to five, the discriminant accuracy correspondingly increases.

Predictive and content validity were further tested by correlating the 2–5-channel QEEG discriminant scores with performance on a series of neuropsychological tests in the same subjects (Thatcher *et al.*, 2001a). Table 11.3 shows the correlation of different EEG TBI discriminant functions with neuropsychological test scores in the same group of TBI patients as in Figure 11.3. As the number of EEG channels increases from two leads to five leads, the strength of correlation to neuropsychological test performance increases. This is what is expected if a measure has predictive validity and is cross-validated by correlation with clinical measures, such as a neuropsychological test (content validity).

TABLE 11.3   Two-to five-channel EEG discriminant functions and correlations to neuropsychological test scores in mild TBI patients (N = 63).

NeuroPsych Tests	Pearson Product-Moment Correlation			
	5 LEADS	4 LEADS	3 LEADS	2 LEADS
WAIS TEST-Scaled Scores				
Vocabulary	0.285	0.235	0.173	0.094
Similarities	0.475	0.432	0.339	0.253
Picture arrangement	0.398	0.38	0.243	0.094
Performance	0.249	0.198	0.142	0.29
Digit symbol	0.454	0.281	0.212	0.188
Boston Naming Test				
# of spontaneous correct responses	0.360	0.366	0.252	0.132
Word Fluency Test—total correct words				
COWA	0.496	0.519	0.604	0.457
Animals	0.501	0.501	0.514	0.372
Supermarket	0.599	0.531	0.465	0.495
Attention Test—raw scores				
Trail Making A—Response Time	−0.526	−0.545	0.44	−0.274
Trail Making B—Response Time	−0.469	−0.475	0.376	−0.296
Stroop—Word	0.256	0.229	0.157	0.149
Stroop—Color	0.464	0.416	0.315	0.373
Stroop—Color + Word	0.249	0.199	0.064	0.11
WISC Test—executive functioning—raw scores				
Perseverative responses	−0.404	−0.47	0.369	0.17
% Concept. level responses	0.289	0.303	0.293	0.28
Categories completed	0.265	0.273	0.28	0.273
Design—Fluency — # originals	0.193	0.178	0.18	0.112
Design—Fluency — # rule violations	−0.166	−0.058	0.043	0.079

Sig. level P < 0.05 > = or = < 0.246
Sig. level P < 0.01 > = or = < 0.318
Sig. level P < 0.001 > = or = < 0.399
Sig. level P < 0.0002 > = or = < 0.441

The use of a small number of QEEG leads is important because a simpler, easier-to-apply and easier-to-use methodology is desirable. For example, the use of Blue-Tooth wireless technology with field effect transistors and amplifiers inside of a football helmet is possible. Such technology is inexpensive, and can be used to evaluate an individual's response to TBI and rapid acceleration/deceleration forces in real-time, and can lead, therefore, to more accurate assessments and a more complete understanding of the consequences of an injury.

XI. EXAMPLES OF CONTENT VALIDITY OF QEEG AND TBI EVALUATION

Content validity is defined by the extent to which an empirical measurement reflects a specific domain of content. For example, a test in arithmetic operations would not be content valid if the test problems focused only on addition, thus neglecting subtraction, multiplication and division. By the same token, a content-valid measure of cognitive decline following a stroke should include measures of memory capacity, attention, and executive function, etc.

There are many examples of the clinical content validity of QEEG in ADD, ADHD, schizophrenia, compulsive disorders, depression, epilepsy, TBI, and a wide number of clinical groupings of patients as reviewed by Hughes and John, (1999). As mentioned previously, there are 258 citations to the scientific literature in the AAN rebuttal review by Hughes and John (1999), and there are approximately 1,672 citations to peer reviewed journal articles in which a quantitative EEG was used to evaluate traumatic brain injury.

Content validity of QEEG is also demonstrated by strong correlations with magnetic resonance imaging (MRI) which provides much more than just a structural picture by which the spatial location of EEG generators can be identified (Thatcher *et al.*, 1994; Thatcher, 1995). For example, the spectroscopic dimensions of the MRI can provide information about the biophysics of protein/lipid water exchanges, water diffusion, blood perfusion, cellular density, and mitochondrial energetics (Gilles, 1994). The marriage of QEEG with the biophysical and structural aspects of MRI offers the possibility of much more sensitive and specific diagnostic and prognostic evaluations, not to mention the development and evaluation of treatment regimens in TBI. A recent series of studies has helped pioneer the integration of QEEG with the biophysical aspects of MRI for the evaluation of TBI (Thatcher *et al.*, 1997, 1998a, 1998b). These studies have provided MRI with quantitative methods to evaluate the consequences of rapid acceleration/deceleration and to integrate the MRI measures with the electrical and magnetic properties of the QEEG as they are affected by TBI (Thatcher *et al.*, 1998a, 1998b, 2001b).

Figure 11.4 shows an example of the relationship between gray matter damage, as measured by MRI T2 relaxation time, and the QEEG in which there is a negative linear relationship between the magnitude of injury and the amplitude of the QEEG at higher frequencies (Thatcher *et al.*, 1998a). This same study showed that damage to the cerebral white matter as measured by MRI T2 relationship was positively related to the magnitude of the injury and to the magnitude of delta or low frequency activity of the EEG. In a subsequent study, the inverse relationship between T2 relaxation time and EEG amplitude was demonstrated for the alpha frequency band (Thatcher *et al.*, 2001b).

Other examples of QEEG and content validity in the evaluation of TBI can be found in a recent study by Korn *et al.* (2005) which showed a strong correlation between QEEG and SPECT (content validity). Consistent with other TBI studies,

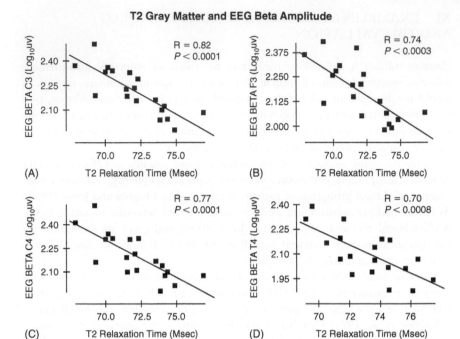

FIGURE 11.4   T2 gray matter and EEG beta (13–22 Hz) frequency scattergrams. Representative scattergrams between the log$_{10}$ EEG amplitude in the beta frequency band on the y-axis and T2 relaxation time on the x-axis. A, B, C and D are scattergrams based on different MRI slices. This is an example of content validity in which there is a strong relationship between EEG and a different clinical measure, in this case the MRI (from Thatcher *et al.*, 1998a).

Korn *et al.* (2005) found reduced power in alpha and increased power in the delta frequency band in mild TBI patients which was evident many months post-injury. As mentioned previously, lesions of the white matter as well as MRI T2 relaxation time deviations from normal in the white matter are correlated with increased delta activity in the QEEG (Gloor *et al.*, 1968, 1977; Thatcher *et al.*, 1998a).

XII.   QEEG CURRENT SOURCE LOCALIZATION AND TBI

Figure 11.5 shows the axial, coronal and sagital views of the current sources of the QEEG in a TBI patient. This is just one of many examples in which the QEEG provides an inexpensive and accurate neuroimage of the focal source of

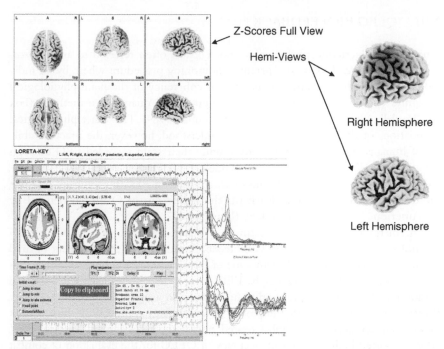

FIGURE 11.5   Example of the use of Low Resolution Electromagnetic Tomography (LORETA) to evaluate the effects of TBI involving a patient hit with a bat on the near right parietal lobe. The lower left panel is the digital EEG and QEEG that are simultaneously available for the evaluation of the EEG with the Key Institute LORETA control panel superimposed on the EEG. The upper and right panels are examples of the location of Z-score deviations from normal, which were confined to the right parietal and right central regions and are consistent with the location of impact (see color plate).

abnormal EEG patterns in a patient who was hit by a blunt object in the right parietal region. In Fig. 11.5, the focal location of the injury is clearly evident, and is validated by the CT scan in which a right hemisphere epidural hematoma developed following the injury. The method of source localization called Low Resolution Electromagnetic Tomography (LORETA) developed by Pascual-Margui et al. (1994) is a well-established and inexpensive neuroimaging method based on QEEG (it is free at: http://www.unizh.ch/keyinst/NewLORETA/Software/Software.htm), which is also helpful in the evaluation of coup contra-coup patterns.

The use of LORETA as a QEEG neuroimaging tool for the evaluation of mild TBI has also been published by Korn et al. (2005). In this study the generators for abnormal rhythms in mild TBI patients were closely related to the anatomical locations as measured by SPECT, thus providing additional concurrent validation of QEEG and TBI.

XIII. QEEG BIOFEEDBACK

Quantitative electroencephalographic biofeedback, often referred to as *neurofeedback* or *EEG biofeedback*, is an operant conditioning procedure where by an individual modifies the amplitude, frequency or coherency of the neurophysiological dynamics of their own brain using a computer and quantitative methods (Fox and Rudell, 1968; Black, 1973; Lubar and Lubar, 1984). The exact physiological foundations of this process are not well understood, however, the practical ability of humans and animals to directly modify their scalp recorded EEG through feedback is well established (Fox and Rudell, 1968; Hetzler *et al.*, 1977; Sterman, 1996). Because computers and transforms are used in EEG biofeedback training, the designation QEEG biofeedback fits the definitions of QEEG as defined by the American Academy of Neurology (Nuwer, 1997).

An emerging and promising treatment approach is the use of quantitative EEG technology and computerized EEG biofeedback training for the treatment of mild to moderate TBI (Thatcher, 1999b). One of the earliest QEEG biofeedback studies was by Ayers (1987) who used alpha EEG training in 250 head injured cases, and demonstrated a return to pre-morbid functioning in a significant number of cases. Peniston *et al.* (1993) reported improved symptomology using QEEG biofeedback in Vietnam veterans with combat-related post-traumatic disorders. Trudeau *et al.* (1998) reported high discriminant accuracy of QEEG for the evaluation of combat veterans with a history of blast injury. More recently, in a biofeedback study of 14 TBI patients Hoffman *et al.* (1995) reported that approximately 60% of mild TBI patients showed improvement in self-reported symptoms and/or in cognitive performance as measured by the MicroCog assessment test after 40 sessions of QEEG biofeedback. Hoffman *et al.* (1995) also found statistically significant normalization of the QEEG in those patients that showed clinical improvement.

Subsequent studies by Hoffman *et al.* (1996a, 1996b) confirmed and extended these findings by showing significant improvement within 5–10 sessions. A similar finding of QEEG normalization following EEG biofeedback was reported by Byers (1995), Tinius and Tinius (2001), Bounias *et al.* (2001, 2002), Wing (2001), Laibow *et al.* (2001), and Schoenberger *et al.* (2001). Ham and Packard (1996) evaluated EEG biofeedback in 40 patients with post-traumatic head ache. They reported that 53% showed at least moderate improvement in headaches, 80% reported moderate improvement in ability to relax and cope with pain, and 93% found biofeedback helpful to some degree. Thornton and Carmody (2005) reported success in using QEEG biofeedback for attention deficit disorders in children with a history of TBI. An excellent review of the QEEG biofeedback literature for the treatment of TBI can be found in Duff (2004).

A recent advancement in EEG biofeedback is the use of real-time Z-scores to guide the biofeedback protocol (Thatcher, 1998, 1999a, 2000a, 2000b). The central clinical concept in the design of Z-score biofeedback is "individualized" EEG biofeedback or non-protocol-driven EEG biofeedback. The idea of linking patient symptoms and complaints to functional localization in the brain as evidenced by "deregulation" of neural populations is fundamental to individualized biofeedback. For example, deregulation is recognized by significantly elevated or reduced power or network measures such as coherence and phase within regions of the brain that sub-serve particular functions that can be linked to the patient's symptoms and complaints.

The use of Z-scores for biofeedback is designed to "re-regulate" or "optimize" the homeostasis, neural excitability and network connectivity in particular regions of the brain. The functional localization and linkage to symptoms is based on modern knowledge of brain function as measured by fMRI, PET, penetrating head wounds, strokes, and other neurological evidence acquired over the last two centuries (see Heilman and Valenstein, 1993; Braxis *et al.*, 2007 see the Human Brain Mapping database of functional localization at: http://hendrix.imm.dtu.dk/services/jerne/brede/index_ext_roots.html).

The concept is to link symptoms and complaints, and then monitor improvement or symptom reduction during the course of treatment. For head injury patients, a careful inventory of the client's personality style, neuropsychological profile, tests of memory and attention, etc. are first obtained. Then a QEEG analysis is run using a minimum of 19 electrode locations according to the International 10/20 system of electrode placement. Identification of the deviant frequencies and locations, and coherence and phase measures are then obtained by comparing the patient with a well-constructed and FDA registered normative database.

Linkage of the patient's symptoms to functional localization of deviant activity is further enhanced by three-dimensional source localization (e.g., low resolution electromagnetic tomography or LORETA) (Pascual-Marqui *et al.*, 1994; Thatcher *et al.*, 2005a, 2005b). Then, the practitioner attempts to link the patient's clinical symptoms and complaints to functional localization as expressed by "deregulation" of deviant neural activity that may be subject to change. A Z-score biofeedback protocol is then implemented with careful monitoring of the patient's progress as well as pre-treatment vs. post-treatment statistical analyses.

XIV. SUMMARY

In summary, QEEG is a reliable, objective, clinically-sensitive, and inexpensive method to evaluate the effects of rapid acceleration/deceleration injuries to the brain. Reduced EEG power in the higher frequencies, and frontal and temporal changes in coherence and phase are the most consistently reported changes in the QEEG following traumatic brain injury. Clinical correlations between the QEEG and neuropsychological test performance, length of coma, Glasgow coma score, post-traumatic amnesia, and MRI biophysical measures are all convergent and systematic, and can be relied upon to help determine the degree of brain injury and likely affects on cognitive functioning.

Repeat QEEG testing does not result in a "learning effect" as occurs with repeated neuropsychological testing, and repeat QEEG testing can be nearly in real-time. Follow-up QEEG measures can help evaluate the rate and extent of recovery from trauma in paralyzed and immobile patients. Finally, QEEG biofeedback is a procedure that is increasingly used to ameliorate the effects of brain injury, especially mild TBI. Neuropsychological and other clinical measures are important, and integration with other imaging modalities is encouraged and made easy using high speed desktop computers (Thatcher *et al.*, 1994).

QEEG biofeedback is a treatment regimen that marries the basic science of QEEG and TBI with a cost-effective method of symptom amelioration. The fact that the effects of mild TBI can be detected with 2–5 electrodes emphasizes the practical and cost-efficient aspect of this technology in the evaluation of athletes (see Figure 11.3 and Table 11.3). For example, Blue Tooth technology and amplifiers inside of a football helmet can evaluate the neurological status of a head-injured athlete in real-time, and combined neuropsychological and QEEG measures thus can be used to ameliorate the effects of brain injury as well as to understand the long-term consequences and rates of recovery from TBI. Similar head-mounted electrode helmets in active duty military personnel can be used to evaluate the extent and nature of traumatic brain injury on the battle field itself, or in nearby medical facilities.

REFERENCES

Arruda, J. E., Weiler, M. D., Valentino, D. and Willis, W. G. (1996). Guide for applying principal-components analysis and confirmatory factor analysis to quantitative electroencephalogram data. *Int. J. Psychophysiol.*, **23(1–2)**, 63–81.

Ayers, M. E. (1987). Electroencephalographic neurofeedback and closed head injury of 250 individuals. In *National Head Injury Syllabusxxxx*, ed.), pp. 380–392. Washington, DC: Head Injury Foundation.

Barth, J., Macciocchi, S. and Giordani, B. (1983). Neurospsychological sequelae of minor head injury. *Neurosurgery*, **13**, 529–537.

Berger, H. (1929). Uber das Electrenkephalogramm des Menschen. *Archiv. Fur. Psychiatrie und Neverkrankheiten,*, **87**, 527–570.

Berger, H. (1932). Uber das Electrenkephalogramm des Menschen. Vierte Mitteilungj. *Archiv. Fur. Psychiatrie und Neverkrankheiten,* **97**, 6–26.

Berger, H. (1934). Uber das Electrenkephalogramm des Menschen. Neunte Mitteilungj. *Archiv. Fur. Psychiatrie und Neverkrankheiten,* **102**, 538–557.

Black, A. H. (1973). The operant conditioning of the electrical activity of the brain as a method for controlling neural and mental processes. In *Psychophysiology of Thinking* (F. J. McGuigan and R. Schoonover, eds), pp. 35–68. New York: Academic Press.

Bounias, M., Laibow, R. E., Bonaly, A. and Stubblebine, A. N. (2001). EEG-neurobiofeedback treatment of patients with brain injury: Part 1: Typological classification of clinical syndromes. *Journal of Neurotherapy*, **5(4)**, 23–44.

Bounias, M., Laibow, R. E., Stubbelbine, A. N., Sandground, H. and Bonaly, A. (2002). EEG-neurobiofeedback treatment of patients with brain injury Part 4: Duration of treatments as a function of both the initial load of clinical symptoms and the rate of rehabilitation. *Journal of Neurotherapy*, **6(1)**, 23–38.

Burgess, A. and Gruzelier, J. (1993). Individual reliability of amplitude distribution in topographical mapping of EEG. *Electroencephalogr. Clin. Neurophysiol.*, **86(4)**, 219–223.

Byers, A. P. (1995). Neurofeedback therapy for a mild head injury. *Journal of Neurotherapy*, **1(1)**, 22–37.

Carmines, E. G. and Zeller, R. A. (1979). *Reliability and Validity Assessment*. Sage University Press.

Cooper, R., Osselton, J. W. and Shaw, J. G. (1974). *EEG Technology*. London: Butterworth & Co.

Corsi-Cabrera, M., Solis-Ortiz, S. and Guevara, M. A. (1997). Stability of EEG inter- and intrahemispheric correlation in women. *Electroencephalogr Clin. Neurophysiol*, **102(3)**, 248–255.

Cronbach, L. J. (1971). Test Validation. In *Educational Measurement* (R. Thorndike, ed.), pp. 443–507. Washington, DC: American Council on Education.

Duff, J. (2004). The usefulness of quantitative EEG (QEEG) and neurotherapy in the assessment and treatment of post-concussion syndrome. *Clin. EEG Neurosci.*, **35(4)**, 198–209.

Duffy, F. H., Hughes, J. R., Miranda, F., Bernad, P. and Cook, P. (1994). Status of quantitative EEG (QEEG) in clinical practice. *Clin Electroencephalogr.*, **25(4)**, VI–XXII.

Fox, S. S. and Rudell, A. P. (1968). Operant controlled neural event: formal and systematic approach to electrical codifing of behavior in brain. *Science*, **162**, 1299–1302.

Gasser, T., Bacher, P. and Steinberg, H. (1985). Test–retest reliability of spectral parameters of the EEG. *Electroencephalogr. Clin. Neurophysiol.*, **60(4)**, 312–319.

Gillies, R. J. (1994). *NMR in Physiology and Biomedicine*. San Diego: Academic Press.

Gloor, P., Kalaby, O. and Giard, N. (1968). The electroencephalogram in diffuse encephalopathies: Electroencephalographic correlates of grey and white matter lesions. *Brain*, **91**, 779–802.

Gloor, P., Ball, G. and Schaul, N. (1977). Brain lesions that produce delta waves in the EEG. *Neurology*, **27**, 326–333.

Ham, L. P. and Packard, R. C. (1996). A retrospective, follow-up study of biofeedback-assisted relaxation therapy in patients with post-traumatic headache. *Biofeedback Self Regul.*, **21(2)**, 93–104.

Hamilton-Bruce, M. A., Boundy, K. L. and Purdie, G. H. (1991). Interoperator variability in quantitative electroencephalography. *Clin. Exp. Neurol.*, **28**, 219–224,.

Harmony, T., Fernandez, T., Rodriguez, M., Reyes, A., Marosi, E. and Bernal, J. (1993). Test–retest reliability of EEG spectral parameters during cognitive tasks: II. Coherence. *Int. J. Neurosci.*, **68(3–4)**, 263–271.

Hellstrom-Westas, L. and Rosen, I. (2005). Electroencephalography and brain damage in preterm infants. *Early Hum Dev.*, **81(3)**, 255–261.

Hetzler, B. E., Rosenfeld, J. P., Birkel, P. A. and Antoinetti, D. N. (1977). Characteristics of operant control of central evoked potentials in rats. *Physiol. Behav.*, **19**, 527–534.

Hoffman, D. A., Stockdale, S., Hicks, L., *et al.* (1995). Diagnosis and treatment of head injury. *Journal of Neurotherapy.*, **1(1)**, 14–21.

Hoffman, D. A., Stockdale, S., Van Egren, L., *et al.* (1996a). Symptom changes in the treatment of mild traumatic brain injury using EEG neurofeedback. *Clinical Electroencephalography (Abstract)*, **27(3)**, 164.

Hoffman, D. A., Stockdale, S., Van Egren, L., *et al.* (1996b). EEG neurofeedback in the treatment of mild traumatic brain injury. *Clinical Electroencephalography (Abstract)*, **27(2)**, 6.

Hoffman, D. A., Lubar, J. F., Thatcher, R. W., *et al.* (1999). Limitation of the American Academy of Neurology and American Clinical Neurophysiology Society Paper on QEEG. *Journal of Neuropsychia. and Clin. Neurosciences,*, **11(3)**, 401–407.

Hughes, J. R. and John, E. R. (1999). Conventional and quantitative electroencephalography in psychiatry. *Neuropsychiatry*, **11(2)**, 190–208.

Korn, A., Golan, H., Melamed, I., Pascual-Marqui, R. and Friedman, A. (2005). Focal cortical dysfunction and blood-brain barrier disruption in patients with Postconcussion syndrome. *J. Clin. Neurophysiol.*, **22(1)**, 1–9.

Laibow, R. E., Stubblebine, A. N., Sandground, H. and Bounias, M. (2001). EEG neurobiofeedback treatment of patients with brain injury: Part 2: Changes in EEG parameters versus rehabilitation. *Journal of Neurotherapy*, **5(4)**, 45–71.

Lubar, J. F. and Lubar, J. O. (1984). Electroencephalographic biofeedback and neurological applications. *Biofeedback and Self-Regulation*, **9**, 1–23.

Lund, T. R., Sponheim, S. R., Iacono, W. G. and Clementz, B. A. (1995). Internal consistency reliability of resting EEG power spectra in schizophrenic and normal subjects. *Psychophysiology*, **32(1)**, 66–71.

Malmivuo, J. and Plonsey, R. (1995). *Bioeletromagnetism: Principles and applications of bioelectric and biomagnetic fields*. New York: Oxford University Press.

Mas, F., Prichep, L. S. and Alper, K. (1993). Treatment resistant depression in a case of minor head injury: an electrophysiological hypothesis. *Clin. Electroencephalogr.*, **24(3)**, 118–122.

McLean, A. J. (1995). Brain injury without head impact?. *J. of Neurotrauma,*, **12(4)**, 621–625.

Nuwer, M. R. (1997). Assessment of digital EEG, quantitative EEG and EEG brain mapping report of the American Academy of Neurology and the American Clinical Neurophysiology Society. *Neurology*, **49**, 277–292.

Niedermeyer, E. and Da Silva, F. L. (1995). *Electroencephalography: Basic principles, clinical applications and related fields*. Baltimore: Williams & Wilkins.

Nunez, P. (1981). *Electrical Fields of the Brain*. Cambridge: Oxford Univ. Press.

Nunez, P. (1995). *Neocortical dynamics and human EEG rhythms*. New York: Oxford Univ. Press.

Nunnally, J. C. (1978). *Psychometric Theory*. New York: McGraw-Hill.

Ommaya, A. K. (1968). The mechanical properties of tissues of the nervous system. *J. Biomech.*, **2**, 1–2.

Ommaya, A. K. (1995). Head injury mechanisms and the concept of preventive management: A review and critical synthesis. *J. Neurotrauma*, **12**, 527–546.

Ommaya, A. K. and Hirsch, A. E. (1971). Tolerances for cerebral concussion from head impact and whiplash in primates. *J. Biomechanics*, **4**, 13–21.

Packard, R. C. and Ham, L. P. (1994). Promising techniques in the assessment of mild head injury. In *Seminars in Neurology* (R. C. Packard, ed.), **14**, 74–83.

Pascual-Marqui, R. D., Michel, C. M. and Lehmann, D. (1994). Low resolution electromagnetic tomography: A new method for localizing electrical activity in the brain. *Internat. J. of Psychophysiol.*, **18**, 49–65.

Peniston, E. G., Marrianan, D. A. and Deming, W. A. (1993). EEG alpha–theta brainwave synchronization in Vietnam theater veterans with combat-related post-traumatic stress disorder and alcohol abuse. *Adv. in Med. Psychotherapy*, **6**, 37–50.

Pollock, V. E., Schneider, L. S. and Lyness, S. A. (1991). Reliability of topographic quantitative EEG amplitude in healthy late-middle-aged and elderly subjects. *Electroencephalogr. Clin. Neurophysiol.*, **79(1)**, 20–26.

Rappaport, M., Hall, K., Hopkins, B. S., *et al.* (1982). Disability rating scale for severe head trauma: Coma to community. *Arch. Phys. Med. Rehabil.*, **63**, 118–123.

Rimel, R., Giodani, B., Barth, J., Boll, T. and Jane, J. (1981). Disability caused by monor head injury. *Neurosurgery*, **9**, 221–223.

Roche, R. A., Dockree, P. M., Garavan, H., Foxe, J. J., Robertson, I. H. and O'Mara, S. M. (2004). EEG alpha power changes reflect response inhibition deficits after traumatic brain injury (TBI) in humans. *Neurosci. Lett. 13*, **362(1)**, 1–5.

Ruijs, M. B., Gabreels, F. J. and Thijssen, H. M. (1994). The utility of electroencephalography and cerebral computed tomography in children with mild and moderately severe closed head injuries. *Neuropediatrics*, **25(2)**, 73–77.

Salinsky, M. C., Oken, B. S. and Morehead, L. (1991). Test-retest reliability in EEG frequency analysis. *Electroencephalogr. Clin. Neurophysiol.*, **79(5)**, 382–392.

Sano, K., Nakamura, N. and Hirakaws, K. (1967). Mechanism of and dynamics of closed head injuries. *Neurol. Mediochir.*, **9**, 21–23.

Schoenberger, N. E., Shif, S. C., Esty, M. L., Ochs, L., and Matheis, R. J. Flexyx neurotherapy system in the treatment of traumatic brain injury: an initial evaluation. *J. Head Trauma Rehabil.*, **16(3)**, 260–274.

Slewa-Younan, S., Green, A. M., Baguley, I. J., Felmingham, K. L., Haig, A. R. and Gordon, E. (2002). Is 'gamma' (40 Hz) synchronous activity disturbed in patients with traumatic brain injury? *Clin. Neurophysiol.*, **113(10)**, 1640–1646.

Slobounov, S., Sebastianelli, W. and Simon, R. (2002). Neurophysiological and behavioral concomitants of mild brain injury in collegiate athletes. *Clin. Neurophysiol.*, **113(2)**, 185–193.

Sterman, M. B. (1996). Physiological origins and functional correlates of EEG rhythmic activities – implications for self-regulation. *Biofeedback and Self Regulation*, **21**, 3–33.

Tebano, M. T., Cameroni, M., Gallozzi, G., *et al.* (1988). EEG spectral analysis after minor head injury in man. *EEG and Clin. Neurophysiol.*, **70**, 185–189.

Thatcher, R. W. (1995). Tomographic Electroencephalography and Magnetoencephalography. *Journal of Neuroimaging*, **5**, 35–45.

Thatcher, R. W. (1998). EEG normative databases and EEG biofeedback. *Journal of Neurotherapy*, **2(4)**, 8–39.

Thatcher, R. W. (1999a). EEG database guided neurotherapy. In *Introduction to Quantitative EEG and Neurofeedback* (J. R. Evans and A. Abarbanel, eds). San Diego: Academic Press.

Thatcher, R. W. (1999b). QEEG and traumatic brain injury: Present and future. *Brain Injury*, **12**, 13–21.

Thatcher, R. W. (2000a). EEG Operant Conditioning (Biofeedback) and Traumatic Brain Injury. *Clinical EEG*, **31(1)**, 38–44.

Thatcher, R. W. (2000b). An EEG Least Action Model of Biofeedback. *8th Annual ISNR conference*, St. Paul, MN. September

Thatcher, R. W. (2006). Electroencephalography and mild traumatic brain injury. In *Foundations of Sport-Related Brain Injuries. Foundations of Sport-Related Brain Injuries* (S. Slobounov and W. Sebastianelli, eds). Springer-Verlag.

Thatcher, R. W. and John, E. R. (1977). New Jersey: Erlbaum Assoc.

Thatcher, R. W., Krause, P. and Hrybyk, M. (1986). Corticocortical associations and EEG coherence: a two compartmental model. *Electroencephalography and Clinical Neurophysiology*, **64**, 123–143.

Thatcher, R. W., Walker, R. A., Gerson, I. and Geisler, F. (1989). EEG discriminant analyses of mild head trauma. *EEG and Clin. Neurophysiol.*, **73**, 93–106.

Thatcher, R. W., Cantor, D. S., McAlaster, R., Geisler, F. and Krause, P. (1991). Comprehensive predictions of outcome in closed head injury: The development of prognostic equations. *Annals New York Academy of Sciences*, **620**, 82–104.

Thatcher R. W., Hallet M., Zeffiro T., John E.R. and Huerta M., (eds) (1994). *Functional Neuroimaging: Technical Foundations*. New York: Academic Press.

Thatcher, R. W., Camacho, M., Salazar, A., Linden, C., Biver, C. and Clarke, L. (1997). Quantitative MRI of the gray-white matter distribution in traumatic brain injury. *J. Neurotrauma*, **14**, 1–14.

Thatcher, R. W., Biver, C., Camacho, M., McAlaster, R. and Salazar, A. M. (1998a). Biophysical linkage between MRI and EEG amplitude in traumatic brain injury. *NeuroImage*, **7**, 352–367.

Thatcher, R. W., Biver, C., McAlaster, R. and Salazar, A. M. (1998b). Biophysical linkage between MRI and EEG coherence in traumatic brain injury. *NeuroImage*, **8(4)**, 307–326.

Thatcher, R. W., Moore, N., John, E. R., Duffy, F., Hughes, J. R. and Krieger, M. (1999). QEEG and traumatic brain injury: Rebuttal of the American Academy of Neurology 1997. Report by the EEG and Clinical Neuroscience Society. *Clinical Electroenceph.*, **30(3)**, 94–98.

Thatcher, R. W., North, D., Curtin, R., *et al.* (2001a). An EEG Severity Index of Traumatic Brain Injury. *J. Neuropsychiatry and Clinical Neuroscience*, **13(1)**, 77–87.

Thatcher, R. W., Biver, C. L., Gomez-Molina, J. F., *et al.* (2001b). Estimation of the EEG Power Spectrum by MRI T2 Relaxation Time in Traumatic Brain Injury. *Clinical Neurophysiology*, **112**, 1729–1745.

Thatcher, R. W., Biver, C. and North, D. (2003). Quantitative EEG and the Frye and Daubert Standards of Admissibility. *Clinical Electroencephalography*, **34(2)**, 39–53.

Thatcher, R. W., North, D. and Biver, C. (2005a). EEG inverse solutions and parametric vs. non-parametric statistics of Low Resolution Electromagnetic Tomography (LORETA). *Clin. EEG and Neuroscience*, **36(1)**, 1–9.

Thatcher, R. W., North, D. and Biver, C. (2005b). Evaluation and Validity of a LORETA normative EEG database. *Clin. EEG and Neuroscience*, **36(2)**, 116–122.

Thatcher, R. W., North, D. and Biver, C. (2005c). EEG and Intelligence: Univariate and Multivariate Comparisons Between EEG Coherence, EEG Phase Delay and Power. *Clinical Neurophysiology*, **116(9)**, 2129–2141.

Thompson, J., Sebastianelli, W. and Slobounov, S. (2005). EEG and postural correlates of mild traumatic brain injury in athletes. *Neurosci. Lett.* **4**, **377(3)**, 158–163.

Thornton, K. (1999). Exploratory investigation into mild brain injury and discriminant analysis with high frequency bands (32–64 Hz). *Brain Inj.*, **13(7)**, 477–488.

Thornton, K. (2003). The electrophysiological effects of a brain injury on auditory memory functioning. The QEEG correlates of impaired memory. *Arch. Clin. Neuropsychol.*, **18(4)**, 363–378.

Thornton, K. and Carmody, D. P. (2005). Electroencephalogram biofeedback for reading disability and traumatic brain injury. *Child Adolesc. Psychiatr. Clin. N. Am.*, **14(1)**, 137–162.

Tinius, T. P. and Tinius, K. A. (2001). Changes after EEG biofeedback and cognitive retraining in adults with mild traumatic brain injury and attention deficit disorder. *Journal of Neurotherapy*, **4(2)**, 27–44.

Trudeau, D. L., Anderson, J., Hansen, L. M., *et al.* (1998). Findings of mild traumatic brain injury in combat veterans with PTSD and a history of blast concussion. *J. Neuropsychiatry Clin Neurosci.*, **10(3)**, 308–313.

Tryer, L. (1988). *Biochemistry*. New York: W. H. Freeman and Company.

von Bierbrauer, A., Weissenborn, K., Hinrichs, H., Scholz, M. and Kunkel, H. (1993). Automatic (computer-assisted) EEG analysis in comparison with visual EEG analysis in patients following minor cranio-cerebral trauma (a follow-up study). *EEG EMG Z Elektroenzephalogr Elektromyogr Verwandte Geb.*, **23(3)**, 151–157.

Niedermeyer E. and da Silva F. L. EEG and Neuropharmacology (2005). *Electroencephalography: Basic Principles, Clinical Applications and Related Fields*, 5th edition, p. xxx. Baltimore, MD: Williams & Wilkins.

Wing, K. (2001). Effect of neurofeedback on motor recovery of a patient with brain injury: A case study and its implications for stroke rehabilitation. *Topics in Stroke Rehabilitation*, **8(3)**, 45–53.

Woody, R. H. (1966). Intra-judge Reliability in Clinical EEG. *J. Clin. Psychol.*, **22**, 150–159.

Woody, R. H. (1968). Inter-judge Reliability in Clinical EEG. *J. Clin. Psychol.*, **24**, 251–261.

CHAPTER 12

Neurofeedback for the treatment of depression: Current status of theoretical issues and clinical research

D. Corydon Hammond, Ph.D., ECNS, QEEG-D, BCIA-EEG[1] and Elsa Baehr Ph.D.[2]

[1]*University of Utah School of Medicine, Salt Lake City, Utah, USA*
[2]*Baehr & Baehr Ltd, Chicago, Illinois, USA*

I. INTRODUCTION

Interest in the relationship between neural functions and emotions has focused particularly on comparisons of activation in the left and right dorsolateral frontal cortices. Beginning with the investigations of Davidson and colleagues (Davidson *et al.*, 1985, 1989, 1990a; Davidson, 1992), the alpha EEG frequency has been used as a measure of hypoactivity, and there has been general agreement among researchers that mood is more positive when the right dorsolateral prefrontal cortex is more hypoactive than the left dorsolateral prefrontal cortex.

A practical application of this theoretical approach was developed when Dr. J. Peter Rosenfeld and colleagues designed an experiment in which they demonstrated that cortical asymmetry (A-score) could be modified in normal subjects by using a simple operant conditioning program (Rosenfeld *et al.*, 1995). Their findings, in which nine of 13 subjects were successfully trained, were replicated by Allen *et al.* (2001). Encouraged by these results, neurofeedback protocols were developed to try with a small group of clinical patients who were suffering from various mood disorders (Baehr and Baehr, 1997; Baehr *et al.*, 1997), (Hammond, 2000, 2005a, 2005b).

In this chapter we will review the extensive theoretical literature that has been published since Davidson's original investigations. We will review the results of the Baehr group's first study, and present follow-up data from one to 10 years post-therapy. In addition, we will report on studies (Baehr *et al.*, 1999) utilizing the asymmetry protocol to study shifts in mood (Baehr, 2000), and on studies of asymmetry changes in women who suffer from premenstrual dysphoric disorder (Baehr *et al.*, 2004). We will also report on other asymmetry protocols designed to alleviate depression (Hammond, 2000, 2005a, 2005b).

Introduction to QEEG and Neurofeedback, Second Edition
ISBN: 978-0-12-374534-7

II. A REVIEW OF THE LITERATURE

A. Frontal EEG asymmetry and emotions

The development of a theory regarding cortical frontal asymmetry and emotions, proposed by Davidson and colleagues (Davidson *et al.*, 1985, 1989, 1990a; Davidson, 1992), evoked the interest of the scientific community worldwide. An approach—avoidance model, developed by Davidson 1993, 1998a, 1998b; Davidson *et al.*, (1990b, 1999a, 1999b), was based on studies demonstrating that hyperactivity in the left frontal cortex was associated with approach behavior and positive mood, while hyperactivity in the right prefrontal cortex was associated with avoidance behavior and negative mood. (Sutton and Davidson, 1997). An advantage of this model was that it provided a way of assessing both normal affective behavior, and also pathological states such as depression.

A scale designed to measure behavioral inhibition and behavioral activation (Carver *et al.*, 1994) provided an objective way to test Davidson's theoretical approach. While data supported a significant relationship of left frontal activation and the behavioral activation scale (BAS), no statistically significant relationship between right frontal activation and the behavioral inhibition scale (BIS) was found (Harmon-Jones and Allen, 1997; Coan and Allen, 2003). The possibility that hypoactivity in the right frontal cortex may be related to the BIS was not considered in this study. Davidson (2004) suggests that there is a relationship between the activity of the prefrontal cortex (PFC) and affect. He states that activity in the PFC is related to its ability to inhibit its input from the sub-cortical centers. In a complicated circuitry involving the amygdala, the hippocampus, the cingulate, the left and right dorsolateral cortex, and other structures, he explains that the influx of negative stimuli can be modulated in this way.

In 2003 and 2004 Coan and Allen reviewed over 80 articles published since Davidson's original work, basically supporting the findings that there is a relationship between resting EEG asymmetry in the frontal cortex and in emotions or emotion-related constructs. They re-examined the many existing studies for the purpose of investigating state and trait features of frontal cortical asymmetry and then, in the later study, looked at activation in the right frontal cortex in terms of influencing behavior. While many studies supported Davidson's results (e.g., Allen *et al.*, 2004a; Harmon-Jones, 2000; McFarland *et al.*, 2006; Pizzagalli *et al.*, 2005; Sutton and Davidson, 1997; Tomarken and Davidson, 1994), not all researchers were able to replicate them (Allen *et al.*, 2004a, Hagemann *et al.*, 1998; Hagemann *et al.*, 1999; Hagemann *et al.*, 2001; Debener *et al.*, 2000; Reid *et al.*, 1998; Allen *et al.*, 2004b; Davidson, 1998; Hagemann, 2004; Coan and Allen, 2004).

The consensus is that a number of factors may contribute to the discrepancies, such as comorbidities, differences in referencing (Cz, linked ears or an average reference), artifacting, statistical methods, montage, methodology (EEG, MRI, Petscan, Glucose Metabolism, blood flow), selection of subjects (Davidson's criteria for inclusion was for subjects who had extreme or stable asymmetry over time), and individual differences in response to the testing situation (Coan and Allen, 2006, Harmon-Jones, 2006, Papousek and Schulter, 2006).

A new approach to studying the functional aspects of frontal asymmetry was developed to resolve some of the inconsistent findings. Coan and Allen (2006) proposed a capability model of individual differences in frontal EEG asymmetry. They point out that all of the studies to date have depended upon resting (inherent) asymmetry that might be classified as dispositional models of personality. The implication is that basic traits will determine how an individual will behave in different situations. The capability model on the other hand is an alternative, interactive way to look at approach and avoidance states when the individual is confronted with an emotionally significant task. By presenting emotional challenges to an individual one can determine the degree to which individuals may utilize approach and avoidance responses. EEG correlations with affect were most significant when subjects were presented with emotions of fear and sadness. The reactions to emotional manipulation were so clear that issues of reference schemes were minimized.

B.   Frontal EEG asymmetry and mood disorders

In citing research on stroke patients where the severity of depression was related to the location of a lesion (left frontal pole lesions were associated with greater negative feelings than lesions near the right frontal pole) a theory was developed regarding left frontal hypoactivation and depression (Robinson et al., 1984; Henriques and Davidson; 1991, Gotlib et al., 1998). Numerous studies have explored the ramifications of this theoretical construct. Inheritability and stability of the asymmetry trait have been studied (Coan, 2003). Developmental studies showed that infants with right frontal activity reacted more to maternal separation than did those with left frontal activation (Tomarken et al., 1990), and adult studies demonstrated that right frontal activity was associated with negative responses to film clips (Tomarken et al., 1990; Allen et al., 2001).

Brief mood shifts brought about by happy and sad thoughts resulted in changes in frontal asymmetry in both depressed and normal control subjects (Baehr, 2002). Daily changes in frontal alpha asymmetry were shown to correlate with changes in affect in therapy sessions (Rosenfeld et al, 1996). Right frontal activation measured in a resting state was found in adults with current, remitted and past depressions (Henriques and Davidson, 1990, 1991; Gotlib et al., 1998). Right frontal activation was found in non-depressed adolescent daughters of depressed mothers (Tomarken et al., 2004). The frontal asymmetry has also been found in infants under the age of one that were born to depressed mothers (Dawson et al., 1992a, 1992b), even as young as at 3–6 months (Field et al., 1995) and at one month of age (Jones et al., 1997).

This may result from either a genetic predisposition to depression that has been passed on, and/or it may result from an over- or underactivation of brain areas that mediate different emotions in the infant whose frontal lobe begins to be increasingly active at about 8 months of age. However, genetic studies of twins provided only limited evidence of heritability of frontal asymmetry patterns (Smit et al., 2006; Anokhin et al., 2006). For the most part, these studies imply that right frontal cortical

EEG may predict both state and trait individual differences in affect, although not all studies confirm these results (Debener et al., 2000, Allen et al., 2004; Vuga, et al., 2006).

Allen et al., (2003) studied subjects over an 8- to 16-week period. They acknowledged that while trait-like aspects of alpha asymmetry were characteristic of depressed individuals, state changes also occurred. Changes were not related to changes in the severity of the depression. However, Askew (2001) found a strong correlation between alpha asymmetry scores and the Beck depression inventory ($P < 0.0001$), and on the MMPI-II depression scale ($P < 0.0001$).

The roles of early experiences and plasiticity as factors in patterns of asymmetry were explored by Davidson (1994). Vuga et al., (2006) studied long-term stability for frontal EEG asymmetry in adults with a history of depression, and non-depressed controls. They found that resting asymmetry reflected a moderately stable condition in adults. Deldin and Chiu (2005) found that depressed persons could respond to a brief cognitive restructuring task, with positive changes also occurring in alpha asymmetry.

An asymmetry with more fast-frequency activity in the right hemisphere has even been found to remain in the architecture of sleep in depression (Armitage et al., 1992, 1993, 1995). Research has further suggested that the right hemisphere may be specialized for processing negative affect (Ahern and Schwartz, 1985; Joseph, 1999; Ladavas et al., 1984; Schwartz et al., 1975).

Along with the frontal electrophysiology findings in depression there also seems to be an inverse relationship between frontal alpha asymmetry and parietal asymmetries. More specifically, depressed patients without significant anxiety appear to have decreased right parietal activation (more alpha at P4 than at P3) (Allen et al., 1993; Bruder et al., 1995; Davidson et al., 1985; Henriques and Davidson, 1990, 1997; Schaffer et al., 1983; Tenke et al., 1993). These findings are also congruent with neuropsychological test findings that have consistently identified right parietotemporal deficits in functioning in depressed subjects (Bruder, 1995; Heller et al., 1995; Jaeger et al., 1987). Recent research (Bruder et al., 2007) has also verified an inverse parietal alpha asymmetry in grandchildren of depressed parents and grandparents, compared with controls without a parental and grandparental depression history.

In summary, in spite of inconsistencies there is overwhelming support for theories relating EEG frontal cortical asymmetry (state and/or trait dependent) and emotions, both normal and pathological. These studies have provided a substantial theoretical basis for research, and for the development of clinical EEG biofeedback protocols designed to train depressed subjects to alter their brainwave patterns.

III. CLINICAL USE OF ASYMMETRY PROTOCOLS FOR TREATMENT OF DEPRESSION: BAEHR/ ROSENFELD STUDIES

There are assessments (as opposed to treatment outcome studies) that have used the Rosenfeld protocol. Eleven non-depressed age-matched controls and 13 depressed patients participated in a study to compare frontal alpha asymmetry mean for a baseline session with the percentage of time in the session when asymmetry scores were greater than zero. It was found that the percent index was a better discriminator of the two groups than was the asymmetry score (Baehr et al., 1998). An A-score of 58% is the cut-off point between depressed and non-depressed subjects. As mentioned, Askew (2001) also provided further validation for this measure in finding a strong correlation between alpha asymmetry scores and the Beck depression inventory and the MMPI-II depression scale.

The phenomenon of brainwave asymmetry and emotions has been further explored by Baehr and colleagues (Baehr et al., 2000). Twenty-two subjects, including 14 patients being treated for depression and 8 non-depressed subjects, were asked to think of a happy or sad thought while alpha asymmetry measures were being taken at cortical sites F3 and F4, referenced to CZ. Sixty-three percent of the subjects demonstrated the ability to change their frontal alpha asymmetry in accordance with voluntarily produced thought change. The remaining 37% of the subjects remained either in the positive alpha asymmetry range (R > L), or in the negative alpha asymmetry range (L > R).

In a study of premenstrual dysphoric disorder (Baehr et al., 2004) evidence was found of changes of frontal asymmetry during the luteal phase of the menstrual cycle that was consistent with severe mood swings. They observed two monthly cycles for five women diagnosed as having PMDD, and one monthly cycle for five non-PMDD control subjects. They found that the asymmetry percent scores for the five PMDD women, and for the five control subjects, before and after the Luteal phase were typically within the normal non-depressed range. However the asymmetry scores for the PMDD group fell into the negative range during the Luteal period while the control subjects remained stable.

A. Replication studies

A single case study of an adolescent patient who was treated for depression using the EEG asymmetry biofeedback protocol replicated our results (Earnest, 1999). In a study of 18 women using the asymmetry protocol, John Allen et al. (2001), demonstrated that frontal asymmetry could be manipulated to train subject's left or right frontal alpha asymmetry. Self-reported emotional responses to film clips and facial EGG were consistent with expressions predicted from the EEG training efforts.

Two other papers (Hammond, 2000, 2005b) have been published on the neurofeedback treatment of depression, both of which built on the same robust foundation of frontal asymmetry research. Hammond (2000) utilized a protocol designed to increase left frontal beta activity (15–18 Hz and 12–15 Hz) in the left frontal cortex at electrode sites FP1 and F3 in a successful single case study. He later reported (Hammond, 2005b) on the successful treatment of seven of eight subjects using the same protocol.

Baehr *et al.* (1999) presented the results of a pilot study in a previous edition of this book A review of that research along with follow-up data will be presented, followed by a detailed review of Hammond's research.

B. Review of previous research

In 1994 Baehr and Rosenfeld introduced their protocol to five depressed patients who were being treated with psychotherapy, and a sixth patient who was seen in another clinic. (Detailed case studies are presented in Chapter 8 of the previous edition of this book [Baehr *et al.*, 1999]). They agreed to participate in a study to assess the effectiveness of this approach. (Baehr *et al*, 1997, Baehr *et al.*, 1999).[1] Using the alpha asymmetry protocol, they assessed and trained depressed patients to reallocate brainwave amplitude so that the amplitude of alpha was greater in the right frontal cortex then in the homogolous left frontal cortex. The application of this protocol requires scalp electrodes at two active sites, F3 and F4, a reference at Cz, and the ground at Fz. (Most of the above reported studies have used a standard EEG montage utilizing 19 or more sites).

C. Procedures

The Beck depression index (BDI) and the Minnesota multiphasic personality inventory-2 (MMPI-2) were administered to assess emotional functioning before and after a series of approximately 30 sessions of EEG asymmetry training designed to increase the difference between right and left alpha magnitude.[2, 3] Prior to neurofeedback training the patients were trained to use diaphragmatic breathing exercises and autogenic suggestions such as "I feel quite relaxed", and "warmth is flowing down my arms into my hands and fingers" to promote relaxation and hand warming. This technique serves to reduce EEG artifacts caused by muscle tension. The patients were also encouraged to focus their thoughts on pleasant, unemotional imagery during EEG training sessions. They sat in a reclining chair with their feet elevated, and were encouraged to maintain a relaxed state, closing their eyes and moving as little as possible.

[1]We thank Carolyn Earnest for providing us with data for one client in this study. This is a different subject than the one reported in a replication study (Earnest, 1999).

[2]The Baehr/Rosenfeld protocol utilized the index $([R - L]/[R + L])$ X 100 as the asymmetry index or A-score, where R and L represent right and left frontal alpha magnitude (microvolts) respectively. The higher the value of this index, the less depressed the patient is assumed to be (see earlier parts of this chapter and Rosenfeld, 1997).

[3]One patient who was initially diagnosed Bipolar remained in therapy for several years after the study terminated. She will be presented later in this chapter.

The patients were seen once or twice a week for hour-long sessions for an average of 30 sessions that consisted of approximately 50% brainwave biofeedback followed by 50% psychotherapy. During biofeedback, scalp sites F3 and F4, referenced to Cz, were recorded. Impedances were 5 ohms or less, as measured by an EIM electrode impedance meter. The threshold was set at zero so that A-scores below zero represented greater left than right alpha magnitude, and A-scores above zero represented the reverse asymmetry. Alpha rhythm reflects cortical hypoactivity; therefore an increase in left frontal activation corresponds to decreased alpha and a positive change in the asymmetry score. To assess significant A-score change, we rely on our previous study (Baehr *et al.*, 1998), in which we found that A-scores >58% of time over threshold were typical of non-depressed normal control subjects, while A-scores <58% of the time were representative of the depressed population.

The EEG data for A-score training were recorded either on a four-channel unit or on a neurosearch 24-channel unit (both by the Lexicor Corp). Fast fourier transforms (FFTs) were derived on Blackman-Harris windowed analog signals over 1-second epochs (Harris, 1978). This device also outputs the mean value over the entire session each day as a mean asymmetry score, which is manifested as a positive or negative asymmetry score, and as a mean percentage score, reflecting the percentage of time that the difference between the right and left alpha magnitude is greater than zero (A-score >0). A bell tone or a clarinet tone that fluctuates in pitch (the greater the A-score, the higher the tone) was used as a reinforcement when the asymmetry score exceeded zero.

D. Results

Each subject was his own control in this study that utilized pre- and post-treatment data. Five of the six subjects were able to increase their percent of time over threshold to the normal range. The sixth subject, whose depression was diagnosed as non-endogenous, increased her asymmetry score but fell just short of reaching the cut-off score of <58%. Four of the six subjects showed significant improvement on the BDI and on the MMPI. A comparison of the patients = pre- and post-MMPI-2 depression scales indicate a significant change. For three patients the pre- to post-depression score differences exceeded two times the standard error of measurement, (SEm), and for one patient, one (SEm) Table 12.1.

Five of the six subjects scored above 9 on the BDI, while four of the six scored below 9 in the post-test (in Table 12.1 scores below 9 on the BDI are considered to be within the normal range).

E. Longitudinal data

Five of the six subjects were available for follow-up. In our first longitudinal study three subjects (Bob, Celia, and Ann Rose in Table 12.2) were evaluated one to five

TABLE 12.1   Pre- and post-alpha asymmetry training measure of depression for the MMPI-2 and BDI, and the percentage of time asymmetry is greater than zero scores

Subjects	MMPI-2 Pre-alpha	MMPI-2 Post-alpha	BDI Pre-alpha	BDI Post-alpha	A% Pre-alpha	A\% Post-alpha
Bob	76	54[a]	21	03	48	84
Celia	74	62[b]	40	04	57	80
Katy	n/a[c]	n/[a]	07	25	50	69
Ann Rose	64	47[a]	n/a	01	49	69
Catherine	62	36[a]	11	01	59	64
Diedre	n/a	n/[a]	34	18	36	55

Reprinted from Baehr, E. *et al.* (1999)
[a]Two SEM p $>$ 0.0005
[b]One SEM p $>$ 0.0025
[c]N/A, tests were not administered

TABLE 12.2   5-year follow-up: The Beck depression inventory (BDI) scores*, and the percentage of time asymmetry is greater than zero (PTAA) scores are shown for three subjects before and immediately after termination of therapy

Subject	BDI Before therapy	BDI After therapy	BDI Follow-up one to five years later	PTAA Before therapy	PTAA After therapy	PTAA Follow-up one to five years later
Bob	31	03	03 (1 year)	48%	84%	86% (1 year)
Celia	40	04	04 (3 years)	57%	86%	66% (3 years)
Ann Rose	n/a	02	03 (5 years)	49%	69%	69% (5 years)

Reprinted from: Baehr, E. *et al.* (2001)
*BDI score $<$ 9, and PTAA scores $>$ 58 are in the non-depressed range

years after therapy (Baehr *et al.*, 2001). All subjects maintained asymmetry scores and Beck depression scores in the normal range (Table 12.2).

Three subjects were available for evaluation 10 years after finishing therapy. One of these subjects, Ann Rose, participated in both follow-up studies. Katie was the formerly bi-polar patient, and Catherine was formerly diagnosed as having unipolar depression. All subjects maintained asymmetry scores in the normal range, and all had Beck depression scale scores in the normal range (Table 12.3).

F. Treatment of a bipolar patient

Research has found that bipolar disorder quite commonly has a different EEG pattern than unipolar depression, where alpha is often reduced (Knott and Lapierre, 1987;

TABLE 12.3   10-year follow-up: The Beck depression inventory (BDI) scores★, and the percent of time asymmetry is greater than zero (PTAA) scores are shown for three subjects before and immediately after termination of therapy

Subject	BDI Before therapy	BDI After therapy	BDI Follow-up 10 years later	PTAA Before therapy	PTAA After therapy	PTAA Follow-up 10 years later
Katy	7	25	02	50%	69%	75%
Catherine	11	01	02	59%	64%	72%
Ann Rose	n/a	01	02	49%	69%	61%

★BDI score < 9, and PTAA scores > 58 are in the non-depressed range

Clementz *et al.*, 1994), beta elevated (John *et al.*, 1988; Prichep and John, 1986), and where manic and depressive phases may be characterized by different EEG patterns (Flor-Henry and Koles, 1984; Koek *et al.*, 1999).

Thus, while we may wish to view the Baehr/Rosenfeld asymmetry protocol as a significant treatment innovation for mood disorders, it is apparent that it does not work in the same way for everyone. For example, in the case of the person diagnosed with bipolar depression, improvement occurred in terms of eliminating mood swings, but the patient remained in a dysphoric state at the end of the 30 sessions of treatment. This case also was complicated by reactions to psychotropic medications. She remained in neurotherapy and psychotherapy therapy for an additional five years. Her asymmetry eventually normalized, and at a 10-year follow-up she reported that she was neither bipolar nor dysphoric. Her asymmetry ratio was within the normal range, >58%, (Baehr, 1998) as was her BDI score of 2. She continues to use a minimal amount of medication.

G. Adjunctive treatments with the Baehr/Rosenfeld asymmetry protocol

Training Breath and Heart Rate Variability

Since the first Baehr study, they have refined the relaxation techniques prior to training with the Asymmetry protocol. All of the sessions begin with 10 minutes of training to balance the sympathetic and parasympathetic activity of the autonomic nervous system, as described by Elliott and Edmonson (2006). Using a combination of programs, patients are trained to use breathing to regulate heart rate variability (Elliott and Edmonson, 2006; Childre and McCraty, 1999). When successful, patients report that they feel calmer and in better control of responses to stress and depression. Validation of this technique has been reported in two new studies: Rotenberg *et al.*, (2007) found a relationship between major depressive respiratory sinus arrhythmia, and Karavodas *et al.* (2007) found that improvement in symptoms of major depressive disorder occurred with short-term biofeedback treatment to increase heart rate variability.

Other Adjunctive Therapies

The Baehr group considers neurofeedback training for depression as one part of a comprehensive treatment protocol, which may also include entrainment devices, nutritional counseling, exercise programs, and ongoing psychotherapy. The lab setting where the neurofeedback treatment occurs, and the alliance with the therapist, also may be important factors, as yet unanalyzed, in the treatment situation. Some question is raised as to whether the positive effects observed would also occur in a lab setting where a therapist was not present.

This group is currently assessing alpha asymmetry in a normative population. They believe that the crucial next step for their research is to demonstrate that appropriate control cases do not improve clinically as much as clinical cases who are administered the asymmetry protocol.

IV. THE HAMMOND DEPRESSION PROTOCOL

Hammond (2000) used the Baehr/Rosenfeld protocol described above for three sessions with a case of medication-resistant depression accompanied by anxiety and obsessional rumination. The patient's score on the protocol was 36.1, representing a severe asymmetry. However, as chance would have it, the patient had considerable difficulty in changing his asymmetry score, which was actually worsening in his scores in sessions 2 and 3. Hammond was familiar with the frontal asymmetry EEG research, as well as neuroimaging research (e.g., Baxter et al., 1985, 1989; Bench et al., 1992, 1993; George et al., 1994; Liotti et al., 2000), and evidence from work by Sterman (1999, also later published in Sterman and Kaiser, 2001) suggesting that the area anterior to electrode site F3 also appears to be hypoactive in depression. Therefore, he considered what other neurofeedback treatment strategy might address this asymmetry.

It was decided to reinforce beta activity while inhibiting alpha and theta activity in the left frontal area at electrode sites Fp1 and F3. Within one session the patient reported sensing an improvement. At the completion of treatment the MMPI depression scale had improved from 97 T-scores to 56 T-scores. Somatic symptoms (gastritis, headaches, achiness, and preoccupation with health) dramatically improved, as did his overemotionality, anxiety and rumination, and fatigue. MMPI and reports from the patient demonstrated that he had become less withdrawn, more active, sociable, and less distrustful. There literally was more "approach" behavior, and the changes were maintained at an 8½ month follow-up.

As a result of this successful case outcome this protocol continued to be used. Clinical experience demonstrated that occasionally a patient reported becoming overactivated from the reinforcement of 15–18 Hz beta, reporting feeling some-what more irritable, anxious, and having some difficulty falling asleep. Therefore, the protocol was modified so that while inhibiting alpha and theta activity, 15–18 Hz beta was reinforced for 20–22 minutes, and then the reinforcement band was changed to 12–15 Hz for the last 8–10 minutes. No further overactivia-tion side effects were seen after that modification. On occasion a patient was also found to demonstrate considerable delta activity in the left frontal area, in which case delta might also be inhibited.

Following other successful clinical experiences, Hammond (2005b) reported on another case series of nine consecutive patients with a primary presenting complaint of depression, which was confirmed on the Minnesota multiphasic personality inventory (MMPI). The only other selection criterion was that each patient had a screening assessment of three 2-minute samples with the Baehr/Rosenfeld protocol to ascertain the presence and degree of the frontal asymme-try (predisposition to depression). As reviewed earlier in this chapter, percentage scores greater than 60 suggest that there is not a predisposition to depression, while percentage scores of 58 or less suggest the presence of a predisposition. The mean percentage score for this sample was 40.05, and their mean score on the MMPI depression scale was 93.75 T-scores—a serious level of depression. Whereas patients in medication studies are often moderately depressed, seven of the eight patients in this series were judged to be seriously to severely depressed, with only one being moderately depressed. Cases cited by Baehr *et al.* (1997, 2001) involved relatively mild depression in the 62–64 T-score range on the MMPI, with an aver-age asymmetry protocol score of 51.3.

The outcomes reported by Hammond (2005b) differed in four ways from the Baehr/Rosenfeld cases. Firstly, the sample was significantly more depressed. Secondly, the Fp1 and F3 protocol was different. Thirdly, treatment duration was only approximately two-thirds the length. And finally, concurrent psychotherapy and relaxation training was purposely not provided to better determine treatment effects from purely the neurofeedback, without contamination from relaxation or cognitive therapy. Eight of the patients completed training, requiring an average of approxi-mately 21 thirty-minute sessions (10+ hours) of neurofeedback, with no other psy-chotherapy provided. Seven of eight patients made very substantial improvements, and one other patient dropped out after five sessions because he was "too busy." The patient who prematurely terminated showed signs of questionable motivation from the beginning, seeming to be in treatment primarily to please his wife and daughter. Many of the patients were on medication at the time of initial testing, but were no longer on medication at the completion of treatment.

Pre–post changes on the MMPI may be seen in Figure 12.1. There was a mean decrease in the depression scale of 28.75 T-scores. One patient showed improve-ment from severely depressed to normal, and two improved from being seriously depressed to normal. Three showed improvement from severe to mild depression, and one showed improvement from moderately depressed to mildly depressed.

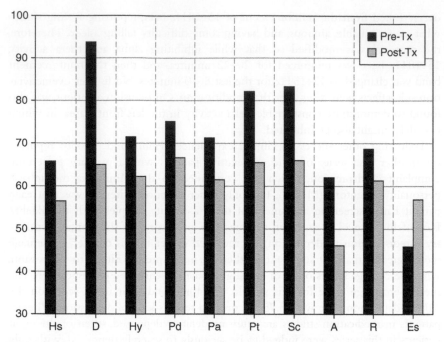

FIGURE 12.1   Hammond depression protocol: Average MMPI pre–post changes for eight cases.

One case who was severely depressed only showed mild improvement. This was an individual who had lost his wife to cancer a year earlier, and issues surrounding this loss seemed likely to need to be addressed; he was referred for psychotherapy for these issues. Classifying this last case, and including the drop-out as failures, this represents 77.8% of cases who made significant improvements. The average length of follow-up for these cases was about 1 year, with a range from 2 years in two cases, to 4 months in the case of the individual who only mildly improved.

It is fortunate that the MMPI was used as an outcome measure, rather than only a measure of depression. MMPI results (see Figure 12.1) have commonly found not only decreases in depression, but also in other scales measuring anxiety, obsessive rumination, withdrawal, and introversion, while ego-strength has improved. The decreases in being withdrawn are congruent with what we would expect when an approach motivation area of the brain is being activated.

In total Hammond has treated at least three-dozen depression cases using this depression protocol, with consistently positive results in an estimated 75–80% of cases. Anecdotal reports from other clinicians using this protocol have also been positive. In ongoing clinical practice, other psychotherapeutic techniques (self-hypnosis training, respiration biofeedback training, cognitive therapy, bibliotherapy) are often added to treatment, but by far the largest component of treatment has remained the use of the Hammond depression protocol. Occasionally the protocol has been done eyes-closed when a patient was simply producing too much eye movement artifact and, in each case where this alteration has occurred, the outcomes remained positive. It should be added that clinical experience in the treatment of obsessive-compulsive disorder (Hammond, 2003, 2004), supported by research (Maihofner et al., 2007) implicating the left frontal area in OCD, has also been suggestive that this protocol may prove helpful as one of the modules in OCD treatment with neurofeedback.

V.   OTHER NEUROFEEDBACK STUDIES WITH DEPRESSION

A unique form of neurofeedback, the Low Energy Neurofeedback System (LENS) (Hammond, 2007b; Ochs, 2006) has also been used with mood disturbances. LENS training differs from other forms of neurofeedback in that it introduces a tiny radio frequency signal which is only about the intensity of the output coming from a watch or radio battery, i.e., far, far weaker than the input you receive from simply holding a cell phone to your ear. This very low intensity input is introduced down the electrode wires for only a few seconds (e.g., often just 1–7). Its frequency varies depending on the dominant brain wave frequency from moment-to-moment, and it is designed to gently nudge the brain to become more flexible and self-regulating, reducing excess amplitude and variability of the brain waves. Larsen et al. (2006) recently reported on a case series of 20 patients where over the course of 20 sessions there was a significant decrease in self-ratings of depression. Ratings decreased from an initial average of almost 8 (on a 0–10 scale) to less than 5 in just six sessions, and to less than 3½ at the end of 20 sessions.

Neurofeedback training to increase alpha and theta, while inhibiting faster beta frequencies, has also been found to produce significant improvements in depression in alcoholic and post-traumatic stress disorder populations—in randomized, control group studies (Peniston and Kulkosky, 1990; Peniston et al., 1993) as well as in a case series (Saxby and Peniston, 1995)—populations where one may expect an excess of fast beta activity to often be prominent, and which is quite different from the EEG patterns usually seen in depression.

Research in Europe (Hardman et al., 1997; Kotchoubey et al., 1996; Rockstroh et al., 1990) using neurofeedback to alter slow cortical potentials has also demonstrated that it can be used to alter hemispheric asymmetries, and thus may also hold potential for use in the treatment of depression.

VI.   SUMMARY AND CONCLUSIONS

A robust body of research has validated that there is a biological predisposition to depression (and to becoming withdrawn) which is associated with a frontal asymmetry wherein there is less activity in the left frontal area. Although pharmacologic treatment for depression is widespread, reviews (e.g., Antonuccio *et al.*, 1999; Greenberg *et al.*, 1992; Hammond, 2007; Kirsch *et al.*, 2002; Kirsch and Sapperstein, 1998; Moncrieff, 2001) have documented that antidepressants, on average, only have an 18% effect over and above placebo effects, and yet they are associated with significant side effects such as sexual dysfunction, insomnia, increased suicide risk, diarrhea, nausea, anorexia, bleeding, forgetfulness, and withdrawal syndromes.

Thus alternatives are needed to the invasive treatments commonly utilized by "biological psychiatry," namely medication, electroconvulsive therapy, transcranial magnetic stimulation, and neurosurgery, which are commonly associated with side effects. Studies (e.g., Elkin *et al.*, 1989; Hollon *et al.*, 1992; Hollon, *et al.*, 1991) that have compared psychotherapy with medication have found that treatment outcomes are generally comparable or better than pharmacologic treatment, and when drop-out rates are taken into account drug treatment alone produces worse outcomes than psychotherapy.

However, the authors have found that neurofeedback offers an additional non-invasive treatment alternative with depression. While more controlled research is certainly needed, neurofeedback that is targeted to altering the frontal asymmetry found in depression has consistently produced favorable results in a majority of clinical cases. LENS neurofeedback, slow cortical potentials training, and the use of alpha/theta neurofeedback training with an alcoholic or PTSD population also appear promising in the treatment of depression.

REFERENCES

Ahern, G. L. and Schwartz, G. E. (1985). Differential lateralization for positive and negative emotion in the human brain: EEG spectral analysis. *Neuropsychologia*, **23**, 745–756.

Allen, J. J., Iacono, W. G., Depue, R. A. and Abrisi, M. (1993). Regional electroencephalographic asymmetries in bipolar seasonal affective disorder before and after exposure to bright light. *Biological Psychiatry*, **33**, 642–646.

Allen, J., Harmon-Jones, E. and Cavender, J. (2001). Manipulation of frontal EEG asymmetry through biofeedback alters self-reported emotional responses and facial EMG. *Psychophysiology*, **38**, 685–693.

Allen, J. J. B., Urry, H. L., Hitt, S. K. and Coan, J. A. (2004a). The stability of resting frontal electroencephalographic asymmetry in depression. *Psychophysiology*, **41**, 269–280.

Allen, J. J. B., Coan, J. A. and Nazarian, M. (2004b). Issues and assumptions on the road from raw signals to metrics of frontal EEG asymmetry in emotion. *Biological Psychology*, **67**, 183–218.

Anokhin, A. P., Heath, A. C. and Myers, E. (2006). Genetic and environmental influences on frontal EEG asymmetry: A twin study. *Biological Psychiatry*, **71(3)**, 295–298.

Antonuccio, D. O., Danton, W. G., DeNelsky, G. Y., Greenberg, R. P. and Gordon, J. S. (1999). Raising questions about antidepressants. *Psychotherapy & Psychosomatics*, **68**, 3–14.

Armitage, R., Roffwarg, H. P., Rush, A. J., Calhoun, J. S., Purdy, D. G. and Giles, D. E. (1992). Digital period analysis of sleep EEG in depression. *Biological Psychiatry*, **31**, 52–68.

Armitage, R., Roffwarg, H. P. and Rush, A. J. (1993). Digital period analysis of EEG in depression: Periodicity, coherence, and interhemispheric relationships during sleep. *Progress in Neuropsychopharmacology & Biological Psychiatry*, **17**, 363–372.

Armitage, R., Hudson, A., Trivedi, M. and Rush, A. J. (1995). Sex differences in the distribution of EEG frequencies during sleep: Unipolar depressed outpatients. *Journal of Affective Disorders*, **34**, 121–129.

Askew, J. H. (2001). The diagnosis of depression using psychometric instruments and quantitative measures of electroencephalographic activity. Unpublished doctoral dissertation, University of Tennessee.

Baehr, E. (2002). Frontal Asymmetry and Brief Mood Shifts in Normal and Depressed Subjects. Unpublished paper, *Society for Neuronal Regulation, 10ᵗʰ Annual Conference. Scottsdale, AZ.*

Baehr, E. and Baehr, R. (1997). The use of brainwave biofeedback as an adjunctive therapeutic treatment for depression: Three case studies. *Biofeedback*, **25(1)**, 10–11.

Baehr, E., Rosenfeld, J. P. and Baehr, R. (1997). The clinical use of an alpha asymmetry neurofeedback protocol in the treatment of depression: Two case studies. *Journal of Neurotherapy*, **293**, 10–23.

Baehr, E., Rosenfeld, J. P., Baehr, R. and Earnest, C. (1998). Comparison of two EEG asymmetry indices in depressed patients and Normal controls. *International Journal of Psychophysiology*, **31**, 89–92.

Baehr, E., Rosenfeld, J. P., Baehr, R. and Earnest, C. (1999). Clinical use of an alpha asymmetry neurofeedback protocol in the treatment of mood disorders. In *Introduction to Quantitative EEG and Neurofeedback* (J. R. Evans and A. Arbarbanel, eds), pp. 181–203. New York: Academic Press.

Baehr, E., Rosenfeld, J. P. and Baehr, R. (2001). Clinical use of an alpha asymmetry protocol in the treatment of mood disorders; follow-up study one to five years post therapy. *Journal of Neurotherapy*, **4(4)**, 11–18.

Baehr, E., Rosenfeld, J. P., Miller, L. and Baehr, R. (2004). Premenstrual Dysphoric Disorder and changes in frontal alpha asymmetry. *International Journal of Psychophysiology*, **52(2)**, 159–167.

Baxter, L. R., Phelps, M. E., Mazziotta, J. C., Guze, B. H., Schwartz, J. M. and Selin, C. (1987). Local cerebral glucose metabolic rates in obsessive-compulsive disorder: A comparison with rates in unipolar depression and in normal controls. *Archives of General Psychiatry*, **44(3)**, 211–218.

Baxter, L. R., Schwartz, J. M., Mazziotta, J. C., et al. (1988). Cerebral glucose metabolic rates in non-depressed patients with obsessive-compulsive disorder. *American Journal of Psychiatry*, **145(12)**, 1560–1563.

Bench, C. J., Friston, K. J., Brown, R. G., Scott, L. C., Frackowiak, R. S. J. and Dolan, R. J. (1992). The anatomy of melancholia: Focal abnormalities in cerebral blood flow in major depression. *Psychological Medicine*, **22**, 607–615.

Bench, C. J., Friston, K. J., Brown, R. G., Frackowiak, R. S. J. and Dolan, R. J. (1993). Regional cerebral blood flow in depression measured by positron emission tomography: The relationship with clinical dimensions. *Psychological Medicine*, **23**, 579–590.

Bruder, G. E., Tenke, C. E., Stewart, J. W., Towey, J. P., Leite, P. and Voglmaier, M. (1995). Brain event-related potentials to complex tones in depressed patients: Relations to perceptual asymmetry and clinical features. *Psychophysiology*, **32**, 373–381.

Bruder, G. E., Tenke, C. E., Warner, V. and Weissman, M. M. (2007). Grandchildren at high and low risk for depression differ in EEG measures of regional brain asymmetry. *Biological Psychiatry*, **62**.

Carver, C. S. and White, T. L. (1994). Behavioral inhibition, behavioral activation, and affective responses to impending reward punishment: The BIS/BAS scales. *Journal of Personality and Social Psychology*, **67**, 319–333.

Childre, D. and Martin, H. (1999). *The HeartMath Solution*. Harper-Collins.

Clementz, B. A., Sponheim, S. R., Iacono, W. G., et al. (1994). Resting EEG in first-episode schizophrenia patients, bipolar psychotic patients, and their first-degree relatives. *Psychophysiology*, **31**, 486–494.

Coan, J. A. and Allen, J. J. B. (2003). Frontal EEG asymmetry and the behavioral activation and inhibition systems. *Psychophysiology*, **40**, 106–114.

Coan, J. A. and Allen, J. J. B. (2004). Frontal EEG asymmetry as a moderator and mediator of emotion. *Biological Psychology*, **67**, 7–49.

Coan, J. A., Allen, J. J. B. and McKnight, P. E. (2006). A capability model of individual differences in frontal EEG asymmetry. *Biological Psychology*, **72(2)**, 198–207.

Davidson, R. J. (1992). Anterior cerebral asymmetry and the nature of emotion. *Brain and Cognition*, **20**, 125–151.

Davidson, R. J. (1993). Cerebral asymmetry and emotion: Conceptual and methodological conundrums. *Cognition and Emotion*, **7**, 115–138.

Davidson, R. J. (1994). Asymmetric brain function, affective style and psychopathology: The role of experience and plasticity. *Development and Psychopathology*, **6**, 741–758.

Davidson, R. J. (1998a). Affective style and affective disorders: Perspectives from affective neuroscience. *Cognition and Emotion*, **12(3)**, 307–330.

Davidson, R. J. (1998b). Anterior electrophysiological asymmetries, emotion, and depression: Conceptual and methodological conundrums. *Psychophysiology*, **35**, 607–614.

Davidson, R. J. (2004). What does the prefrontal cortex "do" in affect: perspectives on frontal EEG asymmetry research. *Biological Psychology*, **67**, 219–233.

Davidson, R. J., Schaffer, C. E. and Saron, C. (1985). Effects of lateralized presentations of faces on self-reports of emotion and EEG asymmetry in depressed and non-depressed subjects. *Psychophysiology*, **22**, 353–364.

Davidson, R. J., Chapman, J. P., Chapman, L. J. and Henriques, J. B. (1990a). Asymmetrical brain electrical activity discriminates between psychometrically-matched verbal and spatial cognitive tasks. *Psychophysiology*, **27**, 528–543.

Davidson, R. J., Ekman, P., Saron, C. D., Senulis, J. A. and Friesen, W. V. (1990b). Approach-withdrawal and cerebral asymmetry: Emotional expression and brain physiology. *International Journal of Personality and Social Psychology*, **58**, 330–341.

Davidson, R. J., Abercrombie, H., Nischke, J. B. and Putnam, K. (1999a). Regional brain function, emotion and disorders of emotion. *Current Opinion in Neurobiology*, **9**, 228–234.

Dawson, G., Grofer Klinger, L., Panagiotides, H., Hill, D. and Spieker, S. (1992). Frontal lobe activity and affective behavior of infants of mothers with depressed symptoms. *Child Development*, **63**, 725–737.

Dawson, G., Grofer Klinger, L., Panagiotides, H., Spieker, S. and Frey, K. (1992). Infants of mothers with depressed symptoms: Electroencephalographic and behavioral findings related to attachment status. *Development & Psychopathology*, **4**, 67–80.

Debener, S., Beauducel, A., Nessler, D., Brocke, B., Heilemann, H. and Kayser, J. (2000). Is resting anterior EEG alpha asymmetry a trait marker for depression? Findings for healthy adults and clinically depressed patients. *Neuropsychobiology*, **41(1)**, 31–37.

Deldin, P. J. and Chiu, P. (2005). Cognitive restructuring and EEG in major depression. *Biological Psychology*, **70(3)**, 41–151.

Earnest, C. (1999). Single case study of EEG asymmetry biofeedback for depression and independent replication in an adolescent. *Journal of Neurotherapy*, **3**, 28–35.

Elkin, I., Shea, T., Watkins, J. T., *et al.* (1989). National Institute of Mental Health treatment of depression collaborative research program: General effectiveness of treatments. *Archives of General Psychiatry*, **46**, 971–982.

Elliott, S. and Edmonson, D. (2006). The New Science of Breath, Coherent Breathing, for Autonomic Nervous System Balance, Health, and Well-Being, 2nd edition. Allen, TX: Choerence Press.

Field, T., Fox, N., Pickens, J. and Nawrocki, R. (1995). Relative right frontal EEG activation in 3- to 6-month-old infants of "depressed" mothers. *Developmental Psychology*, **26**, 7–14.

Flor-Henry, P. and Koles, Z. J. (1984). Statistical quantitative EEG studies of depression, mania, schizophrenia, & normals. *Biological Psychology*, **19**, 257–297.

George, M. S., Ketter, T. A., Perekh, P., *et al.* (1994). Spatial ability in affective illness: Differences in regional brain activation during a spatial matching task. *Neuropsychiatry, Neuropsychology and Behavioral Neurology*, **7**, 143–153.

Gotlib, I. H., Ranganath, C. and Rosenfeld, J. P. (1998). Frontal EEG alpha asymmetry, depression, and cognitive functioning. *Cognition and Emotion*, **12**, 449–478.

Greenberg, R. P., Bornstein, R. F., Greenberg, M. D. and Fisher, S. (1992). A meta-analysis of antidepressant outcome under "blinder" conditions. *Journal of Consulting & Clinical Psychology*, **60**, 664–669.

Hagemann, D. (2004). Individual differences in anterior EEG asymmetry: methodological problems and solutioins. *Biological Psychology*, **67**, 157–182.

Hagemann, D., Naumann, E., Becker, G., Maier, S. and Bartussek, D. (1998). Frontal brain asymmetry and affective style: A conceptual replication. *Psychophysiology*, **35**, 372–388.

Hagemann, D., Naumann, E., Lürken, A., Becker, G., Maier, S. and Bartussek, D. (1999). EEG asymmetry, dispositional mood and personality. *Personality and Individual Differences*, **27**, 541–568.

Hagemann, D., Naumann, E. and Thayer, J. F. (2001). The quest for the EEG reference revisited: A glance from brain asymmetry research. *Psychophysiology*, **38**, 847–857.

Hammond, D. C. (2000). Neurofeedback treatment of depression with the Roshi. *Journal of Neurotherapy*, **4(2)**, 45–56.

Hammond, D. C. (2003). QEEG-guided neurofeedback in the treatment of obsessive-compulsive disorder. *Journal of Neurotherapy*, **7(2)**, 25–52.

Hammond, D. C. (2004). Treatment of the obsessional subtype of obsessive compulsive disorder with neurofeedback. *Biofeedback*, **32**, 9–12.

Hammond, D. C. (2005a). Neurofeedback treatment of anxiety and affective disorders. *Child & Adolscent Psychiatric Clinics of North America*, **14**, 105–123.

Hammond, D. C. (2005b). Neurofeedback treatment of depression and anxiety. *Journal of Adult Development*, **12(2/3)**, 131–137.

Hammond, D. C. (2007a). Hypnosis, placebos, and systematic research bias in biological psychiatry. *American Journal of Clinical Hypnosis*, **50(1)**, 37–47.

Hammond, D. C. (2007b). *LENS: The Low Energy Neurofeedback System*. Binghampton, NY: Haworth Press.

Hardman, E., Gruzelier, J., Chessman, K., *et al.* (1997). Frontal interhemispheric asymmetry: Self-regulation and individual differences in humans. *Neuroscience Letters*, **221**, 117–120.

Harmon-Jones, E. (2000). Relationship between anger and asymmetrical frontal cortical activity. *Psychophysiology*, **S18**.

Harmon-Jones, E. (2006). Unilateral right–hand contractions cause contralateral alpha power suppression and approach motivational affective experience. *Psychophysiology*, **43**, 598–603.

Harmon-Jones, E. and Allen, J. J. B. (1997). Behavioral activation sensitivity and resting frontal EEG asymmetry: Covariation of putative indicators related to risk for mood disorders. *Journal of Abnormal Psychology*, **74**, 1310–1316.

Harris, F. J., (1978). On the use of windows for harmonic analysis with the discrete Fourier transformation. *Proc. IEEC*, **16**, 51–84.

Heller, W., Etienne, M. A. and Miller, G. A. (1995). Patterns of perceptual asymmetry in depression and anxiety: Implications for neuropsychological models of emotion and psychopathology. *Journal of Abnormal Psychology*, **104**, 327–333.

Henriques, J. B. and Davidson, R. J. (1990). Regional brain electrical asymmetries discriminate between previously depressed and healthy control subjects. *Journal of Abnormal Psychology*, **99**, 22–33.

Henriques, J. B. and Davidson, R. J. (1991). Left frontal hypoactivation in depression. *Journal of Abnormal Psychology*, **100**, 535–545.

Henriques, J. B. and Davidson, R. J. (1997). Brain electrical asymmetries during cognitive task performance in depressed and nondepressed subjects. *Biological Psychiatry*, **42**, 1039–1050.

Hollon, S. D., Shelton, R. C. and Loosen, P. T. (1991). Cognitive therapy and pharmacotherapy for depression. *Journal of Consulting and Clinical Psychology*, **59**, 88–99.

Hollon, S. D., DeRubeis, R. J., Evans, M. D., *et al.* (1992). Cognitive therapy and pharmacotherapy for depression: Singly and in combination. *Archives of General Psychiatry*, **49**, 774–781.

Jaeger, J., Borod, J. C. and Peselow, E. (1987). Depressed patients have atypical biases in perception of emotional faces. *Journal of Abnormal Psychology*, **96**, 321–324.

John, E. R., Prichep, L. S., Fridman, J. and Easton, P. (1988). Neurometrics: Computer assisted differential diagnosis of brain dysfunctions. *Science*, **293**, 162–169.

Jones, N. A., Field, T., Fox, N. A., Lundy, B. and Davalos, M. (1997). EEG activation in 1-month-old infants of depressed mothers. *Developmental Psychopathology*, **9**, 491–505.

Joseph, R. (1999). Frontal lobe psychopathology: Mania, depression, confabulation, catatonia, perseveration, obsessive compulsions, and schizophrenia. *Psychiatry*, **62**, 138–172.

Karavidas, M. K., Lehrer, P. M., Vaschillo, E., *et al.* (2007). Preliminary results of an open label study of heart rate variability biofeedback for the treatment of major depression. *Applied Psychophysiology and Biofeedback*, **32**, 19–30.

Kirsch, I., Moore, T. J., Scoboria, A. and Nicholls, S. S. (2002). The emperor's new drugs: An analysis of antidepressant medication data submitted to the U.S. Food and Drug Administration. *Prevention & Treatment*, **5**. Article 23. http://www.journals.apa.org/prevention/

Kirsch, I. and Sapperstein, G. (1998). Listening to Prozac, but hearing placebo? A meta-analysis of antidepressant medication. *Prevention & Treatment*, **1**. Available on the internet at: http://www.journals.apa.org/prevention/

Knott, V. J. and Lapierre, Y. D. (1987). Computerized EEG correlates of depression and antidepressant treatment. *Progress in Neuropsychopharmacology in Biological Psychiatry*, **11**, 213–221.

Koek, R. J., Yerevanian, B. I., Tachiki, K. H., Smith, J. C., Alcock, J. and Kopelowicz, A. (1999). Hemispheric asymmetry in depression and mania: A longitudinal QEEG study in bipolar disorder. *Journal of Affective Disorders*, **53**, 109–122.

Kotchoubey, B., Schleichert, H., Lutzenberger, W., Anokhin, A. P. and Birbaumer, N. (1996). Self-regulation of interhemispheric asymmetry in humans. *Neuroscience Letters*, **215**, 91–94.

Ladavas, E., Nicoletti, R., Umilta, C. and Rizzolatti, G. (1984). Right hemisphere interference during negative affect: A reaction time study. *Neuropsychologia*, **22**, 479–485.

Larsen, S., Harrington, K. and Hicks, S. (2006). The LENS (Low Energy Neurofeedback System): A clinical outcomes study of one hundred patients at Stone Mountain Center, New York. *Journal of Neurotherapy*, **10(2–3)**, 69–78.

Liotti, M., Mayberg, H. S., Brannan, S. K., McGinnis, S., Jerabek, P. and Fox, P. T. (2000). Differential limbic–cortical correlates of sadness and anxiety in healthy subjects: implications for affective disorders. *Biological Psychiatry*, **48**, 30–42.

Maihofner, C., Sperlling, W. and Kaltenhauser, M. (2007). Spontaneous magnetoencephalographic activity in patients with obsessive-compulsive disorder. *Brain Research*, **1129**, 200–205.

McFarland, B. R., Shankman, S. A., Tenke, C. E., Bruder, G. E. and Klein, D. N. (2006). Behavioral activation system deficits predict the six-month course of depression. *Journal of Affective Disorders*, **91(2–3)**, 229–234.

Moncrieff, J. (2001). Are antidepressants overrated? A review of methodological problems in antidepressant trials. *Journal of Nervous and Mental Disease*, **189(5)**, 288–295.

Ochs, L. (2006). The Low Energy Neurofeedback System (LENS): Theory, background, and introduction. *Journal of Neurotherapy*, **10(2–3)**, 5–37.

Papousek, I. and Schulter, G. (2006). Individual differences functional asymmetries of the cortical hemispheres, revival of laterality research in emotion and psychopathology. *Cognition, Brain, Behavior*, **X**, 269–298.

Peniston, E. G. and Kulkosky, P. J. (1990). Alcoholic personality and alpha–theta brainwave training. *Medical Psychotherapy*, **2**, 37–55.

Peniston, E. G., Marrinan, D. A., Deming, W. A. and Kulkosky, P. J. (1993). EEG alpha–theta brainwave synchronization in Vietnam theater veterans with combat-related post-traumatic stress disorder and alcohol abuse. *Advances in Medical Psychotherapy*, **6**, 37–50.

Pizzagalli, D. A., Sherwood, R. J., Henriques, J. B. and Davidson, R. J. (2005). Frontal brain asymmetry and reward responsiveness: A source-localization study. *Psychological Science*, **16**, 805–813.

Prichep, L. S. and John, E. R. (1986). Neurometrics: Clinical applications. In Clinical Applications of Computer Analysis of EEG and Other Neurophysiological Variables. Volume 2, Handbook of Electroencephalography and Clinical Neurophysiology. (F. H. Lopes da Silva, W. Storm van Leeuwen, and A. Remond, eds), pp. 153–170. Amsterdam: Elsevier.

Reid, S. A., Duke, L. M. and Allen, J. J. B. (1998). Resting frontal electroencephalographic asymmetry in depression: inconsistencies suggest the need to identify mediating factors. *Psychophysiology*, **35**, 389–404.

Robinson, R. G., Starr, L. B. and Price, T. R. (1984). A two year longitudinal study of mood disorders following stroke: prevalence and duration at six month follow-up. *British Journal of Psychiatry*, **144**, 256–262.

Rockstroh, B., Elbert, T., Birbaumer, N. J. and Lutzenberger, W. (1990). Biofeedback-produced hemispheric asymmetry of slow cortical potentials and its behavioral effects. *International Journal of Psychophysiology*, **9**, 151–165.

'Rosenfeld, 1997' is cited in footnote 2 – pls list here or delete in footnote.

Rosenfeld, J. P., Cha, G., Blair, T. and Gotlib, I. (1995). Operant biofeedback control of left-right frontal alpha power differences. *Biofeedback Self-Regulation*, **20**, 241–258.

Rosenfeld, J. P., Baehr, E., Baehr, R., Gottlieb, I. H. and Ranganath, C. (1996). Preliminary evidence that daily changes in frontal alpha asymmetry correlate with changes in affect in therapy sessions. *International Journal of Psychophysiology*, **23**, 137–141.

Rottenberg, J., Clift, A., Bolden, S. and Salomon, K. (2007). RSA fluctuation in major depressive disorder. *Psychophysiology*, **44**, 450–458.

Saxby, E. and Peniston, E. G. (1995). Alpha–theta brainwave neurofeedback training: An effective treatment for male and female alcoholics with depressive symptoms. *Journal of Clinical Psychology*, **51(5)**, 685–693.

Schaffer, C. E., Davidson, R. H. and Saron, C. (1983). Frontal and parietal electroencephalogram asymmetry in depressed and nondepressed subjects. *Biological Psychiatry*, **18(7)**, 753–762.

Schwartz, G. E., Davidson, R. J. and Maer, F. (1975). Right hemisphere lateralization for emotion in the human brain: Interactions with cognition. *Science*, **190**, 286–288.

Smit, D. J. A., Posthuma, D., Boomsma, D. I. and DeGeus, E. J. C. (2006). The relation between frontal EEG asymmetry and the risk for anxiety and depression. *Biological Psychology*, **74(1)**, 26–33.

Sterman, M. B. (1999). *Atlas of Topometric Clinical Displays: Functional Interpretations and Neurofeedback Strategies*. Los Angeles: Sterman-Kaiser Imaging Laboratory.

Sterman, M. B. and Kaiser, D. (2001). Comodulation: A new QEEG analysis metric for assessment of structural and functional disorders of the central nervous system. *Journal of Neurotherapy*, **4(3)**, 73–83.

Sutton, S. K. and Davidson, R. J. (1997). Prefrontal brain asymmetry: A biological substrate of the behavioral approach and inhibition systems. *Biological Psychological Science*, **8(3)**, 204–210.

Tenke, C. E., Bruder, G. E., Towey, J. P., Leite, P. and Sidtis, J. (1993). Correspondence between ERP and behavioral asymmetries for complex tones. *Psychophysiology*, **30**, 62–70.

Tomarken, A. J. and Davidson, R. J. (1994). Frontal brain activation in repressors and nonrepressors. *Journal of Abnormal Psychology*, **103(2)**, 339–349.

Tomarken, A. J., Davidson, R. J. and Henriques, J. B. (1990). Resting frontal brain asymmetry predicts affective responses to films. *Journal of Personality and Social Psychology*, **59**, 791–801.

Tomarken, A. J., Diehter, G. S., Garber, J. and Simien, C. (2004). Resting frontal brain activity linages to maternal depression and socio-economic status among adolescents. *Biological Psychology*, **67**, 77–102.

Vuga, M., Fox, N. A., Cohn, J. F., George, C. J., Lenenstein, R. M. and Kovacs, M. (2006). Long-term stability of frontal electroencephalographic asymmetry in adults with a history of depression and controls. *International Journal of Psychophysiology*, **59(2)**, 107–115.

CHAPTER 13

Neurofeedback and attachment disorder: Theory and practice

Sebern F. Fisher, M.A., BCIA

Private practice, Northampton, Massachusetts, USA

I. INTRODUCTION

Reactive attachment disorder (RAD), the focus of this chapter, is a condition of unremitting terror that disrupts the development of the self and renders "the other" unrecognizable. Empathy and trust cannot emerge. It is a disorder that has been refractory to treatment as it has been all but impossible to address the psychic programing of fear and distrust with standard psychotherapy. This chapter will argue that neurofeedback can and does rewrite this program, first in the brain and, over time, in the mind.

RAD can be seen as a discrete diagnosis. However, as attachment dynamics and their effects on brain development are better understood, it is becoming increasingly clear that early unrepaired attachment disruption is implicated in a wide range of severe disorders. It is a central premise of this chapter that where attachment issues prevail, the core affect is fear. Neurofeedback quiets fear. In doing so, it enriches the capacity for attachment and the ability to engage in meaningful relationships, including psychotherapy. It may be possible to generalize the efficacy of neurofeedback, then, in enhancing the treatment of any disorder that has attachment disruption at its root and fear as its aftermath. Attachment theory and the imperative of attachment in human beings offer practitioners a central ethical principle to guide their practice. Neurofeedback providers must understand the primacy and process of attachment, assess for attachment breaks, and pursue the repair of attachment.

Through neuronal regulation, neurofeedback has the potential to promote the human birthright of attachment, love, empathy and trust.

II. REACTIVE ATTACHMENT DISORDER: CASE STUDY

Sammy was three years old when he arrived at Rob and Judy's home for emergency placement. He had been in foster care for a year, and this was his fourth placement. He had been removed from his former foster home after attempting to set a fire, and from the placement before that after a serious attempt on the life of his 17-month-old sister. Judy and Rob were not parents, and had never intended to become foster parents. They were not prepared for how their quiet life was about to change. Few would be.

Sammy had been diagnosed with reactive attachment disorder, post-traumatic stress disorder, ADHD, and dissociation. He had been hospitalized on at least one occasion for failure to thrive, and on another after he fell or was dropped from a third floor window. His birth parents were themselves foster children who had met in residential care. Sammy had reportedly been left alone in a crib for days at a time. He had been physically and sexually abused. He was malnourished. With the exception of several graphic expletives and "no," he was essentially non-verbal. He responded, when he chose to, with one of these words or a gesture. He hoarded food and ate it under the table. Every night at bedtime he screamed and fought until he finally fell into an exhausted sleep around midnight, a sleep riddled with night terrors. He crawled on his hands and knees crying, "No, no, no." He awoke at 5 A.M., and was in constant motion throughout the day. He defecated on the floor; he masturbated incessantly, and made explicit sexual gestures when he was diapered at night. He screamed, arched his back, attempted to bite, and sobbed in heart-wrenching terror when he was held or restrained. It was not hard to understand why the Department of Social Services saw Sammy as the most troubled child in their custody.

Within a week of coming to live with Judy and Rob, Sammy began neurofeedback. His foster parents had to hold him in the chair to get through even 10 minutes of training. However, the night after the first session, he slept for 12 hours, without night terror. Initially, Sammy trained 5 days a week and he was, in very short order, able to cooperate with playing the game. Within 6 weeks, Judy reported the following changes.

"Sammy is eating normally, not trying to grab our food and not overeating. He is no longer preoccupied with food. He is slowly gaining weight. He's sleeping 12 hours a night. He still needs frequent 'holding sessions,' but he has also begun to ask for them. He seems surprised at himself when he does. He is more cooperative and less clingy. He has many fewer episodes of rage and, with prompting, will make eye contact. He has remorse and he's not so selfish. He seems to be getting cause and effect. And he is able to play calmly and asks us to read him books!"

A few weeks later, she told me about an interchange between them. "We'd had a long and rough day. I asked him why he thought it was so tough. He started to cry, real, wet tears, and said, 'I want you!'" After 3 months, now training two to three times a week, Sammy was becoming an emotionally expressive child. He could still go dark behind the eyes, but he no longer went blank. He was no longer dissociating. He was becoming, increasingly, spontaneously, relational. All sexual gesturing had stopped. He was listening, and doing what was asked of him. He was no longer hoarding food. and at times was even able to share it. He was toilet-trained. His speech was still seriously delayed but it was improving.

He was using simple sentence structure, and working cooperatively with his parents to learn articulation. After 6 months, Rob and Judy began the adoption process.

Sammy is now 10 years old, and Rob and Judy's adopted son. He continues neurofeedback training at home. He still exhibits self-defeating (non-aggressive) control battles at school, and requires a one-to-one aide to keep him focused. I was surprised to learn that he had failed a recent reading test. Months earlier, I'd run into the family at the supermarket. As we waited to check out, I picked up a magazine on the brain and said, "Sammy, this could be about you." He took it and read the beginning of the article aloud, with few mistakes. When I asked him why he'd failed that test when he could read so well, he shrugged. He didn't know. Control battles are inherent to attachment disorder. They are the remnants of fighting for survival. He rarely gets into these battles with his parents. These are adults that he has begun to trust. But, given the terrible reality of his first 3 years, trusting, and generalizing that trust, will not come easily. His default belief is that he will be left, and he may never entirely believe otherwise. (The experience of neurofeedback providers with these children and adults supports the growing awareness in the field of psychology that the effects of abandonment and neglect outweigh the effects of trauma.)

Attachment theory as it stands today goes a long way in helping us understand the terrible emotional turmoil and troubling behaviors of a boy like Sammy. The work of Allan Schore (1994, 2003a, 2003b) and Daniel Siegel (1999) on the effects of attachment on brain development and, in turn, on affect regulation, further elucidates the nature of Sammy's profound terror. Sammy's response to neurofeedback provides another vital piece of information. It strongly suggests that attachment disorder is encoded in the frequency domain of the brain, and that it can be addressed with biofeedback to the brain in that domain. Sammy's ability to gain regulation with training is not unique. His response, and that of many like him, takes attachment theory and treatment into a new realm—the electrical realm of the brain, the realm of neurofeedback.

III.   AN OVERVIEW OF ATTACHMENT THEORY

John Bowlby (1988) could be considered the "father of mothering." He was a British psychoanalyst, and a contemporary of Anna Freud and Melanie Klein. Although most of the reigning theorists of his time acknowledged that the mother–infant relationship was important, Bowlby was pretty much alone in maintaining that the quality of this early attachment set the developmental course for the infant into adulthood. He advanced the idea that the child's early attachment experience is central to healthy development as well as to our understanding of the development of psychopathology. In his book of collected lectures, *A Secure Base* (1988), Bowlby states his premise with simplicity and common sense.

> Briefly, it seems clear that sensitive loving care results in a child developing confidence that others will be helpful when appealed to, becoming increasingly self-reliant

and bold in his explorations of the world, co-operative with others, and also – a very important point – sympathetic and helpful to others in distress. Conversely, when a child's attachment behavior is responded to tardily and unwillingly and is regarded as a nuisance, he is likely to become anxiously attached, that is apprehensive lest his caregiver be missing or unhelpful when he needs her and therefore unwilling to leave her side, unwillingly and anxiously obedient, and unconcerned about the troubles of others. Should his caretakers, in addition, actively reject him, he is likely to develop a pattern of behaviour in which avoidance of them competes with his desire for proximity and care, and in which angry behaviour is apt to become prominent. (Bowlby, 1988)

It may be difficult to understand how such a thesis could be challenged, but it was vigorously rejected by most of Bowlby's contemporaries and, in some quarters, continues to be challenged today. Only one of his contemporaries, Ronald Fairbairn, agreed with Bowlby. As discussed by Karen (1994), Fairbairn believed that the fundamental drive in human beings was not "pleasure seeking" but "person-seeking," and he too argued that psychopathology originated in disruptions in early relationships. The British Psycho-Analytic Society, the think tank of psychological theory in post-war England, marginalized them both. But Bowlby persisted, and in 1954 Mary Ainsworth, a developmental psychologist, designed the research model that would provide the data to substantiate his theory. She was to make a profound contribution to the understanding of the role of attachment in human development.

While living in Uganda, Ainsworth developed the test that would come to be known as the Strange Situation (Ainsworth, 1954). She sought to understand if a baby's separation from its mother was harmful, as Bowlby's theory predicted, and, if so, under what circumstances. The Strange Situation tests the security of the baby's attachment to its mother by placing mother and baby in a playroom new to the baby, and assessing the baby's response to the entrance of a kindly stranger, to the mother's leaving, to the stranger's leaving, and to the mother's return. She was able to discern patterns of infant response to the mother and, from this, to establish categories of attachment. The Strange Situation has since been replicated thousands of times. It is a reliable and cross-culturally valid measure of attachment.

On the basis of its responses to its mother in the Strange Situation, a baby (age 12–14½ months) can be assigned to one of four categories that best describe the tenor of its attachment. The categories are secure; insecure, ambivalent; insecure, avoidant; and, the fourth, based on more recent work by Mary Main and Judith Solomon (1986), disorganized/disoriented, or, as it has come to be known, the "D" type.

The securely attached [seek] their mother when distressed, [seem] confident of her availability, [are] upset when she leaves them, eagerly greet her upon her return, and warmly [accept] and [are] readily comforted by her soothing embrace. The avoidantly attached [seem] to depend less on their mother as a secure base; sometimes [attack] her with a random act of aggression; [are] far more clingy and demanding than the secure children in the home environment; and, despite in some cases being just as openly upset by the mother's departure in the Strange Situation, [show] no interest in her when she return[s]. The ambivalently attached [tend] to be the most overtly anxious; like the avoidant children, [are] also clingy and demanding at home; like the secure, [are] upset when abandoned by the mother in the Strange Situation; but who, despite wanting her desperately when she return[s], arch away angrily or [go] limp in her embrace, so that they could not be soothed." (Karen, p. 176, 1994)

The "D" children show no clear strategy to manage either the separation from or the reunion with the mother. Eighty percent of those in this category have a confirmed history of abuse. A child suffering disorganized attachment might, on the mother's return, stare into space or approach her walking backwards. This seminal research begun by Ainsworth supported Bowlby's hypotheses that attachment patterns could be observed and generally categorized, and that these patterns were of significance in the development of children.

IV. ADULT ATTACHMENT CATEGORIES

The effects of the mother–infant attachment seem to be enduring. A longitudinal study led by Alan Sroufe (1995), in progress in Minneapolis, Minnesota, continues to find highly significant correlations between categories assigned during infancy and the child's developmental course. Main's research suggests the same continuity. Along with Carole George and Nancy Kaplan, Mary Main designed the Berkeley adult attachment interview (1986), a psychological assessment equivalent to the Strange Situation for babies.

Main's adult categories are "secure–autonomous," "dismissing of attachment," and "preoccupied with early attachment." She found that "secure–autonomous" adults described having at least one parent who provided them with a secure base during childhood. They talked about their parents coherently and realistically. There were some in this category who had had less than happy attachment histories. These people seem to have come to terms with their histories, and generally showed little evidence of self-deception. Those who fell in the category "dismissing of attachment," did just that. They often had little memory of their childhoods, and felt little inclination to talk about this time in their lives. They were the avoidant children, grown up.

The preoccupied group tended to speak of their childhoods as if they were living them with hurt and anger still fresh and unresolved. They had the hallmarks of the ambivalently attached child. They cannot, as it were, "leave the side" of their pasts. The correlations are robust. Furthermore, attachment histories seem to be transmitted from parent to child. Peter Fonagy, an attachment researcher in London, was able to predict infant classifications in the Strange Situation with 75% accuracy based on pre-natal interviews with the mothers.

Most attachment researchers take pains to emphasize that attachment categories are not diagnoses, and that poor attachment is not, in and of itself, pathology. Nonetheless, as Schore, Siegel and others are exploring extensively, and as Bowlby knew in his bones, early attachment disruption is a central issue in most serious psychological disorders. Without appropriate early intervention, insecure and disorganized attachments present a significant risk factor for some forms of personality, conduct or affective disorders.

There are still developmental theorists who dispute the centrality of attachment in human development. Some prefer to highlight inborn temperament as the critical factor in an individual's course over time. Others feel that attachment theory gives insufficient weight to events or relationships later in life. They tend to emphasize the importance of fate. But to borrow from Winnicott, there is no infant without a mother. It is very difficult, if not impossible, to understand the infant, and the adult that infant becomes, outside of the relationship with the mother. There is no doubt that each baby arrives with some unique aspects of self in wait, but that "self" will be expressed, perhaps even at the genetic level, through the baby's relationship with its parents, most profoundly with its mother.

The seemingly endless debate of nature versus nurture that is embedded here, may, over time, be put to rest through the practice of neurofeedback. Inherently, the success of neurofeedback suggests the hypothesis that both the baby's nature and its nurture are etched in the circuitry of its brain, and that the baby lives by the rules of both as they interact within him or her. It seems clear that these rules also largely govern how a baby will respond to the uncertainties of fate.

V. ALLAN SCHORE AND THE NEUROBIOLOGY OF AFFECT REGULATION

Three years after Bowlby's death, with debate still raging, Allan Schore published his first seminal work on attachment, *Affect Regulation and the Origin of Self: The Neurobiology of Emotional Development* (1994). Throughout his work, Schore weaves a tapestry of attachment theory, psychoanalytic theory, brain development, and affect regulation. He argues in his first book, and two subsequent ones (*Affect Dysregulation and Disorders of the Self* [2003a] and *Affect Regulation and the Repair of the Self* [2003b]), as does Siegel in *The Developing Mind* (1999), that attachment patterns affect not only the developing psychology of the infant but also his developing brain, particularly, and most importantly, the right hemisphere.

The right hemisphere is the first to develop and it does so, preferentially over the left, for the first 18–24 months of life. It is the part of the brain primarily responsible for the regulation of affect. The amygdala of the right hemisphere comes on line during the fifth month in utero. This part of the limbic brain is devoted to the organism's survival through the encoding of fear memory. Schore calls the right orbital-frontal cortex (ROC) "the greater amygdaloid area" because of the number of interconnections between these two parts of the brain. He goes on to say that, "most significantly, in the cortex, the orbitofrontal region is uniquely involved in social and emotional behaviors, and in the homeostatic regulation of body and motivational states" (Schore, p. 195, 2003b).

One of the primary roles of the ROC is to inhibit the amygdala, and to mediate the impulses it generates neuroelectrically, neurochemically and behaviorally. When the ROC fails to develop normally, the amygdala dominates brain response. Fear and rage can flood the circuits, and direct the motivational system of the individual. Fear rises as the first response to most situations, even to those that for others, with adequate ROC development, would not evoke fear. In attachment disorder and its most pathological sequela, sociopathy, fear is often far from evident, but it is there. Fear, in fact, may well be the affect that underlies the development of most if not all personality disorders.

Schore makes the case that the critical development of the right prefrontal cortex depends on "good-enough" attachment between mother and baby. The mother's ability to regulate her baby's affect in the cradle of attunement, expressed through eye contact, facial expression, holding, vocal tone and prosody, and the song of her voice, depends on the mother's right prefrontal cortex, the part of the brain that maintains her capacity to "autoregulate" her own emotional state. With such capacities intact, the mother is able to attune to her baby, to quiet the storms of distress, amplify the experiences of delight, and allow periods of rest, relaxation and quietude. Schore argues convincingly that through these interactions, the mother is developing the baby's right prefrontal cortex, making it increasingly possible for the baby to regulate the full spectrum of affect as he or she grows and matures.

> The orbitofrontal regions are not functional at birth. Over the course of the first year, limbic circuitries emerge in a sequential progression, from the amygdala to anterior cingulate to insula and finally to orbitofrontal. (Schore, p. 41, 2003b)
> ... as a result of attachment experiences, this system enters a critical period of maturation in the last quarter of the first year, the same time that working models of attachment (The Strange Situation) are first measured." (Schore p. 42, 2003b)

The mother's capacity to regulate herself builds her baby's brain structure, particularly the ROC, and with it her baby's ability to internalize her.

Perfect attunement is impossible. Life, mood and circumstances impinge on even the most gifted and well-adjusted mother. When misattunements occur, the mother who is able to autoregulate can and does make emotional repair. This repair allows the baby to regain his regulation. The mother's capacity for regulation in turn permits her awareness of misattunements and her capacity for emotional repair. "The internal working model" (Bowlby) becomes one that includes the restoration of the relationship after it has been stressed. Many patients in psychodynamic therapy, particularly those with challenging attachment histories, discover that they lack any belief that relationships, once broken, can be repaired.

Schore concludes that *the prefrontal cortex of the mother becomes the prefrontal cortex of the baby*. The regulation of the right hemisphere, where all primary affect is housed, promotes brain growth, and with it a coherent and stable unconscious internal working model of relatedness. When the mother is reliable, predictable and empathic, the baby develops a reliable sense of self and other. This sense of self emerges from healthy right hemisphere development and the affect regulation it affords; with it a sense of the other, the one who has been engaged with him or her in the process of learning affect regulation, also emerges. This is the essence of the title of Schore's first book, *Affect Regulation and the Origin of Self*. Daniel Stern also describes this beautiful dance of emergence in his book, *The Interpersonal World of the Infant* (1985). The self can only develop in the presence of the other, and can only truly and wholly develop in the embrace of an attuned, regulating mother—the secure base.

When the mother is not emotionally and physically present, and there is no other who takes up the vital relationship as wholeheartedly and single-mindedly as the "good-enough" mother, the baby's working model of relationships becomes chaotic. The underdeveloped ROC cannot inhibit limbic firing, and the psyche is overwhelmed by the amygdaloid storms of fear and aggression. Whatever model is set down in the crucial early stage of right hemisphere development will become a central aspect of the template for all future relationships.[1]

Schore is almost single-handedly responsible for rescuing attachment theory from years of psychodynamic and psychoanalytic neglect. Not only did he salvage the work of many long-suffering attachment theorists and researchers who preceded him, he has been able to locate these dynamics within the structures and biology of the brain. Neuroimaging is for him what Ainsworth and the Strange Situation were to Bowlby. These studies are beginning to bear them both out.

Schore brought Bowlby into the millennium of the brain. Brain development depends on good enough mothering. When an infant suffers prolonged attachment breaks that are left unrepaired, he or she runs a substantial risk of severe psychopathology.

VI. REACTIVE ATTACHMENT DISORDER AND A HISTORY OF TREATMENT FAILURE

Reactive attachment disorder (RAD) is a profound relational disorder that develops before age 5 (DSM IV). It is highly refractory to treatment, and without treatment can and often does lead to antisocial personality in adulthood. In addition to symptoms described in the DSM IV, those working with this disorder list the following behaviors and incapacities as typical of attachment disorder in children and adults:

- Lack of cause-and-effect thinking
- Lack of remorse or regret

---

[1] The child too contributes to the quality of attachment with its mother. This is most clearly seen in children diagnosed with autism, PDD and Asperger's Syndrome. These children also suffer from right hemisphere over arousal but come by it neurologically not interpersonally.

- Lack of empathy
- Blaming others
- Superficially charming
- Poor eye contact
- Chronic nonsensical lying
- Repetitive useless questions
- Cruelty to animals and/or children
- Poor peer and family relationships
- Lack of ability to give and receive affection
- Demanding and clingy
- Learning disabled
- Speech problems
- Controlling and bossy
- Preoccupied with blood, fire, gore and knives
- Abnormal eating patterns
- Stealing
- Destructive—particularly to others and to material things
- Provoking anger in others
- False allegations of abuse.

These symptoms are understood psychodynamically as a fundamental lack of trust and as attempts to control the behavior of others, and, clearly, they are. They are also highly suggestive of right hemisphere damage, damage that, in this disorder, is interpersonally caused. In neurofeedback cosmology, they are all symptoms of overarousal that strongly suggest the need for right hemisphere training.[2]

Given the severity of symptoms and, even more importantly, the lack of realness of "the other" to the person with RAD, it is easy to understand why therapists have reported routine failure in treating these patients. The initial endeavor of psychotherapy does not necessarily require that a patient care about their treatment or about themselves. It does require that the patient in some way care about the therapist and the therapist's response to him or her. Using this criterion, RAD is self-defining as a disorder that cannot be treated. The RAD patient by definition lacks the capacity to care about the therapist. The therapist barely exists and when he or she does, it is as a needs-gratifying object or as a thin cognitive trace against a stark, usually unrecognized, backdrop of absence. This patient cannot care about the other because there is no other. The patient lives within the darkly mirrored reflection of the original infant state, one in which they had no experience of mother and, as a result, no experience of the reality of self and other. Since the

[2]Studies have shown that the right hemispheres of habitual criminals are up to 25% smaller than those of non-habitual criminals. Attachment disorder, and for that matter its most common adult outcome, antisocial personality, is not only seen in those identified as criminals but in all strata of society, including executives of major corporations whose relationships with their employees and customers is entirely instrumental.

therapist does not materialize in this mind, the therapist and the therapy have no impact. Therapy with the unattached is like boxing with ghosts.

All traditional approaches to therapy have failed with this population, and the non-traditional therapies, particularly those that use holding techniques, have come under assault. "Holding therapy" is, in its best practice, an attempt to reach the wildly aroused brain of the unattached child through containing his or her highly agitated body. For most of these children, holding evokes a deeply encoded yearning so laced with fear that is expressed either as active rage, with kicking, biting, shrieking, spitting and arching the back, or as passive rage, in the form of going limp and averting the eyes. These are the behavioral expressions of the amygdala with no cortical inhibition.

Although "holding" can help these children by providing both a sense of neurological containment and with it the experience of the physical reality of the other, these gains often come at great cost to the parents and the therapists trying to use it. It is exhausting for everyone to try to contain this level of terror, rage and anguish. But conscientious therapists were up against their failures to help these children without having any other way to directly impact their arousal. These patients cannot participate meaningfully in either play or talk therapy. Medications are rarely of much help. And the consequences of treatment failure with this population are devastating: to the RAD individual (although he rarely perceives this), to his family, and to society as a whole. Prisons, many political systems, and all too much of corporate culture are built to house the unattached adult.

VII.   NEUROFEEDBACK AND THE TREATMENT OF REACTIVE ATTACHMENT DISORDER

RAD is routinely misdiagnosed. (I am using the diagnosis *reactive attachment disorder* throughout this chapter somewhat reluctantly. Bessel van der Kolk and others are attempting to change this diagnosis and to broaden it to *developmental trauma disorder*, a more accurate and hopefully less controversial diagnosis.) This condition can be labeled as ADHD, bipolar disorder, conduct disorder, explosive disorder or even Aspergers. Learning disabilities and speech problems that are usually co-morbid with RAD can further confound the diagnostic process. Although both speech and learning are associated with the left hemisphere, their ontological roots lie in the right. Speech develops from the song of prosody, sung in motherese. The left hemisphere adds words to the song when it begins its developmental surge late in the second year.

Learning depends on cause-and-effect thinking, the "cognition" of the right hemisphere, mediated by the ROC. A baby learns cause-and-effect through reliable, predictable parental responses to its needs: a baby is hungry, it cries, and it is fed. This interaction repeated over and over, reliably, provides the underwriting of cause-and-effect thinking. Without it, all subsequent learning is greatly impaired.

If we haven't learned this already as psychotherapists, we quickly see in our practice of neurofeedback that no diagnosis is as discreet as it appears in the DSM IV and, further, that a diagnosis does not always help us in our protocol decision process. As we will see, however, the diagnosis of attachment disorder should always take us to its source—the right hemisphere.

Schore writes, "... current brain research...indicates that the capacity for experience-dependent plastic changes in the nervous system remains throughout the life span. In fact, there is very specific evidence that the prefrontal limbic cortex, more than any other part of the cerebral cortex, retains the plastic capacities of early development" (Schore, p. 202, 2003b). This is the very capacity that neurofeedback exploits.

Although neuronal plasticity is now recognized and accepted, it remains vaguely defined. It is often assumed the plasticity means change in brain structure that allows an uninjured part of the brain to take up the duties and responsibilities of an injured part. Joseph describes it this way:

> ... experience acts to organize neuronal interconnections and the establishment of not just synapses but *vast neural networks* [italics mine] subserving a variety of complex behaviors and perceptual activity. Indeed, the brain is exceedingly plastic and is capable of undergoing tremendous functional reorganization not just over the course of evolution, but within a few years, months, or even weeks of a single individual's lifetime. (Joesph, p. 663, 1996)

In talking about brain development in children who grow up in neglectful or abusive homes, he goes on to say:

> Given the immature state of not just the neocortex but various limbic nuclei, it may well be expected that a failure to receive proper stimulation may result in a significant reduction of those neurons, dendrites and axons and their *associated neural circuits* [italics mine], which subserve 'normal' social-emotional intellectual development. Moreover, given that abnormal experience, including emotional and sexual trauma, also act to stimulate the brain, it is likely that abnormal experiences would result in the establishment of abnormal neural circuits. (Joseph, p. 664, 1996)

When Joseph speaks of "associated neural circuits," he is not speaking metaphorically. He is, without making it explicit, suggesting that the brain organizes itself through its electrical mechanisms (its circuitry). When we train the brain with neurofeedback, we are, it appears, appealing to the frequency-dependent properties of neuronal plasticity. We seem to be discovering that the brain has a "functional neuronal plasticity," and that this plasticity resides in the frequency domain of the brain. Once we see that neurofeedback can promote functional plasticity, and we recognize that attachment disorder lies in the part of the brain that remains the most plastic—the right hemisphere and particularly the right orbital cortex—we can see how neurofeedback can enhance the treatment of RAD when it is integrated into relational psychotherapy.

As we have seen through Schore's work, Bowlby's internal working model forms in the right hemisphere. As we have seen in the field of neurofeedback, it is etched there in the circuitry of the brain. All children and adults who have had serious attachment problems show an inability to quiet their arousal. Survival fear drives them. Among the most important of its functions, neurofeedback regulates affect. More specifically, and most importantly, it quiets fear. Just as Schore's theory would predict, as baseline fear is calmed, the self and other begin to emerge.

The unique contribution of neurofeedback to the treatment of attachment disorder is the reorganization and stabilization of the affect. As speculated, these plastic capacities lie primarily in the frequency domain of the brain. When we train the right hemisphere to reduce high arousal, we observe that the trainee responds to their life with less reactivity and with less fear. In both children and adults, I have witnessed a positive impact on every symptom of attachment disorder listed above. As arousal quiets, one sees less agitation and anger, better judgment, more empathy, greater capacity for remorse, and a generalized capacity for pro-social behavior. These patients begin to grasp cause-and-effect and, with this, have an increasing ability to learn. They report less fear. Therapy is now possible because the self begins to organize and recognize not only itself but also the actuality of the other.

A case study will help to illustrate this process. A 60-year-old man who had grown up with a drunken mother and an abusive, distant father came to me for treatment. He reported returning from school and routinely finding his mother passed out in the living room of his suburban home. He had been hospitalized with severe asthma for weeks at a time every year of his childhood. As an adult he was hated at his work place, he thought his mother was actively scheming to make his life miserable, he had hostile and distrustful relationships with his children, he described his third marriage as a "workable partnership," and he said he had never felt any emotion other than anger.

Within three sessions of neurofeedback training at the right temporal area, he was "awed" by the changes he felt in himself. His neuronal and emotional plasticity were unmistakable. By the time he stopped after 40 sessions, he was well liked in his new position in the company, and he had separated from his emotionally damaged and damaging wife. He commented frequently on "the new universe" that was opening to him. He felt things. His paranoid view of his mother dissolved, and he was able to adopt a more sophisticated understanding that she did the best she knew how to do. He forgave his father, and he reconnected with his children. Before beginning to train, we had worked together for a year in psychodynamic psychotherapy. He had not been able to understand forgiveness as a concept, much less be able to actually forgive. His logics were forged in fear, and he believed them. But as fear subsided with neurofeedback training, he was able to feel attachment to others and a new sense of self. His case suggests that Schore is correct—that plasticity endures and with it the latent capacity for attachment. When fear no longer engulfs them, even those with drastic attachment histories can rediscover the capacity for interpersonal connection within themselves.

There is a growing consensus that all effective therapy relies on affect regulation. Through the work of Marsha Linehan (1993) and her well-validated treatment, dialectical behavior therapy, affect regulation has become a central tenet in behavior therapy. As we have seen, it is the heart and soul of Schore's honing of psychoanalytic theory and his expansion of attachment theory, and Siegel's exploration of the developing mind. Regulation of affect is what neurofeedback does best, particularly heightened or fear-based arousal. It is what right hemisphere training does. It follows then that neurofeedback training of the right hemisphere may well increase the effectiveness of all therapies for disorders where overarousal is a critical problem.

VIII.   PROTOCOLS

I enter the discussion of protocols with caution. Neurofeedback training is a dynamic, evolving process, engaged with a dynamic, emerging system: the brain in relation to itself; the brain in relation to another brain; the brain in relation to mind; and the developing mind in relation to the mind of another. Although all theory and most neurofeedback practice direct us to the right hemisphere with disorders of attachment, all protocols are designed for the individual, not for the diagnosis.

The experience to date in training those with attachment disorders, whether as children or adults, suggests that training at T4, P4, T4-P4, T4-F4 and T4-AF4 at reward frequencies from 10–13 Hz and lower, while inhibiting 0–6 Hz, are the most effective and generally well-tolerated protocols. I have encountered those who have met criteria for this disorder who have had difficulty with temporal lobe training but who did well at C4 and C4-P4. In these cases, it appeared that the contraindication for temporal lobe training may have been head injury at this or the contralateral site. In addition, there have been reports that some children with RAD, those that don't respond well to right hemisphere training, will experience better results with a brief amount of C3-C4 protocol added to the right side training. (Personal conversation with Catherine Rule, 2004).

To date, most of the QEEG data related to RAD suggest that T6 and FZ might also be useful sites. T6 sits over the fusiform gyrus, the part of the brain that specializes in facial recognition and understanding of facial expression. Q findings may well reflect one of the central issues in the development of attachment disorder, i.e., the lack of reciprocal gaze and the interplay of faces that typify the attachment dance between mother and infant:

> ... excessive developmental cell death in specific groups of face processing neurons in the developing right fusiform gyrus, the area that decodes facial stimuli would be associated with ... the psychopath's mindblindness to fearful faces. (Schore, p. 300, 2003a)

In exploring this site to date, I have not found significant benefit over T4 and other T4 based bipolar protocols. But Schore and these Q findings suggest we more fully explore the potential of training at T6. The argument for T4 and, as we will see, for FPO2, is that they may provide a more geographically direct appeal to the regulation of the amygdala, and therefore provide more quieting of fear. FZ too has a geographical advantage. It sits above the anterior cingulate cortex (ACC), a structure that inhibits the amygdala. In most cases, rewarding FZ at 5–8 Hz or lower has significantly quieted fearfulness with the added benefit of easing the perseveration so typical of those with attachment problems.

It is important to note here that I have not found it necessary to use a QEEG to diagnose or address the symptoms and regulation issues of RAD. In the great majority of cases to date, training has been straightforward: right side, low-frequency reward, with over 150 sessions to be expected. I do recommend a "Q" in those cases where the patient does not stabilize, where you suspect seizure activity or brain injury, or when you see negative and unexpected effects from training. In this, I am not recommending against a QEEG, as many of these patients will have histories of confirmed or presumptive head injury and/or seizure.[3] I am, instead, bowing to the pragmatics of cost and availability of QEEG, and reporting that I have not in my practice found it necessary to effectively treat the high arousal of these patients.

A. Negative effects

Using left hemisphere training is likely to evoke negative training effects in people who meet criteria for attachment disorder. This was brought home to me, early in my career, after several left side beta sessions with a young Aspergers patient. She liked how it made her feel: bold and confident. After several weeks of this training, she reluctantly confessed that she had begun a life of petty crime at her school, stealing both food and money. She had not done this before, and she was not drawn to doing it again—after we changed the training back to the right hemisphere. She recognized the sociopathic element in her and she felt, as I do, that this element was promoted by left hemisphere training.

In looking at training outcomes and phenomena, it is important not to be confounded by diagnosis. Aspergers, like autism and like RAD, is a severe disorder of affect regulation marked by heightened emotional arousal and requires most, if not all, training on the right hemisphere. RAD can be conceptualized as an "emotional autism." I have seen similar effects in attempting to address left hemisphere deficits in the RAD population. When I tried training Sammy on the left side for his speech difficulties, he got sneaky and hurt the cat. A woman with a terrible and unresolved attachment history who had been warming up to her infant son, withdrew from him. I started to call these responses "left hemisphere effects."

This preliminary data led me to think that the left hemisphere of these individuals belonged in jail. Scheming replaces cause-and-effect; coldness replaces warmth. In all of these cases I was rewarding in the beta range, and these effects

---

[3]In personal conversation, Jay Gunkleman estimated 10% of this population will have seizure activity, and Ed Hamlin estimated a number as high as 20%.

may have been driven as much by frequency as by site. There is emerging clinical data that claims we can train the left hemisphere as needed, at much lower frequencies, and not encounter negative reactions. But the caution remains.

I have seen similar problematic outcomes with interhemispheric homologous site protocols, regardless of the reward frequency. Even patients without a presumptive history for RAD have exhibited flatness, coolness, rigidity, anger, and lack of empathy with overuse of these protocols. Unlike those with RAD who would not notice these effects, and wouldn't mind them if they did, many of these patients have recognized them and have subsequently stopped or limited the duration of interhemispheric training. I have found these effects training interhemispherically at all homologous sites from the sensory motor strip to the prefrontal poles. To date, I have not seen them with interhemispheric training posterior to the central strip, but I look for them.

Interhemispheric protocols seem to be particularly helpful in conditions such as migraine. When these conditions occur in those with attachment disorder and they must be addressed, the practitioner is cautioned to pay close attention to the effects that interhemispheric protocols have on the patient's capacity for interpersonal connection, and adjust training duration accordingly. In my experience so far, as little as 3 minutes of interhemispheric training can stabilize the brain against migraine without negatively affecting attachment.

B. Alpha–theta training

In addition to these concerns about left hemisphere and interhemispheric protocols, I want to add a note of caution about the use of alpha–theta training with this population. A case in point is a young woman who spent the first year of her life in a poor and understaffed third world orphanage. She was adopted at age one. She had her first serious emotional breakdown after visiting the orphanage as a young adult. She had had many problems growing up, including many on the symptom list for RAD, and came to me directly from a long-term psychiatric hospitalization. She was diagnosed with ADHD, post-traumatic stress disorder, bipolar illness, learning disability, and alcoholism. Even with this highly presumptive history and symptom formation, she had never been diagnosed with attachment disorder.

She stabilized quickly with eyes-open, right hemisphere training. Within 3 months of training two to three times a week, she was off lithium, out of a day treatment program, back at work part-time, and headed back to college. At about this juncture in the training, which was now integrated into meaningful talk therapy, she said something that could become a neurofeedback koan: "I have never been more myself and never known less who I am." As her right hemisphere organized, her identity was emerging. Without the internalized mother, however, she lacked a mirror, and found herself hard to recognize. Part of my function as her therapist was to become "the mirror," the attuned other, who could reflect her, back to her.

She was doing well when we decided to see if we could deepen her recovery through the introduction of alpha–theta training. She had tried some sessions several months earlier, and reported only that she heard moaning or chanting. This time she had done six sessions over a weekend. At the end of this time, she refused to do neurofeedback in any form. She had always come to her sessions beautifully dressed and well groomed. Her appearance was an important issue for her. After this long weekend, she arrived slightly disheveled. She did not like how she felt, which was difficult for her to describe, and she was angry and withdrawn from me. The struggle to regain our therapeutic alliance lasted weeks.

One day she told me that her dog was sick. Her only ongoing and secure attachment was with her dog; she loved him. This was a crisis. I asked her about his illness, and she told me that she hadn't been feeding him regularly! She also told me that she hadn't had the garbage collected for two months, since that weekend of alpha–theta training. I was struck by the enormity of emotional replay that she was engaged in. It seemed as though alpha–theta training had left her in a place that she knew as an infant. She seemed to be back at the orphanage; a place filled with garbage, where innocent and powerless children went hungry, where no mother cared for her.

Another patient with a history of profound neglect, poverty and trauma initially felt some relief with alpha–theta training, but kept her visualizations tightly controlled and scripted. She was unable to abandon herself to state, out of fear. A young patient who was diagnosed with dissociative identity disorder, and whose mother had suffered the same diagnosis, repeatedly tried alpha–theta training but, each time, pulled the electrodes off within minutes, in a state of indescribable, uninhabitable fear. Although not strictly or solely attachment disordered, both of these women had suffered absolute abandonment as infants. They were, I think, both attempting to shut down access to the unbearable state of "no mother."

It is unlikely that alpha–theta training creates a de novo state. The experience one has is probably one already known to the brain/mind, and recalled in this deep state training. If this speculation proves to be accurate, then we might assume that states of bliss and oneness, often reported by those training in alpha–theta, relate to early blissful fusion experiences between mother and infant. My adult adoptee had had no such experience nor had the two women who were raised in homes that echoed with the psychological absence of their mothers, and with all the chaos that ensues from neglect. They did not, as it were, have this default position. Secure attachment in the first 2 years may then be a critical factor in alpha–theta outcomes.

At the same time, I recognize that many colleagues report successful alpha–theta training with people who have poor attachment histories. These differing outcomes pose an interesting question. Might it be the case that the history and expectation of trainer has both subtle and powerful effects on outcomes? Might it be that the density of "no mother" in the experience of the trainer, coupled with that of the trainee, is powerful enough to overwhelm a positive outcome? Since so much of what we are observing and experiencing in the alpha–theta training seems to be occurring in the realm of subtle energies, this seems a credible hypothesis. This is a topic for further study and speculation elsewhere. For now, these cases should serve as a caution. Alpha–theta training may not be indicated for this population.

C. FPO2 training

LeDoux (1996) agrees with Schore about the importance of the prefrontal cortex in quieting fear. "Humans with prefrontal damage become oblivious to social and emotional cues and some exhibit sociopathic behavior. This area receives inputs from sensory processing systems…and is also intimately connected with the amygdala and the anterior cingulate region" (LeDoux, p. 278, 1996). According to LeDoux, the amygdala has two primary pathways: one thalamic and one cortical.

> Information about external stimuli reaches the amygdala by way of the direct pathways to the thalamus (low road) as well as by the pathways from the thalamus to the cortex to the amygdala. The direct thalamo–amygdala path is a shorter and thus a faster transmission route… However, because the direct pathway bypasses the cortex, it is unable to benefit from cortical processing…This can be very helpful in dangerous situations. However, its utility requires that the cortical pathway be able to override the direct pathway. (LeDoux, p. 164, 1996)

He uses the example of walking along a wilderness path and seeing a snake. The amygdala activates the prefrontal cortex and we flee or freeze, before we have time to process that this snake is in fact a rope left behind by a careless hiker. The correct identification is an example of the cortical override. As we have seen, a well-functioning ROC allows this override function. Without it, our wilderness explorer will continue to react to the rope as if it were a snake. Even when he knows better, it is difficult to communicate the reality to the non-verbal and powerful amygdala. We see this kind of "kindling" as a central to post-traumatic stress disorder, but it is a liability in all fear-based disorders.

In 1998, I began to explore the efficacy of training the prefrontal cortex at the site that I named FPO2. This site is off the 10–20 system and lies in the corner of the right eye, beneath the ridge of the orbital socket, where the eyebrow and the bridge of the nose meet. This is the endpoint of amygdala's projection, and seems to be as close to the amygdala as we can get on the cranium. I began the exploration at 8–11 Hz with a 2–7 inhibit, and presently train at frequencies as low as 3–6 Hz and lower, generally with a 0–6 Hz inhibit. The hope was to exploit the limited afferent pathways to the amygdala, to quiet its reactivity. Clinical anecdotal evidence now abounds that training FPO2 reduces fear, and appears to impact fear memory. When FPO2 training is effective, people no longer believe or act on their post-traumatic impulses.

One colleague told me the following story. Several years before our encounter, he had been badly injured when a drunk driver, traveling in the wrong lane, crashed headlong into his car. He had been so traumatized by this accident that he had avoided taking that route ever since, even though this made his commute considerable longer. Two days after I trained him briefly at FPO2, he was driving home late and saw the headlights of a car coming directly at him on the wrong side of the highway. He swerved, pulled off and avoided the collision. He was amazed both at how calm he had been and that his old fear had not ignited. He had responded to the fear-inducing stimuli appropriately, but the event apparently did not create a post-traumatic kindling of the amygdala, a part of the brain quite prone to this terrible cascade.

A patient of mine, however, did suffer this exact cascade during FPO2 training. She has a history of severe emotional, physical, and sexual assault as a child in the context of profound parental absence. By the age of 30 she had suffered a stroke and had seizure and migraine, as well as severe PTSD. Within 3 minutes of FPO2 training she felt twitching in her face, a symptom that signaled the onset of seizure, and she was alarmed. We stopped the training and she did not go into seizure. Instead, over the next 2 weeks she regained memory of 9 years of her childhood that had not been available to her before that FPO2 training. We had, it appeared tapped directly into fear-based memory. Needless to say, our therapy was then turned to processing and integrating these memories.

This was a challenging epoch for her and I recently asked her, a year or so after this episode, whether she would ever train at FPO2 again. She said, "Oh, definitely. It was very rough, but it gave me a large part of my life back." The scope of this chapter allows only a brief discussion of the role of the therapist, but this case study suggests how important therapeutic competence is when working at this level with neurofeedback. Neurofeedback practitioners must be present for what comes up, must recognize what they see, and then be able to work it through, interpersonally and therapeutically.

We don't always trigger fear memory. In fact, in my experience to date, we usually do not. After training at FPO2, my young Aspergers patient reported her first "experience of moral compunction." She read her stepfather's face in response to her threatening behavior and felt, for the first time, that she "just could not do that to him." FPO2 training softened the response of an RAD mother to her toddler, and he responded quickly and warmly to her new presence.

Perhaps the most profound case is that of a mother in her thirties with a history of incest, neglect, and physical abuse who became pregnant with her third child after the onset of training. Although she was a devoted mother who had already addressed a lot of her past in psychotherapy, her two older children suffered the effects of her history and their father's with disregulation of their own. She had suffered severe post-partum depressions after both births. When fetal movement began in this pregnancy, she described the baby as "almost aggressive," kicking her hard, doing somersaults, rarely quiet and then for only short periods. Such activity in pregnancy can be predictive of rapid cycling bipolar disorder in children (Papolos and Papolos, 2000).

I introduced FPO2 as a regular part of the mother's training during the fifth month. During the training, she reported that the fetal movement quieted significantly, something it had not done at T4 earlier in the session. Over the next month, with FPO2, fetal movement became graceful and fluid. The mother reported that there was no more aggressive kicking, and no more somersaulting. She felt bonded to the baby in utero in a way that she had never known was possible. After birth, her baby demonstrated remarkable levels of self-regulation. She didn't fuss, she slept well, she was weaned easily from the breast, she didn't use pacifiers or suck her fingers, and she rarely needed soothing. Her mother suffered no post-partum depression. The baby remains friendly and happy as her baseline mood, and she attracts people to her.

I can only begin to speculate on the method of action. It might be as straight-forward as quieting the mother's fear, and her high stress level quieted the baby. It is clear that the effect on fetal movement was specific to FPO2. It seems fair to assume some correlation between this level of fetal activity and hyper-arousal in the prenatal infant. It is the case that the amygdala comes on line in the fetal brain at 5 months in utero, the same time that fetal movement begins. Although we were training the mother to quiet her amygdala activity, perhaps this directly signaled the baby's to quiet as well. It was a clear and undeniable in-session effect that deepened over the course of training in the next 4 months.

We will only be able to know the effects of the training on this mother and baby as the child grows up. Even if the benefits were unequivocal, such a case would clearly have to be replicated and validated before we can know if there is widespread application of FPO2 in helping mothers to bond to their babies, and for the babies to achieve such levels of self-regulation. This I have to leave for the researchers.

Given the present levels of insecure attachment in the US, this is vital research. But maternal infant bonding is not only a priority in the US; it is or should be a priority worldwide. Neglected, abandoned and orphaned children are at great risk of attachment disorder, and the subsequent development of sociopathic personality. There are 35 million AIDS orphans alone. What does this portend for our common welfare?

IX. THE ROLE OF THE THERAPIST

The scope of this chapter does not permit a full discussion of the role of the therapist who uses neurofeedback. This topic stirs controversy in the field ,and requires a chapter of its own to adequately begin to explore the implications for the therapy and for the therapist once neurofeedback is introduced. But in brief, this chapter postulates that neurofeedback enables affect regulation, thereby enhancing the patient's capacity for attachment. Neurofeedback, however, cannot provide the patient with someone to attach to. This is the role of the therapist: new attachment object, interpreter, and guide, someone who can accurately discern the effects of training and teach the patient to do the same, ultimately becoming a companion on the brain/mind journey. (For attachment disordered children, this is primarily the job of the parents.)

For patients who have suffered unrepaired attachment disruption, neurofeedback does not obviate the need for psychotherapy; it makes psychotherapy possible. The attuned presence of the therapist is needed as much if not more than it ever has been. The therapist's primary role, however, has changed. He or she is no longer the patient's primary affect regulation system. There is a new clinical challenge. Now the therapist needs to discern and understand the changes in state, trait, and even identity that are likely to occur and, as mentioned earlier, to mirror and validate these changes as they happen.

A brief case study will illustrate this new therapeutic challenge. My Aspergers patient was struggling with feelings she was having about her brother's situation at school. After listening for a while, I told her that those feelings were empathy. She smiled, relieved and said, "So, that's what empathy feels like. Now I know." There are pragmatic implications as well. Because I believe that neurofeedback is about creating the capacity for attachment, I am always in the room with my patient, and I set my system up so that I can look at them, as well as at the screen, while they are training. In addition my sessions are often longer than an hour and, as needed, I will talk with patients during training.

X. CONCLUSION

Neurofeedback cannot by itself address the problem of attachment disorder, but attachment disorder is nearly impossible to treat without it. Neurofeedback offers hope to children and adults who have suffered the devastating personal circumstances that lead to this disorder, something as subtle as maternal depression, or as horrifying as the parental neglect and abuse that Sammy endured. Neurofeedback optimizes right hemisphere frequency properties that permit the regulation of affect and, as Bowlby highlights, most importantly allows the unattached to become "sympathetic [empathic] and to help others in distress." When fear, the affect of attachment disorder, is reduced, the self and the other emerge in empathic engagement with one another.

Optimally, neurofeedback will be used within the holding environment of an attuned therapist or, in the case of a child, an attuned parent. (Neurofeedback can also help the parent and the therapist achieve this attunement). We are hard wired to relate to each other, and to seek out others who enhance our sense of connection and well-being. Therapeutic settings, unfortunately, are not readily available in most of the world, but the entire world needs its citizens to be securely attached. I would argue that right hemisphere training could go a long way toward achieving that goal even when used in institutional settings. It would be far better than nothing at all.

In summary, good enough attachment underwrites brain development that in turn gives rise to affect regulation. To the extent that affect regulation fails, the human being fails. Because the attachment disordered lack the capacity for empathy, trust and love, they cannot establish healthy peer relationships or marriages, and cannot raise secure children. My experience training those with attachment disorders suggests an ontological approach to neurofeedback. As in the developing brain, and in the optimal first relationship between mother and infant, the first order of business should be affect regulation and the enhancement of attachment.

Attachment disorder may be the worst human tragedy. It degrades or destroys the elemental humanity of its victim, and propagates disaster in every realm it touches—the family, the school, the group, the institution, and the society. Neurofeedback addresses attachment disorder. It makes interpersonal therapies possible, which in turn allow other secure relationships to develop.

Neurofeedback is a relational technology. When used properly, brain wave training effectively quiets fear and reactivity, the greatest barriers to the ability to love. The first goal of our work as neurofeedback practitioners should be to secure and deepen human attachment. This is the ethical imperative of our field.

REFERENCES

Ainsworth, M. D. S., Blehar, M. C., Waters, E. and Wall, S. (1978). *Patterns of Attachment: A Psychological Study of the Strange Situation*. Hillsdale, NJ: Erlbaum.

Bowlby, J. (1988). *A Secure Base*. New York: Basic Books.

Joseph, R. (1996). *Neuropsychiatry, Neuropsychology, and Clinical Neuroscience*, 2nd edition. Baltimore: Williams and Wilkins.

Karen, R. (1994). *Becoming Attached*. New York: Warner Books.

LeDoux, J. (1996). *The Emotional Brain*. New York: Touchstone.

Linehan, M. (1993). *Cognitive Behavior Therapy for Borderline Personality Disorder*. New York: Guilford.

Main, M. and Solomon, J. (1986). *Discovery of an insecure-disorganized/disoriented attachment pattern*. In *Affective Development in Infancy* (T. B. Brazelton and M. W. Yogman, eds). Norwood N. J.: Ablex Publishing.

Papolos, D. and Papolos, J. (2000). *The Bipolar Child*. New York: Broadway Books.

Schore, A. (1994). *Affect Regulation and the Origin of the Self*. New Jersey: Erlbaum.

Schore, A. (2003a). *Affect Dysregulation and Disorders of the Self*. New York: Norton.

Schore, A. (2003b). *Affect Regulation and the Repair of the Self*. New York: Norton.

Siegel, D. (1999). *The Developing Mind*. New York: Guilford.

Solomon, J. and George, C. (1999). *Disorganized Attachment*. New York: Guilford.

Sroufe, L. A. (1995). *Emotional Development: The Organization of Emotional Life in the Early Years*. New York: Cambridge University Press.

Stern, D. N. (1985). *The Interpersonal World of the Infant*. New York: Basic Books.

CHAPTER 14

QEEG and neurofeedback for assessment and effective intervention with attention deficit hyperactivity disorder (ADHD)

Lynda Thompson, Ph.D. and Michael Thompson, M.D.

ADD Centre and Biofeedback Institute of Toronto, Mississauga, Ontario, Canada

I. INTRODUCTION

As a scientist who has worked for many years in the field of neurofeedback and who has published numerous papers on this topic in respected scientific journals, I am convinced that this method is as effective as any, and far more benign than most, in achieving improved functional regulation in the human brain.

M. Barry Sterman

Sterman's words, taken from the introduction he wrote for *The A.D.D. Book: New Understandings, New Approaches to Parenting Your Child* (Sears and Thompson, 1998) sum up the content of this chapter. It provides an overview of how individuals with attention deficit hyperactivity disorder (ADHD) can learn better regulation of their brain function. After reviewing briefly the current status and history of the diagnosis, there are guidelines to help practitioners develop effective neurofeedback (NFB) interventions for people with this disorder. Using quantitative electroencephalography (QEEG) for assessment, then combining that assessment data with knowledge about the client's symptoms and how they correspond to known functional neuroanatomical areas of the brain, the NFB provider can customize an intervention that can directly improve brain function in a way that is harm-free and lasting.

Note that the emphasis here is on approaches that have published research behind them. NFB came out of research labs, and is based on learning theory and on neurophysiology. It is important to honor that tradition and collect data to track learning curves within and across sessions, and to also collect outcome data, whether the practitioner is working in clinical or research settings. Joel and Judy Lubar, whose theta–beta training model for intervention with ADHD is the accepted standard in the field, are exemplars of successful clinician scientists. They combine a rigorous scientific approach with exquisite therapeutic skills while remaining open to innovation. Joel published the first paper about using NFB in the treatment of a hyperactive child more than 30 years ago (Lubar and Shouse, 1976). He is still extending the field through teaching other professionals, through the work of those who have been his graduate students at the University of Tennessee, and through the development of newer approaches, such as his current interest in LORETA-based NFB.

While this chapter deals primarily with NFB, the reader must keep in mind that interventions for ADHD should utilize a multi-modal approach, and be individualized according to each client's profile and needs. Training the brain will not readily transfer to better classroom performance if the teenager stays up till 2 A.M. playing video games, sleeps in, skips breakfast, and arrives late to class with homework incomplete. Common sense dictates that approaches that encourage sensible diet, good sleep hygiene, and regular exercise will enhance neurofeedback results. That is why *The A.D.D. Book* (Sears and Thompson, 1998) contains advice on all those matters in addition to sections on diagnosis, behavior management, medications, ways to promote learning, and the legal entitlements of children with the diagnosis of ADHD. A chapter on neurofeedback is tucked in there, too, which helps parents recognize that it should be considered one of the options for helping their child.

Combining NFB with concurrent coaching in learning strategies appears to be helpful for clients with ADHD (Thompson and Thompson, 1998). Thus a whole chapter in *The Neurofeedback Book* (Thompson and Thompson, 2003) is devoted to metacognition, which involves awareness of how one learns and remembers things so that one can consciously apply strategies to guide performance. Though no specific research has been conducted about the additional benefit of devoting some of each NFB training session to learning strategies, it has been part of the Lubars' methods from the beginning. We concur with their view that it helps with the acquisition and generalization of the skill of paying attention while doing schoolwork if some of the training is done while the client is maintaining their focus (as indicated by auditory feedback contingent upon reduced theta and increased beta) while concurrently doing reading, writing or math tasks.

Increasingly, the synergistic effect of combining NFB and regular biofeedback (BFB) is being utilized (Thompson and Thompson, 2007). The central nervous system that we are influencing with NFB has numerous and complex interconnections both within the brain and with other systems in the body. In particular, areas of the mid-brain and the brain stem connect with structures and functions influenced by the sympathetic nervous system and the various branches of the vagus, the well-named "wandering nerve," as discussed by Stephen Porges in publications about his polyvagal theory (Porges, 2003, 2004).

Oscillatory phenomenon, like respiration and heart rate variability, are of particular relevance when the goal is to achieve calmer functioning, as is the case with those who are hyperactive and impulsive, or in those who have co-morbidity with anxiety. The importance of heart rate variability training is evident, with the Spring 2008 edition of the magazine *Biofeedback* (Volume 36, Number 1) dedicated to this topic. A fuller discussion of these factors, and of how to combine NFB and BFB, is found in Chapter 15 of this book. Here, it suffices to say at the outset that the bigger mind–body picture needs to be kept in mind even though this chapter focuses on cortical functions as reflected in EEG activity.

II. BACKGROUND TO ADHD

A. Etiologies

Multiple causes can produce the symptoms of ADHD but there is no question about heredity playing the largest role in this neurologically-based disorder. Barkley's review of numerous twin studies found the genetic contribution ranged from 50–95%, and averaged 80% or higher. He notes that this makes ADHD about as heritable as height. Environment can play a role in how the symptoms are expressed, but child-rearing styles do not produce ADHD. Toxic exposure increases the risk of a child developing ADHD, including maternal smoking or alcohol use, increased lead levels in infant and toddler years, and, in some vulnerable individuals, streptococcal infections. With strep infections an immune response of antibodies may sometimes destroy cells in the basal ganglia (reviewed by Barkley, 2006).

Diet can play a role in some children but is not a factor for most of them. Food dyes and additives are most often the culprit, not sugar. Observations concerning adverse behavior after ingesting sugar are likely due to reactions to the other ingredients in the sweet treats consumed by children. Consumption of high fructose corn syrup has sky-rocketed in the American diet as it gets added to so many processed foods, and corn is one of the top seven foods that produce allergic reactions. An elimination diet can be helpful in some cases of ADHD in establishing food–mood connections, and it makes sense to have children take a multivitamin, mineral, and an omega-3 essential fatty acid supplement, such as fish oil (Sears and Thompson, 1998).

Lifestyle factors (TV viewing and computer games) are not the source of ADHD but can exacerbate the symptoms, especially since the hyper-focus characteristic of those with ADHD (found in both the "inattentive" and the "combined" sub-types) is often displayed by being "glued to the screen." Violent themes have been shown to increase aggression in children so excessive exposure could contribute to co-morbidity with oppositional defiant disorder and conduct disorder.

B. Prevalence

Currently, the most frequent pediatric application of NFB (also known as *EEG biofeedback*) is for ADHD (Gruzelier and Egner, 2005). It is also the condition for which there is the most published research relating to NFB, as can be readily seen by scanning the bibliography maintained by psychologist Cory Hammond on the web site of the International Society for Neurofeedback and Research (www.isnr.org). In early 2008 there were 84 citations under the heading ADD/ADHD, Learning and Development Disabilities, and Academic Cognitive Enhancement. This burgeoning amount of research is not surprising given that ADHD, the most prevalent diagnosis treated by child psychiatrists, currently represents the biggest market for NFB services.

Prevalence rates are high for ADHD—7.4% of school-aged children were considered to have this disorder in studies using DSM-IV criteria in the United States and Australia. Use of that 1994 version of the *Diagnostic and Statistical Manual* of the American Psychiatric Association (American Psychiatric Association, 1994) yields higher prevalence rates than were found in earlier studies using DSM-III or DSM-III-R, as is thoroughly reviewed by Russell Barkley (2006). Whether this is due to changing criteria, greater awareness of the condition among physicians and the public, a true increase in incidence, or some combination of these factors is unclear.

Usually male to female ratios are about 3:1 in children. Using parental reports of symptoms rather than a doctor's diagnosis, prevalence rates are even higher; for example, a telephone survey covering 3,082 children for the National Health and Nutrition Examination Survey found 9% of the children age 8–15 qualified for a diagnosis of ADHD with 11.8 % of the boys and 5.4% of the girls meeting the criteria. (This would extrapolate to 2.4 million children in the USA, not counting children age 7 and younger, or teens above age 15.) Parents were asked about symptoms between 2001 and 2004. With respect to medical management, 39% were on medications for ADHD at the time of the survey, and 48% had received treatment in the last year. The poorest children had the highest rates of symptoms but were the least likely to be treated with medications. In 2000, 3% of the school-aged population in the USA was taking prescribed stimulant medication (American Academy of Pediatrics, 2000).

Rates in adults are also high (about 5%), and it is estimated that 66% of people diagnosed in childhood will continue to have the traits and a degree of impairment in adulthood (Barkley, 2006; Wender, 1995). This disorder has a high media profile, in part due to the publication of popular books on the subject, like Edward Hallowell and John Ratey's *Driven to Distraction* (Hallowell and Ratey, 1994). They are both Harvard trained physicians who, after becoming psychiatrists, realized they themselves had ADHD. Their book increased awareness and reduced the stigma of adult ADHD when it appeared in 1994. Thom Hartmann's books have also been a boon, starting with *Hunters in a Farmer's World*, as they highlight the positive aspects of creativity, high energy, and tenacity found in those with ADHD.

An ADHD industry has evolved encompassing books, magazines, videos, medications, dietary supplements, local and national organizations, ADHD coaches, and neurofeedback practitioners. Increased awareness is in part due to the education of physicians and the general public by drug companies, especially since direct to consumer advertising of drugs was legalized. With fewer than 10% of adults with ADHD being actively treated for their disorder, it was estimated in 2003 that the $2-billion-a-year market for drug treatments for ADHD could double if affected adults sought treatment (*Business Week*, 2003).

There is increasing concern within the British Medical Association, (Magnus, 2008), about the use of stimulants by people without ADHD who want to increase alertness, such as truckers, athletes, poker players, and students. The BMA's medical ethics committee is looking at the question of the use of stimulants for performance enhancement. The article by Magnus mentions that more than 16% of students on some campuses are using methylphenidate (Ritalin) without a prescription, according to the *Journal of American College Health*. The United States consumes 90% of all methylphenidate produced, with Britain ranking second, and Canada third. This is not surprising given that response to a stimulant is very similar whether one has ADHD or not.

The non-specificity of stimulant effects was first established in NIMH studies by Rapaport and his colleages (Rapaport *et al.*, 1978, 1980) with the first study dealing with children, and the second reporting on adults who received dextroamphetamine. A study with Ritalin was done more recently (Spencer *et al.*, 1995), and it too indicated that adults with and without ADHD respond in the same manner. These studies are reviewed in the final chapter of a detailed book that presents the state of knowledge at the turn of the century concerning ADHD and medications, (Solanto, Arnsten, & Castellanos, 2001). This text also has, as an appendix, a reprint of Charles Bradley's classic 1937 paper describing the first use of stimulants in behavior-disordered children.

C. Interventions

Ritalin (trade name for methylphenidate) has been used in the treatment of ADHD since 1955, and is considered a safe drug, though it does have frequent side effects, particularly appetite suppression (14%), abdominal pain (11%), insomnia (8%), and headache (13%). (Rates are from pooled data of four clinical trials reviewed by Connor [2006].) Ritalin is no longer under patent, and a number of new delivery systems for methylphenidate have been brought to market with an emphasis on slow release products that allow once a day dosing, such as Concerta and Biphentin (available in Canada). Adderall, a mixture of amphetamine salts, has even higher rates of the symptoms of anorexia (22%) and insomnia (17%).

Amphetamines are stronger than methylphenidate in terms of mg/Kg effects and, in children who respond to both, the Ritalin dose is typically twice as high to have equal efficacy.

Sudden death occurred in 12 children and adolescents taking Adderall XR between 1999 and 2003, which prompted Canadian authorities to take it off the market. It was allowed back on the market after about 8 months, with the proviso that its "black box" warning include the caution that it not be used in children with cardiac defects because all stimulants increase heart rate and blood pressure. The manufacturer successfully argued that, although the risk of sudden death existed with Adderall, it was no greater than the risk with other stimulants. Deaths with prescribed Ritalin have mainly been associated with the concomitant use of Clonidine, which reduces blood pressure as a side effect, especially if one of the medications was abruptly withdrawn.

With respect to non-stimulants, Canadian authorities took Cylert (pemoline) off the market after the death of a teenager from liver failure. In the USA the manufacturer just stopped producing the medication without the FDA taking any official action. As there is concern about the use of stimulants, drug companies are responding by bringing new non-stimulants to market for the treatment of ADHD, such as Strattera (atomoxetine). But none of the drugs are without side effects. About 25% of children and 50% of adults are non-responders when a stimulant is prescribed and, even when drugs do work, the effect is lost as soon as the drug wears off (Bradley, 1937; Wender, 1995).

A large review of the literature was done in the early 1990s concerning the effects of stimulants on children with ADHD. By that time there were over 2,000 research publications on the topic so James Swanson at the University of California, Irvine, who coordinated the review, decided to make the task manageable by just reviewing review articles. There was research support for stimulant medication being effective for the short-term management of behavior. Evidence is still scant for broader gains, such as in academic ability (Swanson et al., 1993; Connor, 2006). Neurofeedback, on the other hand, is associated with behavioral, cognitive, and academic gains (Lubar and Lubar, 1984; Lubar, 1991, 1997; Lubar et al., 1995; Linden et al., 1996; Thompson and Thompson, 1998) and the results appear to last (Lubar, 1995).

The largest study to date of interventions for ADHD which did not include a NFB group, and which did not follow up on drug-treated children after medication was discontinued, concluded that medication was the most effective intervention. Combining drugs with behavior modification improved the percent of cases with successful treatment, but not to a statistically significant degree. Behavior modification alone was effective to a degree, but the limitation of that approach is that it does not generalize. Behavior only improves in settings where the contingencies are in place (Barkley, 2006).

This book by Barkley is the definitive review of all the research on ADHD, and it updated the literature review to cover the nearly 1,000 papers that had appeared on ADHD since the second edition done in 1998. Yet NFB receives not a single entry in the subject index in this otherwise very thorough book. There is brief mention of QEEG as an aid in diagnosis, which concludes that it is "showing some promise in accurately distinguishing children with ADHD from nondisabled children." Barkley views ADHD as a disability with no redeeming features, and he rejects the idea that it is associated with creativity. His books and research deal only with the "combined type" of ADHD, not the "inattentive type", and he sees a lot of children who have ADHD plus co-morbidity with oppositional defiant disorder (ODD) or conduct disorder (CD), which may contribute to this more negative view.

NFB practitioners, on the other hand, usually are working with motivated families willing to invest time and money in their child's improvement, which typically is associated with less ODD and CD. The most common co-morbidity seen at our ADD Centre is with learning disabilities in children, and with anxiety and/or depression in adults. Though people with ADHD are never easy to work with, neurofeedback practitioners may have a slightly easier time in terms of client characteristics than do child psychiatrists. NFB must always be carefully, indeed painstakingly, done but the observation that NFB response rates can be higher than medication response may be due to less co-morbidity. Lubar mentions 70–90% positive outcomes (Lubar and Lubar, 2001). Medication response rates are typically 70–75% to a single drug, and patient physicians with patient patients can get drug response rates up higher if they try different drugs, such as alternate stimulants, anti-depressants, and anti-seizure medications.

It is perhaps natural that long-term researchers like Russell Barkley and Keith Conners, who have had much of their work funded by drug companies and thus are steeped in double-blind, placebo-controlled studies as the gold standard, do not embrace NFB, which they regard as "scientifically unproven." More important for the growth of the field, however, is the observation that non-medication approaches have high appeal with parents. In a study done in southern Germany (Fuchs *et al.*, 2003), for example, parents could choose between methylphenidate and NFB as treatments, and 22 out of 34 selected to have their children in the NFB group. The study thus had the weakness of lack of randomization, but respecting parental choice is also part of ethical practice, and must be considered when doing research in clinical settings. NFB can, of course, be combined with medication.

Since stimulant medication has been shown to be the most effective intervention for ADHD, then NFB should logically be considered the most promising non-medication approach because there are a number of studies that show efficacy of NFB to be equal to that of methylphenidate in terms of reduction of ADHD symptoms (Fuchs *et al.*, 2003; Monastra *et al.*, 2002; Rossiter, 2004; Rossiter and LaVaque, 1995). Unlike stimulant medications, whose effects last only as long as the child has the drug in their system (Bradley, 1937; Swanson *et al.*, 1993), NFB has the added advantage that the results do not disappear when training stops

(Lubar, 1995; Monastra *et al.*, 2002). Additionally, stimulants are effective only for the short-term management of behavior (Swanson *et al.*, 1993; AMA, 1998) whereas NFB has been shown to be associated not only with decreased symptoms but also to be associated with better performance on academic and intellectual functioning measures (Linden *et al.*, 1996; Lubar *et al.*, 1995; Thompson and Thompson, 1998).

Those doing NFB need not be anti-medication since clearly medication is helpful, especially in very hyperactive children. It is easier to do quality feedback in a child who can sit still. Using pills while training skills makes sense for some children. Most often the child can be weaned to a lower dose or completely off the drug with enough training.

III. DIAGNOSIS OF ADHD

A. DSM-IV criteria

ADHD is a neurological disorder yet it has traditionally been diagnosed on behavioral criteria. The DSM-IV criteria are well known and available elsewhere Barkley (2006); Sears and Thompson (1998). DSM-IV-Text Revision lists symptoms in three areas: inattention, hyperactivity, and impulsivity. The symptoms must be present (six out of nine symptoms of inattention and/or six out of nine hyperactive–impulsive symptoms) "to a degree that is maladaptive and inconsistent with developmental level." Symptoms must occur across two areas (such as home and school), must cause significant impairment in functioning, be present before the age of seven, and not be due to any other diagnosis, such as pervasive developmental disorder.

There are three sub-types: 314.00 ADHD, inattentive type; 314.01 ADHD, hyperactive-impulsive type; and 314.01 ADHD, combined type. Medications work best for the combined type, and that group receives most of the research. The hyperactive–impulsive type is rarely diagnosed since most children who are hyperactive and impulsive are also inattentive so they meet the criteria for combined type. NFB is effective for both inattentive and combined type (deBeus, Ball, *et al.*, 2006).

DSM criteria are largely developed by and for researchers. Prior to 1994 the categories were attention deficit disorder, either with hyperactivity or without hyperactivity. Those terms make more sense to parents. In particular, parents of daydreamers (ADHD, inattention) never understand why "hyperactivity" appears in their child's diagnosis. Today one often finds the designations ADD (for ADHD, inattentive type) and ADHD (for ADHD, combined type) used. Historically the terms *hyperkinetic disorder of childhood* and *minimal brain dysfunction* were used.

DSM-IV guidelines make diagnostic criteria clear but one still has to be vigilant about other conditions that can mimic the symptoms. These include medical problems such as thyroid disease, allergies/food sensitivities, nutritional problems, chronic ear infections, and sleep apnea. There is also the large issue of co-morbidities, and whole books have been written on that topic (Brown, 2000). The most common co-morbidity in children is learning disabilities. If oppositional defiant disorder is present it increases the chance that conduct disorder will develop, and that leads to a poor prognosis for outcome. Other neurological problems that have overlap with ADHD symptoms include Tourette's syndrome, Asperger's disorder, Bipolar disorder, post-traumatic stress disorder, obsessive-compulsive disorder, generalized anxiety disorder, and personality disorders.

B. EEG patterns

The most common pattern found in ADHD is excess slow wave activity in the frontal regions. That finding parallels documentation of less activation using imaging techniques, including positron emission tomography (PET) that reflects metabolism, single photon emission computed tomography (SPECT) that reflects perfusion (blood flow), and functional magnetic resonance imaging (fMRI). Another way of assessing brain activation—event-related potentials (ERPs)—also indicates differences in ADHD, especially lower amplitude and delayed P300 responses (Kropotov et al., 2007).

There are numerous ways of looking at sub-types of ADHD based on EEG patterns. Excess theta activity is the most common type, as reflected in theta–beta ratios using single channel QEEG that have 98% specificity and 86% sensitivity (Monastra et al., 1999, 2001). There can also be excess alpha activity, usually in the lower alpha range (8–10 Hz), and Lubar mentions excess 'thalpha' (6–10 Hz) being seen in older clients (adolescents and adults). Another pattern, identified by Clarke, is excess beta. Clarke and his colleagues in Australia have published a great deal on this subject (Clarke et al., 2001). They use a very broad frequency range for beta (above 12 Hz and going up to about 25 Hz), which makes it harder to determine what mental state the excess beta group represents. It may be consistent with our own observations of spindling beta occurring in narrow frequency ranges above 20 Hz (the range specific to each person), which we named "busy-brain" (Thompson and Thompson, 2006).

IV. NEUROFEEDBACK FOR ADHD

A. History

The practice of neurofeedback for ADHD has three main streams of influence that have joined to form a larger river that meanders but has one main direction. The first of the streams was the work of Joe Kamiya, who learned about EEG from William Dement, the sleep researcher who started the first sleep clinics in America. Kamiya started research concerning alpha frequencies (8–12 Hz) at the University of Chicago in the 1950s, and established that subjects could tell when they were producing alpha. The work was not published till the 1960s, and by that time he was in California and continuing research that included the relationship between alpha and relaxation and, more generally, the exploration of consciousness (Kamiya, 1979).

Kamiya's influence is still apparent, and he continues to remind our field of our link with the origins of psychology in the late 1800s when it was closer to philosophy and there was an emphasis not only on the measurement of phenomenon but also on personal introspection. When we encourage a client to figure out what mental activity is associated with increasing particular frequencies, such as ruminating being found in conjunction with "busy-brain" beta frequencies above 20 Hz, we are utilizing things learned from that early work.

The next stream was a torrent of research from the labs of M. Barry Sterman. Now professor emeritus at UCLA, and still very active in clinical work and innovative in QEEG analysis with his SKIL database, he was primarily a sleep researcher doing animal studies involving EEG in the 1960s when he noticed, while training cats, that there was a momentary stillness before the "performance" of a bar press for food. During those alert yet still periods there were bursts of spindle-shaped, synchronous EEG activity occurring across the sensory and motor areas of the cortex. This could be seen clearly with recordings from implanted electrodes. He labeled this very specific rhythmic pattern *sensorimotor rhythm* or *SMR*, and its peak frequency was at 14 Hz. (The range used today is usually 13–15 Hz in adults, and 12–15 Hz in children since frequency ranges move a little higher with age.)

It was a specific brain wave signature associated with being motorically motionless and mentally vigilant, ready to perform. He established that these spindle-like bursts of activity originated in the thalamus and projected to the areas of the cortex located across the sensorimotor strip, and he showed that the cats could learn to voluntarily increase that activity if given a food reward contingent upon its production. Sterman and one of his graduate students were the first to publish on operant of conditioning of brain wave activity (Wyrwicka and Sterman, 1968). These findings led to further research that established that increasing SMR activity correlated with a decrease in the frequency, duration, and severity of seizures that have a motor component.

His research group subsequently moved from pure animal research to include work with humans, teaching individuals with epilepsy how to use the SMR to control seizures. Sterman later used the same EEG measurement techniques to assess mental functioning, in particular the ability to pay attention, in air force personnel, including top-gun pilots. Sterman's work is the bedrock of the practice of neurofeedback because it emphasizes the application of learning theory, and the importance of tracking data. He also foreshadowed the range of applications

of NFB by studying EEG in both serious medical disorders and optimal performers. The first lecture he gave in Canada, in Banff in 1993 at a meeting of the
Northwestern Biofeedback Society, was entitled "From tonic-clonic to Top Gun."

The third stream, and the one most directly linked to NFB for ADHD, came
from the hills of Tennessee where Joel Lubar, already a full professor at the
University of Tennessee at age 28, got a prestigious grant to study in Sterman's
labs for a few months, and then built on the observation that epileptics treated
with NFB not only showed reduced seizure activity but also became less restless
and hyperactive. He did careful studies concerning NFB for epilepsy (including
one with an ABA design that established the specific effects of uptraining versus
downtraining SMR), and pioneered using SMR and other EEG states to teach
individuals with ADHD how to achieve behavioural stillness and improve attentional states.

He was the first to publish on the successful training of a hyperactive child
(Shouse and Lubar, 1976), and he and his wife, Judith Lubar, have published
and taught extensively about neurofeedback since that time. For an overview of
Lubar's work concerning ADHD, see Lubar (2003) and his now classic Lubar
(1991).

The river that is now meandering has some currents and eddies that are not
mainstream, such as doing bipolar training across the hemispheres. These may
prove to be very helpful approaches but are not discussed in this chapter due to
lack of published outcome data. For a readable journalist's review of the field, see
Jim Robbins' *A Symphony in the Brain* (1998). It was carefully researched, and a
new edition is soon to be published. The important thing to remember from the
history is that EEG biofeedback is a discipline that has its origins in research labs,
and it is still firmly planted in applied neuroscience, not belief systems.

V.   SCIENTIFIC BASIS OF USING NFB

A.   Theta/SMR and theta/beta approaches

While recognizing that there exists a range of approaches to providing NFB services, this chapter presents only approaches for which there is published research.
Thus approaches based on the pioneering work done by Joel Lubar, who first
published on the successful treatment of a hyperkinetic child in 1976, are advocated. Decreasing theta and increasing faster activity, SMR or beta, while also
inhibiting higher frequencies most influenced by muscle artifact, is central to
Lubar's training methods. Other important components include doing part of the
training sessions on task (for example, while reading or listening), and tracking
learning curves both within and across sessions.

There will also be mention of successful, research-supported interventions
based on training slow cortical potentials, as done by Nils Birbaumer, Ute Strehl

and their colleagues at the University of Tuebingen in southern Germany (Leins et al., 2007). An excellent recent study compared outcomes with SCP training and theta/beta neurofeedback. Although SCP work is much fussier to do, as evidenced by the fact that the head psychologist in the group did that training with the children whereas the NFB group's training was done by graduate students, both groups had successful outcomes, and they did not differ statistically. This is a pleasing finding since NFB is easier to do. A third approach to treating ADHD that has shown measured results is that used by Juri Kropotov and his group in St. Petersburg, Russia (Kropotov et al., 2007). Their training stresses beta enhancement without theta suppression. Perhaps the most impressive new entry into the research field is the husband and wife team of Mario Beauregard and Johanne Levesque at the Université de Montreal, who have used fMRI as the outcome measure to establish changes in brain function after NFB training for ADHD.

The objective of NFB training is that the client gain self-regulation skills with respect to their brain function; for example, being able to recognize different cognitive states, such as daydreaming or focused attention. More importantly, as they do sufficient training, clients should be able to produce the mental state appropriate for the task at hand. At our ADD Centre we do progress testing at no charge after 40 sessions have been completed, usually on a twice a week schedule. If it is determined that further training is needed (progress is being made but goals are not yet reached on some measures), sessions are typically tapered to once a week.

Lubar is still advocating the careful theta–beta work at central locations that he pioneered in the mid-seventies; this reportedly produces consistently good results in 70–90% of cases (Lubar and Lubar, 1999). The higher rates are achieved when there is appropriate patient selection, and enough sessions are done to learn the task, which is to shift EEG activation towards a normal, age appropriate pattern. Exclusion criteria mentioned by the Lubars include family dysfunction (unless therapy is done concomitantly), young age (longer attention span is not yet expected), lower intelligence, primary diagnosis of depression (not just reactive to the problems of having ADHD), and non-prescription drug use.

With respect to intelligence, Tanju Surmeli in Istanbul has done work with lower functioning children, including some with Down's syndrome, and has reported on increased IQ scores as well as improved attention (Surmeli, 2007). Of 17 subjects in a series of 8- to 15-year-olds with severe learning problems, 13 had below normal IQ scores. NFB training was done with the Lexicor Biolex software, and was based on QEEG assessment data analyzed using E. Roy John's NXLink normative database. Retesting on the WISC-R after 6 months showed significant improvement in all 17 children, and post-test scores on the TOVA were significantly improved in nine children (Surmeli and Ertem, 2007).

There is both a conscious component to the learning, dependent on a degree of introspection, and unconscious learning that takes place during neurofeedback training. The unconscious learning is associated with changes in brain activation; for example, Sterman documented increases in sleep spindle density at night, and smoother transitions during sleep stages when daytime training for increased SMR was done. Unlike general biofeedback where changes are not maintained unless there is ongoing practice, changes with NFB training do appear to last.

Joel Lubar, who has done so much of the ground-breaking work concerning NFB for ADHD, has reported on a retrospective study with 52 students who received training when they were in elementary school, and were then followed for up to 10 years. He found that, in those who showed the desired changes in EEG patterns, gains were maintained into the college years, particularly with respect to school performance, completion of tasks, and better peer and family relationships (Lubar, 1995). He stresses that it is important to see EEG changes that indicate that learning has taken place. When they did a study using 19-lead QEEG before and after training with 17 subjects, the 11 subjects who showed that they had learned the task by exhibiting a greater than 30% reduction in their theta–beta ratios showed changes in their brain maps, whereas the six subjects without significant reductions did not (Lubar *et al.*, 1995).

B. Assessment

The EEG assessment is done in the context of a broader evaluation that includes history taking, current symptoms, medical information, discussion of diet, sleep and exercise, and goals of training. There will also likely be a continuous performance test, such as the test of variables of attention (TOVA), the integrated visual auditory (IVA), continuous performance test (CPT), or the Conners' CPT. Psycho-educational assessment with intellectual testing using the Wechsler scales (WISC-IV for children and the new WAIS-IV for adults at the present time), and academic screening for basic subjects is also helpful, both for knowing the client's strengths and needs when it comes to strategies, and in order to facilitate pre–post comparisons.

With respect to EEG, our recommendation is to always do a single-channel assessment at CZ to start, and then determine what other information is needed with respect to EEG for that client. At the ADD Centre NFB intervention is based on parameters determined by assessment findings rather than the application of a protocol. This approach considers a triad of factors, and all three should supply convergent data. We have referred to this as the *decision-making triangle* (Thompson and Thompson, 2003) where the three corners represent:

1. The client's problems and objectives.
2. The EEG pattern observed
3. Understanding of the functions of the cortical area where EEG findings differ from expected values.

If a 19-lead QEEG is done (quantitative electroencephalographic assessment) it yields considerable additional data about communication between different cortical sites (coherence) that can also be considered. Note that you are using quantitative EEG as soon as you put numbers to your EEG measurements. QEEG can be done with a single channel, two channels, 19 channels, or even dense arrays of over 200 channels. The cover of *National Geographic* for March 2005 shows a dense array of electrodes on a Tibetan monk, an indicator of how interested the general public is becoming in neuroscience.

In an ideal setting where time and money were not issues, one would want to do a 19-lead assessment on every client. In practice, one can often proceed with straightforward cases of ADHD with a single-channel assessment at the vertex. The findings with respect to theta–beta power ratios can be compared to the norms from the multi-site study coordinated by Vince Monastra and Joel Lubar (Monastra *et al.*, 1999; Monastra *et al.*, 2001). They measured theta (4–8 Hz) and a wide range beta (13–21 Hz), and calculated power ratios in picowatts (the square of the microvolt ratios). The Pw measure was used to provide larger numbers: it is more impressive to reduce a ratio from to 9 to 4 in picowatts than from 3 to 2 in microvolts. This incredibly helpful work allows the practitioner to set goals and realistic time lines for the client based on how deviant their initial score is. Training at CZ has a number of advantages. In addition to norms being available for that location, it is relatively free of eye movement and EMG artifact as compared to sites closer to the eyes of jaws. It straddles the frontal and the sensorimotor cortex so it is a good reflection of where the problems are with ADHD, which is primarily a frontal lobe disorder (though influenced by deeper structures, such as the striatum).

Neurologists, on the other hand, primarily look at wave forms without quantifying how much activity there is at particular frequencies. They want to identify wave forms that are abnormal, such as spike and wave activity that indicates epileptiform activity. With respect to assessment of ADHD, physicians do not generally recommend referral to a neurologist. Nevertheless, Small (1993) found that in studies of children with ADHD 30–60% showed abnormal findings, including generalized and/or intermittent slowing. In a paper reviewing the clinical utility of QEEG in childhood attention and learning disorders, E. Roy John's group in the Psychiatry Department at New York University School of Medicine mention that the most comprehensive study found 48.5% of a group of 66 hyperactive children had EEG abnormalities. Findings included focal slowing, and also 14-Hz and 6-Hz spiking.

These statistics need to be kept in mind because people doing neurofeedback are not expert in abnormal brainwaves. We are dealing with more subtle differences in terms of how much of a particular activity there is at a particular location, and whether it is an amount appropriate for the person's age and the condition (eyes-open, eyes-closed, on task). But we have to be able to recognize abnormalities and make an appropriate referral to a neurologist if we see anything unusual that might require medical intervention, such as activity indicative of a seizure.

VI. SETTING UP AN INDIVIDUALIZED NEUROFEEDBACK TRAINING PROGRAM

The details of deciding on the parameters for training depend on the complexity of the case, and whether you have single-channel, two-channel or 19-channel assessment data to use. In the simple cases of ADHD without co-morbidity in which you just need a single-channel assessment at CZ, you will see a pattern when you look at a spectral array that averages your assessment data. You determine which frequency range shows the excess slow wave activity, and whether the dip is more in the SMR or beta 1 (15–18 Hz) range.

Symptoms get correlated with the EEG profile; for example, low SMR in association with a child who is restless, fidgeting, and gets distracted if his sock is not on straight, is a clear cut case. You will want to set the parameters to enhance SMR activity because that is associated with more appropriate inhibition in the brain: essentially reducing the sensory input and reducing the motor output by affecting thalamo-cortical pacemakers. Just like the cats in Sterman's early experiments, the child will need to find the mental state associated with being motorically still yet mentally vigilant. (Sterman also did experiments in which he rewarded cats for reducing SME and they became twitchy cats with tails and ears flicking.) As a bonus, sleep will probably improve, given Sterman's early finding of increased sleep spindle density, correlated with smoother transitions between stages of sleep and greater sleep efficiency, when SMR is increased.

Concurrent with SMR enhancement you will set two inhibits: one for slow waves and one for EMG artifact. The slow waves will be the frequencies that are high for that individual so it will vary across clients: 2–5, 3–7, 4–8, 4–19, 6–10, or whatever applies. Make sure the slow frequencies are real EEG, and not eye blink, by carefully artifacting your sample. (For more details on artifacts see *The Neurofeedback Book* (Thompson and Thompson, 2003), *The Art of Artifacting*, and articles by Lubar.

With EMG you choose higher frequencies that are most affected by muscle tension in the jaws, neck, and shoulders. EMG can affect frequencies down into the alpha range so you want to monitor it so that you are not fooled into thinking you are seeing increased SMR or beta when really the child is just tensing their jaw or pushing their tongue against their palate. If you have seen a busy-brain pattern, which is common in adults and can be seen in some children, usually ones who have anxiety as part of the symptom picture, then use 23–35 Hz as your inhibit (Thompson and Thompson, 2006). Monastra suggests suppressing 22–30 Hz while enhancing SMR for ADHD, H-I sub-type (Monastra, 2006; Monastra *et al.*, 2005).

If the child has no hyperactivity, and SMR is not too low, then you will again have slow-frequency inhibits in the theta to low alpha range, and an EMG inhibit (or busy-brain inhibit that doubles as an EMG inhibit), but the enhance frequencies will more likely be 15–18 Hz for beta activation. In terms of placement, both could be done at CZ. Some people advocate doing SMR at C4 if there is hyperactivity, and the beta at C3. There is a review of protocols used in research studies in an article by Monastra (2006). A very detailed account of how training is done at the ADD Centre, including such things as how to set thresholds, is found in the methods section of our 1998 case series review of outcomes in 111 cases of ADHD (98 children and 13 adults) (Thompson and Thompson, 1998). There is also an excellent review in the Lubars' chapter in the first edition of *Introduction to Quantitative EEG and Neurofeedback*. The question of referential (monopolar) versus sequential (bipolar) is covered there.

Recently, a detailed treatment of the question of the most appropriate montage for different situations appeared, done by two highly respected and experienced people, Les Fehmi and Tom Collura, which is worth reading (Fehmi and Collura, 2007). Essentially it comes down to understanding that you are measuring a potential difference between the two electrodes. If one is over an active site and the other over a relatively neutral site, like an ear lobe, then you can assume that the activity you are measuring is from the scalp location. With sequential placement, usually at FCz and CPz (either side of CZ), you still have a potential difference but the amplitude will be smaller due to common mode rejection. This is helpful sometimes in reducing artifact that is in common, such as EKG or EMG from the jaws. The downside is that you do not really know what is changing at either site: it could be one site increasing, one decreasing, or a change in the phase relationship of the activity at the two sites. Lubar notes sequential placement may give the brain more ways to learn the task.

This chapter is not a how-to manual but a guide to NFB for ADHD. For details of how to do this work see Thompson and Thompson (2003), the methods section of our 1998 paper, papers written by Lubar (1984; 1991; 2003; 2008) over the years, or papers by Vince Monastra (1999; 2001), and Gruzelier and Egner (2005). The chapter by Joel and Judy Lubar in the first edition of *Quantitative EEG and Neurofeedback* covers issues such as: tracking learning curves; training on task; determining length of training and termination criteria; adjunctive techniques; follow-up, and the appropriateness of refresher sessions when needed.

VII.   EVIDENCE-BASED PRACTICE, RESEARCH DESIGN, AND COMBINED TREATMENTS

At the present time, ADHD is one of the two NFB applications for which there is enough research to meet the criteria for efficacious treatment status according to standards approved by the Association for Applied Psychophysiology and Biofeedback; that is, there are a sufficient number of controlled studies published in peer reviewed journals to establish Level 4 efficacy. Efficacy means there is evidence of benefit in controlled research, especially randomized controlled trials. For the exact criteria and details see Yucha and Gilbert (2004), which can be downloaded at no charge from www.aapb.org. The other condition with established efficacy is epilepsy, which was the first disorder treated clinically after Sterman's work involving operant conditioning of brain wave activity in cats indicated that increasing sensorimotor rhythm (SMR) made the cats resistant to seizures. For an understanding of this work, which provides a scientific basis for the use of NFB to reduce hyperactivity and increase sustained attention, read Sterman's original paper (Wyrwicka and Sterman, 1968) and his review article in the January 2000 issue of the journal *Clinical EEG* (Sterman, 2000), a volume devoted to neurofeedback interventions.

Laurence Hirshberg and the other guest editors of an issue of *Child and Adolescent Psychiatric Clinics of North America* that was devoted to "Emerging Interventions" reviewed the less stringent guidelines for measuring evidence-based treatments published in 2002 by the American Academy of Child and Adolescent Psychiatry. Those journal editors concluded that

> Specific recommendations based on the body of empirical evidence currently available suggest the EBF [EEG biofeedback] be considered by clinicians and parents as a first-line treatment for ADHD when parents or patients prefer not to use medication and as an empirically supported treatment choice when significant side effects or insufficient improvement occurs with medication (Hirshberg *et al.*, 2005).

They note further that EBF may be used in combination with psychopharmacology or psychotherapy. With respect to cost-benefit ratio, they remark that the initial cost is high, especially since insurance companies may not cover the treatment, but there might be a cost advantage over long-term use of medication if results last. Finally, they point out that finding a practitioner and judging their competence may be difficult. That problem is often discussed in the professional organizations devoted to biofeedback, and all maintain member lists on their web sites to help the public find providers (www.aapb.org, www.bcia.org, www.isnr.org, www.applied-neuroscience.org). To keep up to date with skills, and thus enhance the image of NFB, practitioners should join at least one organization and seek credentialing by the Biofeedback Institute of America. BCIA now offers certification based on experience for "old hands" in the field in addition to the usual route of didactic course work, multiple-choice written examination, self-training, and supervised practice.

Note that the web site for the National Resource Center on AD/HD, a program of CHADD, has an information sheet that critiques NFB as an alternative treatment for AD/HD. It notes that the CHADD Professional Advisory Board (PAB) rates NFB at Level 2 Efficacy ("possibly efficacious") on the APA scale, and also just at the second level "Option" according to the AACAP guidelines. It mentions that some researchers rate the efficacy higher. The PAB is clearly more stringent. And there is the comment that, even if efficacy were established, NFB is costly and cumbersome. The article reviews eight controlled studies concerning NFB, and finds them all flawed in one way or another: lack of control group; if a waiting list control were used then criticism that it was not a sham control; and lack of randomization in four of the studies. The two randomized, blind studies with credible control groups were cited: video games designed to improve attention and cognition in the Orlandi and Greci study (2004), and sham feedback in the deBeus *et al.* study (2006). The criticism for those two was that the studies were presented at meetings so "Neither of these has yet undergone peer reviewed publication". Clearly CHADD is going to hold NFB to a very high standard, but at least it is being mentioned.

As contrasted to efficacy, which requires controlled research, effectiveness can be established through evidence of usefulness in clinical settings. In real-life settings it is recognized that interventions are combined, and so measurement of outcomes in everyday clinical practice are used in effectiveness research. A good model for this kind of research in the NFB field is the paper by Monastra *et al.* (2002) that studied 100 students who received combined community care interventions (medication, parent counseling, school consultation) with 51 of the families choosing to also have neurofeedback training for their child. Half thus received the intensive community care interventions plus about 40 sessions of neurofeedback (range 34–50 sessions). There was no random assignment to groups.

After a year, both groups were tested on and off medications. Both groups showed equivalent improvements as measured by TOVA scores. The encouraging finding for those in the NFB field was that parents and teachers rated the neurofeedback group as more attentive and less hyperactive/impulsive. Even more impressive was the finding that, when medication was removed (a one-week wash-out period), those gains in parent and teacher ratings were maintained. Additionally, when the students were retested on the TOVA, improvements were still there in the NFB group but those who had not received NFB lost their gains and went back to baseline.

As Charles Bradley had observed in his 1937 study (Bradley, 1937) using benzedrine for children with behavioral problems in an in-patient setting, the beneficial effects of administration of a stimulant are apparent within hours of administration of the drug, and disappear as soon as the drug is out of the child's system. Most encouraging was follow-up after 2 and 3 years post-treatment, with the NFB group maintaining their superior results on the TOVA and still showing the EEG changes. Additionally, 70% in the NFB group had reduced their medications by at least half whereas 85% in the other group had increased the dose.

By way of comparison with the Monastra *et al.* study (1999), the largest controlled study of interventions for ADHD ('combined type' only) done to date, is the 14-month multi-modal treatment study of ADHD (MTA Cooperative Group). It included community comparison (CC) as one of the four groups. In fact, the CC group was an active treatment group with 67% of the children receiving medication. The intensive medication management group (MedMgt) differed in that they had their methylphenidate carefully titrated for optimal dose using double-blind, placebo-controlled medication trails, three times per day dosing, and intensive monthly follow-up with parents. The other two groups were behavior management alone (Beh), and combined medication plus behavior management (Comb).

Of the 289 subjects assigned to the MedMgt and Comb groups 11% did not complete titration of medications. Of the 89% who did, 68.5% received methylphenidate with an average starting dose of 30.5 mg per day. Non-responders to methylphenidate (n = 26) were placed on dextroamphetamine, and a further 32 children did not receive medication because they had done best on placebo. At the end of the 14-month active treatment phase the average daily dose was 31.2 in the Comb group, 37.7 for MedMgt, and just 22.6 mg/day for CC. At the conclusion of the 14 months of active treatment the best outcomes were in the Comb group (68% successful outcomes based on a DSM-IV rating scale) but improvement was not statistically better than MedMgt (56% successful). Both were significantly better than Beh (34%) and CC (25%).

Success was defined as a score of 1 or less on the SNAP-IV questionnaire where symptoms rated "not at all" receive 0, "just a little" receive 1, "pretty much" gets 2, and "very much" gets 4. The total score is divided by the number of items, so a 1 means the symptoms are mild. At 24-month follow-up, however, benefits were less apparent in the two groups who had received intensive medication management with success rates of 48%, 37%, 32% and 28% respectively. Results at 36 and 48 months are pending. One question of interest will be longer-term effects on growth, since the results to date determined there was a bit more than 1 cm/year reduction in height gain, and about 2.5 kg/year less weight gain in children on methylphenidate.

Management with medication is the accepted standard of care for ADHD and, rather than comparing to a placebo, the World Medical Association in their Declaration of Helsinki advocates comparing a new treatment to a proven treatment if one exists. Writing from Paris where the WMA is based, Peter O'Neil (2008) recently reported on proposed revisions to that document. It was last revised in 2000 with guidelines designed to limit placebo trials after controversy developed regarding a placebo-controlled study involving HIV-positive women in the developing world. Half were given azidothymidine to see if shorter-course treatment would be as effective as the proven longer-course treatment, and the other half were given placebo.

The women had entered the study hoping that they would not pass their illness on to their babies, yet half were relegated (with random assignment to have a proper design) to an increased chance of their children dying of AIDS. Some ethicists defended the study, arguing that the women would likely have received no treatment had the trial not been conducted, and the drug industry and some academics opposed the Declaration, saying that restrictions on placebos were impractical and would impede research. Double-blind placebo-controlled studies continued to be the gold standard, although there has been further articulate criticism from some quarters, including the book *The Truth about the Drug Companies* written by a former editor of the *New England Journal of Medicine*, Marcie Angell

(2005). She sides with the WMA guidelines, and points out that the main benefit of placebo-controlled studies is that they allow drug companies to bring copy-cat drugs to market and increase their profits; examples would be new, expensive forms of methylphenidate, like Concerta and Biphentin, that became popular once Ritalin was no longer under patent.

In studies like the early one by Rossiter and LaVaque (1995), and the more recent one done in southern Germany by Fuchs and his colleagues (Fuchs *et al.*, 2003), neurofeedback has been compared to medication and found to have equivalent effectiveness. They thus meet the ethical guidelines of the WMA. Those studies can be criticized for lack of random assignment but the data should not be ignored. Beauregard and Levesque (2006) did do random assignment in a comparison of NFB and medication in subjects with ADHD. The NFB group had significantly better performance on Digit Span (an auditory working memory task), on a continuous performance test, and on Stroop interference. The Conners' parent rating forms showed significant reduction in inattention and hyperactive-impulsive sub-scales compared to the group receiving stimulant medication.

This study by Beauregard and Levesque performed with random assignment showed even stronger results than the other comparisons of NFB versus medication in that NFB was not just equivalent to, but actually superior to, treatment with stimulant medication. One of the most impressive aspects of the work done in Montreal by Marcus Beavregard and Johanne Levesque is that they have used fMRI as a pre–post measure. In a study comparing those who received NFB with a wait list control group, only those in the active treatment group showed changes in activation patterns using fMRI after 40 sessions of NFB done three times a week. The areas affected were the left caudate, lateral prefrontal cortex, and right anterior cingulate. These are all areas that have been shown, in other research using a variety of brain-imaging techniques, to differ in those with ADHD.

The above studies and 11 others using neurofeedback for treatment of ADHD that were found through a PubMed review covering the period March 1981 to May 2007 were reviewed by Maggie Toplak of the Psychology Department of York University in Toronto (Toplak *et al.*, 2007). She and her colleagues also reviewed six studies involving cognitive behavioral therapies, and six involving cognitive therapies (such as working memory training). With respect to NFB they concluded, "There is good reason to continue rigorous experimental investigations using neurofeedback, as the evidence is demonstrating some amelioration of performance on both cognitive and behavioral outcome measures." They commented further that ADHD is a disorder where we should be trying to create a strong multi-modal approach addressing all the components of ADHD.

Multi-modal approaches have always been advocated by leaders in the neurofeedback field, as evidenced by Joel and Judy Lubar's (1999) in which they note that NFB is not a stand-alone therapy. They mention specifically that it can be combined with medication. The Lubars also include advice concerning the importance of family assessment (including Judy's specialty of genograms), family therapy if there is dysfunction, and intervention for co-morbidities such as depression.

The A.D.D. Book (Sears and Thompson, 1998), which was the first book written for parents that had a chapter on neurofeedback, includes chapters on medications and diet as well as lots of information on behavior management and learning strategies in sections that give advice on setting up for success at home and school. Vince Monastra (2004) similarly covers multi-modal interventions in the publication, *Parenting Children with ADHD: 10 lessons that medicine cannot teach*. His book, which is published by the American Psychological Association, makes favorable mention of NFB in passing, but does not dwell on it because the emphasis is on approaches like diet and management techniques that parents can implement themselves.

People practicing neurofeedback should not feel in competition with other approaches, or be anti-medication. Sometimes it is pills *and* skills that are needed. Sometimes medication can be reduced, or avoided entirely, if self-regulation skills are adequately learned, but the goal is always to acquire self-regulation, not to stop medication, though that is a bonus in the view of most parents. We reported on a case series of 111 consecutive clients with ADHD treated with NFB (Thompson and Thompson, 1998), and 29 of the 98 children in that study (30%) were taking methlyphenidate (Ritalin) when they started NFB. About 80% (23 children) had discontinued the medication by the time they completed 40 sessions of training, five more reduced the dose they were taking, and one was on the same dose. Vince Monastra counsels parents to watch for worsening behavior as the child taking stimulants proceeds in their training because they may start to show overdose effects once NFB is producing changes.

We encourage practitioners to add other biofeedback modalities to NFB with older adolescent and adult clients to enhance self-regulation, with respiration and heart rate variability training among the most promising. Some children are also suitable candidates but others would fidget more with sensors on their fingers, or a breathing belt/respiration sensor. You can teach diaphragmatic breathing to children without actual biofeedback measurements by just teaching them to do belly breathing with their hand on their stomach as they pretend they are inflating a balloon in their tummy as they breathe in, and deflating it as they breathe out.

Functional neuroanatomy supports a systems theory of neural synergy whereby various components augment one another, such as SMR enhancement and diaphragmatic breathing both influencing muscle spindles as used in a case of a woman with advanced Parkinson's disease (Thompson and Thompson, 2002), or listening exercises, such as SAMONAS sound therapy and heart rate variability training both influencing the strapesius muscle in the inner ear so that it responds appropriately to sounds and voices. One should always be on the lookout for the right combination of interventions for a particular client to maximize positive outcomes. Just as medication should not be used as a sole intervention, NFB can be the core approach for empowering people with ADHD to manage their symptoms, but it should not be the only one.

VIII. THE INTERNATIONAL SCENE AND FUTURE DIRECTIONS

There is international research that is exciting and ongoing from areas as geographically diverse as England, Australia, Austria, Germany, and Russia. In London final data analysis is being done on an ADHD study initiated by John Gruzelier that used Captain's Log cognitive training as a control group. Gruzelier and his graduate students are responsible for doing research that answers many of the fundamental questions in the NFB field, things that had been assumed but not explicitly tested. John Gruzelier and Tobias Egner (2005) review much of this work. For example, studies done at Imperial College London using healthy subjects supported the hypothesis that enhancing SMR over sensorimotor cortex will reduce impulsive behavior. One study involved giving music students ten 15-minute sessions of increasing beta 15–18 Hz at C3, and SMR 12–15 Hz at C4. Reduction in commission errors on a continuous performance test correlated with positive success at increasing SMR.

Training to enhance SMR and beta did not, in a different study, enhance musical performance. Musicality in students at the Royal College of Music was significantly enhanced only by alpha–theta training. Gruzelier postulates that increasing theta may have had beneficial effects on memory as well as producing a state of deep relaxation that might enhance feelings of relaxation and well-being. Of interest to those doing NFB for ADHD is that high level music students would have the opposite EEG profile to people with ADHD—they would produce lots of beta and be capable of being very still for long periods of time. Thus the training that benefitted music students was to help them access states that come naturally to those with ADHD; that is, more theta. The main point of the various studies is that training is both site-specific and frequency-specific in its effects. Gruzelier has now moved on to Goldsmiths College, after 25 years at Imperial College, and his research is shifting to include virtual reality.

In Sydney, Adam Clarke's group at the University of Wollongong have collaborated with pediatricians in Sydney to produce interesting papers, including a few about the beta excess sub-type of ADHD. Also based in Australia, the Brain Resource Company continues to build an impressive database correlating EEG with other parameters. At the University of Salzburg, which hosted the Biofeedback Foundation of Europe meeting in 2008, Wolfgang Klimesch's group has done work that includes studies on peak individual alpha and enhanced cognitive performance.

Juri Kropotov's group in St. Petersburg has designed QEEG equipment (Mitsar), and created a database that includes not only Russian subjects but 200 Swiss schoolchildren. Kropotov's innovative work with ADHD emphasizes uptraining beta. They are reluctant to do theta inhibit protocols due to the possibility of decreasing hippocampal theta around 6 Hz that is linked to memory. Their studies are notable for including ERP data (event-related potentials) in addition to QEEG data. In a recent study involving 86 children ages 9–14 years they compared good and poor performers (as determined by performance during training sessions) on a GO/NOGO task, and found that only the good performers showed changes in their ERP responses. The changes were in the frontal-central area, and appeared to reflect increased activation that was associated with 15–22 sessions of beta training. Each session had consisted of 20 minutes of enhancing the ratio of power in the 15–18 Hz range with power in the rest of the spectrum with C3-Fz placements, and then doing 7–10 minutes of training to increase the ratio of 12–15 Hz compared to the rest of the spectrum with C4-Pz placements.

On the horizon is a proposed international study on ADHD. Also drawing interest to training the brain is work showing that one can do feedback using fMRI (DeCharms *et al.*, 2004). People have been showing EEG changes after training for decades, and Sterman showed operant conditioning of brain waves back in 1968 with cats as the subjects. However, medical people are more likely to be impressed with training brain activation using high tech and very expensive equipment. EEG work continues to be the less expensive, less invasive procedure, and it has the best temporal resolution. The fMRI would have greater spatial resolution, but the calculations involved before giving feedback mean it is a slower process, even though DeCharms uses the phrase "real time fMRI" in his title.

Another possibly fruitful avenue is QEEG-based coherence training. This involves two-channel work, and is based on coherence abnormalities (either hypercoherence or hypocoherence) found when analyzing data from 19-lead EEG recordings. There is no set coherence abnormality established for people with ADHD but this work is, in any event, always individualized. Coherence training may be particularly helpful for people who have co-morbidity with learning disabilities (Walker and Norman, 2006), or for those who have acquired attentional problems due to head injuries (Walker *et al.*, 2002).

Many people are excited about the possibilities of Z-score training. This approach uses database information about the degree of deviation from the database mean (a Z-score has a mean of 0 and a standard deviation of 1), and allows goals to be set for the individual according to how much they deviate from the mean at a particular site (say CZ) for a particular frequency. The goal is normalization so one might choose a feedback parameter of being within the range of plus or minus 1.5 when using Z-scores. (If using T-scores with a mean of 50 and an s.d. of 10, the equivalent range would be 35–65. If using standard scores with a mean of 100 and an s.d. of 15 it would be 77.5–122.5.) A more stringent criterion would be plus or minus 2, which would encompass two-thirds of a normally distributed population. Due to its newness, there are no published reports regarding outcomes of treatment but there are anecdotal reports concerning Z-score training being helpful. Manufacturers of biofeedback equipment and practitioners have invested considerable money into the development of Z-score feedback.

Finally, there is low resolution electromagnetic tomography (LORETA)-based feedback. Joel Lubar has been experimenting with this, and feels it has great potential. The idea is that the source of abnormal activity measured on the scalp can be identified by the mathematical calculations of LORETA, developed by Roberto Pascual-Marqui at the KEY Institute in Zurich (Pascual-Marqui *et al.*, 2002). This allows feedback to be done while this source localization program is actively running. It may also allow NFB to influence deeper cortical structures more directly. Being able to train more directly the activity of the cingulate gyrus, which is often identified as the source of dysfunction, may prove to be key. The biggest challenge is that LORETA analysis has to be done on artifact-free data and, obviously, when running continuous EEG there is going to be artifact—from eye movements, muscle contractions, EKG, and so on. Thus feedback must be inhibited in the presence of artifacts so that you are not training something false. Lubar is currently refining such methods (Lubar, 2008).

IX. CONCLUSION

Studies have supported the observation that neurofeedback can be as effective as stimulant medication in reducing the symptoms of ADHD (Rossiter and LaVaque; 1995; Fuchs *et al.*, 2003; Monastra *et al.*, 2002). There is also evidence of significant improvements in measures of intelligence, academic performance, and behavior (Lubar and Lubar, 1984; Lubar, 1991, 1997; Lubar *et al.*, 1995; Linden *et al.*, 1996; Thompson and Thompson, 1998). Even as we await further research meeting stringent criteria regarding random assignment of subjects, and more follow-up studies regarding maintaining gains, NFB has established itself as a key component in the treatment of ADHD that adds to positive outcomes. It is not easy work and it needs to be done carefully, always keeping in mind that there should be evidence of learning, as measured by EEG parameters as well as transfer of the self-regulation skills to everyday life.

Neurofeedback fits into the twenty-first century Zeitgeist concerning health maintenance and self-regulation; that is, skills, not just pills. The real power of NFB, and the reason it should become the preferred intervention for ADHD, is that it empowers the child, or adult for that matter, to achieve changes through their own efforts, and thus gain the means and motivation to realize their full potential.

REFERENCES

American Academy of Pediatrics Committee on Quality Improvement and Sub-committee on Attention-Deficit/Hyperactivity Disorder (2000): Clinical Practice Guidelines. *Pediatrics*, **105(5)**, 1159–1170.
American Psychiatric Association (2000). *Diagnostic and Statistical Manual of Mental Disorders.* American Psychiatric Association, Arlington, VA.

Baehr, E., Rosenfeld, J. P., Baehr, R. and Earnst, C. (1999). Clinical use of an alpha asymmetry neu-rofeedback protocol in the treatment of mood disorders. In *Introduction to Quantitative EEG and Neurofeedback* (J. R. Evans and A. Abarbanel, eds), San Diego: Academic Press, pp. 181–203.

Barkley, R. A. (2006). *Attention-Deficit Hyperactivity Disorder: A Handbook for Diagnosis and Treatment*, 3rd edition. New York: Guilford Press.

Beauregard, M. and Levesque, J. (2006). Functional magnetic resonance imaging investigation of the effects of neurofeedback training on the neural bases of selective attention and response inhibition in children with attention-deficit/hyperactivity disorder. *Applied Psychophysiology and Biofeedback*, **31(1)**, 3–20.

Bradley, C. (1937). The behavior of children receiving Benzedrine. *American Journal of Psychiatry*, **94**, 577–585.

Brown, T. E. (2000). *Attention-Deficit Disorders and Comorbidities in Children, Adolescents and Adults*. Washington, D.C: American Psychiatric Press.

(2003). Attention deficit: Not just kid stuff. *Business Week*, 27 October.

Chabot, R. J., di Michele, F., Prichep, L. and John, E. R. (2001). The clinical role of computerized EEG in the evaluation and treatment of learning and attention disorders in children and adolescents. *Journal of Neuropsychiatry and Clinical Neuroscience*, **13(2)**, 171–186.

Clarke, A. R., Barry, R. J., McCarthy, R. and Selikowitz, M. (2001). EEG-defined subtypes of children with attention-deficit/hyperactivity disorder. *Clinical Neurophysiology*, **112**, 2098–2105.

Connor, D. F. (2006). Stimulants. In *Attention-Deficit Hyperactivity Disorder: A handbook for diagnosis and treatment* (R. A. Barkley, ed.), 3rd edition, pp. 608–648. New York: Guilford Press.

DeBeus, (2006). Progress in efficacy studies of EEG biofeedback for ADHD. Annual Meeting of the American Psychiatric Association.

DeCharms, R. C., *et al.* (2004). Learned regulation of spatially localized brain activation using real time fMRI. *Neuroimage*, **21**, 436–443.

Fehmi, L. G. and Collura, T. (2007). Effects of electrode placement upon EEG biofeedback training: The monopolar-bipolar controversy. *Journal of Neurotherapy*, **11(2)**, 45–62.

Fuchs, T., Birbaumer, N., Lutzenberger, W., Gruzelier, J. H. and Kaiser, J. (2003). . *Applied Psychophysiology and Biofeedback*, **28(1)**, 1–12.

Gruzelier, J. and Egner, T. (2005). Critical validation studies of neurofeedback. *Child and Adolescent Psychiatric Clinics of North America*, **14(1)**, 83–104.

Hallowell, E. and Ratey, J. (1994). *Driven to Distraction*. New York: Random House.

Hartmann, T. (1995). Hunters in a Farmers World. In *Attention Deficit Disorder: A Different Perception*. Grass Valley, CA: Underwood Books.

Hirshberg, L. M., Chiu, S. and Frazier, J. A. (2005). Emerging brain-based interventions for children and adolescents: overview and clinical perspective. *Child and Adolescent Psychiatric Clinics of North America*, **14(1)**, 1–19.

Kropotov, J. D., Grin-Yatsenko, V. A., Ponomarev, V. A., Chutko, L. S., Yakovenko, E. A. and Nikishena, I. S. (2005). ERP correlates of EEG relative beta training in ADHD children. *Internatioanl Journal of Psychophysiology*, **55**, 21–54.

Kropotov, J. D., Grin-Yatsenko, V. A., Ponomarev, V. A., Chutko, L. S., Yakovenko, E. A. and Nikishena, I. S. (2007). Changes in EEG specrograms, event-related potentials and event-related desynchroniza-tion induced by relative beta training in ADHD children. *Journal of Neurotherapy*, **11(2)**, 3–11.

Leins, U., Goth, G., Hinterberger, T., Klinger, C., Rumph, M. and Strehl, U. (2007). Neurofeedback for children with ADHD: A comparison of SCP and theta/beta protocols. *Applied Psychophysiology and Biofeedback*, **32(12)**, 73–88.

Linden, M., Habib, T. and Radojevic, V. (1996). A controlled study of the effects of EEG biofeedback on cognition and behavior of children with attention deficit disorder and learning disabilities. *Biofeedback and Self-Regulation*, **21(1)**, 35–49.

Lubar, J. F. (1991). Discourse on the development of EEG diagnostics and biofeedback treatment for attention deficit/hyperactivity disorders. *Biofeedback and Self-Regulation*, **16**, 202–225.

Lubar, J. F. (1997). Neocortical dynamics: implications for understanding the role of neurofeedback and related techniques for the enhancement of attention. *Applied Psychophysiology and Biofeedback*, **22(2)**, 111–126.

Lubar, J. F. (2003). Neurofeedback for the management of attention deficit disorders. In *Biofeedback: A practitioner's guide* (M. S. Schwartz and F. Andrasik, eds), 3rd edition, pp. 409–437. New York: Guilford Press.

Lubar, J. (2008). *Update on neurofeedback for AD/HD*. Presentation at the annual meeting of the Society for the Advancement of Brain Analysis (SABA). St. Petersburg, FL, May, 2008.

Lubar, J. F. and Lubar, J. O. (2001). Neurofeedback intervention for treatment of attention deficit/hyperactivity disorder. *Molecular Psychiatry*, **6(57)**, Suppl. 1, Feb.

Lubar, J. F. and Lubar, J. O. (1999). Neurofeedback assessment and treatment for attention deficit/hyperactivity disorder. In Evans, J. R. and Abarbanel, A. eds. *Quantitative EEG and Neurofeedback*, San Diego, CA, pp. 103–146.

Lubar, J. O. and Lubar, J. F. (1984). Electroencephalographic biofeedback of SMR and beta for treatment of attention deficit disorders in clinical settings. *Biofeedback and Self-Regulation*, **9(1)**, 1–23.

Lubar, J. F. and Shouse, M. N. (1976). EEG and behavioral changes in a hyperkinetic child concurrent with training of the sensorimotor rhythm (SMR): A preliminary report. *Biofeedback and Self-Regulation*, **1(3)**, 293–306.

Lubar, J. F., Swartwood, M. O., Swartwood, J. N. and O'Donnell, P. H. (1995). Evaluation of the effectiveness of EEG neurofeedback training for ADHD in a clinical setting as measured by changes in T.O.V.A. scores, behavior ratings, and WISC-R performance. *Biofeedback and Self-Regulation*, **20(1)**, 83–99.

Magnus, B. (2008). Academic athletes. *Canadian Medical Association Journal*, **178(8)**, 989.

Monastra, V. J. (2004). *Parenting children with ADHD: 10 lessons that medicine cannot teach*. Washington, D.C.: American Psychological Association.

Monastra, V. J. (2005). Electroencephalographic biofeedback (neurotherapy) as a treatment for attention deficit hyperactivity disorder. Rationale and empirical foundation. *Child and Adolescent Psychiatric Clinics of North America*, **14(1)**, 55–82.

Monastra, V. J., Lubar, J. F., Linden, *et al.* (1999). Assessing attention deficit hyperactivity disorder via quantitative electroencephalography: An initial validation study. *Neuropsychology*, **13(3)**, 424–433.

Monastra, V. J., Lubar, J. F. and Linden, M. (2001). The development of a quantitative electroencephalographic scanning process for attention deficit hyperactivity disorder: Reliability and validity studies. *Neuropsychology*, **15(1)**, 136–144.

Monastra, V. J., Monastra, D. M. and George, S. (2002). The effects of stimulant therapy, EEG biofeedback, and parenting style on the primary symptoms of attention-deficit/hyperactivity disorder. *Applied Psychophysiology and Biofeedback*, **27(4)**, 231–249.

Monastra, V. J., Lynn, S., Linden, M., Lubar, J. F., Gruzelier, J. and LaVaque, T. J. (2005). *Journal of Neurotherapy*, **9(4)**, 5–34.

O'Neil, P. (2008). Ethics guidelines for clinical trials to be revised. *Canadian Medical Association Journal*, **178(2)**, 138.

Pascual-Marqui, R. D., Esslen, M., Kochi, K. and Lehmann, D. (2002). Functional Imaging with Low Resolution Electromagnetic Tomography (LORETA): A review. *Methods & Findings in Experimental & Clinical Pharmacology*, **24C**, 91–95.

Pfeifer, J. H., Jacoboni, M., Mazzalotta, J.C. and Dapretto, M. (2007). Mirroring others' emotions relates to empathy and interpersonal competence in children. *Neuroimage*, **39(4)**, 2076–2085.

Porges, S. W. (2003). Social engagement and attachment: A phylogenetic perspective. *Annals of the New York Academy of Sciences*, **1008**, 31–47.

Porges, S. W. (2004). The Vagus: A mediator of behavioral and physiologic features associated with autism. In *The Neurobiology of Autism* (M. L. Bauman and T. L. Kemper, eds), pp. 65–78. Baltimore: Johns Hopkins University Press.

Rossiter, T. R. (2004). The effectiveness of neurofeedback and stimulant drugs in ADHD: Part I. Review of methodological issues. Part II. Replication. *Applied Psychophysiology and Biofeedback,* **29(2)**, 135–140.

Rossiter, T. R. (2005). The effectiveness of neurofeedback and stimulant drugs in ADHD: Part II. *Replication. Applied Psychophysiology and Biofeedback,* **29(4)**, 233–243.

Rossiter, T. R. and LaVaque, T. J. (1995). A comparison of EEG biofeedback and psychostimulants in treating attention-deficit/hyperactivity disorder. *Journal of Neurotherapy,* **1**, 48–59.

Sears, W. and Thompson, L. (1998). *The A.D.D. Book: New Understandings, New Approaches to Parenting Your Child.* New York: Little, Brown & Co.

Shouse, M. N. and Lubar, J. F. (1979). Sensorimotor rhythm (SMR) operant conditioning and methylphenidate in the treatment of hyperkinesis. *Biofeedback and Self-Regulation,* **4**, 299–311.

Smith, B. H., Barkley, R. A. and Shapiro, C. (2006). Combined Child Therapies. In *Attention-Deficit Hyperactivity Disorder: A Handbook for Diagnosis and Treatment* (R. A. Barkley, ed.) 3rd edition. New York: Guilford Press.

Solanto, M., Arnsten, A. and Castellanos, F. (2001). *Stimulant Drugs and ADHD: Basic and Clinical Neuroscience.* Guilford Press, NY, US and Oxford University Press, Great Britain.

Spencer, T., Wilens, T., Biederman, J., Faraone, S., *et al.* (1995). A doubleblind, crossover comparison of methylphenidate and placebo in adults with childhood-onset attention-deficit hyperactivity disorder. *Archives of General Psychiatry,* **52(6)**, 434–443.

Sterman, M. B. (2000). Basic concepts and clinical findings in the treatment of seizure disorders with EEG operant conditioning. *Clinical Electroencephalography,* **32(1)**, 45–55.

Surmeli, T. and Ertem, A. (2007). Post WISC-R and TOVA improvement with QEEG guided neurofeedbacktraining in learning problems: 17 cases. Abstract of the paper presented at the 11th Annual Meeting of the Biofeedback Foundation of Europe, Berlin, Germany, February 2007. Published in *Applied Psychophysiology and Biofeedback,* **32(3–4)**, 215.

Swanson, J. M., McBurnett, K., Wigel, T., Pfiffner, L. J., Williams, L., Christian, D. L., *et al.* (1993). The effect of stimulant medication on children with attention deficit disorder: A "review of reviews". *Exceptional Children,* **60(2)**, 154–162.

Thompson, L. and Thompson, M. (1998). Neurofeedback combined with training in metacognitive strategies: Effectiveness in students with ADD. *Applied Psychophysiology and Biofeedback,* **23(4)**, 243–263.

Thompson, M. and Thompson, L. (2002). Biofeedback for Movement Disorders (Dystonia with Parkinson's Disease): Theory and Preliminary Results. *Journal of Neurotherapy,* **6(4)**, 51–70.

Thompson, M. and Thompson, L. (2003). *The Neurofeedback Book: An introduction to basic concepts in applied psychophysiology.* Wheat Ridge, CO: Association for Applied Psychophysiology and Biofeedback.

Thompson, L. and Thompson, M. (2005). Neurofeedback Intervention for Adults with ADHD. *Journal of Adult Development,* **12(2–3)**, 123–130.

Thompson, M. and Thompson, L. (2006). Improving Attention in Adults and Children: Differing Electroencephalograhy Profiles and Implications for Training. *Biofeedback,* **34(3)**, 99–105.

Thompson, M. and Thompson, L. (2007). Neurofeedback for Stress Management. In *Principles and Practice of Stress Management* (P. Lehrer, R. Woolfolk and W. Sime, eds), 3rd edition, pp. 249–291. New York: Guilford Publications.

Toplak, M. E., Connors, L., Shuster, J., Knezevic, B. and Parks, S. (2007). Review of cognitive, cognitive-behavioral, and neural-based interventions for Attention-Deficit/Hyperactivity Disorder (ADHD). *Clinical Psychology Review,* doi:10.1016/j.cpr.2007.10.008

Walker, J. F., Weber, R. and Norman, C. (2002). Importance of QEEG guided coherence training for patients with mild closed head injury. *Journal of Neurotherapy,* **6(1)**, 31–42.

Walker, J. E. and Norman, C. A. (2006). The Neurophysiology of Dyslexia: A Selective Review with Implications for Neurofeedback Remediation and Results of Treatment in Twelve Consecutive Patients. *Journal of Neurotherapy,* **10(1)**, 45–55.

Wender, P. H. (1995). *Attention-Deficit Hyperactivity Disorder in Adults*. Oxford, UK and NewYork: Oxford University Press.

Wyrwicka, and Sterman, M. B. (1968). Instrumental conditioning of sensorimotor cortex EEG spindles in the waking cat. *Physiology and Behavior*, **3**, 703–707.

Yucha, C. and Gilbert, C. (2004). Evidence Based Practice in Biofeedback and Neurofeedback. Wheat Ridge, CO: Association for Applied Psychophysiology and Biofeedback.

CHAPTER 15

Asperger's syndrome intervention: Combining neurofeedback, biofeedback and metacognition

Michael Thompson, M.D. and Lynda Thompson, Ph.D.

ADD Centre and Biofeedback Institute of Toronto, Mississauga, Ontario, Canada

I. INTRODUCTION

The goal of this chapter is to broaden practitioners' understanding of Asperger's syndrome (AS), a disorder along the continuum of autistic spectrum disorders (ASD). AS is becoming a relatively common diagnosis in schoolchildren who are very bright intellectually but totally inept socially (Nash, 2002). They are usually initially misdiagnosed as having attention deficit hyperactivity disorder (ADHD). This chapter emphasizes how to use neurofeedback (NFB) plus biofeedback (BFB), in conjunction with coaching in learning strategies (metacognition) to address the major symptoms observed in AS. We are developing an understanding of how feedback can improve a person's cognitive, emotional, and even physical functioning, and have named this a systems theory of neural synergy (STNS). The name underscores the fact that NFB plus BFB influence dynamic circuits, and emphasizes that no matter where we enter the nervous system with an intervention the larger system adjusts as it seeks a new balance. If the intervention is done correctly, the new equilibrium will bring out the individual's potential.

This chapter is divided into four sections. Section I gives a general overview of Asperger's syndrome including background, a historical note, information on prevalence, and a description of symptoms that includes the authors' clinical observations. Section II correlates symptoms with functional neuroanatomy and electroencephalographic (EEG) findings. Four key groups of symptoms are discussed in the order that they are usually addressed using NFB intervention, namely:

1. ADHD symptoms of inattention and impulsivity.
2. Anxiety and affect modulation.
3. Empathy, affect interpretation and expression, and social interaction.
4. Executive function difficulties.

Introduction to QEEG and Neurofeedback, Second Edition
ISBN: 978-0-12-374534-7

Section III further highlights brain areas found to be dysfunctional in ASD, and cites research findings for each of seven key regions that are repeatedly found to differ when compared to people with typical development. They are:

- Prefrontal cortex
- Hippocampal gyrus
- Amygdala with its connections to the orbital and medial frontal areas of the brain
- Fusiform gyrus
- Superior temporal gyrus containing the auditory cortex
- Anterior insula and the anterior cingulate (both part of the limbic system or emotional brain), and
- Frontal and parietal-temporal mirror neuron areas.

Lack of normal functioning in these critical areas of the brain can be seen using the quantitative electroencephalogram (QEEG). A comparison to database norms can be combined with low resolution electromagnetic tomography (LORETA) to ascertain which cortical area is the source of abnormal EEG activity measured on the surface of the scalp. LORETA is a mathematical procedure developed by Roberto Pascual-Marqui of the Key Institute in Zurich. In addition, this section briefly summarizes theories to explain the functional neuroanatomical findings in ASD.

Section IV is concerned with intervention. It provides an overview of the use of NFB plus BFB for managing the symptoms of AS. It provides a summary of what to do, and a discussion of why it is effective. A review of results with clients diagnosed with AS seen at the authors' centre is summarized, with pre- and post-training testing results. An important observation from this review is that the significant results were not due to a small number of cases with very dramatic improvements skewing the results but, rather, were obtained with virtually every case improving in one or more key areas.

II.   SECTION I: BACKGROUND, HISTORICAL NOTE, PREVALENCE, AND SYMPTOMS

A.   Background

Clinicians in North America have been paying increasing attention to people with Asperger's disorder since it became recognized as a diagnosis by the American Psychiatric Association (2004). These children and adults show qualitative impairments in social interaction plus restrictive, repetitive and stereotyped patterns of behaviors, interests, and activities. These difficulties produce significant impairment in functioning in everyday life, despite the person having normal to very high intelligence, and without a history of cognitive or language delay. A somewhat broader range of symptoms is associated with Asperger's syndrome (AS), as will be described below.

Since the first author was diagnosing AS before the DSM-IV was developed, and also because the criteria for AS fit better with clinical experience, and because it is more widely used internationally, Asperger's syndrome is the nomenclature chosen for this chapter. Similarly, we prefer referring to the autistic spectrum of disorders as described by Lorna Wing (2001) rather than using the DSM-IV category of pervasive developmental disorders, the grouping under which Asperger's disorder falls.

B. Historical note

In 1944, the Viennese pediatrician Hans Asperger published a description of a group of boys with an unusual constellation of symptoms. They were like little professors with advanced knowledge in their special areas of interest, but they were socially inept. Asperger used the term *autistischen Psychopathen* (*autistic psychopathies*), borrowing the term *autism* from Bleuler (1911), and using *psychopathy* to indicate a personality disorder rather than a psychiatric illness. When his work eventually became more widely known, it was referred to as *Asperger's syndrome* (Wing, 1981; Wing and Gould, 1979).

Lorna Wing, a British psychiatrist and autism expert who was largely responsible for bringing this interesting diagnosis to the attention of English-speaking professionals, set out the following criteria for Asperger's syndrome (Wing, 2001). Those with AS have well-developed language skills that are, nevertheless, a bit odd with respect to the use of pedantic language, and a lack of normal prosody (rhythm, intonation, and pitch). They show impaired social interaction, and have limited non-verbal communication with little facial expression or use of gesture. They show resistance to change and like routines, repetitive activities, and spending time learning about their special interest areas. They have excellent rote memory for things of interest. They show poor motor coordination, and often have an odd gait and posture. Asperger noted that they did not fit in socially, made their parents' lives miserable, and drove their teachers to despair (Cumine *et al.*, 1998). These continue to be the problems that bring them to the attention of mental health professionals today.

Asperger died in 1980 without ever meeting Wing, and before his astute observations and eponymous diagnostic grouping really became known in Britain or the USA. His original work was eventually translated into English, and published in a textbook about Asperger's syndrome and autism written by Ute Frith (1991) (Asperger, 1991). It was 50 years after Asperger's initial paper was published that the disorder bearing his name was officially recognized in the USA through inclusion in the DSM-IV. By the time Tony Attwood (2007) was writing his second book about AS, however, there were over 2000 publications and 100 books on the subject.

C. Prevalence

Estimates of prevalence of AS range from 2 per 10,000 in school-aged children (Fombonne and Tidmarsh, 2003) to a higher estimate of 36 per 10,000 people (Ehlers and Gillberg, 1993). The Autism Society in Canada estimates that there are 15,000 people diagnosed with AS, which would translate into a prevalence of roughly 5 per 10,000 people. The condition is much more frequent in boys (Gillburg and Billstedt, 2000); indeed, Hans Asperger's original sample was all boys. Recent estimates place the male to female ratio at 4:1, which was the ratio found in the Ehlers and Gillberg survey, and also the ratio found by Tony Attwood (2007), an Australian psychologist specializing in AS, when he reviewed hundreds of cases he has assessed in his clinic in Brisbane.

Among engineers, computer specialists, and eccentric, "absent-minded professors," prevalence seems to be much greater, though this has not been formally measured. In Silicon Valley, California, the rates are particularly high, and AS was dubbed the "geek syndrome" in an article in *Time* magazine (Nash, 2002). This makes sense because vocations which require logical, sequential thinking without much emotional content or social understanding suit people with AS, and they are experts in their areas of intense special interests. Here is an example of a future professor.

A high school student was brought by his mother for assessment because of suspected learning disabilities and attention deficit disorder. He could not pass ninth grade English, despite his mother being a teacher. Reading comprehension (at least, for reading assigned in English class) was weak, he seemed to be daydreaming in class, and organizational skills were terrible. In the first interview he was diagnosed with Asperger's. The AS presumably came from his father, a dairy farmer totally engrossed in cows who actually tried to disinheret his son because of his lack of bovine interests. The boy's obsession was dinosaurs. He read papers from the *Acta Paleontologica Polenska* avidly, and corresponded with university professors about issues of classification, especially concerning winged dinosaurs. After NFB training combined with coaching in strategies (including how to deal with Romeo and Juliet so he could pass Grade 9 English), he was eventually able to graduate high school and go on to university studies in paleontology. His mother called only once to discuss a concern after his training was completed: now that he was being invited to parties, she wondered how to handle the possibility of teenage drinking.

When one looks at data for the wider grouping of autistic spectrum disorders (ASD) the numbers being diagnosed have become very high indeed. Coben (2007) cites the most recent prevalence estimates from the Centers for Disease

Control and Prevention in the United States to be 1 in 150 for ASD. The same principles that are developed in this chapter for intervening with AS apply to ASD, and so we will include case examples of children with diagnoses of autism in this chapter.

D.   Asperger's syndrome traits: The authors' observations

The following description of AS traits is culled from both reading about AS and the clinical experience of the authors. Anecdotes are gleaned from history-taking done with clients, and parents of clients, over the past 15 years (1993–2008).

Clients with AS are a heterogeneous group. None have all of the traits, and some show opposite patterns to the common ones mentioned here. For example, although most children with AS are proficient in language areas, there is the occasional child with AS who is mathematically inclined, excels in spatial reasoning rather than language, loves LEGO or other building toys, and dislikes reading. In a similar vein, Alvarez (2004) noted that the way personality interacts with the symptomatology of the disorder and deviance, and with the developmental delay, is exceedingly complex. Most people we have seen with AS have rather high IQs. Perhaps this should not surprise us, since most of the Wechsler Intelligence Scale subtests can be done using verbal mediation and logical left hemisphere skills. Nevertheless, AS traits can be found in conjunction with all levels of intelligence (Wing, 2001) and there can also be co-morbidity with specific learning disabilities. Superb verbal skills, for example, constitute a main feature of those with AS but, in rare cases, there is a coexisting learning disability in the language area.

Although unusual, there are a few clients with Asperger's who are great artists. The vast majority whom we have assessed, however, showed reluctance when asked to draw a person (d-a-p). We think that this may be related to their problems in reading people. Often clients with AS would produce a drawing with facial features hidden, or draw a detailed train or airplane with the person just a tiny head in the window. We have found that, after NFB intervention, there are quite dramatic changes in the d-a-p task. This has proven to be an interesting and reliable way to gauge clinical improvement.

Those with AS tend to be endearingly honest (no social lies and sometimes too open about personal topics), and one often feels they would have a smoother time if the world were a better place; that is, if people would say what they mean (clear communication without confusing figures of speech, pretence or sarcasm), keep to rules and routines, and be kind. There are some differences in their speech, such as pedantic phrases, and a tone of voice that lacks prosody and is monotone. When upset, they can be very loud. Their temper tantrums will be inappropriate for their age, and may be triggered by things that seem trivial to others. Though usually they show flat affect, when upset they will overreact.

A boy who did not cry after his grandfather died, explaining that Grandad was old and old people are expected to die, burst into tears when his mother put the wrong kind of jam in his sandwich.

Yelling, anger and impatience are all counter-productive when dealing with someone with AS. If a client with Asperger's is out of control and digging in their heels, one usually finds that they are trying to control the situation to reduce anxiety. The clinician should therefore teach the parents how to be flexible, and model for the child the calmness that one wants to see, not escalate the confrontation.

Children with AS can often interact well with those younger than themselves and with adults. If you ask the mother of a young child with AS what happens when he goes out on the playground, she will usually tell you that her little boy wants to have friends. He will go immediately over to others and begin talking, but he does not seem aware of the social rules of how to enter a conversation. He launches immediately into his special area of interest. The other children simply do not understand where he is coming from, and soon they just start playing with each other as if he were not even there.

Six-year-old Matthew's special interest was Superman. The other children were choosing teams for a game of baseball. Matthew ran over to them, pushed one boy to get his attention, and began talking about kryptonite, a substance lethal to Superman. The other children looked at him as if he had just arrived from outer space, and then went on with their game.

In this example, the other children listened a bit, and then simply ignored Matthew. However, this difficulty in reading social cues and responding appropriately can have more detrimental effects to the child's self-esteem if the other children not only ignore him, but tease him, bully him, and ostracize him from the group. Maintaining friendships with AS is very difficult for the child with AS. One hears repeatedly that the child makes friends quickly but cannot keep friends. On the other hand, when Matthew was with children who were a couple of years younger, it was a different story. Then he was able to dominate and control the activities, getting them to play games about superheroes.

Another example of not realizing that a personal special interest may not be important to others, and inappropriately forcing this interest on to other people, comes from Stephen.

Steven, age 12, had a special interest in cars. When he first arrived for training he would burst into an office and barrage the client and trainer sitting there with questions about their make of car and license plate number. He would go from office to office doing this until he was brought under control. If the client was obviously upset when he burst in, it made no difference to his behavior. This boy had a previous diagnosis of attention deficit hyperactivity disorder before coming to the ADD Centre, and such behavior was seen as impulsive. From the perspective of AS functioning, it can be viewed as an attempt to feel more comfortable in a new situation by introducing something familiar—talking about cars.

After about 20 sessions of neurofeedback Steven's hyperactive and impulsive behavior was greatly decreased, and his behavior became calm. After 40 sessions our staff, his parents, and the schoolteachers had all noticed that his social awareness had shifted. He was actually thinking of the reaction of others before he did things. In the clinic, instead of interrupting one staff after another, he would arrive and, if he wanted to ask permission to do something, he would silently stand by the author's open door and wait until he was asked what he would like, which was often permission to make a cup of tea if he had arrived early for his session.

In addition to their inappropriate initiation of interaction with peers, most people with AS demonstrate motor clumsiness (Weimer *et al.*, 2001) and a lack of interest in competitive sports. Disinterest in team sports may be due both to skill deficits and to spatial awareness problems that make it hard for them to get a sense of the game. Avoidance of sports is another factor that makes normal social interaction with their peer group difficult, especially as they get into adolescence and a lot of their peers' main interest will be sports. (Hint: those with AS sometimes like bowling.) Certainly they do better in individual rather than team sports, and often benefit from private rather than group instruction.

Despite their impressive vocabularies, those with AS can have communication problems because they tend to be literal and have difficulty with figurative language. They will follow instructions to the letter. This may get them in trouble, particularly at school. If a boy with AS is asked if he would like to do math now, he may just continue reading his book, believing he was being given a choice. Two more examples of taking things literally follow.

Six-year-old Michael, told by his teacher in first grade that she did not want to see him out of his seat, kept the seat of his chair pressed to his buttocks when he got up. Another first-grader named Sam, given the same admonition, went under the desks to get to the pencil sharpener. Both these children were confused when sent to the office. Each thought that the teacher did not see him out of his seat, and that he had sincerely tried to do as he was told.

Although they may be excellent readers and have prodigious memories for facts, students with AS have problems reading social cues, and thus struggle with reading comprehension when it involves emotional insight, innuendo, or inference. Words with double meanings can be very confusing, too. Given the sentence, "Mary tore up the letter and shed a tear." the child might wonder how you can shed a tear (reading 'tear' as the present tense of 'tore').

Mathematics is frequently the weakest subject due to weak spatial reasoning skills. Most people with AS just do not see the relationships in the number patterns so necessary for understanding many aspects of math. They also have trouble with money concepts, time concepts, and reading the clock. In this respect there is overlap in symptoms between AS and non-verbal learning disorder (NVLD), a learning style in which verbal IQ is much higher than performance IQ. Spatial reasoning weaknesses also mean they will have great difficulty with organizing themselves and their things. Though they may be obsessively tidy about their own collections of things of interest, be it model cars or Yugioh cards, you cannot just tell them to tidy their room because they will not know where to begin. Their desk or their locker will also be messy, and papers get lost in backpacks.

There is also overlap with pragmatic language disorder (PLD) since the speech and language differences are in practical applications; such things as holding conversations (they talk about their interests too much and fail to read non-verbal cues), tone of voice (loud or monotone), or failure to keep the other person's viewpoint in mind when explaining things.

John, an adolescent, spoke of a female teacher he enjoys, and his trainer remarked in a pleasant tone that Miss X. sounded like a nice person. When John described something nasty a male teacher did, the clinician used a different tone of voice and said, in a very sarcastic tone while shaking his head, "Boy! He's a nice guy!" John, missing the sarcasm in the trainer's voice, was completely confused as to why anyone would call this terrible man a nice guy.

Tony Attwood (2007) considers non-verbal learning disorder and pragmatic language disorder to be diagnoses equivalent to AS, just looked at from a particular perspective—that of a learning disabilities specialist, and that of a speech and language pathologist. We do differentiate, because those with NVLD usually have better social skills (though they may have problems with boundaries and invading other people's space), and those with PLD also have better social skills and do not have the motor clumsiness, such as difficulty tying shoelaces. Nor do they have the same emotional differences, such as having "melt-downs" if routines are changed, or the intense special interests.

In comparison to autism, there is an increased likelihood of seeking social interaction (Khouzam et al., 2004) and, as noted previously, some aspects of speech and language may be advanced in those with AS but are delayed or absent in those with autism.

For the most part, individuals with AS are very honest, and take people at their word. Perhaps this is a reflection of their being quite concrete and literal. They do not understand the unwritten rules of a social hierarchy. A third grade student with AS matter-of-factly told the supply teacher that she was not allowed to yell in the classroom. They may talk to a teacher as if they were equals rather than showing appropriate deference. They do not understand that there are sometimes exceptions to the rule.

> Jane fell and sprained her ankle in the school corridor. The strict rule at the school was that you never put your books on the radiator. Sam saw Jane fall, put his armful of books on the radiator, then helped Jane to stand up. John, a student with AS, was very upset and went into a tirade about Sam putting his books on the radiator.

The child with AS may appear bossy, may act like a little policeman, and may be called a *tattle-tale*. When others break the rules it upsets the person with AS. One boy in kindergarten was very well behaved except that he would cry when other children broke the rules. In general they are sweet, socially naïve children who do not present many problems in their pre-school years, but who have difficulty with peer interactions once they start school. They become more withdrawn, and often seem depressed in their teen years due to increasing social isolation and awareness of not "fitting in".

In contrast to their difficulties in initiating and maintaining peer group relationships, the mothers of AS clients often relate how good their child is with adults. She may tell you that he is polite and quite talkative, and that adults are often impressed by his verbal facility. With some of the brighter children you may note how they present like the "little professors" described by Asperger in his original paper. Although many, as adults, have problems with employment because their social skills lag so far behind their intellectual abilities, some will develop their special interests into careers, and may even become professors in a field where they possess vast, arcane knowledge. From a historical point of view, there has been a retrospective diagnosis of AS in Jonathan Swift, author of *Gulliver's Travels*, and the eccentric Dean of St. Patrick's Cathedral in Dublin (Fitzgerald, 2000).

Emotionally, AS clients appear to lack fine-tuning when reading and expressing emotion, and do not show the usual gradations of emotions. They do not react to situations where one would normally expect emotions but may overreact at other times, going quite suddenly from a placid stance to extreme anger or tears if upset by something, including things that seem trivial to others. They are very egocentric in their responses, and may appear to lack empathy. Sometimes sudden emotional changes or their odd behavior will get them labeled aggressive, and they may then be designated as behavioral problems. They make easy victims for teasing, bullying or extortion. They may copy behavior from books or television, not realizing it is inappropriate outside of that context. Since they lack street smarts, they are the ones "left holding the bag." With the promise of "I'll be your friend if you…" others can set them up to do things that get them laughed at or in trouble.

> Seven-year-old Michael was dared by the other boys to kiss Jane. He did, and was suspended from school for sexual harassment.

Those with AS have intense special interests, and are soothed by doing them, reading about them, or carrying around something related to them. Retreating into a special interest area is a way to cope and feel less anxious.

> One five-year-old, whose special interest was weather, took over the interview that had started with a remark about the rainy day and explained what a barometer was. Then he gave instructions for making one. Instead of cartoons on television, he watched the weather channel. Though only in kindergarten, he could read at a third grade level; he scanned the shelf full of attractive story books and then looked in the science section for something on meteorology.
> Fourteen-year-old Jason had a fascination with guns and could tell you the ballistic details of virtually any model, from rifles to handguns. He felt less anxious if he had his special toy, a miniature water pistol, in his pocket. This resulted in him being suspended from school for carrying what appeared to be a weapon into the classroom.

Unusual behavior is often the product of anxiety, or simply not knowing what the correct behavior is in a new situation.

> Eight-year-old Matt was taken to the airport to meet his grandparents. As soon as they appeared he was so excited that he broke away from his parents, ran up to his grandmother, and spat on her.

A change in routine may be very difficult, and they have trouble with transitions.

> Trevor had an older brother who would be dropped off first at his school and then Trevor was dropped off. When his older brother had a dentist appointment

and Mother tried to take Trevor to school first, he refused to get out of the car. Trevor became so upset and clearly anxious that finally mother had to drive around and drop the older brother off at his school, take Trevor to his school, and then drive back to get his brother to take him to the dentist.

Change or ambiguity is difficult and anxiety provoking for those with AS, and they have trouble making choices. Other students love field trips but those with AS dislike the change in routine. At our training center we have a large cabinet with all kinds of toys that can be purchased with the tokens earned during a child's training sessions. These children just cannot seem to make a choice. They save up an extremely large number of tokens, and may finally decide to get a certificate to purchase something at the mall, thus delaying making a choice even longer.

The attire of the person with AS may set them apart because they wear what is comfortable, rather than what is fashionable. (Tactile sensitivity plus anxiety in new situations means getting electrodes on the first time can be very difficult.) The teenager who wears sweat-pants to school when everyone else wears jeans likely has AS. This lack of sartorial acumen is due to a combination of sensory sensitivity and not reading fashion cues.

John was an adult who came to his first appointment with his baggy, unkempt, much too large trousers hitched up with braces. His first comment to the author was that she had made syntax errors when writing "The A.D.D. Book," which he had been perusing in the waiting room. He came for training because he wanted to improve his concentration for playing bridge, which he taught and played competitively. About 2 years after he finished his neurofeedback training he returned dressed so well he could have been a model for Brooks Brothers clothing. He had brought a magazine that featured his byline. Now, in addition to teaching bridge, he was writing a column on the social aspects of bridge for a glossy publication.

To get more of the flavor of people with this syndrome, read Tony Attwood's books *Asperger's Syndrome: A Guide for Parents* (1998) and *Asperger's Syndrome: The Complete Guide* (2007), or read anything by Lorna Wing. For a more informal rendition of the symptoms, rent the movie "About a Boy" starring Hugh Grant, enjoy the novel *The Curious Incident of the Dog in the Night-time* (Haddon, 2002) or the autobiographies *Pretending to Be Normal* (Willey, 1999) and *Born on a Blue Day* (Tammet, 2007).

III.   SECTION II: SYMPTOM CORRELATION WITH FUNCTIONAL NEUROANATOMY AND EEG FINDINGS

A.   Inattention and impulsivity: ADHD symptoms and signs

In our clinical experience (especially in the 1990s before AS was being broadly recognized), virtually all the children, and a majority of the adults, who were diagnosed with AS originally came for treatment due to ADHD symptoms that parents, partners, and others felt were seriously affecting their ability to progress in school or function at work or home (Simpson, 2004). A British study found that children, on average, were first diagnosed as having AS at age 11, and that they had had three previous assessments, usually with a diagnosis of ADHD, before they were diagnosed correctly (Wing, 2001). Other studies have confirmed the presence of ADHD symptoms in Asperger's syndrome (Corbett and Constantine, 2006). A person with AS is more in their own world, and demonstrates difficulties with attention span when expected to pay attention to something someone else thinks is important. Difficulties are both in sustaining attention and in filtering out extraneous data and shifting attention appropriately. Impulsivity, hyperactivity and hyper-focus on a personal area of interest are also symptoms that are often seen in both AS and ADHD clients. Steven barging in and asking about people's cars, mentioned above, was a good example of symptoms that overlap between the two disorders.

In the early years of doing NFB we were always careful to recognize the ADHD symptoms that had been responsible for the parents coming to the Center. We could reassure parents that we could identify specific EEG patterns associated with ADHD (Jantzen et al., 1995; Lubar, 1991; Mann et al., 1992), and suggest to the parents that, given the publications that have demonstrated the success of NFB to improve attention span, it was reasonable to expect an improvement in this area (Fuchs et al., 2003: Linden et al., 1996; Rossiter and LaVaque, 1995; Thompson and Thompson, 1998). It was also discussed with parents that, in our experience, improved attention span appeared to result in an improved ability to de-center; that is, see things from another's perspective, and focus on needs and feelings that others were expressing. Although we just aimed for improved attention, when children and adults with AS underwent NFB training, people also noted a change in their ability to socialize appropriately. In addition, the children appeared much more confident, and free of their former anxiety.

These observations led us to further investigate what was known about the pathophysiology of Asperger's, and to review where we had been placing the active electrode, and what frequency bands we had been enhancing and inhibiting when our primary objective in these early years had only been to decrease the co-morbid symptoms of ADHD. We were asking the question of what, neurophysiologically, was in common to both ADHD and Asperger's and, further, what was in common to both these disorders and anxiety?

B. Brain regions that underlie ADHD symptoms, and appropriate NFB training

Beauregard and Levesque (2006) reviewed the literature showing abnormal functioning of the anterior cingulate cortex (ACC), the prefrontal cortex, and the caudate in children with ADHD during tasks involving selective attention. They demonstrated that neurofeedback can normalize these areas as shown by pre- and post-functional magnetic resonance imaging (fMRI) in 15 students diagnosed with ADHD who received neurofeedback training as compared to five control subjects. The anterior cingulate has also been implicated in AS because it is involved in appropriate shifting and fixating of attention.

In one study, Landry and Bryson (2004) showed that children with ASDs, when compared to normal children, and even to children with Down's syndrome, have a distinct difficulty with attention. They demonstrated that, once attention was first engaged on a central fixation stimulus, persons with autistic spectrum disorder had a marked difficulty in disengaging their attention in order to shift attention to a second stimulus. Belmonte's group (Belmonte and Yurgelun-Todd, 2003) studied visual selective attention comparing autistic subjects with normals. They noted that, in autism, physiological indices of selective attention are abnormal even in situations where behavior is intact. They used functional magnetic resonance imaging (fMRI) while subjects performed a bilateral, visual-spatial attention task. In normal subjects, the task evoked activation in a network of cortical regions including the superior parietal lobe. The subjects with ASD differed from normal activation patterns.

These studies parallel our EEG observations that clients with AS show EEG differences from the normal data base, and that the source of the abnormal activity, as determined by LORETA, is similarly in those locations: the anterior cingulate gyrus, the superior temporal gyrus, and the parietal cortex.

The use of NFB to train the brain to sustain attention has been well established, starting with the work of psychologists M. Barry Sterman and Joel Lubar in the early 1970s. Sterman in the late 1960s established that operant conditioning of brain wave activity in cats was possible. Cats could be trained to increase spindles of 12–15 Hz activity. He named this activity *sensorimotor rhythm* (SMR) because it was seen across the sensorimotor cortex, and was associated with diminished sensory input and motor output; that is, seen in an alert, still cat that was waiting for a signal before making a response. The SMR activity originated in the thalamus, and projected to the sensorimotor cortex.

The thalamus is the major source of rhythmic activity, including alpha (8–12 Hz), theta (4–8 Hz), and SMR (12–15 Hz). These frequency ranges are key ones used in NFB training paradigms, particularly those that address ADHD and seizure disorders. More recently, high amplitude, high frequency beta (>20 Hz usually) has also been implicated in the symptoms of inattention (Chabot and Serfontein, 1996; Chabot *et al.*, 2001; Clarke *et al.*, 2001; Thompson and Thompson, 2006). We also frequently observe this high frequency beta in clients with AS and other ASDs. Beta spindling refers to spindle-like bursts of high amplitude, synchronous beta in a very narrow (often single Hz) frequency band in the beta range. Beta spindling appears to be a cortical phenomenon that may signal cortical instability (Gibbs and Knott, 1949; Gibbs and Gibbs, 1950). However, it also appears in clients who complain of ADHD plus anxiety, or show manic or ASD symptoms. In these persons it correlates with a busy brain that may interfere with attention span; that is, they are distracted by inner worries or ruminations, or they get stuck on things.

Often we note a dip in amplitude around 14 Hz over the central area of the cortex. When this is observed we have acted on the hypothesis, following Sterman's work, that it may correlate with reduced sensorimotor rhythm (SMR) being produced by the thalamus. We have used NFB as a method for assisting the client to raise the average amplitude of the 13–15 Hz frequency band over the sensory-motor cortex. The result has been a decrease in impulsivity and hyperactivity. It also is associated with less tactile sensitivity and less distractibility. In addition, we have emphasized using NFB to raise SMR in those clients who presented with very high amplitude high frequency beta (the so-called *busy-brain pattern*) and a high (>1.55) 23–35 Hz /13–15 Hz ratio (Thompson and Thompson, 2006). These clients improved.

It appears possible that one method for improving the stability of the cortex may be this SMR training (Sterman, 2000a). In addition, pairing the NFB training with BFB methods to reduce sympathetic drive, and thus normalize the limbic-cortical-hypothalamic-adrenal axis has been effective. In particular, respiration and heart rate variability training appear to accelerate the acquisition of self-regulation skills in clients who present with the combination of ADHD and anxiety symptoms. The combination of NFB, BFB and strategies improves client performance in sessions and, eventually, in everyday life. (More of this is discussed below under the topic of anxiety.)

Some clients with ADHD exhibit very low arousal in relatively boring situations. They can actually fall asleep in the classroom or at work. In sessions when they suddenly feel sleepy (usually in association with having work of a boring or difficult nature to do) their electrodermal response (EDR) level drops dramatically. In this group we have used EDR feedback (also called SC for skin conductance). They have learned to sustain their normal awake and aroused EDR level while also maintaining other biofeedback measurements at a healthy level, such as heart rate variability (HRV) levels that indicate that they are calm and relaxed. For excellent explications concerning heart rate variability read recent publications by Gevirtz (2007), and by Gevirtz and Lehrer (2005).

There is one caveat to increasing SMR. When doing EEG feedback, we have been careful not to reward the 13–15 Hz activity at Cz or FCz if our assessment at these sites already demonstrated a very high amplitude 14 Hz. This has been observed in some clients who have co-morbidity of depression and ADHD. It can be a very high amplitude spindling beta rather than true SMR, and this has also been observed in a small number of both adults and children who were very impulsive. This is an unusual finding but, when present, rewarding 14–15 Hz can rather rapidly make these clients much worse. We had made the assumption that this beta was not really SMR originating from the thalamus and, indeed, in recent years when the assessment included LORETA, we found that this beta or spindling beta originated from Brodmann area 24 in the anterior cingulate gyrus. Clearly these complex clients with spindling beta also had anxiety symptoms, and this leads us into the next section.

C. Anxiety and the modulation of affect responses

Although anxiety is often mentioned as a common co-morbidity with ADHD, especially in adults, in AS it is even more important. It is a central symptom. Usually there is a combination of anxiety and a deficiency in the ability to modulate affective responses to what appear to others to be minor stressors. In part, anxiety may be related to difficulty in distinguishing abstraction, innuendo and social meaning, which results in defensive withdrawal from emotionally laden social situations. That would be the psychodynamic explanation but, in terms of brain function, there appears to be atypical activation in areas of the brain related to anxiety such as the anterior cingulate gyrus. Attempts to cope with anxiety may result in other presentations of symptoms, as seen in disorders that have anxiety at their core, for example obsessive-compulsive disorder (OCD) and social anxiety disorder.

Having observed the overlap between anxiety, worry with ruminations, and ADHD symptoms in both adults and children, we looked for EEG patterns at Cz (children) and/or FCz (adults) associated with these symptoms, and found that it was beta, often a spindling beta, at frequencies above 19 Hz with the particular band width being specific to each client. When we reviewed the records of those clients who had also had a LORETA analysis of their 19-channel EEG we found a consistent pattern. The anterior cingulate gyrus, Brodmann area 24 was the source of the high frequency beta activity that was outside the Neuroguide database norms. Frequently the bursts of beta in the surface EEG appeared to be beta spindling (high amplitude, narrow frequency range, synchronous beta), which we named a *busy-brain pattern* (Thompson and Thompson, 2006).

Whenever high amplitude, high frequency beta is observed we recommend that the client discover what mental state is associated with increasing it, and then decrease it. Most clients find that decreasing it using NFB at FCz is associated with a calm state without anxiety and ruminations. Clients who show this activity are not necessarily AS; it is also helpful for athletes who engage in negative self-talk or people coming in for stress management (Thompson and Thompson, 2007).

Figure 15.1 is an example of beta spindling in a child with moderate Asperger's syndrome plus ADHD symptoms. He was an anxiously polite boy. The spindling beta in this nine-year-old boy's record, seen at Cz, was consistently at 20 Hz.

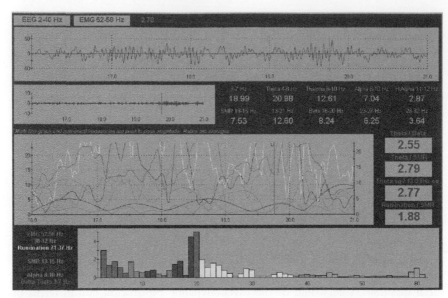

FIGURE 15.1   Beta spindling, 20 Hz; eyes-open is seen using the Infiniti instrument (Thought Technology) and the "Clinical Success" assessment screen (Thompson and Thompson, 1995) (see color plate).

This boy trained down both the 20 Hz beta at Cz and his 4–8 Hz theta while increasing SMR (13–15 Hz). Clinically he improved during training. Interestingly his draw-a-person, always an interesting aspect of our pre- and post-assessment, changed from a tiny almost stick person to a full smiling figure. His theta/beta power ratio $(4–8)^2/(13–21)^2$ ratio dropped from 8.23 to 5.57. His attention quotient on the integrated visual auditory continuous performance test (IVA) improved from a standard score of 80 before training to 100 (mid-average) on testing done after 40 sessions.

That reducing spindling beta, whose source is in the anterior cingulate (AC), helps people with AS should not be any surprise given the functions associated with the AC. Devinsky and his colleagues in 1995 did an excellent summary of the functions and the connections of the anterior cingulate, that banana shaped structure that wraps around the upper side of the corpus callosum. He and others have noted that the AC appears to be central to affect regulation and control. It has executive functions, and it is critical in areas of attention and concentration (Devinsky et al., 1995). But the AC is also well connected to areas in the limbic network including: amaygdala, periaqueductal gray, autonomic brain stem motor nuclei, ventral striatum, orbitofrontal and anterior insular cortices, and to the mirror neuron system (Carr et al., 2003).

The amygdala can assess the motivational content of, and assign emotional valence to, internal and external stimuli, while the medial frontal cortex controls the behavioral responses. The AC may be thought of as the 'hub' of affective control, and of decision-making. The AC regulates context-dependent behaviors.

It regulates emotional responses and behavior through the autonomic nervous system (ANS), endocrine functions, and conditioned emotional learning. The mirror neuron system in conjunction with the limbic cortex is key to our understanding of the autistic spectrum disorders that include Asperger's syndrome.

The amygdala-hypothalamus-pituitary-adrenal (AHPA) axis (see *The Neurofeedback Book*, Thompson and Thompson, 2003b, pp. 106–108) controls the automatic and unconscious aspects of the stress response. This response system is controlled by interaction between brain stem nuclei (including autonomic nervous system nuclei and the locus coeruleus) and the limbic-hypothalamus-pituitary-adrenal axis (LHPA). The frontal lobes and hippocampus have a major influence on this axis through connections to the anterior cingulate, amygdala and hypothalamus. These are the neuroanatomical connections of the cingulum and the uncinate fasciculus.

Cz and FCz are the surface sites that best reflect activity in "affective" areas of the AC. Interestingly, we had been having success in lowering both ADHD symptoms and symptoms related to anxiety when we used a Cz or FCz site to train down frequencies that were high amplitude compared to the rest of the client's EEG (typically theta 3–7 Hz or low alpha 8–10 Hz, and/or high frequency beta in the range 20–35 Hz), and train up sensorimotor rhythm (12–15 or 13–15 Hz, depending on the client's profile). Other symptoms, such as obsessive thinking, also decreased. In some clients this was related to anxiety, and at times a diagnosis of obsessive-compulsive disorder (OCD) was made. The reader should refer to the work of E. Roy John and Leslie Prichep for more about EEG patterns in OCD (Prichep *et al.*, 1993; Prichep and John, 1992).

In clients with AS, they all have intense special areas of interest, and that symptom may also relate to the AC and its connections. The training that we were doing not only decreased the symptoms of ADHD and anxiety-related symptoms but it improved the AS client's ability to modulate their affective responses. The example of Steven above is a good one. Instead of racing from office to office and immediately demanding that people answer questions related to his special area of interest (i.e., cars), he was able to enter the Center calmly and wait patiently until the trainer was ready for him. He even seemed to understand subtle social cues, which leads to the next area for discussion.

D.   Empathy and affect interpretation and expression

Clients with AS display both sensory and motor aprosodia. Sensory aprosodia refers to an inability to correctly interpret social innuendo, either verbal or non-verbal; that is, they do not get the messages conveyed by tone of voice or gestures. Sensory aprosodia resulting from neurological damage has been reviewed by Ross (1981). Like AS clients, these individuals often cannot copy emotional tones of sadness or happiness. Motor aprosodia refers to an inability to use emotionally appropriate vocal tones in conversation. Research has demonstrated the difficulties adolescents have with humorous materials. Emerich found that the ability of adolescents with Asperger's syndrome to comprehend humorous material, such as picking funny endings for cartoons and jokes, was significantly impaired (Emerich *et al.*, 2003).

At our Center, a study was done to compare children with AS to a normal school group in terms of reactions to reading happy stories. The Asperger's group, as measured by self-report using an adjective check list describing their mood, done before and after reading the passage, did not show a shift towards positive emotion. It was found that, after NFB training, the children with Asperger's did identify more adjectives that signified positive mood in the same way as matched normal controls (Martinez, 2003). An example of these difficulties in an AS client was 19-year-old Brian.

In his early sessions Brian would watch people and, if someone told a joke, he would see others smiling and laughing, and then he would burst into a forced laugh. After 40 neurofeedback sessions to decrease high frequency beta activity originating in the anterior cingulate at Brodmann area 24 (seen with LORETA analysis of the 19-channel QEEG and observed in the surface EEG at FCz), Brian not only picked up on humor and laughed appropriately, but he was also telling truly funny stories and jokes. Interestingly, staff were independently commenting to the author that they actually felt that Brian was showing empathy, and truly understanding of how others were feeling. His parents also noted this.

Theoretically the FCz NFB might have influenced both the anterior cingulate and the medial prefrontal frontal cortex. Certainly this training would have addressed the beta spindling observed at FCz. The electrode was referenced to the right ear because Brian, similar to the majority of our AS clients, demonstrated high amplitude, low frequency alpha at T6 compared to T5. Our assumption has been that this high amplitude alpha (in some clients it will be low amplitude beta 14–17 Hz) corresponded to relative inactivity at this site in the right hemisphere—an area involved in processing the emotional tone of language and gestures as well as spatial information.

But how would training at a central location account for the success of NFB at these right hemisphere sites that relate to the primary symptoms of sensory and motor aprosodia? A decrease in the symptoms of sensory aprosodia (right temporal-parietal cortex dysfunction), which is a key dysfunction in Asperger's, might have a relatively simple explanation. We had been referencing to the right ear (or right mastoid) in some of the overanxious AS clients. All training with a referential montage ("bipolar") is done with the assumption that the ear reference electrode will show minimal EEG activity. Could it be that the very high amplitude slow waves in the T6 region were picked up by the ear electrode (through volume conduction), and were being inhibited by our training, albeit without us initially intending to have this effect?

However, this would not explain the changes observed in emotional tone (motor aprosodia). An alternative, or perhaps complementary, explanation is that we were normalizing the AC's EEG activity, and that this had effects on many areas of the cortex, including the parietal temporal junction, and even the right frontal area where dysfunction corresponds to motor aprosodia. Note that this area in the right frontal lobe may also be a mirror neuron area.

Recent work on mirror neurons (Iacoboni and Dapretto, 2006) notes the strong connections of these neurons to the limbic system, including the AC. Frontal cortex mirror neurons (emphasis on imitation and on intention and goal of actions) are found in the pars opercularis. The dorsal portion of the pars opercularis has a "mirror" function while the ventral portion may correlate with prediction of the sensory consequences of a motor action. This area is in the posterior inferior frontal cortex (the homologous site in the left hemisphere would be posterior Broca's area near F5) and the adjacent ventral prefrontal cortex. Parietal mirror neurons (emphasis on motoric description of action) are found in the rostral portion of the inferior parietal lobule.

The visual input (description of action, matching of imitation plan to the description of the observed action) to the mirror neuron system (MNS) comes from the posterior sector of the superior temporal sulcus. The MNS system is at the core of social learning, and appears to be responsible for the imitation of appropriate social interactions as well as for understanding the behavior and intentions of others. An fMRI study demonstrated that activity of the MNS is correlated with empathic concern and interpersonal competence (Pfeifer *et al.*, 2005).

The importance of imitation in social learning has been well described (Meltzoff and Prinz, 2002). Imitation can be directly linked to the MNS. Structural abnormalities have been found in the MNS system in autistic spectrum disorders and are significant in understanding ASD (Hadjikhani *et al.*, 2006). Delayed conductivity in the MNS for imitation has been found in ASD (Nishitani *et al.*, 2004). It has also been shown that children with ASD have reduced activity in MNS regions during tasks that require the child to mirror facial expressions of different emotions (Dapretto *et al.*, 2006). Given these findings it is not surprising that deficiencies in this system are being hypothesized to be a core deficit in ASD.

Given the clear relationship of the MNS to ASD, it seems reasonable to hypothesize that normalizing what we have termed the *hub* of the affective nervous system, the AC, may have been responsible for the normalizing of the sensory aprosodia symptoms in clients with Asperger's who did training at our Center. It may also explain why resolution of ASD symptoms takes longer (60–80 or more sessions) than resolution of ADHD (40–60 sessions) because the influence over the involved area of the cortex is less direct. Perhaps the NFB has had its positive effects by changing the responsiveness of the MNS. We postulate that this may be

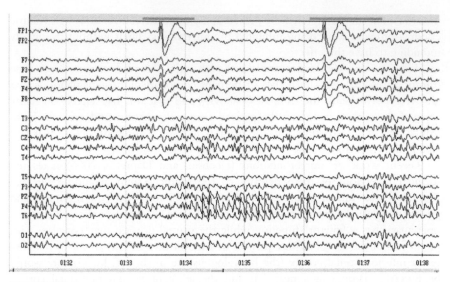

FIGURE 15.2   (Eyes-open, linked-ear reference, 19-channel EEG) T6 and P4 show bursts of high amplitude slow wave 10 Hz activity. Contrast these sites with T5 and P3 where this resting activity is not observed.

why, in most cases, we have not had to use NFB to directly activate the T6 area to ameliorate sensory aprosodia, F6 to assist in treating motor aprosodia, or F5 to more directly improve empathy.

Figure 15.2 is an example of the slowing so often seen in the right temporal-parietal area when 19-lead EEG assessments are done in people with AS.

In addition to the high amplitude theta (3–7 Hz) or low frequency alpha (8–10 Hz) activity frequently observed at T6, another observation that may help us identify some Asperger's clients could be the "mu" rhythm response. Mu occurs in the same frequency range as alpha but has a slightly different morphology: one end of the waveform will be pointed rather than rounded, and it is sometimes called a *wicket rhythm* due to this shape. Recent research involving mirror neurons suggests that mu may prove to be a helpful index of MNS impairment in ASD (Ramachandran and Oberman, 2006). In ASD there is a reduction in mu rhythm suppression during action observation (Oberman *et al.*, 2005). Although lack of appropriate mu suppression may be a helpful indicator of difficulty copying others, because mu is typically measured at C3 and C4 it is not often observed when the training is done at the vertex (CZ) as described above. That training has been successful. Thus, for the present, mu has not become a target for NFB training at our Center, which has a clinical focus and thus stays with interventions that have shown their effectiveness, though mu will doubtless prove an interesting focus for research centers.

Figure 15.3 schematically, although simplistically, illustrates relationships between ADHD symptoms, anxiety, Asperger's symptoms, and the anterior cingulate.

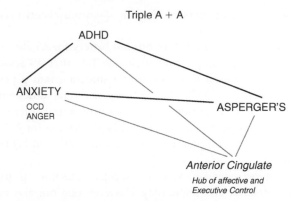

FIGURE 15.3   This figure emphasizes the central importance of the anterior cingulate in disorders that have in common clinically significant anxiety symptoms.

E.   Executive function difficulties

Executive functioning requires the individual to integrate sensory information inputs, inhibit what might be immediate responses, and take the time to evaluate the inputs, formulate a plan of action that best uses all the available information, shift mental set to view the information from different points of view, initiate a response, and then monitor and evaluate the results of that response. All of this requires a good working memory, an intact frontal lobe, and good communication between parietal and frontal regions. The reader will note that a number of these functions are subsumed under the rubric of cingulate gyrus function by Devinsky, as discussed above (Devinsky *et al.*, 1995). Others are considered functions of the dorsolateral frontal cortex.

AS clients do not seem to integrate all of these functions together easily, and executive functioning may be impaired in many clients with AS. One test that seems to address a number of the functions subsumed under the term *executive functioning* is the Tower of London (ToL), (or Tower of Hanoi) test. This test is difficult for those with ASDs. The ToL requires the subject to move colored rings that are placed over three pegs of progressively shorter height, to match the arrangement on the examiner's pegs. The test requires the subject to inhibit immediate response, plan, shift mental set, use working memory, initiate a response, and then monitor and evaluate the results of that response. The required cognitive functions all depend on good prefrontal functioning. Interestingly, this prefrontal area is one that is also seen to be outside EEG database norms in our clients with Asperger's.

This dysfunction is not unique to autistic spectrum clients, but is also found in clients with other frontal lobe problems including head trauma, ADHD, obsessive-compulsive disorder (OCD), and Tourette's syndrome. Another test that is also difficult is the Wisconsin card-sorting test. This requires the subject shift mental set mid test, and try sorting the cards according to a new "rule" (from sorting by, say, shape, to sorting by color or number). Autistic spectrum clients perseverate, and find it very difficult to shift mental set.

We have started to include the ToL in our test battery for AS clients, and a pilot study has shown significant improvements in the ToL after 40 sessions of NFB training. (Reported by Bojana Knezevic in her student award paper at the ToL annual meeting, September, 2007). The NFB was the same as described above at Cz for the children, and FCz for the adults. At least three studies have reported IQ gains of 10–12 points in people who received NFB training for ADHD (Linden *et al.*, 1996; Lubar, 1991; Thompson and Thompson, 1998), and IQ tests certainly tap executive functions.

Perhaps the improvement on tests of executive functions is partly due to improvements in attention and impulsivity. However, one can also posit that the improvements seen in ADHD symptoms are, to a large part, due to improved executive functioning and/or decreased anxiety. It has to always be acknowledged how little we really know. However, although we will remain theorizing about the 'why,' the results of NFB plus BFB and metacognitive strategies are becoming indisputable. Clients who complete their training and demonstrate EEG changes improve by self report, by parent questionnaires, and on objectively measured parameters such as: ToL, WISC (or WAIS), wide range achievement test, and the test of variables of attention (TOVA). This same measured improvement has not been demonstrated with other treatment modalities, such as combinations of medications, psychotherapies, educational intervention, and behavior modification for clients with AS.

IV. SECTION III: REGIONS OF THE BRAIN IDENTIFIED AS DYSFUNCTIONAL IN AS

In the foregoing discussion of the major groups of symptoms addressed using NFB we touched upon different brain areas that might be responsible for the observed symptoms. Here we will briefly expand on those discussions and suggest that, if there is a common axis of disturbed functioning in addition to the anterior cingulate, this axis probably includes the seven areas listed in the introduction. In our clients with AS, using QEEG assessment and LORETA, one or more of these seven areas has shown frequency band activity outside the database norms using Robert Thatcher's Neuroguide program (Neuroguide Delux, 2.3.7, 2007).

In the recent research literature on autistic spectrum disorders, the seven areas of the brain that are repeatedly found to differ when compared to people with typical development are:

A. Prefrontal cortex (the medial and orbital surfaces).
B. Hippocampal gyrus.
C. Amygdala with connections to the orbital and medial frontal areas of the brain.
D. Fusiform gyrus.

E. Superior temporal gyrus containing the auditory cortex.

F. Anterior insula and the anterior cingulate, Brodmann areas (BA) 24 or 25 for affect gating (both are part of the limbic system, the emotional brain).

G. Frontal and Parietal-Temporal Mirror Neuron areas.

Our practical interest in these findings, which come from research using a variety of imaging techniques, is that the lack of normal functioning in these critical areas of the brain can also be seen using a QEEG assessment with LORETA.

A. Prefrontal cortex

Shamay-Tsoory and colleagues note that prefrontal lesions resulted in significant impairment in irony and faux pas. The important areas are the orbito-frontal and/or ventromedial areas of the prefrontal cortex (but not the dorsolateral areas) (Shamay-Tsoory *et al.*, 2005). In contrast to the patient who has damage to the amygdala, who cannot correctly understand the significance of another person's anger or aggressive behavior, the patient with orbital-frontal damage recognizes the significance of other people's emotions but may fail to modulate their behavior as the social situation changes. This kind of impairment, when combined with amygdala dysfunction, could lead to difficulty in correctly recognizing the intentions of others and, theoretically, this could lead to inappropriate behavior (Bachevalier and Loveland, 2006).

Wing notes that, as early as 1966, a positron emission tomography (PET) study demonstrated that, unlike normal subjects, those with Asperger's syndrome did not show activity in the left medial prefrontal cortex during tasks that required them to consider what might be going on in another person's mind (Wing, 2001). This finding corresponds to our discussion above on decreased empathy. Nikolaenko (2004) found that problems in metaphorical thinking are associated with decreased right hemisphere functioning. Frontal lobe dysfunction in Asperger's was also noted by Shelley Channon (2004). In her research she finds that impairments in real-life problem-solving is associated with left anterior frontal lobe lesions. Her findings fit our discussion on deficiencies in executive functioning.

B. Hippocampal cortex—medial temporal cortex

Salmond and his colleagues (2005) have noted that studies of mnemonic function in high functioning autistic spectrum disorders (ASD) have suggested a profile of impaired episodic memory with relative preservation of semantic memory. Such a pattern is consistent with a hippocampal abnormality. In these subjects imaging studies have measured gray matter density in the junction area involving the amygdala, hippocampus, and entorhinal cortex. Differences from normal were found that corresponded to this type of impaired mnemonic function. This might also be consistent with our common EEG findings of uncus, amygdala, and/or hippocampus being the source for activity that registers extreme compared to the normative database.

Structural abnormalities were also seen in these studies in the medial temporal lobes. Gunkelman notes that intense negative experiences increase cortisol release from the adrenal cortex, and that this can adversely affect the hippocampus, which has immune receptors. Because the hippocampus also functions as a memory comparator, which is required for both comprehension and recall, learning may be severely affected by stress (Johnstone *et al.*, 2007). We have noted above the importance of recognizing the effects of stress and anxiety in Asperger's. All these observations appear to support the importance of the hippocampus in ASDs.

In our QEEG evaluations, we consistently find EEG differences from the DBM in the temporal lobe regions, including the hippocampus, in our clients with AS and ASD. It is therefore always of interest to find studies done using other research technologies that implicate this area.

C. Amygdala

Richard Davidson and his group at the Institute for the Study of Emotion, in NIMH-funded studies, have published findings related to the amygdala. This is of great interest because, when using LORETA, we often see the amygdala showing EEG frequency bands being more than two standard deviations from the neuroguide (NG) database mean (DBM). Davidson in one study notes that: "Those in the autism group who had a small amygdala were significantly slower at identifying happy, angry, or sad facial expressions and spent the least time looking at eyes relative to other facial regions. Autistic subjects with the smallest amygdalae took 40% longer than those with the largest fear hubs to recognize such emotional facial expressions." Furthermore, "the autism subjects with small amygdala had the most non-verbal social impairment as children" (Nacewicz *et al.*, 2006).

Studies have also shown that irrational social behavior and social disinhibition result from amygdala damage (Adolphs, 2003), and that the human amygdala is critical for the retrieval of socially relevant knowledge on the basis of facial information (Adolphs *et al.*, 2005).

D. Fusiform gyrus

Using LORETA we often see abnormal EEG amplitudes in the right and/or left fusiform gyrus. This area has been implicated in face recognition. Davidson's research has shown that autistic subjects have reduced activation of this face-processing area on both sides of their brains while performing a face-processing task, whereas their well siblings showed this difference only on the right side. Davidson and his colleagues feel that this suggests an "intermediate pattern" in the siblings (Dalton *et al.*, 2005).

E. Temporal-parietal junction and the auditory cortex

We have discussed this area when referring to sensory aprosodia above. Anatomically this area at the junction of the parietal and temporal lobes includes part of the angular gyrus and, in the right hemisphere, it is a site homologous to Wernicke's area in the left hemisphere. It corresponds in part to Brodmann area 39. The angular gyrus merges with the supramarginal gyrus, and is at the junction of visual, auditory and touch centers. It is known to contain cells with mirror neuron properties (Ramachandran and Oberman, 2006). The auditory cortex's function is in part to integrate diverse pieces of auditory information. In the left hemisphere dysfunction of the auditory cortex in the superior temporal lobe could lead to difficulties integrating diverse inputs into one meaningful whole.

F. Anterior insula and the anterior cingulate

The anterior insula and the anterior cingulate are both part of the limbic system (the emotional brain). We have discussed the importance of this area in both ADHD and anxiety symptoms, and noted Devinsky's summary in 1995 of the functions and connections of the AC in the section above on anxiety (Devinsky, *et al.*, 1995). The involvement of these areas in the mirror neuron system is reported by Carr who states that the AC is well connected to the insula and the amygdala and, with them, to other areas of the limbic network, and to the mirror neuron system (Carr *et al.*, 2003).

G. Mirror neuron areas

The areas described above are all connected to frontal, parietal, and temporal mirror neuron areas in what is called the mirror neuron system (MNS). Mirror neurons are groups of neurons that fire when a person is watching and mentally mirroring the actions of another person. Young children learn to mirror and reflect the behavior and feelings of others, starting with their mother. Think of how intently a baby watches its mother's face; within a few weeks of birth a baby will start to mirror the expressions of the caregiver when held face-to-face in their lap. This mirroring system is crucial for the young child in order to understand the intentions and meanings of other people as expressed through non-verbal communication. The MNS is postulated to be responsible for the imitation of movements, and perhaps also to copying appropriate social interactions, as well as being necessary for understanding the behavior and intentions of others.

F. Other theories to explain AS symptoms

The mirror neuron system deficiencies do not account for some of the other symptoms that are seen in autistic children, such as repetitive movements, the need to maintain sameness, and the hypersensitivity to sounds or to touch. Ramachandran and colleagues have therefore put forth a further theory that they labeled the *salience landscape theory*. They note the importance of the amygdala, and suggest that pathways from the sensory areas of the brain to the amygdala may be altered in ASD, resulting in extreme emotional responses to minimal stimuli. In effect, the individual with an ASD cannot distinguish salient from non-salient aspects of incoming information. They have suggested that self-stimulation might actually dampen these extreme responses and be self-therapeutic for the child (Ramachandran and Oberman, 2006, 2007). At our Center, parietal and amygdala regions are both found to be outside the neuroguide database norms when a 19-channel QEEG and LORETA analysis are done.

British researchers have focused on three functional groupings to cover the symptoms:

1. Theory of mind (really theory of other's minds)
2. Central coherence (not to be confused with EEG coherence)
3. Executive dysfunction (Hill and Frith, 2003).

The theory-of-mind hypothesis proposes that a fault in any component of the social brain can lead to an inability to understand aspects of social communication (Abu-Akel, 2003; Dissanayake and Macintosh, 2003). These children do not "read" the intentions of others, and may be gullible, literal and concrete, as described earlier in this chapter. The examples given in Hill and Frith's paper are also well worth reading (Hill and Frith, 2003). These authors describe possible malfunction in the medial prefrontal cortex, (anterior paracingulate cortex), the temporal-parietal junction, and the temporal poles. These are also areas referred to in the above discussion of mirror neurons. The amygdala may also be involved so there is overlap with the salience landscape theory. They mention findings of less connectivity between the occipital and temporal regions, and that is a finding that we observe using coherence analysis in the EEG. It should be recognized that this theory does not account for the difficulty in recognition of faces that can correspond to deficits in the fusiform gyrus, another area that is often observed to be outside database norms using surface EEG and LORETA.

Weak central coherence refers to a lack of appropriate connectivity between the posterior sensory processing areas of the brain and the more frontal areas that modulate responses to the sensory input ('top-down' modulation). One result of this dysfunction may be piecemeal recall, rather than a recall that shows an understanding of the total context (Brock *et al.*, 2002). Brock's group proposed that this could result from a reduction in the integration of specialized local neural networks in the brain caused by a deficit in temporal binding (synchronized high-frequency gamma activity) between local networks. They feel that temporal binding deficits could also contribute to executive dysfunction in autism, and to some of the deficits in socialization and communication.

Hill states that one cause of this deficit could be a failure of normal developmental 'pruning' in early life, pruning that eliminates faulty brain connections and optimizes the coordination of neural functioning. This could be one neural basis for the apparent perceptual overload experienced by these individuals. This overload may, in turn, be partly responsible for their 'autistic' withdrawal. Withdrawal from social interaction, and focusing on a narrow area of interest, results in a reduction of the quantity of unpredictable sensory inputs.

Executive dysfunction is the third cognitive theory discussed by Hill and Frith (2003). As we noted above, executive functioning appears to be impaired in autistic spectrum clients. One test that seems to address many of the functions subsumed under the term *executive functioning* is the Tower of London (ToL), also called Tower of Hanoi, test. We have previously described how this test requires the client to inhibit initial responses, plan, shift mental set, use working memory, and monitor their moves. It has been shown to be difficult for those with autism or Asperger's. All the required cognitive functions depend on good prefrontal functioning.

G. The polyvagal theory

The polyvagal theory developed by Stephen Porges (2003) provides the context for explaining how social engagement, in general, can go awry, as manifested in a number of disorders. Porges (2004) explains how the vagus, whose name means *wandering nerve*, can be the mediator of behavioral and physiologic features associated with autism. His theory helps in the understanding of the neural underpinnings of the symptoms observed in the continuum of autistic spectrum disorders, including Asperger's syndrome (Dykema, 2006; Porges, 2003, 2004, 2007). This theory emphasizes dysfunction in autonomic regulation, and forces us to move away from our attempts to relate specific deficiencies in AS to specific cortical defects by stressing the complex circuits involved in behavior. Functional neuroanatomy should not become a twenty-first century version of phrenology.

Porges describes how three phylogenic levels of development relate to three autonomic nervous system circuits that are kept inconstant balance. They involve:

1. The primitive, unmyelinated vagus.
2. The ergotropic (energy generating) sympatheic nervous system.
3. The tropotropic (calming down) parasympathetic myelinated vagus.

Porges' theory emphasizes holistic understanding of the human organism as elucidated by Walter Hess, who said in his address when receiving the Nobel Prize for Medicine and Physiology in 1949, "Every living organism is not the sum of a multitude of unitary processes, but is, by virtue of interrelationships and of higher and lower levels of control, an unbroken unity." The challenge is to integrate some understanding of dysfunction in discrete cortical regions, as discussed above, with differences in the client's autonomic nervous system (ANS), both the sympathetic and parasympathetic branches.

Porges' theory helps us look at the feedback loops between the cortical areas discussed previously and the interaction of structures in the diencephalon, corpus striatum, midbrain, and brain stem regions that control the ANS. He has shown how a fundamental deficiency in people along the autism continuum is the misinterpretation of a neutral environment as being threatening. He shows that this deficiency can change normal ANS vagal activity and result in the symptoms observed in the ASDs, such as withdrawal from social interaction.

The polyvagal theory underscores the broader understanding of mind–body connections, and posits that many of the symptoms observed in children with ASD are not to be interpreted as being solely related to cortical deficiencies. That everything is cortically based might be surmised from an emphasis on the mirror neuron system and, in particular, on the anterior cingulate (anxiety and attention, and links to the entire limbic system), the left frontal cortex (F5) involvement in empathy and in understanding the intentions of others, the right parietal temporal junction for an understanding of sensory aprosodia, and the right frontal (F6) area for motor aprosodia. We must now broaden this approach and see that each of these symptoms, and other symptoms such as not "hearing" others (which requires using the strapesius muscle of the middle ear) also involves complex interactions of cortical deficiencies with structures within the diencephalon, corpus striatum, midbrain and brainstem regions, and thus various levels of the ANS.

In our earlier discussions we emphasized how the AC seems central to our understanding in that it connects to the amygdala, and to all of the cortical areas that are involved in the mirror neuron system. The AC also connects to the nucleus ambiguus, giving it control over aspects of the vagal parasympathetic efferents controlling such important physiological functions as heart rate, while it receives vagal afferent feedback from such organs as the heart from connections relayed through the nucleus solitarus in the medulla of the brain stem. Given these two points of emphasis we can better understand why BFB of, for example, HRV, will influence many of the symptoms seen in clients with AS via the vagal afferents to the brain stem. The vagal afferent sensory information is conveyed from the medullary nucleus of the solitary tract to the parabrachial nucleus and the locus coeruleus. These nuclei connect to the forebrain with links to the hypothalamus and amygdala, and thereby providing thalamic connections to the insula, orbito-frontal and prefrontal areas, all of which give feedback to the anterior cingulate.

One of these direct AC connections is to the brain stem nuclei and, in particular, to the nuclei controlling the ANS, such as the nucleus ambiguous and the nucleus of the solitary tract in the medulla. These nuclei control the autonomic nervous system including the parasympathetic myelinated fibers that are linked to the cranial nerves that control facial expression, vocalization, and even listening.

Dysfunction in this parasympathetic system may be an additional way in which we can better understand difficulties that AS clients have with 'hearing' emotional tone, listening to what others are trying to express, showing emotion through facial expression, and demonstrating emotion in their own tone of voice.

There is a balance between the anabolic and calming functions associated with parasympathetic (vagal) system and the catabolic and emergency reactions of the sympathetic system. Neurophysiologically, in response to threat, the central nucleus of the amygdala stimuates the dorsolateral periaqueductal gray, and activates the sympathetic system rostrally for fight or caudally for flight. In a safe environment the fusiform gyrus and the superior temporal gyrus actively inhibit the central nucleus of the amygdala so that the primitive sympathetic defensive systems are not activated, and the parasympathetic system predominates, thus allowing for social behaviors.

When there is dysfunction in the system, however, the result may be that even relatively minimal stress or tension results in a defensive withdrawal from social interaction as was described in the 1950s by child psychiatrist and autism expert Milada Havelkova (Thompson and Havelkova, 1983). More recently, others such as Dykema have connected social behavior withdrawal to this autonomic dysfunction (Dykema, 2006). A major focus of our work with AS clients has been BFB to decrease sympathetic drive and increase parasympathetic tone by encouraging an increase in heart rate variability (HRV). An increase in vagal efferent tone inhibits the inherent high intrinsic rate of the sinoatrial node slowing the heart, increasing HRV and engendering a feeling of 'calm.'

The polyvagal theory provides a coherent explanation of why our work using BFB, in particular heart rate variability training, combined with NFB, with its hypothesized effects on AC function, has been successful in clients with Asperger's syndrome.

V.   SECTION IV: INTERVENTION

Biofeedback is not a stand-alone intervention for AS. It can be combined with diet, medications, psychotherapy, behavior modification, and specialized education. Indeed, psychotherapy, behavior therapy, social training, and medications have reportedly been the most commonly used interventions for children who present with the symptoms of Asperger's syndrome (Jacobsen, 2003). These interventions, plus speech therapy, are also the most commonly tried interventions for ASD (Green et al., 2006). The advice for intervention with AS also largely applies to high functioning autism since there is much overlap in symptoms (Bregman, 2005).

Diet should be discussed during the intake evaluation of clients with AS since there is preliminary evidence that ASD in some individuals may involve the digestive system and the immune system. The group called Defeat Autism Now! (DAN) encourages trying elimination diets that avoid wheat (because of gluten) and dairy products (because of casein), which they believe can have neuroinflammatory effects in susceptible individuals. The basic theory is that some individuals with autistic spectrum disorders have a digestive problem so their bodies cannot handle the proteins found in gluten and casein. The Online Asperger Syndrome Information and Support (OASIS) website has done a Survey on Alternative Treatments and concluded that, although some individuals reported benefits, special diet regimens probably have higher success rates for autism than for AS (Bashe and Kirby, 2005).

Although there is no specific pharmacological treatment for AS or, for that matter, any of the autistic spectrum disorders, psychotropic medications are used to treat symptoms (Sloman, 2005). Many children with AS show hyperactive behavior, and are placed on medications that range from stimulants and antidepressants to antipsychotics. The stimulants target hyperactive behavior, and the commonly used ones are methylphenidate, either Ritalin or the controlled release Concerta, and amphetamines such as Dexedrine and Adderall. Common side effects are appetite suppression and insomnia. Stimulants reduce the seizure threshold, and rates of seizure disorders are higher among people along the autistic spectrum, so that is one reason they should be used with caution. A second reason for caution is that anxiety is a primary symptom in ASDs, and it may be increased with these medications. A third caution is that a reasonable number of the ASD clients we have assessed have previously been given stimulants, and/or selective serotonin reuptake inhibitors (SSRI), and suffered significant side effects including unpredictable outbursts of anger and impulsive behavior.

In our EEG assessments these clients also demonstrated beta spindling in the raw EEG. For now this seeming association between beta spindling and side effects being reported by the client is only conjecture. However this observation would make a good future research study. EEG profiles can be used to better differentiate which medications may or may not be useful for particular symptoms, so choice of medications may prove to be a little easier in future (Prichep et al., 1993; McCann, 2006). Suffin and Emory (1995) have reported on EEG patterns predicting drug response in those with ADHD, and these observations may perhaps be extended to those with AS; namely, frontal excess theta responds best to stimulants, frontal excess alpha responds better to antidepressants, and coherence problems respond best to anticonvulsants (seizure medications).

To this we would add that when beta spindling or excess high frequency beta is observed in the raw EEG, one should be very cautious about using stimulants because they may make the patient's symptoms worse. This is hypothesized to be because stimulant drugs increase beta, and result in a narrow focus that may be on an inner worry. Thus using stimulants for dealing with ADHD symptoms that present in someone with AS may actually worsen behavior. In general, one needs to balance skills and pills. As the person learns self-regulation skills, they should be able to reduce reliance on pills.

Some children with Asperger's have angry outbursts and overreact to frustrations that seem trivial to others. For symptoms of anger, temper tantrums, and aggression, psychiatrists may prescribe Risperdal (risperidone), an anti-psychotic medication with calming properties. This medication is given to decrease agitation and aggressive outbursts, and increase social interaction. Although it has fewer extrapyramidal (Parkinsonian) side effects when compared to other commonly used neuroleptics such as haloperidol and thioridazine, it can cause significant weight gain.

If targeting symptoms of anxiety, panic, obsessive-compulsive behavior, and depression, the psychiatrist usually starts with an antidepressant from the class of selective serotonin re-uptake inhibitors (SSRIs). They may also try mood stabilizers or anticonvulsants like Neurontin and Tegretol; anxiolytics like Ativan and Valium; and antihypertensives like Catapres (clonidine). Sloman notes that most of the psychotropic medications used in children have not gone through the evaluation necessary to establish their efficacy, tolerability, and safety. There is also the limitation that, "Medication does not ameliorate the basic deficits in social interaction and communication" (Sloman, 2005). Nevertheless, a wide range of drugs is prescribed for those with AS when their symptoms bother other people, or when difficulties arise (usually in school settings) where they feel overstimulated or confined.

A. Neurofeedback + biofeedback: What we do and why it is effective

Although we continue to emphasize the importance of diet, sleep, exercise, social skills training, and a good educational and extracurricular program, the primary approach for helping people with AS has become NFB + BFB and cognitive strategies, simply because this has proven most effective.

By combining knowledge of functional neuroanatomy with the foregoing theoretical discussions, a picture has emerged concerning the difficulties experienced, both neuroanatomical and functional, by those with ASD. Quantitative electroencephalographic assessment (QEEG) can pinpoint cortical areas with abnormal activation and abnormal connectivity (coherence) as compared to database norms (Thatcher et al., 2003). These areas and/or connections can then be addressed using the neurofeedback approach. It must be emphasized that what follows are some commonly used sites and frequencies but, in all cases, the initial assessment results, either single-channel or 19-channel assessment, lead to the final decision as to the sites and frequencies to be addressed in order to 'normalize' cortical functioning.

As stated above, we address each of the symptom areas both individually and together. Attention span, impulsivity, and hyperactivity when present, are addressed; firstly, by down-training low-frequency activity between 2 and 10 Hz (whichever range is appropriate for each client, for example, 2–5 Hz, or 3–7 Hz, or 4–8 Hz, and so on) and higher frequency beta, most often somewhere between 19 and 36 Hz at sites that depend on the assessment findings. The most common starting site for clients who have AS is Cz in children, and between Cz and Fz (called FCz in this chapter) in adults. At the same time we frequently up-train SMR at the same site providing, as previously noted, the central site does not evidence high amplitude spindling beta in this frequency range. We may also reward 15–18 Hz beta while the subject is learning and/or carrying out the metacognitive learning strategies that have been taught; for example, while reading and analyzing material that is emotionally descriptive (Thompson and Thompson, 2003a).

Anxiety is addressed by combining biofeedback (BFB) with the NFB. BFB includes heart rate variability training (with diaphragmatic breathing and heart rate monitoring), electromyogram (EMG) feedback, usually over the frontalis or over the trapezius muscle groups, and, when shown to be abnormal with the stress test, peripheral skin temperature and skin conduction (Thompson and Thompson, 2007). The NFB for affect modulation emphasizes down-training the high amplitude, high-frequency beta that often originates in the anterior cingulate and/or the medial prefrontal cortex. The site for this training is based on a 19-channel assessment, and usually includes Fz or FCz. This activity may also be found in the anterior portion of the right frontal lobe and the site trained will, once again, depend on the assessment findings using QEEG.

In many adult clients we will up-train alpha but we are careful not to up-train high-frequency alpha (11–13 Hz) if it is found to be very high compared to the database norms (DBN) on the assessment profile. This avoids actually making the anxiety symptoms more severe (Rice *et al.*, 1993; Thompson and Thompson, 2007), which can occur with alpha training, though usually increasing alpha is associated with a relaxed state. We will usually up-train SMR (13–15 Hz) with a site over the motor cortex (C3, CZ, or C4). This SMR training will reinforce a calm, relaxed state. It may improve sleep by increasing sleep spindle density during sleep (Sterman, 2000b).

The following case example displays the kind of complex findings that often appear in our adult Asperger's clients. The client was a 28-year-old man of high intelligence who was very much into his own areas of interest. He did not 'read' or appear to understand how others were actually feeling about his behavior. The subtleties of social interaction, particularly within his own family, escaped him. He had on several occasions become verbally aggressive and even physically violent with family members when he felt criticized. He was extremely egocentric. The following figures show significant differences from the neuroguide (NG) database mean (DBM) in areas of the brain where the brain functions could correlate with the observed abnormal social behaviors.

Figure 15.4 from LORETA, using the Neuroguide database Z-scores, shows a clear anterior cingulate finding. It shows 4 Hz activity that is 1.86 standard deviations (SD) outside the DBM for his age originating from Brodmann area (BA) 24. This indicates dysfunction in this location. Such dysfunction might be expected to correspond to his socially inappropriate behavior, and to his anxiety. This LORETA finding does correspond to the surface EEG findings.

In Fig. 15.5 LORETA shows 17 Hz beta activity to be 2 SD below the DBM using NG in the right fusiform gyrus and at the parietal-temporal junction. Dysfunction in this location might be expected to correspond to a sensory aprosodia, and to his inability to appropriately pick up cues from facial expressions.

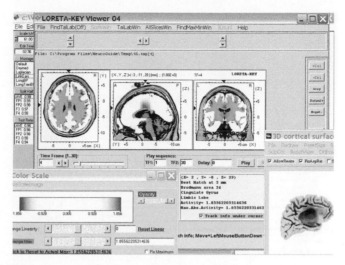

FIGURE 15.4   Image from eyes-open condition, linked-ears reference, using NG. LORETA shows 4 Hz activity at FCz, and is 1.9 SD above the DBM (see color plate).

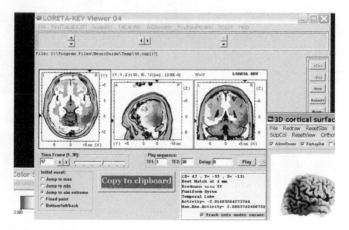

FIGURE 15.5   LORETA image: Z-scores, from eyes-open condition, linked ears reference (see color plate).

In Fig. 15.6, LORETA shows 10 Hz alpha activity in the left prefrontal area to be 1.6 SD below the DBM using NG. Dysfunction in this location might be expected to correspond to his difficulties with impulse inhibition.

In Fig. 15.7 the Z-scores demonstrated > 2 SD at FCz due to beta spindling at 26 Hz. Training to decrease spindling beta at FCz while increasing SMR, and carrying out biofeedback to increase HRV normalized the symptom picture to the degree that we did not have to proceed to other training sites.

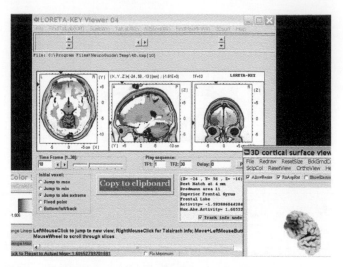

FIGURE 15.6   LORETA image from eyes-open condition, linked-ears reference.

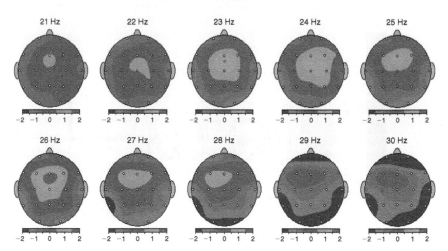

FIGURE 15.7   Brain map, linked-ear reference, eyes-open, showing standard deviations (SD) (see color plate).

Deficiencies in empathy are addressed by increasing the appropriate activity at frontal mirror neuron sites, such as F5, while decreasing spindling beta when present, and normalizing anterior cingulate activity at FCz. Affect and innuendo interpretation is addressed by decreasing slow wave activity or increasing normal 14–17 Hz beta at the T6 parietal-temporal junction, a frequent site for finding slowing, as described above. Motor aprosodia (lack of prosody) may be addressed by normalizing activity at F6. Again, the specific frequencies to be normalized at these sites are chosen after the 19-channel assessment (SKIL, Sterman-Kaiser, 2007; Sterman, 1999).

In addition to specific spatial reasoning, verbal interpretation and comprehension difficulties, executive functioning for clients with AS includes the synthesis, integration, and appropriate modulation of all sensory information input: auditory, visual and kinesthetic. Deficiencies in these executive functions are addressed by careful assessment, and then NFB. The identification of specific verbal and non-verbal learning disorders (NVLD) requires psycho-educational testing. Deficiencies can then be linked to EEG findings. Then an NFB intervention is designed to normalize the electrical activity over the appropriate cortical areas while the client is learning appropriate strategies, and also doing BFB. Usually the EEG feedback involves placement over Wernicke's area for comprehension difficulties, and right parietal areas for NVLD symptoms. The specific frequency ranges for enhance and inhibit are set according to assessment findings for each case.

Whether it be comprehension or NVLD, or whether, as in the autistic child, it appears to be a lack of appropriate cingulate and prefrontal modulation of the sensory input from the parietal areas, the connectivity (coherence and/or comodulation) will usually be outside the database norms. Commonly in Asperger's and in NVLD, we observe a 'disconnect' with hypo-coherence between right parietal-temporal region (T4, T6) and the left frontal lobe (F5) combined with hyper-coherence in the right hemisphere between parietal and temporal, temporal and frontal areas. Thus the differences from the normal database can be either too much or too little communication between specific sites.

Hyper-coherence between regions is an abnormality that is interpreted as resulting from a lack of appropriate differentiation of functioning between regions. This can negatively affect the client's ability to efficiently perform multiple tasks. It can lead to impaired decision-making when fast responses are needed. Hyper-coherence is interpreted as indicating a lack of differentiation (and flexibility) between functional regions. Hypo-coherence, on the other hand, is often interpreted as a 'disconnect' between regions of the brain, i.e. an area of the brain is not communicating as it should with other regions.

Although we cannot efficiently, until LORETA NFB is perfected, address specific findings in the amygdala, orbital-frontal cortex, and the hippocampus, we know that the anterior cingulate is well connected to these areas. Our overall results seem to suggest that we may be affecting these areas by training at the central location to normalize the EEG findings whose source is anterior cingulate activity.

B. Case example

This rather severe case shows some of the findings in a nine-year-old boy diagnosed as autistic. His language development was at a three-year-old's level, and he made little eye contact. He would draw a stick figure if requested, but preferred to draw a repeating pattern he called a train. One of his brain maps is shown in Fig. 15.8.

In Fig. 15.8 each of the circles (labeled 6 to 10 Hz) shows how much electrical power there is at a particular frequency at various sites. The red color means

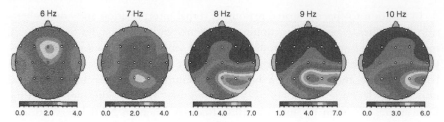

FIGURE 15.8   Brain map, absolute power, linked-ear reference, eyes-open (see color plate).

that there is high amplitude activity at that frequency. It can be seen that 8–10 Hz activity (alpha) is high amplitude at T6. Indeed, it was found that the activity was > 2 standard deviations (SD) above the database mean for boys of his age at this T6 site. As previously explained, this area plays an important role in processing sensory information and reading social cues. This is an important mirror neuron area at the junction of the parietal and temporal lobes. Dysfunction in this area from any cause may cause difficulty interpreting emotions and innuendo, such as the hidden meanings in the other person's tone of voice, or in their gestures.

In addition, at 6 Hz on the left side there is a darkened area between the two frontal lobes at Fz. Using LORETA this slow, 6 cycles per second activity was discovered to come from an important area involved with emotional feelings, attention, and executive functioning, namely, the anterior cingulate. Too much slow wave activity suggests under-activation and, in a child with ASD, this parallels the symptom of not appropriately understanding or expressing emotion.

In other brain maps that were done on this child, other frequencies and sites showed up. Some of these findings are discussed below. The next two pictures are LORETA images. They look like slices through the brain, like the pictures you might expect to see using MRI (magnetic resonance imagery) but these pictures are derived using Low Resolution Electromagnetic Tomography—LORETA for short. The three views are horizontal, sagittal and coronal. Each LORETA image shows the area that was the source of some of the abnormal activity seen on the surface of the cortex in various brain maps.

The LORETA image, shown in Fig. 15.9, shows a darkend area at a very important mirror neuron site in the left frontal lobe. This indicates that the 20 cycles per second activity is far too high compared to the normative database at F5.

This child was unusual in ASD cases in that he had better visual analysis (could do computer games) and verbal tone recognition, yet verbal output was very poor with very little verbal communication.

As described above, recent literature has emphasized dysfunction in a small central nucleus of neurons called the *amygdala*. Dysfunction here can mean that the child cannot correctly interpret the emotions of other people, and it may also mean that they cannot control their own emotional responses. They may ignore things or, on the other hand, they may overreact. In the LORETA view in Fig. 15.10, the amygdala is shown to have far too much of a very slow wave (delta activity).

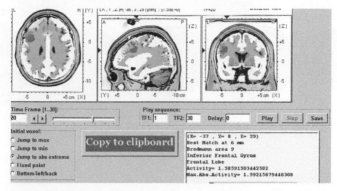

FIGURE 15.9   LORETA image from eyes-open, linked-ears reference showing 20 Hz activity source is in the inferior frontal gyrus, 1.59 SD > DBM in Neuroguide. We saw spindling 20 Hz beta at F5 (MNS) in raw EEG.

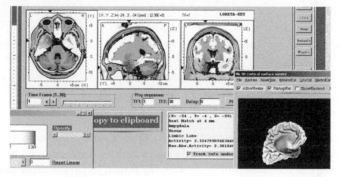

FIGURE 15.10   LORETA image, eyes-open, linked-ears reference showing 1 Hz delta activity, amygdala and Uncus, > 2.3 SD above the DBM in NG.

The next brain map, shown in Fig. 15.11, is a picture we frequently see in terms of a deviation at Pz. Here, 7 Hz activity is far above the normative database for boys his age. The area is at Pz on the surface, and is over important parietal areas needed for the synthesis and integration of all sensory (hearing, vision, kinesthetic) information.

In Figs. 15.8–15.11 it is *not* the frequency (number of waves per second) of the wave that is necessarily important. What is crucial is the area of the brain where the electrical activity differs from normal, the function of that area, and whether the functions of that area correspond to the difficulties that particular child is having.

An early study found significantly increased coherence between hemispheres in autistic children as compared to three different groups: normals, a matched group of mentally handicapped children, and normal toddlers matched for mental age (Cantor *et al.*, 1986). In the coherence patterns shown in Fig. 15.12 (from the same nine-year-old boy with autism whose images are shown above), the red lines

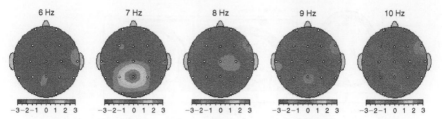

FIGURE 15.11   Brain map, relative power, eyes-open, Laplacian montage.

Before Training:

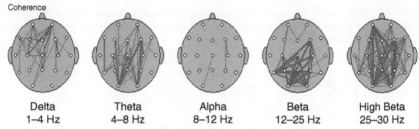

FIGURE 15.12   Coherence map before training: Coherence, eyes-open, linked-ears showing hyper-coherence between many sites (see color plate).

in the far right circle (high beta 25–30 Hz) show that far too many sites in the posterior regions of the brain, especially on the left side, are engaged in the same kind of activity at the same time as areas in the frontal lobes. There are faulty parietal-frontal connections, both in the left hemisphere, which handles most language functions, and in the right hemisphere, which does more emotional processing.

Coben (2007) has also discussed findings of coherence differences in autistic spectrum disorders. Although not observed in these data, which are from a child with autism, a number of our cases of people with Asperger's syndrome show a blue line (disconnect–hypo-coherence) between the right parietal-temporal area and the left frontal region.

The second coherence brain mapping was done at the time of progress testing after 40 sessions of training. Training had mainly emphasized beta and theta amplitude normalization, and then coherence training of theta, alpha and beta was begun. At the time of progress testing he was more focused, as evidenced by normal range scores on the TOVA and IVA (Sanford and Turner, 2002) continuous performance tests, and much less anxious by parental report, including changes in questionnaire ratings. Childhood autism rating scale (CARS) ratings done by his parents have moved from the 'severely autistic' range into the 'mild to moderately autistic' range. He receives special direct instruction in academic areas, and is now doing oral reading at a second grade level, up from a pre-primer (kindergarten) level.

Coherence

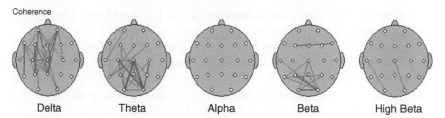

| Delta | Theta | Alpha | Beta | High Beta |

FIGURE 15.13   Coherence map after 40 sessions (see color plate).

The coherence shows particular improvement in theta and beta, especially high beta, bands (Fig. 15.13). Now training will focus on decreasing delta coherence in the left hemisphere (F3-P3 and F7-P7) while also working on strategies for language comprehension. Training will also be done to increase coherence in beta between the two frontal lobes (blue line). Coherence findings are moving towards normal in this nine-year-old boy. His training was twice a week for his first 40 sessions so those gains were made over the course of 5 months; he now does training once a week and continues to improve.

C. Typical training session steps for clients with Asperger's syndrome

The training can be conceptualized as a progression of stages that address different aspects of the AS disorder. These are outlined in point form in five steps below. In many cases not all five steps will be needed. Symptoms may resolve after the initial two or three steps. However the actual work of the trainer during the sessions is more complex. It is described as four overlapping processes following the brief outline of steps.

Training Steps

1. *Address the ADHD symptoms:* Begin by helping the client to be more 'externally' oriented and calm. Decrease the dominant slow wave frequencies, and enhance 13–15 Hz activity. A common placement is at Cz referenced to the right ear, or C4 to the left ear, respectively. For an excellent discussion of electrode placement, monopolar (referential) as compared to bipolar (sequential), see Les Fehmi and Tom Collura's article (2007).
2. *Deal with anxiety, (perseveration when present), and internal ruminative thinking* Decrease high amplitude 19–22 Hz activity (when present). Also, decrease dominant high amplitude beta activity between 23–36 Hz (when present). Usually the electrode is placed at a site that may influence the activity

of the cingulate gyrus, that is, between Fz and Cz. In addition, when beta spindling is also observed at another site (sometimes F6 or F5, and occasionally at Pz) then this beta frequency will be decreased at that site. In all adult clients a stress test is carried out, and biofeedback is added to the training program.

3. *Deal with the sensory aprosodia*: Decrease dominant slow wave activity at P4 and T6, and increase low beta 14–17 Hz. Normalize coherence abnormalities (often hypo-coherence between T6 and F5, and hyper-coherence between parietal and temporal/frontal areas).

4. *Deal with the motor aprosodia*: Decrease dominant slow wave activity at F6.

5. *Deal with language delays (as in autism or AS with language-based LD)*: Decrease dominant slow wave activity and increase 14–17 Hz activity over Wernicke's area and the angular gyrus, and normalize coherence in the left parietal-temporal-frontal axis while doing reading comprehension exercises. Decrease dominant slow wave activity and increase 15–18 Hz activity over Broca's area while reading and answering questions and organizing written work.

For all clients, decisions concerning training sites, bandwidths, and BFB parameters are made using the "decision pyramid" shown in Fig. 15.14. For EEG settings the bottom triangle findings: symptoms—EEG findings—anatomical functions

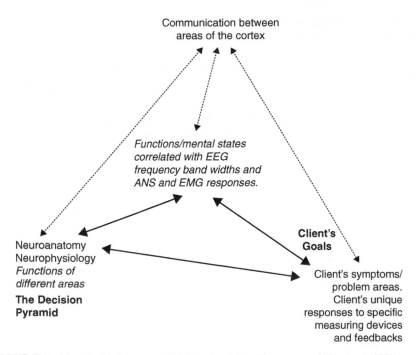

FIGURE 15.14   The "decision pyramid." (Reprinted from Thompson and Thompson, 2003).

of the areas noted to be outside database norms, must all correlate or training is delayed and a reevaluation of all the parameters takes place.

D. The four overlapping processes for training AS

Treatment Stages

We have found that most clients derive benefit from combining NFB with BFB and strategies. Clients get benefit from beginning their training with relaxation techniques and BFB. However, strategies and BFB exercises cannot just be learned in the office—they must be fully and consciously integrated into the client's daily living. NFB is fundamentally different. NFB takes much longer to learn but, when EEG changes are achieved, it appears that they are unconsciously retained, and the corresponding mental state changes are long-lasting. It can be compared in this manner to learning a new skill, such as riding a bicycle, where the "neurofeedback" is from the inner ear to the brain, and the acquisition of the skill of balancing is rapid and permanent.

Our treatment approach is conceptualized in four overlapping stages which overlap, and eventually merge as the person becomes more flexible in mental functioning. With this gain in mental flexibility, shifts to the appropriate mental state for the task at hand become largely automatic.

In the first step the student learns to be able to turn on a mental state of external broad focus, aware of everything in their environment (open awareness) which, in a later stage, they learn to alternate with singular focus. In this mental state the client learns to breathe diaphragmatically at a rate of about six breaths per minute (BrPM). By practicing this, a balance occurs between sympathetic and parasympathetic systems, and there is also balance in natural biological oscillators (heart rate, respiration, blood pressure). The resulting synchrony between heart rate oscillations (heart rate variability [HRV]) and respiration cycles of inhalation and exhalation is termed respiratory sinus arrhythmia (RSA). When breathing at 6 BrPM, HRV will be around 0.1 oscillations per second (that is, 6 per 60 seconds). It will vary a little between individuals, and the breathing rate will be faster in children (about 8 BrPM).

The important emphasis at this stage is that the client's breathing be comfortable. Overbreathing can cause cerebral and cardiac vasoconstriction which, when combined with the Bohr effect (oxygen less easily released from hemoglobin), can decrease oxygenation of the brain and heart by as much as 50% in a short time. In addition, the client must combine this relaxed diaphragmatic breathing with an increase in peripheral skin temperature, and a decrease in muscle tension. As previously noted, we generally initially use EMG sensors on the forehead or the trapezius muscle, but placement will vary depending on the client's characteristic areas of muscle tension under stress. The stress test, as described elsewhere (Thompson and Thompson, 2007), guides our choice of biofeedback modalities, and also helps the client visualize how tension affects their body.

The second step is to use operant conditioning of brain waves in order that the client can train themselves to consciously move from a calm, alert readiness, open awareness, high alpha (11–13 Hz) and SMR (sensorimotor rhythm, 13–15 Hz) state of mind to a focused, concentrating state where they lower their dominant slow wave activity, desynchronize the alpha, and increase beta (15–18 Hz). This may require that they practice consciously shifting in and out of open awareness to this narrowly focused state.

When using Infiniti equipment there is a 'scripted' training session (a series of screens and instructions available from Biofeedback Foundation of Europe, 2007) to practice this control for optimizing performance in executives and athletes, but it also works very well in the client population that has AS. To improve focus they learn to control theta and low frequency alpha. To decrease interfering anxiety and ruminations they decrease high frequency beta. The sites and precise frequency bands are determined by the QEEG assessment either single- or 19-channel. Connectivity is normalized through coherence training. Clients train themselves to control, and perhaps to permanently change, their brain wave pattern. Mental flexibility is the goal.

Here, again, there has to be a caution. As previously mentioned, a small number of clients may show very high amplitude, high-frequency alpha (12–13 Hz), which for them correlates with a brittle emotional state and sudden bursts of very high anxiety (Thompson and Thompson, 2007). Though relatively rare in our practice, it is a concrete finding, and the trainer must actually move in the opposite direction to the training of most clients and train down the high-frequency alpha. Similarly, there is another danger, but this time in the beta range. We emphasize the importance of enhancing SMR. As in Sterman's work and writings concerning seizure disorders, in our experience this seems to stabilize an unstable and easily kindled cortex. However, as previously described, only rarely but quite definitely, we will see a client in whom we observe beta spindling at 14 or 15 Hz.

It is important to note this because it makes it very difficult to reward the enhancement of SMR if beta spindling is present in the same frequency range. However, because spindling beta can be very consistent as to the site at which it is observed, it may be possible to reward SMR over a different part of the motor cortex. It is also possible to make a screen where the very low, general 13–15 Hz SMR can be enhanced, and a strong inhibit come into play if there is a sudden burst of very high amplitude waves in this frequency range. For the most part, these cautions about spindling beta are based on our clinical experience and require research studies. However, the caution concerning alpha is in the literature (Plotkin and Rice, 1981; Rice et al., 1993; Thomas and Sattlberger, 2001).

The third step is to link a desired strategy and activity, such as studying or organizing materials to be learned, with breathing diaphragmatically and relaxing while in an efficient mental state that normalizes the brain wave patterns. This linking of mental state to using cognitive strategies for work is classical conditioning. If the client is working on a cognitive task, they receive continuous auditory reinforcement for sustaining the mental state of externally oriented narrow focus while performing the task. If the feedback stops, the student immediately moves back to the operant conditioning mode of watching the display screen until the desired mental state is again achieved. Training in metacognitive strategies is also used to assist in generalizing the processes learned during the NFB sessions. After this training, which pairs the learned efficient mental state in the patient's brain when he is confronted with an applied strategy, the client will automatically go into an efficient, active, mental state whenever they use cognitive strategies and begin to work.

The fourth step is to train the student in procedures which will help them to generalize this ability to produce calm, relaxed, alert, flexible focusing to home, school and work situations. Breathing techniques and metacognitive strategies are examples of effective methods of doing this. We insist that our adolescent and adult clients pair the diaphragmatic breathing and relaxation, and broad open mental awareness, with routines in their daily living: getting out of bed, getting dressed, brushing teeth, eating breakfast, reading the paper, driving, answering the telephone, and so on. It is of no use to tell your client to practice twice a day for 10 minutes. They simply will not do it. But if they link the 6 BrPM to daily activities it becomes part of their natural routine: the phone rings and they think about doing 6 BrPM, they come to a red light while driving and start their counting for 6 BrPM—4 seconds in and 6 seconds out—while relaxing their shoulders.

E. Adding metacognition to treatment

After doing 30 years of work with Asperger's clients using psychotherapy and behavior therapy, it was sensible to integrate into our current work aspects of these approaches. The most useful appeared to be metacognitive strategies appropriate to the life situation of the particular client. Metacognition refers to thinking about thinking; that is, the client's awareness of his own cognition, of how he perceives things, learns, and remembers things. For a lengthier explanation with examples, see the section on 'Executive Thinking Strategies' in *The A.D.D. Book* (Sears and Thomspon, 1998) or the 56-page chapter on metacognition in *The Neurofeedback Book* (Thompson and Thompson, 2003). Gifted students use metacognitive strategies, whereas less successful students do not (Cheng, 1993).

With many clients with AS they have superb decoding skills but reading comprehension lags. They need reading strategies for analyzing the emotional content of text and pictures. Social stories can be used. Practice in identifying facial expressions may be helpful. For some, where NVLD was a part of the clinical picture, strategies for performing spatial reasoning tasks, especially verbal mediation techniques (talking their way through it), are wonderfully helpful. Tackling these deficiencies could improve self-esteem and accelerate improvements in the Asperger's symptoms as well as the learning difficulties.

For adults, techniques for understanding the needs, emotions and motivations of others can be useful in business as well as socially. For the adolescents and adults, writing down their areas of concerns (the things about which they ruminate) takes very little time or space. If they agree to worry only at one time of day and to only open their book (to make a new entry) when a completely new concern starts to become a rumination, and to immediately stop and divert their thoughts at other times when an old rumination comes into mind, the positive effects can be quite remarkable. We call this little pocket diary book, SMIRB, for "Stop-My-Irritating-Ruminations-Book." Sometimes the simplest methods are the most effective, and this technique has many variations among people who do cognitive behavior therapy. The SMIRB method is formally termed *compartmentalization* of concerns. It is further described in a chapter on stress management in Thompson and Thompson (2007).

F. Review of training results in clients with AS

We are preparing a case review for publication (Thompson *et al.*, in press) that summarizes the results of neurofeedback (NFB) training with more than 149 clients with Asperger's syndrome and nine additional clients with autistic spectrum disorder (ASD) over a 15-year period (1993–2008). All charts were included for review where there was a diagnosis of ASD, and pre- and post-testing (after 40–60 sessions) results were available for one or more of the standardized tests used. NFB was combined with training in metacognitive strategies and, additionally for adolescent and adult clients, with BFB as has been described above.

The most common initial montage was referential placement at the vertex (CZ) for children, and FCz for adults, referenced to the right ear. Metacognitive strategies were taught when the feedback indicated that the client was relaxed, calm, and focused. Trainers shared strategies that typically covered the areas of reading comprehension, understanding/labeling emotions, spatial reasoning, and math. Using 1-tailed T-tests and a Bonferroni correction, significant improvements were found on the following measures:

- Test of variables of attention (TVA).
- Attention quotients on the integrated visual auditory (IVA) continuous performance test.
- Australian scale for Asperger's syndrome (published in Attwood, 1998).
- ADD-Q (published in Sears and Thompson, 1998).
- Conners' Global Index.
- SNAP version of the DSM-IV criteria for ADHD.
- Wide range achievement test.
- Wechsler intelligence scales (WISC or WAIS).

The average gain for the full-scale IQ score was about 9 points. A significant decrease in EEG ratios was also observed for $(4–8)/(16–20)$, and $(3–7\,Hz)/(12–15\,Hz)$. We cannot state precisely what the efficacious treatment components were because it was not a controlled study but the outcomes were impressive, and provide pilot data to encourage further research.

VI. DISCUSSION

ADHD symptoms are a common initial presentation in those with AS. Neurofeedback (NFB) combined with coaching in metacognitive strategies is effective for ADHD (Thompson and Thompson, 1998), and helping people with stress management is facilitated by training using biofeedback (Thompson and Thompson, 2007), so it seemed there was a rationale for working to improve the symptoms associated with AS. What had not been expected was that the training would ameliorate many of the core Asperger's symptoms, occasionally even more rapidly than the ADHD symptoms, and that changes in social interactions, including developing friendships, would be seen. Clients with AS typically take more training sessions than those with attention deficit disorder (60–80 sessions, or more rather than 40–60) but they do respond, often showing quite dramatic positive changes across a wide range of symptoms.

Perhaps our success with clients with Asperger's has been due to (unwittingly in the early years) focusing our NFB work at FCz in adults and Cz in children referenced to the right ear. We were reducing high amplitude theta (3–7 Hz) or low-frequency alpha (8–10 Hz), and high-frequency beta (19–36 Hz) while increasing sensory motor rhythm (13–15 Hz). The high amplitude low-frequency alpha at T6 is close to the right ear electrode, and it may have been reduced due to the reference electrode being placed at that site as previously explained. Beta spindling (narrow frequency band, showing high amplitude, synchronous beta) may correspond to an unstable, easily kindled cortex so reducing this beta (Johnstone et al., 2007) and increasing SMR might be expected to stabilize the cortex (Sterman, 2000b) and improve functioning. However, the most likely reason for the success of NFB was the focus of training being over the anterior cingulate gyrus, which has connections to all the key areas of both the limbic system and the mirror neuron system.

We cannot emphasize too strongly the importance of always including BFB, and in particular heart rate variability training, when doing NFB for people with ASDs. In children the BFB may not be done with sensors attached but they should be taught diaphragmatic breathing techniques. As a clinician, one looks for the combination that best helps a client realize their potential. In real life a brain–body separation is artificial. For our purpose of explaining why neurofeedback plus biofeedback can rebalance, and thus improve, mind–body functioning, we have developed a systems theory of neural synergy (STNS) which emphasizes that, no matter where we enter the nervous system with our interventions, the neural system will adjust to its own new balance and equilibrium.

Whether we train the brain (NFB) or we train the heart (BFB), the neural pathways do connect across the forebrain, the midbrain and the hindbrain as was described under the polyvagal theory above. In particular, the anterior cingulate connects with the brainstem, and that brings all the connections inherent in Porges' polyvagal theory into play. These considerations support the importance of recognizing the interconnectedness of the entire central nervous system and, in our work with Asperger's syndrome, they support the combined use of NFB and

BFB. The NFB works from the top down. The BFB works from the bottom up in terms of CNS connections. The processes synergistically support each other.

VII. CONCLUSION

This chapter describes the core symptoms of AS, and explains how we assess and intervene to help these clients. The rationale for the training is based on research findings concerning brain function combined with observations of what differs in terms of EEG findings. A combined approach is advocated. Neurofeedback is the core intervention that pulls the brain in the direction of typical functioning, using comparisons to database norms to establish the training goals. We are likely affecting many complex cortical loops by training centrally over the anterior cingulate, including links to the mirror neuron systems.

When neurofeedback is augmented by peripheral biofeedback (especially effortless diaphragmatic breathing that enhances heart rate variability), there is a synergistic effect with neural circuits then being influenced not just from the top down (brain changes), but also from the bottom up by way of the complex interactions and connections of the vagal nerve (both its myelinated and unmyelinated fibres). Everything is integrated with complex feedback loops, and thus we explain the results using a systems theory of neural synergy: a change in any part of the system can produce changes elsewhere. When two components of the system are changed in a complementary fashion—as when diaphragmatic breathing is combined with SMR training, for example—the resulting new equilibrium is healthier than if either technique had been learned separately.

The experience to date using neurofeedback is encouraging (Coben, 2007; Jarusiewicz, 2002; Thompson and Thompson, 1995; Thompson et al., in press). The findings of neuroscience research, including recent work on the mirror neuron system, are supportive of an intervention that allows an individual to exercise their brain and move towards normalization of EEG patterns. Training the brain—bringing inactive areas online and improving communication between different areas of the cortex using neurofeedback—and combining that with biofeedback for further self-regulation and calming will likely become an important component of the tool-kit of interventions for autistic spectrum disorders. It is particularly gratifying to work with those with Asperger's syndrome because they so often have high intelligence, and there is great potential that can be realized.

REFERENCES

Abu-Akel, A. (2003). A Neurobiological Mapping of Theory of Mind. *Brain Research Reviews*, **43**, 39–40.

Adolphs, R. (2003). Is the human amygdala specialized for processing social information?. *Annals of the New York Academy of Scences*, **985**, 326.

Adolphs, R., Gosselin, F., Buchanan, T. W., Tranel, D., Chins, P. and Damasio, A. R. (2005). A mechanism for impaired fear recognition after amygdala damage. *Nature*, **433**, 68.

Alvarez, A. (2004). Issues in assessment: Asperger's syndrome and personality. In *The many faces of Asperger's syndrome. The Tavistock clinic series* (M. Rhode and T. Klauber, eds), pp. 113–128. London: Karnac Books.

American Psychiatric Association (1994). Diagnostic and Statistical Manual of Mental Disorders (DSM-IV, code 299.80), 4th edition. Washington, DC.

Asperger, H. (1991). Autistic psychopathy in childhood. In *Autism and Asperger's syndrome* (U. Frith, editor and translator), pp. 37–92. Cambridge, United Kingdom: Cambridge University Press. Originally published as Asperger, H. (1944). Die "Autistischen Psychopathen" im Kindesalter. *Archiv fuer Psychiatrie und Nervenkrankheiten*, **117**, 76–136.

Attwood, T. (1998). *Asperger's Syndrome: A Guide for Parents and Professionals*. London: Jessica Kingsley Publications.

Attwood, T. (2007). *The Complete Guide to Asperger's Syndrome*. London: Jessica Kingsley Publishers.

Bachevalier, J. and Loveland, K. A. (2006). The orbitofrontal-amygdala circuit and self-regulation of social-emotional behavior in autism. *Neuroscience and Behavioral Reviews*, **30**, 97–117.

Bashe, P. R. and Kirby, B. L. (2005). *The Oasis Guide to Asperger Syndrome*. New York: Crown Publishers.

Beauregard, M. and Levesque, J. (2006). Functional Magnetic Resonance Imaging Investigation of the Effects of Neurofeedback training on the Neural Bases of Selective Attention and Response Inhibition in Children with Attention-Deficit/Hyperactivity Disorder. *Applied Psychophysiology and Biofeedback*, **31(1)**.

Belmonte, M. K. and Yurgelun-Todd, D. A. (2003). Functional anatomy of impaired selective attention and compensatory processing in autism. *Cognitive Brain Research*, **17(3)**, 651–664.

Bowler, D. M., Gardiner, J. M. and Berthollier, N. (2004). Source Memory in Adolescents and Adults with Asperger's Syndrome. *Journal of Autism & Developmental Disorders*, **34(5)**, 533–542, Oct.

Bregman, J. D. (2005). Definitions and characteristics of the spectrum. In *Autism spectrum disorders: Identification, education, and treatment* (D. Zager, ed.), , 3rd edition, pp. 3–46. Mahwah: Lawrence Erlbaum Associates.

Brock, J., Brown, C., Boucher, J. and Rippon, G. (2002). The temporal binding deficit hypothesis of autism. *Review of Development & Psychopathology*, **14(2)**, 209–224.

Cantor, D. S., Thatcher, R. W., Hrybyk, M. and Kaye, H. (1986). Computerized EEG analyses of autistic children. *Journal of Autism and Developmental Disorders*, **16**, 169–187.

Carr, L., Iacoboni, M., Dubeau, M. C. and Mazziotta, J. C. (2003). Neural mechanisms of empathy in humans: a relay from neural systems for imitation to limbic areas. *Proceedings of the National Academy of Sciences, USA*, **100**, 5497–5502.

Chabot, R. J. and Serfontein, G. (1996). Quantitative electroencephalographic profiles of children with attention deficit disorder. *Biological Psychiatry*, **40**, 951–963.

Chabot, R. J., di Michele, F., Prichep, L. and John, E. R. (2001). The clinical role of computerized EEG in the evaluation and treatment of learning and attention disorders in children and adolescents. *Neuropsychiatry and Clinical Neuroscience*, **13(2)**, 171–186.

Chan, A. S., Sze, S. L. and Cheung, M. (2007). Quantitative Electroencephalographic Profiles of Children with Autistic Spectrum Disorder. *Neuropsychology*, **21(1)**, 74–81.

Channon, S. (2004). Frontal lobe dysfunction and everyday problem-solving: Social and non-social contributions. *Acta Psychologica*, **115(2–3)**, 235–254.

Cheng, P. (1993). Metacognition and giftedness: The state of the relationship. *Gifted Child Quarterly*, **37(3)**, 105–112.

Clarke, A. R., Barry, R. J., McCarthy, R. and Selikowits, M. (2001). Electroencephalogram differences in two subtypes of attention-deficit/hyperactivity disorder. *Psychophysiology*, **38**, 212–221.

Coben, R. (2007). Connectivity-guided neurofeedback for Autistic Spectrum Disorder. *Biofeedback*, **35(4)**, 131–135.

Coben, R. and Padolsky, I. (2007). Assessment-guided neurofeedback for autistic spectrum disorder. *Journal of Neurotherapy*, **11**, 5–23.

Corbett, B. A. and Constantine, L. J. (2006). Autism and attention deficit hyperactivity disorder: assessing attention and response control with the integrated visual and auditory continuous performance test. *Child Neuropsychology*, **12(4–5)**, 335–348.

Cumine, V., Leach, J. and Stevenson, G. (1998). *Asperger Syndrome: A practical guide for teachers*. London: David Fulton Publishers.

Dalton, K. M., Nacewicz, B. M., Johnstone, T., *et al.* (2005). Gaze fixation and the neural circuitry of face processing in autism. *Nature Neuroscience*, **8(4)**, 519–526.

Dapretto, M., Davies, M. S., Pfeifer, J. H., *et al.* (2006). Understanding emotions in others: mirror neuron dysfunction in children with autism spectrum disorders. *Nature Neuroscience*, **9(1)**, 28–30.

Deruelle, C., Rondan, C., Gepner, B. and Tardif, C. (2004). Spatial Frequency and Face Processing in Children with Autism and Asperger Syndrome. *Journal of Autism and Developmental Disorders*, **34(2)**, 199–210.

Devinsky, O., Morrell, M. and Vogt, B. (1995). Contributions of Anterior Cingulate Cortex to Behavior. *Brain*, **118**, 279–306.

Dissanayake, C. and Macintosh, K. (2003). Mind reading and social functioning in children with autistic disorder and Asperger's disorder. In *Individual differences in theory of mind: implications for typical and atypical development. Macquarie monographs in cognitive science* (B. Repacholi and V. Slaughter, eds), pp. 213–239. New York: Psychology Press.

Dykema, R. (2006). "Don't talk to me now, I'm scanning for danger." How your nervous system sabotages your ability to relate. An interview with Stephen Porges about his polyvagal theory. *Nexis* magazine, March–April, 30–35.

Ehlers, S. and Gillberg, C. (1993). The Epidemiology of Asperger's Syndrome. A Total Population Study. *Journal of Child Psychology and Psychiatry*, **34**, 1327–1350.

Emerich, D. M., Creaghead, N. A., Grether, S. M., Murray, D. and Grasha, C. (2003). The Comprehension of Humorous Materials by Adolescents with High-Functioning Autism and Asperger's Syndrome. *Journal of Autism & Developmental Disorders*, **33(3)**, 253–257.

Fehmi, L. and Collura, T, (2007). Effects of electrode placement upon EEG biofeedback training: the monopolar-bipolar controversy. *Journal of Neurotherapy*, **11(2)**, 45–63.

Fitzgerald, M. (2000). Jonathan Swift: Victim of Asperger's syndrome? *The Canadian Journal of Diagnosis,* May 2000, 31–36.

Fitzgerald, M. (2004). Response to "Features of Alexithymia or features of Asperger's syndrome?". *European Child & Adolescent Psychiatry*, **13(2)**, 123, by M. Corcos.

Fitzgerald, M. and Kewley, G. (2005). Attention-Deficit/Hyperactivity Disorder and Asperger's Syndrome. *Journal of the American Academy of Child & Adolescent Psychiatry*, **44(3)**, 210.

Fombonne, E. and Tidmarsh, L. (2003). Epidemiological data on Asperger's disorder. *Child and Adolescent Psychiatric Clinics of North America*, **12(1)**, 15–21.

Frith, U. (editor and translator Refer msp. 4.) (1991). *Autism and Asperger's syndrome*. Cambridge, UK: Cambridge University Press.

Fuchs, T., Birbaumer, N., Lutzenberger, W., Gruzelier, J. and Kaiser, J. (2003). Neurofeedback treatment for attention-deficit/hyperactivity disorder in children: a comparison with methylphenidate. *Journal of Applied Psychophysiology and Biofeedback*, **28(1)**, 1–12.

Gevirtz, R. (2007). Biofeedback Training to Increase Heart Rate Variability. In *Principles and Practice of Stress Management* (P. M. Lehrer, R. L. Woolfolk and W. E. Sime, eds), 3rd edition. New York: Guilford Publications.

Gevirtz, R. and Lehrer, P. (2005). Resonant Frequency Heart Rate Biofeedback. In *Biofeedback: A Practitioner's Guide* (M. S. Schwartz and F. Andrasik, eds), 3rd edition. New York: Guilford Press, Chapter 11.

Gillburg, C. and Billstedt, E. (2000). Autism and Asperger Syndrome: coexistence with other clinical disorders. *Acta Psychiatrica Scandinavica*, **102**, 321–330. Cited in Fitzgerald, M. and Corvin, A.

(2001). Diagnosis and differential diagnosis of Asperger Syndrome. *Advances in Psychiatric Treatment*, **7**, 310–318.

Gibbs, F. A. and Knott, J. R. (1949). Growth of the electrical activity of the cortex. *Electro-encephalography and Clinical Neurophysiology*, 223–229.

Gibbs, F. A. and Gibbs, E. L. (1950). *Atlas of Electroencephalography*. Reading, MA: Addison-Wesley.

Green, V. A., Pituch, K. A., Itchon, J., Choi, A., O'Reilly, M. and Sigafoos, J. (2006). Internet survey of treatments used by parents of children with autism. *Research and Developmental Disabilities*, **27**, 70–84.

Haddon, M. (2002). *The Curious Incident of the Dog in the Night-time*. Toronto: Doubleday Canada.

Hadjikhani, N., Joesph, R. M., Snyder, J. and Tager-Flusberg, H. (2006). Anatomical Differences in the Mirror Neuron System and Social Cognition Network in Autism. *Cerebral Cortex*, **16**, 1276–1282.

Hess, W. (1949). The central control of the activity in internal organs. Acceptance speech when receiving the Nobel Prize in Physiology and Medicine.

Hill, E. L. and Frith, U. (2003). Understanding Autism: Insights from mind and brain. Theme Issue 'Autism: mind and brain'. *Phil. Trans. of The Royal Society London*, Bulletin **358**, 281–289.

Iacoboni, M. & Dapretto, M. (2006). The mirror neuron system and the consequences of its dysfunction. *Nature Reviews and Neuroscience*, **December**, 942–951.

IVA. Intermediate Visual and Auditory Continuous Performance Test. Available through BrainTrain, 727 Twin Ridge Lane, Richmond, VA 23235.

Jacobsen, P. (2003). *Asperger's Syndrome and Psychotherapy: Understanding Asperger Perspectives*. London: Jessica Kingsley Publishers.

Jantzen, T., Graap, K., Stephanson, S., Marshall, W. and Fitzsimmons, G. (1995). Differences in baseline EEG measures for ADD and normally achieving pre-adolescent males. *Biofeedback and Self-Regulation*, **20(1)**, 65–82.

Jarusiewicz, E. (2002). Efficacy of neurofeedback for children in the autistic spectrum: A pilot study. *Journal of Neurotherapy*, **6(4)**, 39–49.

Johnstone, J., Gunkelman, J. and Lunt, J. (2005). Clinical Database Development: Characterization of EEG Phenotypes. *Clinical EEG and Neuroscience*, **36(2)**, 99–107.

Khouzam, H. R., El-Gabalawi, F., Pirwani, N. and Priest, F. (2004). Asperger's Disorder: A Review of Its Diagnosis and Treatment. *Comprehensive Psychiatry*, **45(3)**, 184–191.

Klin, A. and Miller, K. (2004). When Asperger's Syndrome and a Nonverbal Learning Disability Look Alike. *Journal of Developmental and Behavioral Pediatrics, Special Issue: Challenging Cases in Developmental & Behavioral Pediatrics* (M. T. Stein, ed.) **25(5S)**, S59-S64. (This reprinted article originally appeared in the *Journal of Developmental & Behavioral Pediatrics* **25(3)**, 190–195.

Knezevic, B. (2007). Pilot Project to Ascertain Utility of Tower of London Test (ToL) to Assess Outcomes of Neurofeedback in Clients with Asperger's Syndrome (AS). Student award Presentation, *15th Annual Meeting of the International Society for Neurofeedback and Research*, San Diego, CA, September.

Landry, R. and Bryson, S. E. (2004). Impaired disengagement of attention in young children with autism. *Journal of Child Psychology & Psychiatry and Allied Disciplines*, **45(6)**, 1115–1122.

Linden, M., Habib, T. and Radojevic, V. (1996). A controlled study of EEG biofeedback effects on cognitive and behavioral measures with attention-deficit disorder and learning disabled children. *Biofeedback and Self-Regulation*, **21(1)**, 35–49.

Lubar, J. F. (1991). Discourse on the development of EEG diagnostics and biofeedback treatment for attention deficit/hyperactivity disorders. *Biofeedback and Self-Regulation*, **16(3)**, 202–225.

Mann, C. A., Lubar, J. F., Zimmerman, A. W., Miller, C. A. and Muenchen, R. A. (1992). Quantitative analysis of EEG in boys with attention-deficit/hyperactivity disorder: Controlled study with clinical implications. *Pediatric Neurology*, **8(1)**, 30–36.

Martinez, Y. (2003). University of Waterloo. Unpublished Honours thesis for undergraduate degree in Psychology. Available from the ADD Center.

McCann, J. (2006). REEG – The new image of diagnostic accuracy. *Neuropsychiatry*, **7(8)**.

Meltzoff, A. and Prinz, W. (eds) (2002). *The Imitative Mind: Development, Evolution and Brain Bases*. New York: Cambridge University Press.

Monastra,V.J., Lubar,J. F., Linden, M., *et al.* (1999). Assessing attention deficit hyperactivity disorder via quantitative electroencephalography: An initial validation study. *Neuropsychology*, **13(3)**, 424–433.

Nacewicz, B. M., Dalton, K. M., Johnstone, T., *et al.* (2006). Amygdala volume and nonverbal social impairment in adolescent and adult males with autism. *Archives of General Psychiatry*, **63(12)**, 1417–1428.

Nash, J. M. (2002). The Secrets of Autism. *Time* (Canadian Edition), May 6, **159(18)**, 36–46.

Neuroguide Delux, 2.3.7, (2007). Robert Thatcher, *Applied Neuroscience Inc.* (www.appliedneuroscience.com)

Nikolaenko, N. N. (2004). Metaphorical and Associative Thinking in Healthy Children and in Children with Asperger's Syndrome at Different Ages. *Human Physiology*, **30(5)**, 532–536.

Nishitani, N., Avikainen, S. and Hari, R. (2004). Abnorml imitation-related cortical activation sequences in Asperger's syndrome. *Annals of Neurology*, **55**, 558–562.

Oberman, L. M., Hubbard, E. M., McCleery, J. P., Altschuler, E. L., Ramachandran, V. S. and Pineda, J. A. (2005). EEG evidence for motor neuron dysfunction in autistic spectrum disorders. *Brain Research and Cognitive Brain Research*, **24**, 190–198.

Pascual-Marqui, R. D., Esslen, M., Kochi, K. and Lehmann, D. (2002). Functional Imaging with Low Resolution Electromagnetic Tomography (LORETA): A review. *Methods & Findings in Experimental & Clinical Pharmacology*, **24C**, 91–95.

Pfeifer, H., Iacoboni, M., Mazziotta, C. and Dapretto, M. (2005). Mirror neuron system activity in children and its relation to empathy and interpersonal competence. Accessed in Abstract Viewer/Itinerary Planner. *Society for Neuroscience Abstracts*, **660(24)**.

Plotkin, W. B. and Rice, K. M. (1981). Biofeedback as a Placebo: Anxiety reduction facilitated by training in either suppression or enhancement of brain waves. *Journal of Consulting and Clinical Psychology*, **49**, 590–596.

Porges, S. W. (2003). Social Engagement and Attachment: A Phylogenetic Perspective. *Annals of the New York Academy of Sciences*, **1008**, 31–47.

Porges, S. W. (2004). The Vagus: A mediator of behavioral and physiologic features associated with autism. In *The Neurobiology of Autism* (M. L. Bauman and T. L. Kemper, eds), pp. 65–78. Baltimore: John Hopkins University Press.

Porges, S. W. (2007). The Polyvagal Perspective. *Biological Psychiatry*, **74**, 116–143.

Prichep, L. S. and John, E. R. (1992). QEEG profiles of psychiatric disorders. *Brain Topography*, **4(4)**, 249–257.

Prichep, L., Mas, F., Hollander, E., *et al.* (1993). Quantitative electroencephalographic subtyping of obsessive-compulsive disorder. *Psychiatry Research: Neuroimaging*, **50**, 25–32.

Ramachandran, V. S. and Oberman, L. M. (2006). Broken Mirrors. *Scientific American*, **295(5)**, 62–69. Reprinted in *Scientific American Mind: Scientific American Reports* June, 2007, 21–29.

Rice, K. M., Blanchard, E. B. and Purcell, M. (1993). Biofeedback of generalized anxiety disorder: Preliminary results. *Biofeedback and Self-Regulation*, **18(2)**, 93–105.

Ross, E. D. (1981). The Aprosodias: Functional-Anatomic Organization of the Affective Components of Language in the Right Hemisphere. *Archives of Neurology*, **38**, 561–569.

Rossiter, T. R. (2004). The effectiveness of neurofeedback and stimulant drugs in treating AD/HD: Part II. Replication. *Applied Psychophysiology & Biofeedback*, **29(4)**, 233–243.

Rossiter, T. R. and LaVaque, T. J. (1995). A comparison of EEG biofeedbaclk and psychostimulants in treating attention deficit hyperactivity disorders. *Journal of Neurotherapy*, **1(1)**, 48–59.

Rubin, E. and Lennon, L. (2004). Challenges in Social Communication in Asperger Syndrome and High-Functioning Autism. *Topics in Language Disorders*, **24(4)**, 271–285.

Salmond, C. H., Ashburner, J., Connelly, A., Friston, K. J., Gadian, D. G. and Vargha-Khadem, F. (2005). The role of the medial temporal lobe in autistic spectrum disorders. *European Journal of Neuroscience*, **22(3)**, 764–772.

Sanford, J. A. and Turner, A. (2002). *Integrated Visual and Auditory Continuous Performance Test Manual.* Richmond, VA: Brain Train.

Sears, W. and Thompson, L. (1998). *The A.D.D. Book: New Understandings, New Approaches to Parenting Your Child.* New York: Little, Brown and Co.

Shamay-Tsoory, S. G., Tomer, R., Berger, B. D., Goldsher, D. and Aharon-Peretz, J. (2005). Impaired "Affective Theory of Mind" is associated with right ventromedial prefrontal damage. *Cognitive and Behavioral Neurology*, **18(1)**, 55–67.

Simpson, D. (2004). Asperger's syndrome and autism: Distinct syndromes with important similarities. In *The many faces of Asperger's syndrome. The Tavistock Clinic Series. xviii, 302* (M. Rhode and T. Klauber, eds), pp. 25–38. London: Karnac Books.

SKIL, Sterman-Kaiser Imaging Laboratory, Copyright 2001. Version 3.0 (2007).

Sloman, L. (2005). Medication use in children with high functioning pervasive developmental disorder and Asperger syndrome. In *Children, Youth and Adults with Asperger Syndrome: Integrating Multiple Perspectives* (K. P. Stoddart, ed.), pp. London: Jessica Kingsley Publishers.

Sterman, M. B. (1999). *Atlas of Topometric Clinical Displays: Functional Interpretations and Neurofeedback Strategies*. New Jersey: Sterman-Kaiser Imaging Laboratory.

Sterman, M. B. (2000a). Basic concepts and clinical findings in the treatment of seizure disorders with EEG operant conditioning. *Clinical Electroencephalography*, **31(1)**, 45–55.

Sterman, M. B. (2000b). EEG markers for attention deficit disorder: pharmacological and neurofeedback applications. *Child Study Journal*, **30(1)**, 1–22.

Tammet, D. (2007). *Born on a Blue Day*. London: Free Press.

Thatcher, R. W., Walker, R. A., Biver, C. J., North, D. N. and Curtin, R. (2003). Quantitative EEG normative databases: Validation and clinical correlation. In *Quantitative electroencephalographic analysis (QEEG) databases for neurotherapy: Description, validation, and application* (J. F. Lubar, ed.), pp. New York: Haworth Press.

Thomas, J. E. and Sattlberger, E. (2001). Treatment of Chronic Anxiety Disorder with Neurotherapy: A Case study. *Journal of Neurotherapy*, **7(2)**.

Thompson, M. and Havelkova, M. (1983). Childhood Psychosis. In *Psychological Problems of the Child in the Family* (P. Steinhauer and Quentin Rae-Grant, eds). New York: Basic Books, Inc.

Thompson, L. and Thompson, M. (1995). Exceptional Results with Exceptional Children. *Proceedings of the Society for the Study of Neuronal Regulation, 3rd Annual Meeting*, Scottsdale, Arizona.

Thompson, L. and Thompson, M. (1998). Neurofeedback Combined with Training in Metacognitive Strategies: Effectiveness in Students with ADD. *Applied Psychophysiology and Biofeedback*, **23(4)**, 243–263.

Thompson, M. and Thompson, L. (2003a). Neurofeedback for Asperger's Syndrome: Theoretical Rationale and Clinical Results. *The Newsletter of the Biofeedback Society of California*, **19(1)**.

Thompson, M. and Thompson, L. (2003b). *The Neurofeedback Book: An Introduction to Basic Concepts in Applied Psychophysiology*. Wheat Ridge, CO: Association for Applied Psychophysiology.

Thompson, M. and Thompson, L. (2006). Improving Attention in Adults and Children: Differing Electroencephalograhy Profiles and Implications for Training. *Biofeedback Magazine*, **34(3)**, 99–105.

Thompson, M. and Thompson, L. (2007). Neurofeedback for Stress Management. In *Principles and Practice of Stress Management* (P. M. Lehrer, R. L. Woolfolk and W. E. Sime, eds), 3rd edition. New York: Guilford Publications.

Thompson, M. and Thompson, L. (2007). Setting-up-for-clinical-success: Scripts. *Biofeedback Foundation of Europe*, www.bfe.org.

Thompson, M., Thompson, L., and Reid, A. (in press). Neurofeedback Outcomes in Clients with Asperger's Syndrome. *Applied Psychophysiology and Biofeedback*.

Weimer, A. K., Schatz, A. M., Lincoln, A., Ballantyne, A. O. and Truaner, D. A. (2001). "Motor" impairment in Asperger syndrome: Evidence for a deficit in proprioception. *Journal of Developmental and Behavioral Pediatrics*, **22(2)**, 92–101.

Weitz, P. and Weitz, C. (2002). *About a Boy*.

Willey, L. H. (1999). *Pretending to be Normal*. London: Jessica Kingsley Publishers.

Wing, L. (1981). Asperger's syndrome: A clinical account. *Psychological Medicine*, **11**, 115–129.

Wing, L. (2001). *The Autistic Spectrum: A parents' guide to understanding and helping your child*. Berkeley, CA: Ulysses Press.

Wing, L. and Gould, J. (1979). Severe impairments of social interaction and associated abnormalities in children: Epidemiology and classification. *Journal of Autism and Developmental Disorders*, **9**, 11–29.

CHAPTER 16

Neurofeedback in pain management

**Victoria L. Ibric, M.D., Ph.D. BCIAC[1] and
Liviu G. Dragomirescu, Ph.D.[2]**

[1]*President, Neurofeedback and Neuro Rehab Institute, Inc., Pasadena, California, USA*
[2]*Department of Ecology, University of Bucharest, Romania*

I. INTRODUCTION

Pain is a necessary "evil." To feel pain is to be forewarned that something is wrong in the body. Moreover, when the pain becomes chronic and debilitating, it is definitively related to more than a specific event or body area. It has been demonstrated that the chronic pain patient shows dysfunctional structural and emotional impairment in cortical regions (Acerra and Moseley, 2005). Fox and Raichle (2007) indicate that long-term pain disrupts the balance of the "default mode network: (DMN), producing a widespread impact on overall brain function. These disruptions of the DMN are believed to be related to the associated depression, anxiety, sleep disturbances, and faulty decision-making which plague chronic pain patients." Pain has become one of the most common symptoms for which patients are requesting medical attention (more than 80% of medical visits). This care has cost an excess of $80 billion each year in the US (as reported by the Institute of Medicine (Osterweis *et al.*,1987).

As defined by the International Association for the Study of Pain (IASP), "Pain is unquestionably a sensation in a part or parts of body but is always unpleasant and therefore also an emotional experience" (Merskey 1986). Pain symptoms have been evaluated and addressed variously over time, projecting numerous models for understanding the overall pain experience. From ancient times until Descartes, in the 1700s, pain has been considered a disease condition. Thus, within this "biomedical pain model," pain is considered a symptom associated with physical damage, purportedly having an objective element connected with the sensation. However, identifying physical pathology does not predict severity of pain, intensity or level of disability (Holroyd *et al.*, 1999).

II. PSYCHOLOGICAL PAIN ASSOCIATED WITH PHYSIOLOGICAL CONDITIONS

The first attempt to integrate the physiological with psychological pain aspects was achieved by Melzak and Wall in 1965 through development of the "gate theory" of pain. This theory incorporated the three systems that are involved in pain experience: sensory-discriminative, motivational-affective, and cognitive-evaluative. This model integrates the notions that pain can be somatic as well as psychogenic.

In the light of the gate theory of pain control, one must understand the pathways involved in pain experience. In short, the pain is recorded by specialized peripheral sensory receptors, and the information is brought to the brain through the spinal cord, via afferent pathways. A half century ago, Penfield and Jasper (1954) described these pathways wherein the brain receives the information in specialized centers and performs analysis of the pain's intensity, quality, and the peripheral localization. This information is integrated in other areas as well, such as limbic system memory of pain, and the emotional encounter caused by the pain sensation. The brain and spinal cord also have the capacity for diminishing the pain sensation by sending, via efferent pathways, messages to reduce the pain experience (the pain control "analgesia" systems are described in any neurophysiology manual).

The psychological aspects described by the gate theory were revisited and considered incomplete by others (Sufka and Price 2002). In spite of the limitations of the mechanisms proposed within this theory (Nathan, 1976), the gate theory of control of pain is considered to have provided an extraordinary contribution to the understanding that chronic pain includes brain function. The mechanisms of pain, incorporating peripheral receptors, pain pathways, and cortical and subcortical centers where pain is perceived, have brought emphasis to the importance of the corticalization of pain. Understanding corticalization of pain (Birbaumer et al., 1995), and neuroplasticity (Ramanchandran and Rogers-Ramanchandran, 2000), may explain why neurofeedback is such a valuable technique. Neurofeedback proposes that by teaching self-regulation, a patient can reduce or even eliminate pain sensations. Since the advent of the gate theory, numerous therapeutic modalities have evolved based on the neurophysiological mechanisms of pain (e.g., neurostimulation procedures, pharmacological interventions, behavioral treatments, and neuromodulation techniques through neurofeedback).

There are no two individuals who perceive pain or other physical symptoms similarly. The perception of pain is based partially on an individual's pain tolerance and pain threshold. The bio-psychosocial make-up determines the pain perception of different individuals as well. Often the subjective complaints cannot be corroborated by any objective measurements. To understand chronic pain, we need to understand the distinction between "disease" and "illness." To be "diseased" implies that an individual presents objective anatomic-pathological disturbances in their body, while "illness" represents the "subjective experience" of that individual. Thus chronic pain, as a subjective phenomenon, must be evaluated using the bio-psychosocial model that focuses on illness.

III. THE BIO-PSYCHOSOCIAL MODEL OF PAIN

The intricate interaction among biological, psychological, and social aspects of one's life must be considered. The biomedical model is too limited as a formulation to understand the complexity of chronic pain syndromes. A comprehensive historical perspective of the bio–psychosocial model is thoroughly presented by Gatchel and Turk (1996) and Turk and Gatchel (1999), and also in Craig's statements including the theory on social learning mechanisms (1986).

Operant learning mechanisms of pain, as discussed by Fordyce (1976), represented a unique direction, and were expanded over the years by others such as Cairns and Passino (1977). Pain is a symptom that is acute as a response to an injury. If the pain persists for more than 6 months since the onset, it becomes chronic. Chronicity of pain is based on the respondent learning mechanisms. However, such learning theory approaches ignore the brain/body interface. Not only are the assaults on the body, which first generated the experience of pain, ignored, but the brain's emotional responses to bodily insults are not considered. To accomplish a successful self-regulatory program through the biofeedback/neurofeedback (BF/NF) treatment approach, considerations should be given to evaluate the underlining etiologies of chronic pain syndromes as well as overlapping diagnosis or co-morbidities (see Table 16.1). For example, patients who suffered from chronic pain usually suffer from depression, anxiety, fatigue, sleep disorders, hypertension, and cognitive disabilities, diabetes, etc. (Turk *et al.*, 1995).

The frequent pairing of chronic pain with several other chronic disabilities may not be coincidental. As Baliki *et al.* (2008) demonstrated in chronic pain patients, the default-mode network (DMN) shown by fMRI is imbalanced and shown to be disrupted, and this disruption may account for the development of accompanying diagnostic conditions. Therefore, neurofeedback's effect in restoring the brain functions in general may be based on its contribution to aid in the correction of this cortical disruption. These findings are elaborated in the discussion section of this chapter.

There are various factors perpetuating pain syndromes that contribute to the chronicity of pain, which also need to be addressed (Table 16.2).

Pain is a symptom that affects many people in our society, causing an alarming dependence on pain medications (Kudrow 1982; Mayo Clinic 2007; News-Medical.Net 2007). Chronic pain's effect on perpetuating other disabilities is enormous. According to the 2005 National Survey on Drug Use and Health, the incidence of new non-medical users of pain relievers is now at 2.2 million

TABLE 16.1   Etiology of Chronic Pain of our patients' population and Overlapping Diagnoses of our patients' population

Etiology of Chronic Pain	Overlapping Diagnoses
Head Injuries due to different accidents: STBI, MTBI, CVA	Anxiety and/or Depression
Work related injuries due to repetitive muscle activities	ADHD
Post surgery	Asthma
Post inflammation (ie: post shingles)	Cancer – different localizations
Psychological or Idiopathic	Essential Tremor or Parkinson's
Chronic degenerative diseases	Hypertension
	Sleep Disorders
	Memory impairment

TABLE 16.2   Factors perpetuating and aggravating pain syndromes

1	Mechanical stressors	Structural asymmetry Poor Posture
2	Nutritional deficiencies	Avitaminosis, Poor or imbalanced diet
3	Metabolic and Endocrinologic abnormalities	Hypothyroidism Hypoglycemia Hyperuricemia
4	Secondary Psychosocial Factors	Adjustment Disorder Psychosomatic Disorder Secondary Gain
5	Chronic Infections	Bacterial, viral, fungi, etc Immune Deficit Syndromes
6	Sleep Disorders	Sleep Apnea Bruxism
7	Neurologic Disorders	Radiculopathies Entrapment neuropathies Peripheral neuropathies Multiple Sclerosis
8	Rheumatologic Disorders	Osteoarthritis Rheumatoid arthritis Systemic lupus erythematosus

Americans age 12 and older, surpassing the number of new marijuana abusers (2.1 million). Also, more than 6 million Americans reported current non-medical use of prescription drugs—more than the number abusing cocaine, heroin, hallucinogens, and inhalants combined.

IV.   THE USEFULNESS OF BF/NF WITH CO-MORBIDITIES ASSOCIATED WITH CHRONIC PAIN

It would be erroneous and an oversimplification to suggest that biofeedback/ neurofeedback alone would effectively assist the chronic pain patient to overcome co-morbidities associated with their pain. Other therapies that have been shown to be beneficial in pain management are mentioned in *Mosby's Complementary and Alternative Medicine* (Freeman, 2004). They include behavioral modification techniques (Block *et al.*, 1980), acupuncture (Price and Meyer, 1995) and Chinese medicine, Alexander technique, Bachflower remedies, chiropractic, craniosacral therapy, Feldenkreis, Hellerwork, homeopathy, meditation, physiotherapy techniques such as heat, CES, TENS, ultra sound, laser, and Shiatsu, massage, yoga, etc.

Nonetheless, using BF/NF as a central modality, many of the causes, co-morbidities, and perpetuating factors of pain often have been addressed successfully with BF/NF techniques. These co-morbidities include high blood pressure and cognitive dysfunctions (Ibric and Grierson, 1995), and sleep disorders (Ibric, 2001). NIH recommends the use of BF/NF in pain syndromes and sleep disorders, and the same recommendations also are found in Freeman (2004). The addictive behaviors associated with chronic pain have been addressed with NF, resulting in remarkable success (Ibric 2002; Guyol, 2006). Some of the patients presented in the case study section of this chapter completely renounced their pain medication regimen, as the NF training progressed.

Biofeedback (BF) protocols designed to address the peripheral correlates of arousal, such as temperature (TMP), muscle tension (EMG), sweat gland activity (SCR), and heart rate variability (HRV), indirectly affect pain parameters. By comparison, neurofeedback (NF) directly affects the processing of pain perception. By modifying the electrical activity of the central processing units at cortical and subcortical areas, the pain perception, pain memory and pain affect are modulated, and pain tolerance and pain thresholds enhanced. We also hypothesize that NF produces an enhanced process of analgesia, due to endorphine and enkephaline stimulation (see the discussion section of this chapter).

Over the last 50 years numerous studies reported biofeedback (BF) and relaxation as useful complementary techniques to medical approaches in treating acute and chronic pain syndromes (Arena and Blanchard, 1996). Examples include: headaches (Brown 1974; Budzynski et al., 1973; Tansey 1991); temporomandibular joint (TMJ) pain (Ham and Packard, 1996); neck, shoulder and back pain (Carlsson 1975; Cairns and Passino, 1977); and myofascial pain syndrome (MPS) (Toomim, 1987; Ibric, 1996). Early in its history neurofeedback (NF), or EEG-BF, as a sub-specialty of BF, was reported useful in epilepsy (Sterman 1973), in obtaining a relaxation response (Jacob and Benson 1996) and enhancing creativity (Brown and Klugg, 1974; Budzynski, 1976; Fehmi, 1970; Green, 1972, and Kamiya, 1968), and in attention deficit problems (Lubar, 1985; Tansey, 1993). As the years went by, the applications of NF expanded to psychological and physical dysfunctions, such as migraine in children (Siniatchkin et al. 2000, Kropp et al., 2002), headaches (McKenzie et al., 1974), sleep disorders and pain syndromes (Ibric and Jacobs, 1997, Ibric and Kaur, 1999, Ibric, 2000, 2001, 2002; Donaldson et al., 2004a-d; Othmer, 2001) as well as depression, anxiety, and chronic fatigue (Rosenfeld et al., 1995; Hammond, 2000, 2001).

V. OVERVIEW OF THE COMPLEXITY OF TREATING CHRONIC PAIN

This presentation of our clinic's experience demonstrates the difficulties in stylizing protocols for chronic pain treatment. The co-morbidities often overlap—one person's pain experience itself is very unlike another's, social and home conditions superimpose upon the chronic pain experiences, and the EEG patterns associated with pain demand their own unique training locations and training modifications. Over 10 years of practice, 147 patients were referred to us for biofeedback training for different chronic pain syndromes, ranging from migraine to complex regional pain syndromes (see Table 16.3). These patients had been previously treated with other modalities, but had little resolution of pain.

From the total of 147 patients who were statistically analyzed at the end of this chapter, 10 cases are presented in Table 16.4, and will be detailed below.

TABLE 16.3   Classification of the pain syndromes of our
patient population and the number of patients in each category

Main Pain Diagnostic and/or localization	No. of patients
Headache & Migraines	58 total
(Headaches only)	(19)
Neck & Shoulder Pain	9
Back & Leg Pain	30
MFPS & Fibromyalgia	10
CRPS type I, II	13
Abdominal pain of Different origins	7
Rheumatoid Arthritis (RA)	3
Other (e.g. Cancer pain)	17

TABLE 16.4   The ten cases presented in detail in this chapter

Case Number	Age	Sex	Main Diagnostic	Co-morbidities	#NF sessions
1	52	F	RSD, POST MVA	Depression, Sleep disorders	15
2	67	F	Headaches, Neck spasticity post meningitis, Gait dysfunction	Hypertension, Urinary incontinence	145
3	33	M	Neuropathy post TBI & spinal cord injury due to work accident	Addiction to Pain Killers	82
4	20	F	RSD left foot	NA	20
5	63	M	Idiopathic neuropathy	Hypertension	22
6	62	M	Neuropathy post laminectomy	Bipolar Depression, Addiction to Pain killers	46
7	35	F	Myfascial pain, Headaches, TMJ	PTSD, Bruxism	16
8	51	F	TMJ/ RSD or Fibromyalgia post MVA	Rheumatoid Arthritis	54
9	60	F	Chronic pain, upper/ lower back and legs	Parkinson's Disease, Colon cancer, Leukemia	56
10	42	M	Left inguinal chronic pain post surgery, mTBI	Kidney stones, Addiction to Pain Killers	112

Three longitudinal studies (Case studies 8, 9 and 10) are included among these 10 patients. Case number 10, presented in more detail, demonstrates the progress of NF training and its effects on subjective and objective measures. The QEEG evaluation of the real-time changes on connectivity during NF and HEG modification during a NF session are also shown to indicate the totality of changes of all measurements on the brain. The efficacy study of the NF training in pain syndromes will conclude this chapter.

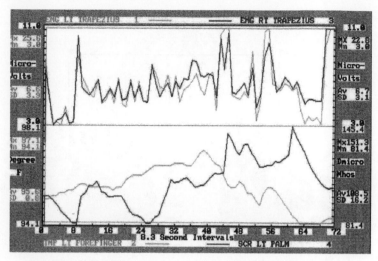

FIGURE 16.1   Psycho–physiological evaluation on Biocomp instrument.

A. Data collection of subjective and objective symptoms

Our clinic's methods of evaluation of chronic pain patients are comprehensive, and include a complete medical history followed by a psycho–physiological profile (PPP) using a Biocomp instrument. The PPP consists of measures of the peripheral level of arousal via electromyography (EMG), of skin temperature (TMP) and sweat gland activity, or skin conductance response (SCR), as patients are engaged in resting, then mental and emotional stress. An example of PPP is presented in Fig. 16.1.

The evaluation process includes objective cognitive tests such as TOVA (test of variables of attention) or IVA (integrated visual and auditory), and the MAS (memory assessment scale). Results of stress tests, depression or CES-D (Radloff 1977), anxiety tests, SCL-90R, and the level of pain evaluated with the chronic pain grade questionnaire (CPG) as VAS (visual analog scale) and/or the McGill questionnaire (Melzack 1975), are very important subjective parameters that aid in measuring progress.

The Electroencephalography (EEG) was obtained with an NF instrument, such as the Neurocybernetics or ROSHI. This provides us with information concerning electrical activity of the brain. We are especially interested in the sensory-motor area corresponding to the Penfield homunculus (Fig. 16.2) (Penfield and Jasper, 1954).

A quantitative EEG (QEEG), using the Lexicor Neurosearch-24, gives us further important and detailed information regarding various parameters such as relative and absolute magnitude, asymmetry, phase, and coherence using various software programs, e.g., Neuro-Guide, Nx–Linx, NeuroRep and LORETA. We are using the QEEG primarily in cases of traumatic brain injuries (TBI). The results obtained guide us more precisely in designing an appropriate protocol to assist in the neuromodulation of the client's pain perception. Recently we introduced the

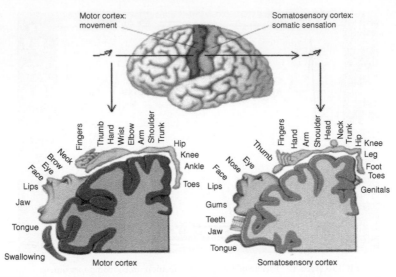

FIGURE 16.2   Penfield's homunculus presenting the sensory and motor cortical areas where we first analyze the EEG, and often where the NF training starts.

Hemoencephalogram (HEG) measurements to monitor the blood perfusion in the NF trained areas in some of our chronic pain patients. (An example is presented in the case studies section.)

B. Training strategies

The specific training strategy chosen is decided primarily by the BF modality that we, and others, have found to produce the best result in lowering the pain perception. In our practice, peripheral BF was useful in correcting the perception of tension headaches, myofascial pain syndromes, some TMJ, and in conducting neuromuscular re-education. Others have reported such BF useful as well, e.g., Sime (2004).

Nevertheless, in our practice NF has been the modality of choice in treating complex chronic pain syndromes, such as fibromyalgia, and RSD or complex regional pain syndrome I, CRPS type I (Ibric, 1996). In certain complex pain syndromes associated with many co-morbidities, the NF training is enhanced by light and/or electromagnetic stimulation, using ROSHI instruments. In short, the ROSHI instrument, designed to aid in the neurofeedback training, uses an algorithm, developed by Chuck Davis, named *complex adaptive modality*. This involves extracting the error aspects of one's EEG (for example, features such as transients) from the wideband EEG, and feeding back to the client non-error features of his or her brain activity in the form of colored LED light flashes and/or electromagnetic pulses, very much in real-time (Ibric and Davis, 2007).

After a comprehensive evaluation (Ibric, 1996), electrodes are placed in positions individualized for each case based on the type or localization of pain, and located according to 10/20 international system (Jasper, 1958).

Patients trained for 20 consecutive NF sessions, 45 minutes long, were then re-evaluated with the same battery of tests as those used at the intake. The number 20, for the number of NF sessions, before first re-evaluation followed the literature (Marzano *et al.*, 2001) that describes the "learning curve" for any learned skill. We also have found and reported earlier (Ibric and Dragomirescu, 2005) that 20 sessions were "necessary and almost sufficient" for the NF to be effective. The results of our statistical analyses on NF efficacy are presented at the end of this chapter.

To monitor progress, stress tests and depression/anxiety scales were used periodically, and the VAS for pain was used pre/post each NF training. NF was done either as "traditional NF" (audio-visual NF) using a Neurocybernetics system, and/or "NF enhanced by light or electromagnetic closed-loop EEG" (CL-EEG), using the ROSHI instrument. For example, we had discovered earlier that myofascial pain syndrome (MFPS) responded well to "traditional NF," versus fibromyalgia, or CRPS (chronic repetitive pain syndrome) that required NF enhanced by light and/or electromagnetic CL-EEG to have positive results. The employment of various light colors (LED or light emitting diodes) in the "eyesets" or goggles, and electromagnetic stimulation, was determined case by case, taking into consideration each person's emotional response to colors. For example, it has been observed that red and indigo colors are useful in cases were pain is accompanied by depression, while green and blue are necessary to reduce associated anxiety. Patients with different pain syndromes required different numbers of NF sessions.

VI.   CASES STUDIES 1–7

Case 1

Patient description: A 52-year-old female with reflex sympathetic dystrophy (RSD) post-MVA, post-neck surgery.

Symptoms: Right side face shoulder/arm, right eyelid spastic ptosis, depression, sleep disorder.

Etiology: MVA 3 years prior to investigating BF.

Other therapies: Neck surgery, physical therapy, electrical stimulator implanted.

Medications: Antidepressants, Vicodin.

NF training: 15 sessions. NF protocols were done mostly at C3 site (where Beta [15–18 Hz] was enhanced while Theta [4–7 Hz] and High Beta [22–30 Hz] suppressed.) Neurocybernetics was the instrument used. The C3 site corresponds to the right eye projection, at the sensory-motor area of the homunculus (see Fig. 16.1 above).

NF results: Patient was able to open the right eye as presented in Figs 16.3a and 16.3b, and have minimal pain over the right face, neck, shoulder and arm. In parallel, after 30 minutes of NF, the EEG activity normalized (Figs 16.3c and 16.3d). After the first session, the eye stayed open for 1 hour. As the NF continued, after each session the same effect occurred as described in the first session, except that it was

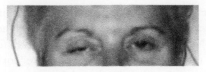

FIGURE 16.3A   Patient with RSD—right eye presents palpebral ptosis—before NF.

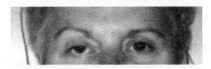

FIGURE 16.3B   Same patient as in Fig. 16.3a after 30 minutes of NF training, on Neurocybernetics instrument trained at the C3 position/Beta (15–18 Hz) enhanced.

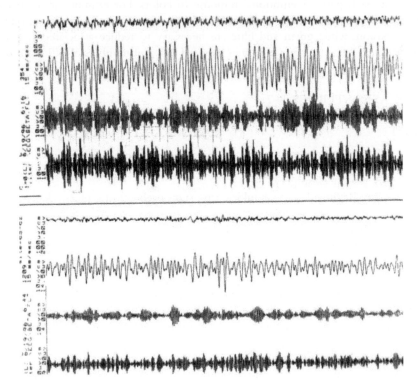

FIGURES 16.3C and 16.3D   EEG presentations of Case 1 (recorded on Neurocybernetics), corresponding to Figs. 16.3A and 16.3B respectively.

sustained for a longer and longer time. After 15 sessions, NF training was terminated due to her family leaving the state. This case was presented at the Myofascial Pain Syndrome Symposium sponsored by Discovery International (Ibric, 1996).

Case 2

Patient description: A 67-year-old retired actress (recently widowed) with chronic headaches, neck and low back pain, spasticity post-meningitis, and hypertension as co-morbidity.

Symptoms: Headaches, right side neck spasticity, gait dysfunction, depression/anxiety, sleep disorders, memory and concentration impairments, urinary incontinence.

Etiology: Three neck surgeries after an MVA that occurred 20 years prior to investigating BF. Last surgery was done a year before BF and that induced meningitis.

Other therapies: Surgery, psychotherapy, physical therapy, acupuncture.

Medications: Lorcet, Neurontin, Elavil, Restoril, Depakote, Norvasc, Baclofen, Hydrochlorothyazide, Duragesic patches, Synthroid, Cardura, Norco 10-350, Vitamin B complex, Vitamin E.

NF training: 145 sessions. Neurocybernetics and ROSHI instruments were used for her NF training. The electrode positioning varied from CZ to C3, or C4, C3-Cz, Cz-C4 and F3/F4, or C3/C4, enhancing either SMR, 15 Hz, or correcting coherence. EEG patterns modified, from a great variability to a more stable activity.

NF results: Pain perception modified and decreased to none, less depressed or anxious, better and more restful sleep, lowered blood pressure, better gait, and better quality of life. Patient was able to enjoy travel, and she was able to move to a new house, which she was unable to do, since her husband died. Able to reduce her meds by half, under her physician's supervision.

Case 3

Patient description: A 33-year-old retired construction engineer, neuropathy post-TBI and spinal cord injury.

Symptoms: Neck, shoulder, upper/lower back, arms and legs pain, spasticity, tremor, gait dysfunction, memory problems, depression, panic attacks, sleep deprivation, neurovegetative deregulation (temperature fluctuations with profuse sweats, paroxysmal tachycardia, blood pressure with large fluctuations!), which were exacerbated by Elavil (discontinued).

Etiology: TBI due to work injury that affected the brain stem (post-16 ft ladder fall).

Medications: Zoloft, Mirapex, Baclofen, Buspar, Vicodin, Sonata, Ambien, Elavil.

NF training: Total of 82 sessions. Protocols on NC (8) and on ROSHI (74).

NF results: Decreased pain, tremor and spasticity reduced, less depression, better sleep, reduced medication.

As an example, the Case 3 protocols were designed following the peripheral symptoms, such as for legs spasticity, and pain; the electrodes were placed over the central sensory motor area over the vertex at the Cz position. The ROSHI training was set for complex adaptive modality (CAM) for the light stimulation, to inhibit high beta frequency over 25 Hz, or HiBeta[I]. The effect was enhanced by using the electromagnetic stimulation, concomitantly. The hands tremor ceased when the electrodes were placed over the C3/C4 positions (where the motor control projection of the hands is located on Penfield's homunculus), and the training was designed to enhance S14 (SMR 14) or SMR, 12–15 Hz (while Theta and HiBeta were discouraged). The sessions done on ROSHI I, monitored and recorded on Neurocybernetics, and the changes in EEG presentation shown in Figs 16.4A and 16.4B.

In both Fig. 16.4A and 16.4B there are three panels. The first, at the top, represents the EEG evaluation at the C3 position; the second, in the middle, is at C4 position and the third, at the bottom, at Cz position. The changes, from before NF (Fig. 16.4A) and after NF (Fig. 16.4B), in the amplitude and the variability of all the frequencies analyzed (Theta, SMR and HiBeta) are obvious.

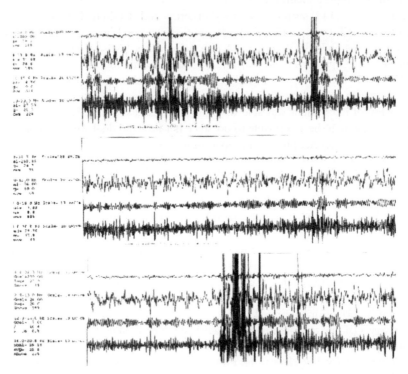

FIGURE 16.4A   Examples of brain waves of case 3 recorded on NC—before NF training on ROSHI.

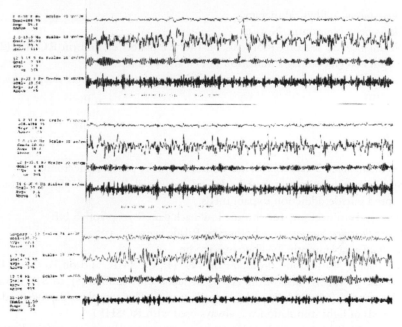

FIGURE 16.4B   Examples of brain waves of case 3 recorded on NC—after NF training on ROSHI.

Case 4

Patient description: A 20-year-old student with RSD left foot.

Symptoms: Chronic pain of left foot migrating to the right, headaches, and cognitive dysfunctions due to meds.

Etiology: A heavy metal object fell on her left foot, 2 years prior to investigating BF.

Other therapies: Physical therapy, acupuncture.

Medications: Various antidepressants, Vicodin, Motrin.

NF training: 20 sessions. Protocols mostly over the central sensory area at the Cz or Cz/C4 positions using the Neurocybernetics (11) followed by the ROSHI (9) NF instruments.

NF results: Pain reduced from 8 (0–10 VAS) to 2–1. Able to return to school.

Case 5

Patient description: 63-year-old retired engineer with idiopathic neuropathy and hypertension as co-morbidity.

Symptoms: Pain in both legs, level 9 (0–10 VAS) anxiety, sleep disorder, hypertension.

Other therapies: Physical therapy.

Medications: Neurontin, Norvasc.

NF training: 22 sessions. Protocols on NC Cz SMR (2), and on ROSHI (20) with light and electromag stimulation F3/F4 alpha inhibit.

Results: Pain reduction down to none, anxiety controlled, better sleep, reduced Neurontin.

Case 6

Patient description: 62-year-old writer with neuropathy post-laminectomy.

Symptoms: Chronic pain low back and legs, level 8 (0–10 VAS), depression, attempted suicide, addiction to pain meds.

Etiology: Laminectomy for chronic low back pain 8 yrs prior to NF.

Other therapies: Surgery, psychotherapy, Palade exercises, yoga.

Medications: Neurontin, Wellbutrin, Vicodin.

NF training: 46 sessions. Protocols on NC (4), Cz SMR, and on ROSHI (42), F3/F4 the protocols varied from AO[I] or alpha only inhibit (8), to S14 reward (4), B16 reward (16), B17 (5) and Sync enhance (9). The complex adaptive modality (CAM) of light stimulation was always used with ROSHI I.

NF results: Pain reduction down to none, no more depression, reduced meds, no more Vicodin.

Seven years after the NF training ended, the learned skills continued to benefit the client, and enhanced his performance.

Case 7

Patient description: A 35-year-old student with MFPS, chronic headaches (multiple origins) and (PTSD), Bruxism.

Symptoms: Headaches due to dental problems or sinus infections or allergies, left TMJ, teeth grinding, depression, anxiety, anger, sleep disorders.

Other therapies: Chiropractic, massage therapy, sinus surgeries, psychotherapy.

Medications: Neurontin, Depakote, Vicodin, Acetaminophen, Motrin, Relafen, Diazepam, Lorcet, Relafen, Baclofen, Tegretol, Serozone, Lidocaine Infusions, Antihistamines (Zyrtec, NavCon-A, Albuterol, as needed).

NF training: 15 sessions. Protocols used as needed at Cz or C4 SMR and C3 Beta (some sessions done with alternation of C3 beta followed by C4 SMR) using Neurocybernetics instrument.

NF results: Headache and TMJ pain reduced from 8–9 to 2–1, and emotional correction of depression. Anxiety reduced from 8 to 2–0. Improved cognitive functioning with the reduction of the meds. Three months post the 15th session the normalization of the brain wave activity sustained, and she was able to resume school.

VII. LONGITUDINAL CASE STUDIES (8–10)

Case 8

Patient description: A 51-year-old teacher with chronic neck/shoulder or N/S pain, and TMJ/RSD; co-morbidity, rheumatoid arthritis.

Symptoms: Severe chronic pain (left neck/shoulder, TMJ, ear), numbness of left hand; sleep disorders—insomnia, teeth grinding; fatigue, nervousness.

Etiology: MVA 4 years prior to investigating BF.

Medications: Relafen, Plaquenil, Prozac, Serozone (Elavil, Zoloft, Sinequal in the past), HRT for menopause.

BF: 2 sessions without any positive results.

NF training: 22 sessions on NC, resumed NF after a 5-month break, then continued to session 51 on NC, followed by three re-evaluations.

NF training: At Cz or C4—SMR enhanced, and theta and high beta discouraged.

NF results: TMJ and neck/shoulder pain level was lowered from 8–9 to 2–4, and was gradually reduced and kept at acceptable levels of 1–3 on the visual analog scale, or VAS (see Figs. 16.5–16.9) for a longer time, even after the NF ended.

The pain reduction for session number (n) was estimated by subtracting from the declared pain at the end, the declared pain at the beginning of each session, or $Post_n$-Pre_n. For every session n, the relative reduction of pain (R_n), compared to the pain perceived before the first session (Pre_1), was calculated by using the formula: $R_n = (Post_n-Pre_n)/Pre_1$. (See for cases 8 and 9, the Figs 16.6 and 16.8, and Figs 16.11 and 16.13, respectively).

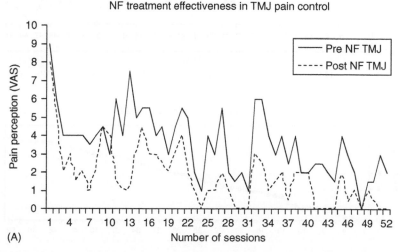

FIGURE 16.5A   TMJ pain, pre and post each NF session in time. Note: Session 22 done after a 5-month break; session 51 marked the end of NF series; session 52 is a re-evaluation.

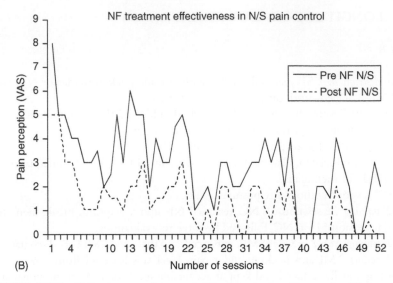

FIGURE 16.5B   N/S pain, pre and post each NF session in time. Note: session 22 done after a 5-month break; session 51 marked the end of NF series; session 52 is a re-evaluation after another year.

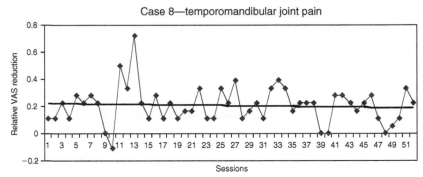

FIGURE 16.6   TMJ pan relative reduction (R_n), based on VAS. $R_n = (Pre_n - Post_n)/Pre_1$. Pre_n and $Post_n$ are VAS values Pre and Post, respectively, in session number n.

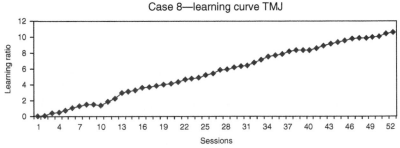

FIGURE 16.7   The learning curve for controlling TMJ pain, following NF training sessions (where $C_1 = R_1$ and $C_n = C_{n-1} + R_n$).

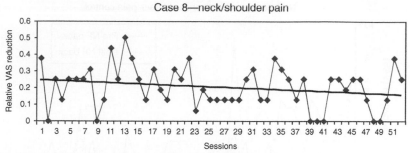

FIGURE 16.8   Neck/shoulder pain relative reduction (R_n), based on VAS. $R_n = (Pre_n - Post_n)/Pre_1$.

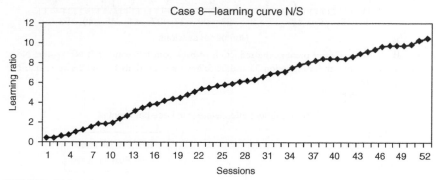

FIGURE 16.9   The learning curve for controlling neck and shoulder (NS) pain, following the NF training sessions (where $C_1 = R_1$ and $C_n = C_{n-1} + R_n$).

To quantify the clients' learned control of pain over n sessions, we constructed the cumalative learning curves presented in Figs 16.7 and 16.9 and 16.12 and 16.14, for cases 8 and 9 respectively. For example, the client, after session one learned to reduce pain in proportion R_1, therefore $C_1 = R_1$. After a second session the client learned from previous session (n−1) plus the current session (n), or $C_n = C_{n-1} + R_n$.

Case 9

Patient description: 60-year-old housewife with chronic pain. Co-morbidities: Parkinson's disease (PD), skin and colon cancer, chronic lymphatic leukemia (CLL).

Etiology: 2 years prior BF fell and injured left knee, diagnosed also with CLL and PD.

Symptoms: Severe lower back and left knee pain, level 8–9 (0–10 VAS), spasticity of left foot, numbness of the left hand, tremor, depression, anxiety, sleep disorder, tinnitus.

Medications: Cinemet, Trazadone, Zoloft, Lodosyn, HRT, Oscal and multivitamins.

NF training: Protocols total of 56 sessions on NC (Session 54 after a 6-month break; session 55 and 56 follow-up evaluations at 1½ and 2½ years after NF ended,

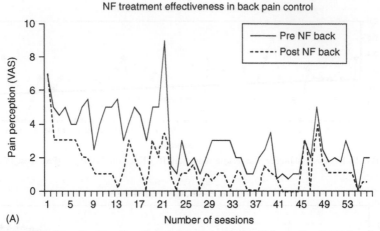

(A)

FIGURE 16.10A   Case 9 presents the reduction of back pain following each NF session. Note: Session 54 after a 6-month break; session 55 and 56 follow up evaluations 1½ and 2½ years after NF ended, respectively.

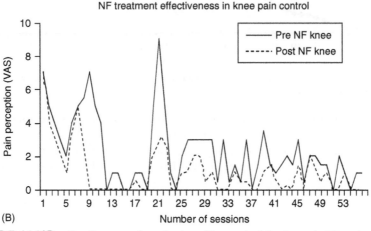

(B)

FIGURE 16.10B   Case 9 presents the reduction of knee pain following each NF session. Note: Session 54 after a 6-month break; session 55 and 56 follow up evaluations 1½ and 2½ years after NF ended, respectively.

respectively.), mostly at Cz position enhancing SMR and reducing high beta and theta.

Results: Spasticity lowered form 8–10 to 3 post 20 sessions, and reduced to none after 50 sessions. Tremor more controlled and better after each session, imperceptible after 50 sessions. Pain reduction to 2–1, anxiety/depression controlled, better sleep, reduced meds (under physician control). Pain continued to be under control even after 1½ or 2½ years, after the NF training ended (see Figs 16.10–16.14).

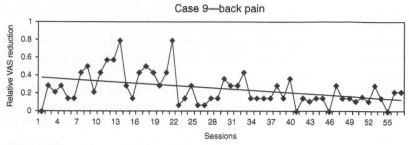

FIGURE 16.11   Back pain relative reduction (R_n), based on VAS. ($R_n = (Pre_n - Post_n)/Pre_1$.

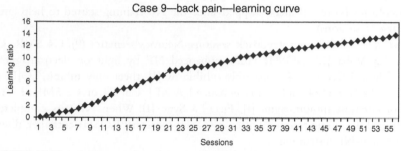

FIGURE 16.12   The learning curve for controlling back pain, following the NF training ($C_1 = R_1$ and $C_n = C_{n-1} + R_n$).

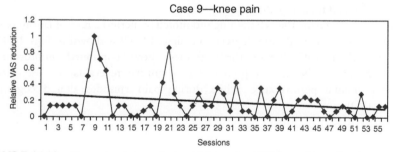

FIGURE 16.13   Knee pain relative reduction (R_n), based on VAS. $R_n = (Pre_n - Post_n)/Pre_1$.

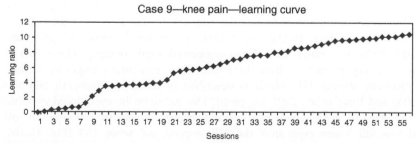

FIGURE 16.14   The learning curve for controlling knee pain, following the NF training ($C_1 = R_1$ and $C_n = C_{n-1} + R_n$).

Case 10

Patient description: A 42-year-old carpenter with left inguinal pain post-surgery and kidney stones (185 over the years), MTBI, chronic colitis, addictions to pain killers/ marijuana and smoking.

Symptoms: Depression/anger, chronic fatigue, left inguinal pain, low back pain.

Etiology: Hernia surgery and epidydimectomy 4 years prior to investigating BF; work injury (hit with a construction wood log of 2 by 4 at the posterior right side of the head).

Other therapies: Acupuncture, chiropractic, herbs.

Medications: Vicodin, Morphin (repeated ER visits), Iboprufen 2400 mg, Epinephrine. Note: All meds stopped since the NF training started to help (after the first 15 sessions).

NF training: 112 neurofeedback sessions. Neurocybernetics (9); C4 SMR, C3 Beta, P3 Alpha [E]; ROSHI (103); enhanced NF by light or electromagnetic closed-loop EEG: F3/F4 alpha only inhibit, AO[I]; theta only inhibit, TO[I], or theta 4, T4[I]; P3/P4, alpha only enhanced, AO[E]; C3/C4 or Cz SMR; F3/F7, synchronization inhibit, Sync [I]; Fp1/T3 Sync [I]. When NF was completed, continued the home training with a pROSHI (personal ROSHI entrainer/disentrainer, non-NF instrument).

NF Results: Pain reduction from 9–10 immobilizing pain to 3–1, and complete elimination of painkillers. Able to go back to work, and produced musical CDs due to enhanced mental performance.

The progress during the NF training monitored by periodic re-evaluations of the stress response, SCL-90R, and depression scale (CES-D) is shown in Figs. 16.15A 16.15B and 16.15C. These three figures show continued improvement of this patient's subjective responses. The cognitive re-evaluation also shows increased mental performance, while during pain episodes altered cognition (Fig. 16.15D).

QEEG

The case's 10 results of the QEEG connectivity map, using NeuroRep program, are presented in Fig. 16.16A, and the response to the ROSHI light enhanced NF is shown in Figs. 16.16B and 16.16C. There are disconnected (blue) areas of the brain and other areas hyper-connected (dark orange). These data are part of an experiment we have done to evaluate real-time changes in the brain connectivity during NF, which is described in detail in Hudspeth and Ibric (2004) and Ibric *et al.*, 2007 (in press). The nZ-score in eyes-closed condition is 335 (Fig. 16.16A), which was lowered during the NF to 179 (Fig. 16.16B,) and was still lower even after the NF stopped, nZ score 169 (Fig. 16.16C). Our interpretation, for the results obtained, is that the lower the nZ score, the

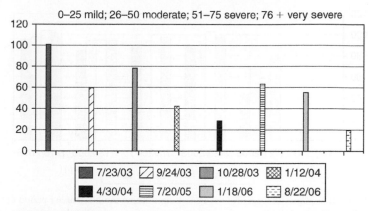

FIGURE 16.15A   Case 10: Stress test evaluations over the years of NF training.

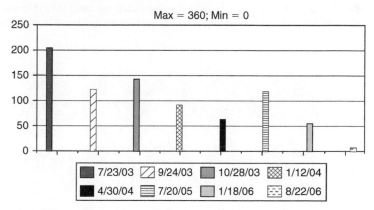

FIGURE 16.15B   Case 10: SCL-90R evaluations over the years of NF training.

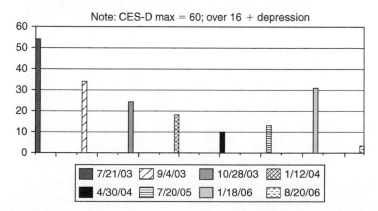

FIGURE 16.15C   Case 10: Depression CES-D evaluations over the years of NF training.

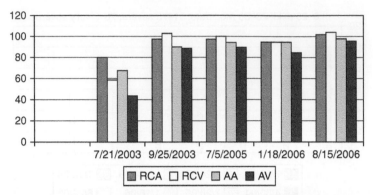

FIGURE 16.15D   Case 10: Cognitive test IVA changes during the NF training period of 3 years since the NF training started. Observe that, due to pain, the first evaluation shows lower values for the response control for auditory (RSA) as well as response control for visual (RCV) processing; even lower values are shown for the attention quotients for auditory (AA) and visual (AV). (Normal values are over 90). NF training produced normalization of the IVA parameters in subsequent measurements.

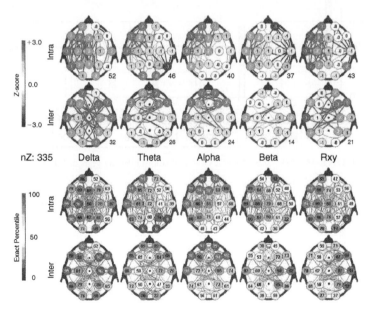

FIGURE 16.16A   Case 10: QEEG—Connectivity map in eyes-closed condition (nZ score 335, shows a high level of disconnection).

better the brain should function. Therefore the NF, by modifying the connectivity parameters, proves to be an effective training tool for patients post-TBI and suffering with chronic pain.

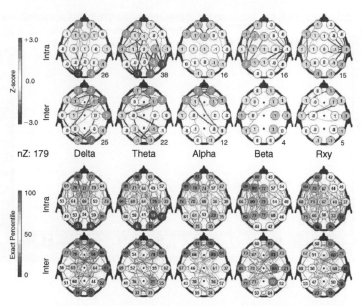

FIGURE 16.16B   Case 10: QEEG—Connectivity map in eyes-closed condition during the ROSHI NF training (nZ score 179 shows a reduction of the disconnection).

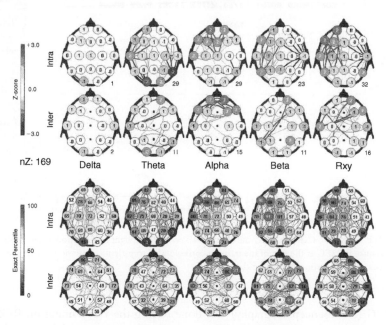

FIGURE 16.16C   Case 10: QEEG—Connectivity map in eyes-closed condition after ROSHI NF training (nZ score 169 shows a continued correction of the connectivity).

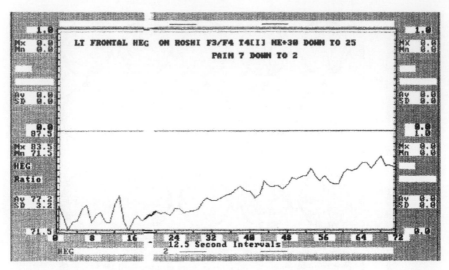

FIGURE 16.17A   Case 10: HEG during the NF on ROSHI NF light enhanced.

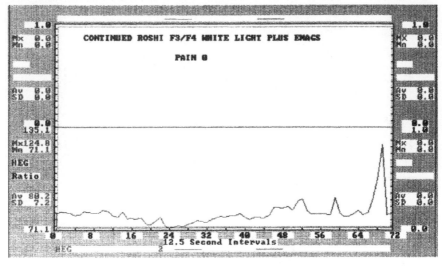

FIGURE 16.17B   Case 10: HEG during the NF on ROSHI, light and electromagnetic enhanced NF. The spike in HEG at the end of the training corresponded to patient's expression of happiness, due to the complete resolution of pain for the first time.

HEG (Hemoencephalography) was done during the NF training on ROSHI instrument. Figs. 16.17A and 16.17B shows that the perfusion of the frontal area increased and corresponded to lowering of the pain perception.

VIII.   STATISTICAL ANALYSIS OF THE NF EFFICACY IN PAIN SYNDROMES

The analysis of the responses to the NF training in our chronic pain patient group offered many interesting results, which are reported here. Firstly, we evaluated the relationship between the number of sessions and the outcome; secondly, we verified the efficacy of NF in cases treated for more than 19 sessions; thirdly, we checked if there is a correlation between the age of our patients to the number of sessions needed; and fourthly, we evaluated the influence of gender on the number of NF sessions needed to correct their pain perception.

Table 16.5 presents the total number of patients (147) used in the study, from which 52 were males and 95 females. The outcomes of the NF training in relationship to the number of NF sessions are presented. It can be seen that there is a direct correlation between the number of sessions and the positive outcome. When the NF training was done only for up to 19 sessions, the rate of success is very reduced (only three cases ameliorated), while in the case of the patients who completed more than 19 sessions of NF, the success rate was evident (68 out of 74 cases with clinical significant improvement (CSI), or 92%, and up to 95% total success if we consider all CSI cases plus two ameliorated).

We chose the value 20 (first number >19) as a minimal limit for the number of NF sessions (CSM), following the literature (Marzano et al., 2001). We also found and reported previously (Ibric and Dragomirescu, 2005) from our patient group, and in particular from Cases 8 and 9 that a minimal number of 20 sessions was necessary to obtain CSI, or to attain 70–80% of the learning curve as Marzano described in his study on students' learning skills.

A.   NF training efficacy relative to number of sessions (NS)

We compared NS for the three types of results obtained: Clinical significant improvement = CSI, Ameliorated = A, and those without any positive results or zero results = 0 results. The results are presented in Tables 16.5 and 16.6.

TABLE 16.5

	No. cases	Positive results
Number of patients with 1 NF session after evaluation	15	0
Number of patients who completed 2–10 NF sessions	33	[1 ameliorated (A)]
Number of patients who completed 11–19 NF sessions	25	[3 A]
Number of patients who completed >19 NF sessions	74	[2 A + 68 CSI* = 70]
Success rate CSI* = 68/74 = 92%		
Success rate of POSITIVE RESULTS = 70/74 = 95%		

*CSI is abbreviation for "Clinical Significant Improvement"

TABLE 16.6 The minimum (Min), maximum (Max) and the three quartiles [lower (Q_1), median (Me) and upper (Q_3)] of NS (# Sessions) for the "0 or no results", (0) ameliorated (A) and clinical significant improvement (CSI) patients

Efficacy Results	Number of NF Sessions (NS)					
	Number of patients	Minimum (Min)	Lower Quartile, Q1 (25%)	Median (Me) (50%)	Upper Quartile, Q3 (75%)	Maximum (Max)
0 results	73	1	2	**6**	13	32
A	6	8	14	**18.5**	25	34
CSI	68	20	27	**35.5**	64.5	250

The differences (Kruskal-Wallis test) between medians 6.0, 18.5, 35.5 are significant ($p < 0.001$). ($H = 104.79, DF = 2, P = 0.000$)

Table 16.6 shows that the "0 results" were obtained in 73 cases, from which some were only evaluated and had a minimum of one session, some with a maximum of 32, and with a median of 6 sessions. Amelioration was obtained in 6 cases only, with a minimum of eight sessions, a maximum of 34, and a median of 18.5 sessions. The lack of success in some of the cases where more than 20 NF sessions were completed may be linked to the complexity, as well as to a large numbers of co-morbidities and the duration of these pain syndromes (see the discussion section below for details regarding the distortion of the Default Mode Network dynamics of the brain). Therefore, it can be seen in Table 16.6 that the NF efficiency results are highly dependent on the number of sessions. In the same table there are other interesting observations. For example, the minimum number to show clinically significant improvement (CSI) is 20. The differences (based on Kruskal-Wallis test) between medians 6.0, 18.5, 35.5 are significant ($p<0.001$). ($H = 104.79, DF = 2, P = 0.000$).

Using the MINITAB program for plotting data presented in Table 16.6, we generated Fig. 16.18 showing that there are statistical outliers in the CSI and the "0 results" categories. These values are outside the $Q_3 + 1/5(Q_3 - Q_1)$ quartile interval in their respective subsets.

TABLE 16.7 Case control study of the Efficacy of NF training for "more than 19 sessions"

NF exposure	Cases—with illness (0 effect)	Controls—without illness (Positive effect)
Exposed to enough NF training (More than 19 sessions)	4	70
Not exposed to enough NF training (1–19 NF sessions)	69	4

From Table 16.7, a case-control study was considered and (Odd Ratio OR) = 0 was obtained. Because one or more expected values are less than 5 we used the exact confidence limits according to the Fisher Exact test, and they are: exact lower 95% confidence limit = 0, and exact upper 95% confidence limit = 0.02. Because OR < 1 and

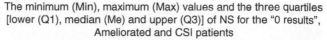

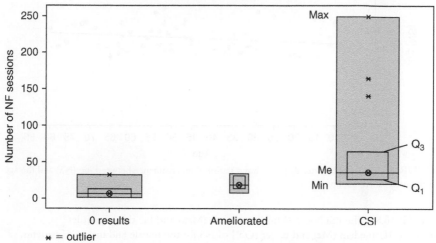

* = outlier

FIGURE 16.18   Boxplot of number of NF sessions for "0 results," ameliorated, and CSI patients. The areas of the boxes are proportional to the sample volumes. (See Table 16.6 for the values.)

the confidence interval (0, 0.02) does not include 1, our data indicate that treatment with more than 19 sessions is a protective factor for chronic pain. This is consistent with other previous reports in the NF literature (Lubar, 1985, Steinberg and Othmer, 2004).

B. Relationship between the patient's age and the number of sessions (NS) of NF

Figure 16.19 shows a scatter diagram of age of our pain patient group versus log (NS). This was done for exploratory purposes only. The cloud of the data points is distributed, approximately, parallel to the horizontal axis. This result shows that there is no correlation between the age of our pain patient group and the number of NF sessions needed, expressed as log (NS).

C. Relationship between the patient's gender and the response to the NS of NF

Table 16.8 presents the quartiles of NS for both sexes from the "CSI" group of patients. According to the Mann–Whintey test, the two median values, 32 and 46.5, for females vs. males respectively, are not significantly different (p < 0.128). This p value is very close to 0.1, which may be significant from some statisticians'

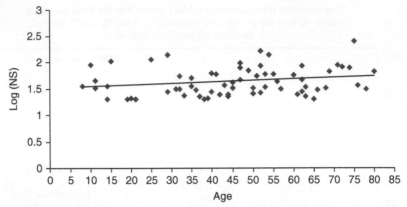

FIGURE 16.19   The scatter diagram shows statistical independence between log (NS) and the age of the pain patient group.

TABLE 16.8   The minimum (Min), maximum (Max) and the three quartiles [lower (Q1), median (Me) and upper (Q3)] of NS for the female and male CSI patients. (See Figure 16.20 for the Boxplot representation).

Sex	Number of sessions (NS)				
	Number of patients	Minimum (Min)	Lower Quartile, Q1 (25%)	Median (Me) (50%)	Upper Quartile, Q3 (75%)	Maximum (Max)
Female	40	20	24.5	32	60	250
Male	28	20	31.5	46.5	73.5	164

The differences (based on Kruskal-Wallis test for two groups equivalent to Mann-Whitney test or Wilcox on Two-Sample Test) between 32 and 46.5 are not significant (H = 2.314, DF = 1, p = 0.128)

standpoint. (Some statisticians accept the value 0.1 as a limit with statistic significance, instead of 0.05. Therefore, the value p = 0.128 we obtained is very close to 0.1. We consider then, if we would have increased the sample number for this analysis, we could possibly obtain a significant difference between the responses of the two sexes in controlling pain through NF training.)

IX.   DISCUSSION

Why is neurofeedback useful in the modulation of pain perception? If we are to follow the localization of the central parameters of pain as mentioned above, we can design protocols that can rather directly address these parameters. For example, for pain intensity, by considering the SI area or the main sensory area over the central SM, and following the homunculus map, we can address the pain intensity for the particular area that needs attention (Tolle et al., 1999). If the emotional issues

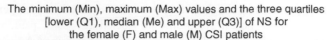

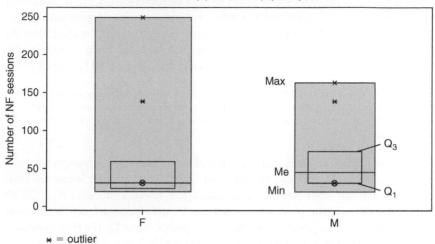

* = outlier

FIGURE 16.20 Boxplot of number of NF sessions for CSI patients: female (F) versus male (M) population. The areas of the boxes are proportionally to the sample volumes. (See Table 16.8 for the values.)

are associated with the pain they are usually feeding the pain; then the area to address with NF training will be the anterior cingulate gyrus (Rainville, 1997).

Insofar as psychological factors are concerned, the cognitive processes of the patient are important to investigate in order to understand pain and disability. Coping mechanisms with chronic pain differ from patient to patient, as mentioned by Hanson and Gerber (1990) and Haythornthwaite et al., 1998. Psychological and social factors impacting on pain may change the level of arousal, and modify body chemistry. Thought effects on sympathetic arousal and muscle tension could be measured with peripheral BF. Thoughts apparently can change the body bio-chemistry, producing endogenous analgesia. For example, Bandura (1987) examined and demonstrated the direct effect of cognitive control of pain on central opiod activity. And Birbaumer et al. (1995) and Maihöfner et al. (2003) showed that the brain changes its functional organization at the level of the somato-sensory cortex in chronic pain patients. Thus, it should not be especially surprising that NF, with its emphasis on volitional control, has been found useful in pain modulation as demonstrated by Ibric (1996) and Donaldson et al. (1998, 2004).

X. CONCLUSIONS

Pain or DOLOR is one of the five symptoms described in any kind of inflamma-tion process. That is why so many anti-inflammatory drugs are administered at the first sign of persistent and debilitating pain. However, when pain persists for longer than 6 months, and the symptoms are labeled as chronic pain, other medications such as morphine or its derivatives tend to be prescribed. A major problem is that often the pain is accompanied by other symptoms such as depression, anxiety, sleep disturbances, and decision-making abnormalities (Apkarian et al., 2004a). As stated by Baliki et al. (2008, p. 1398), "chronic pain hurts the brain, disrupting the default-mode network dynamics (DMN)." Their study, using fMRI, showed that

> the brain of a chronic pain patient is not simply a healthy brain processing pain information, but rather is altered by the persistent pain in a manner reminiscent of other neurological conditions associated with cognitive impairments (Baliki et al. 2008, p. 1402).

In their study, these co-morbidities are found accompanying the pain syndromes, possibly having been produced by disrupted DMN. During a task, there are areas of activation while other areas are deactivated. The research of Baliki et al. (2008) showed that chronic pain patients presented much smaller areas of brain deactivation in several key areas, suggesting widespread disruptions of the DMN, thus indicating that this phenomenon may underlie the cognitive and behavioral impairments.

During the last half century NF has become a state-of-the-art training modality. With each passing year, more sophisticated computer programs have been developed, and improved NF protocols designed based on comprehensive standardized evaluations. Adding QEEG evaluations has played an important role in enhancing NF by guiding training protocol designs. Training strategies evolved as more accurate electrode positioning, and more brainwave enhancement/suppression possibilities became available. Specifically with regard to NF for pain syndromes, training is being dictated by the characteristics of pain and the multitude of overlapping diagnoses.

There are many examples of clinical and research findings of special significance for the understanding and treatment of pain. For example, NF training applied over the frontal cortex has been found to be followed by a change in pain affect as reported by patients with acute or chronic pain syndromes. And this effect correlates with the localization of the unpleasantness of the pain as described by Rainville et al. (1997). Apkarian (2004b), using functional MRI techniques, revealed that chronic back pain appears in a different part of the brain (prefrontal cortex) than the discomfort of burning a finger, for example. The acute sensory pain of the burned finger appears in the sensory part of the thalamus with projection into the cortical homunculus. That may explain why NF may be successful when applied to the areas of the brain corresponding to the peripheral perception of an acute pain. However, chronic back pain shows up in the prefrontal cortex. By contrast, with the acute pain representation, the chronic pain leaves an imprint in the prefrontal cortex; thus, it seems that the longer the suffering of pain, the more activity in the prefrontal area.

QEEG evaluations have provided similar results to fMRIs, and have guided NF practitioners to train the prefrontal cortex in patients who have suffered from chronic pain for a very long time. This "cumulative memory" may be modulated, or erased through NF.

However, NF training in patients with acute or chronic pain syndromes, applied over the contralateral central cortex area corresponding to the peripheral painful regions, can bring significant changes in the perception of pain, expressed as pain threshold and pain tolerance. There are no significant differences between the number of NF sessions and the age of the patient population analyzed in this study. There are no significant differences between the male and female responses to NF training regarding the change in pain perception. Thus, we can conclude that the ages of the pain patient population do not influence the response in modulating the pain perception. The number of NF sessions does influence the outcome. Twenty sessions were "necessary and almost sufficient" to produce some positive effects on the pain perception and affect of our patients.

Due to the relatively small number of cases analyzed in this study, it was hard to determine how the different diagnostic cases responded to NF training. Also, we could not conclude that gender influenced the outcome like others observed (Derbyshire, 2008), since our sample population was too small. As a final conclusion, however, we can say that NF training, if carried out past 19 sessions, can modify pain perception and pain affect, perhaps permanently. Correction of sleep and emotional dysfunctions has also been noted.

NF training directly addresses cortical areas corresponding to pain perception, memory, and affect. NF, based on neuromodulation, achieves its positive and sustained results largely through operant conditioning. However, it also can impinge favorably upon the pain experience indirectly through arousal regulation, as well as through enhanced central nervous system and autonomic nervous system stability, and improved homeostatic control. Commensurate with the neuroplasticity of the nervous system, the localization of pain perception at the central level seems capable of being changed by events at the periphery (see work on the remapping of the brain sensory area in amputees [Ramanchandran and Rogers-Ramachandran, 2000]). The corticalization of pain perception described by Birbaumer et al. (1995), Apkarian et al. (2004 a and b), and Baliki et al. (2008) also helps explain the basis of the pain modulation obtained through NF techniques.

DeCharms et al. (2005), using fMRI, reported that the anterior cingulate is an area involved in pain severity, and found the fMRI imaging to be responsive to feedback control. Since then greater attention has been given to the possibility of using fMRI in pain management. In 2007, the Institute of Medicine's report states that functional imaging is under study and possibly can be used not only to detect brain areas affected by chronic pain, but also act as a therapeutic intervention. However, fMRI used in therapy may not be cost-effective. nfortunately, despite many clinical and research findings regarding EEG correlates of pain, and a great many cases of successful treatment of pain through NF, nothing was mentioned in this report about the promise of NF.

The use of QEEG as the basis for identifying the location and type of brain disturbances, or the efficacy of using neurofeedback for modifying or eliminating pain, should also be considered. The research and clinical cases cited in this chapter attest to the fact that through the application of neurofeedback it is possible for pain patients to extend the brain's natural self-healing powers, and perhaps re-establish a "default mode network" needed for optimal brain function. These non-invasive techniques, QEEG and NF, must continue to be integrated in the medical care for those who suffer with chronic pain.

REFERENCES

Acerra, N. E. and Moseley, G. L. (2005). Dysynchiria: watching the mirror image of the unaffected limb elicits pain on the affected side. *Neurology*, **65**, 751–753.

Apkarian, A. V., Sosa, Y., Krauss, B. R., *et al.* (2004a). Chronic pain patients are impaired on an emotional decision-making task. *Pain*, **108**, 129–136.

Apkarian, A. V., Sosa, Y., Sonty, S., *et al.* (2004b). Chronic Back Pain is Associated with Decreased Prefrontal and Thalamic Gray Matter Density. *J. Neurosci.*, **24**, 10410–10415.

Arena, J. G. and Blanchard, E. B. (1996). Biofeedback and Relaxation Therapy for Chronic Pain Syndromes. In *Psychological Approaches to Pain Management: A Practitioner's Handbook* (R. J. Gatchel and D. S. Turk, eds), pp. 179–230. New York: The Guilford Press.

Baliki, M. N., Geha, P. Y., Apkarian, A. V. and Chialvo, D. R. (2008). Beyond Feeling: Chronic Pain Hurts the Brain, Disrupting the Default-Mode Network Dynamics. *Journal of Neuroscience*, **28(6)**, 1398–1403.

Bandura, A., O'Leary, A., Taylor, C. B., Gauthier, J. and Gossard, D. (1987). Perceived self-efficacy and pain control: Opiod and non-opiod mechanisms. *Journal of Personality and Social Psychology*, **53**, 563–571.

Birbaumer, N., Flor, H., Lutzenberger, W. and Elbert, T. (1995). The Corticalization of Pain. In *Pain and the Brain: From Nociception to Cognition. Advances in Pain Research and Therapy* (B. Desmendt and J. E. Desmendt, eds) **Vol. 22**, pp. 331–343. New York: Raven Press.

Block, A. R., Kremer, E. F. and Gaylor, M. (1980). Behavioral treatment of chronic pain: Variables affecting treatment efficacy. *Pain*, **8**, 367–375.

Brown, B. B. (1974). *New Mind, New Body, Bio-feedback: New Directions for the Mind*. Harper and Row Publishers, New York, Evanston, San Francisco, London.

Brown, B. B. and Klugg, J. W. (1974). Exploration of EEG Alpha biofeedback as a technique to enhance rapport. *Abstract at Proceedings of the Biofeedback Research Society*, **79**.

Budzynski, T. H. (1976). Biofeedback and the twilight states of consciousness. In *Consciousness and Self-Regulation* (G. E. Schwartz and D. Shapiro, eds), p. 1. New York: Plenum Press.

Budzynski, T. H., Stoyva, J. M., Adler, C. S. and Mullaney, D. J. (1973). EMG biofeedback and tension headache: A controlled study. *Psychosomatic Medicine*, **35**, 484–496.

Carlsson, S. G. (1975). Treatment of temporomandibular joint syndrome with biofeedback training. *Journal of the American Dental Association*, **91**, 602–605.

Cairns, D. and Passino, J. (1977). Comparison of verbal reinforcement and feedback in the operant treatment of disability of chronic low back pain. *Behavior Therapy*, **8**, 621–630.

Craig, K. D. (1986). Social modeling influences: Pain in context. In *The psychology of pain* (R. A. Sternbach, ed.), 2nd edition, pp. 67–95. New York: Raven Press.

DeCharms, R. C., Maeda, F., Glover, G. H., *et al.* (2005). Control over brain activation and pain learned by using real-time functional MRI. *Proc. Natl. Acad. Sci. USA*, **102(51)**, 18626–18631.

Derbyshire, S. W. G. (2008). Gender, Pain, and the Brain. *Pain, Clinical Updates* (3). pp. 1–4.

Donaldson, C. C. S., Sella, G. E. and Mueller, H. H. (1998). Fibromyalgia: A retrospective study of 252 consecutive referrals. *Canadian Journal of Clinical Medicine*, **5(6)**, 116–127.

Donaldson, C. C. S., Sella, G. E. and Mueller, H. H. (2004a). The Neural Plasticity Model of Fibromyalgia: Theory, Assessment and Treatment. (Part 1). Practical Pain Management. Glen Mills, PA: PPM Communications. May/June, 12–18.

Donaldson, C. C. S., Sella, G. E. and Mueller, H. H. (2004b). The Neural Plasticity Model of Fibromyalgia: Theory, Assessment and Treatment. (Part 2). Practical Pain Management. Glen Mills, PA: PPM Communications. July/August, 18–25.

Donaldson, C. C. S., Sella, G. E. and Mueller, H. H. (2004c). The Neural Plasticity Model of Fibromyalgia: Theory, Assessment and Treatment (Part 3). Practical Pain Management. Glen Mills, PA: PPM Communications. September/October, 25–31.

Donaldson, C. C. S., Sella, G. E. and Mueller, H. H. (2004d). The Neural Plasticity Model of Fibromyalgia: Theory, Assessment and Treatment. (Part 4). Practical Pain Management. Glen Mills, PA: PPM Communications. November/December, 31–40.

Egner, T., Zech, T. F. and Gruzelier, J. H. (2004). The effects of neurofeedback training on the spectral topography of the electroencephalogram. *Clinical Neurophysiology*, **115**, 2452–2460.

Fehmi, L. G. (1970). Feedback and states of consciousness meditation. In *Proceedings of the Biofeedback Research Society* (B. Brown, ed.), pp. 1–22.

Fordyce, W. E. (1976). *Behavioral methods for chronic pain and illness*. St. Louis, MO: C.V. Mosby.

Fox, M. D. and Raichle, M. E. (2007). Chronic Pain and the Emotional Brain: Specific Brain Activity Associated with Spontaneous Fluctuations of Intensity of Chronic Back Pain. *Nat. Rev. Neurosci.*, **8**, 701–711.

Freeman, L. W. (2004). *Mosby's Complementary and Alternative Medicine (CAM): A research based approach, 2nd edition*. St. Louis: Mosby.

Gatchel, R. J. and Turk, D. C. (eds) (1996). *Psychological Approaches to Pain Management—A Practitioner's Handbook*. New York: Guilford Press.

Green, E. (1972). Biofeedback for mind-body self-regulation: Healing and creativity. In *Biofeedback and Self Control*, Shapiro. *et al.* (eds). Aldine Publishing Co.

Guyol, G. (2006). Neurofeedback: Retraining Brain Waves *Healing Depression and Bipolar Disorder without Drugs. Part II – The Most Effective Nondrug Therapies*, pp. 149–157. NY: Walker and Company. Inc.

Ham, L. P. and Packard, R. C. (1996). A retrospective, follow-up study of biofeedback-assisted relaxation therapy in patients with posttraumatic headache. *Biofeedback & Self-Regulation*, **21(2)**, 93–104.

Hammond, C. (2000). Neurofeedback Treatment of Depression with the ROSHI. *Journal of Neurotherapy*, **4(2)**, 45–55.

Hammond, D. C. (2001). Treatment of chronic fatigue with neurofeedback and self-hypnosis. *NeuroRehabilitation*, **16**, 295–300.

Hanson, L. M. and Ainsworth, K. D. (1990). Self-regulation of chronic pain: Preliminary empirical findings. *Canadian Journal of Psychiatry*, **25(1)**, 38–43.

Hanson, R. W. and Gerber, K. E. (1990). *Coping with chronic pain: A guide to patient self-management*. New York: Guilford Press.

Haythornthwaite, J. A., Menefee, L. A., Heinberg, L. J. and Clark, M. R. (1998). Pain coping strategies predict perceived control over pain. *Pain*, **77**, 33–39.

Holroyd, K. A., Malinoski, P., Davis, M. K. and Lipchik, G. L. (1999). The three Dimensions of Headache Impact: Pain, Disability and Affective Distress. In: Pain, **83(3)**, 571–578.

Hudspeth, W. J. and Ibric, V. L. (2004). qEEG and Behavioral Indices for Neurofeedback Effectiveness. ECNS Symposia [Abstract] in *Clinical EEG and Neuroscience*, **35(4)**, 213–214.

Ibric, V. L. (1996). Components in Long Term, Comprehensive Care of patients with Myofascial Pain Syndrome: Part II – The Usefulness of Biofeedback. In *Contemporary Management of Myofascial Pain Syndrome Symposium*, sponsored by the Division of Continuing Medical Education, Discovery International, IL Beverly Hills, CA, pp. 29–39.

Ibric, V. L. (2000). Neuro-Modulation of Pain Perception through Neurofeedback Training: Long Lasting Effects on Pain Control. *Proceedings at the 25th AAPM Conference,* New Orleans, LA. February 24–26.

Ibric, V. L. (2001). Neurofeedback enhanced by light closed-loop EEG and electromagnetic closed-loop EEG in a case of sleep deprivation post methadone withdrawal. *Poster presented at the 9th Annual Conference of SNR*, Monterrey, CA, October 27–30, pp.

Ibric, V. L. (2001). EEG biofeedback-neurofeedback training in chronic pain. Poster presented at the *International Scientific Conference on Complementary, Alternative and Integrative Medicine Research*, San Francisco, CA. May 17–19.

Ibric, V. L. (2002). Neurofeedback training enhanced by light and/or electromagnetic closed-loop EEG induces analgesia in patients with neuropathic pain syndromes. Poster presented at the 10th World Conference on Pain, IASP, San Diego, CA, *Pain*, Suppl., 439–440 (S1338).

Ibric, V. L. and Grierson, C. (1995). Neurofeedback and High Blood Pressure. *Proceedings of 3rd Annual Conference of SSNR*, Scottsdale, AZ. April 28–May1.

Ibric, V. L. and Jacobs, M. S. (1997). *Neurofeedback Training in Chronic Pain Associated with Post Traumatic Stress Disorder, and Affective Disorders*. San Diego, CA: [Abstract] Second APEA (ECNS) symposium. May 17.

Ibric, V. L. and Kaur, S. (1999). Neuro-Modulation of *Pain* Perception through Neurofeedback Training: Long Lasting Effects on Pain Control. Poster presented at 9th World Conference on Pain, IASP, Vienna, Austria, *Pain*, **82**, (S272).

Ibric, V. L. and Dragomirescu, L. G. (2005). Neurofeedback and Chronic Pain. How to measure progress for research purposes? *BSC Annual Meeting* November 2005, Irvine, CA.

Ibric, V. L. and Davis, C. J. (2007). The ROSHI in Neurofeedback. In *Neurofeedback Applications: Dynamics and Clinical Applications* (J. Evans, ed.), Chapter 8, NY: The Haworth Press, Inc.

Ibric, V. L., Dragomirescu L. G., and Hudspeth, W. J. (2007). Real-time changes in connectivity during Neurofeedback training. *Journal of Neurotherapy* (in press).

www.theInstituteofMedicineoftheNationalacAdemies.org CHRONIC PAIN MEDICAL TREATMENT GUIDELINES, proposed August 8, 2007.

http://www.guideline.gov/summary/pdf.aspx?doc_id = 11026&stat = 1&string =

Jacob, D. and Benson, H. (1996). Topographic EEG mapping of the relaxation response. *Biofeedback and Self-Regulation*, **21**, 121–129.

Jasper, H. H. (1958). The ten twenty electrode system of the international federation. *Electroencephalography and Clinical Neurophysiology*, **10**, 371–375.

Kamiya, J. (1968). Conscious control of brain waves. *Psychology Today*, **1(11)**, 55–60.

Kropp, P., Siniatchkin, M. and Gerber, W. D. (2002). On the pathophysiology of migraine--links for "empirically based treatment" with Neurofeedback. *Appl. Psychophysiol. Biofeedback*, **27(3)**, 203–213.

Kudrow, L. (1982). Paradoxical effects of frequent analgesic use. In *Advances in Neurology: Vol. 33. Headaches: Physiological and clinical concepts* (M. Critchley, A. P. Freidman, S. Gorini and F. Sicuteri, eds), pp. 335–341. New York: Raven Press.

Lubar, J. F. (1985). Changing EEG activity through biofeedback applications for the diagnosis of learning disabled children. *Theory and Practice*, **24(2)**, 106–111.

Maihöfner, C., Handwerker, H. O., Neundörfer, B. and Birklein, F. (2003). Patterns of cortical reorganization in complex regional pain syndrome. *Neurology* **61**, 1707–1715.

Marzano, R. J., Norford, J. S., Paynter, D. E., Pickering, D. J. and Gaddy, B. B. (2001). *A Handbook for Classroom Instruction that Works*. Alexandria, VA, USA: Association for Supervision and Curriculum Development.

Mayo Clinic (2007). http://www.mayoclinic.com/health/prescription-drug-abuse/DSO1079/

McKenzie, R., Ehrisman, W., Montgomery, P. S. and Barnes, R. H. (1974). The treatment of headache by means of electroencephalographic biofeedback. *Headache*, **13**, 164–172.

Melzack, R. and Wall, P. D. (1965). Pain mechanisms: A new theory. *Science*, **50**, 971–979.

Melzack, R. (1975). The McGill Pain Questionnaire: Major properties and scoring methods. *Pain*, **1**, 277–299.

Merskey, H. (1986). Classification of chronic pain: Description of chronic pain syndromes and definitions of pain terms. *Pain*, **(Suppl. 3)**, S1–S225.

Nathan, P. W. (1976). The gate-control theory of pain. A critical review. *Brain*, **99**, 123–158.

News-Medical.Net (2007). National study to treat addiction to prescription pain medications. http:// www.med.nyu.edu/

Osterweis, M., Kleinman, A. and Mechanic, D., (eds) (1987). *Pain and Disability – Clinical, Behavioral and Public Policy Perspectives.* Institute of Medicine, Committee on Pain, Disability and Chronic Illness Behavior, published by Washington, DC: National Academy Press.

Othmer, S. (2001). Neurofeedback: Pain and Suffering. *California Biofeedback*, pp. 14–18. Winter Newsletter.

Penfield, W. G. and Jasper, H. H. (1954). *Epilepsy and the functional anatomy of the human brain.* Boston: Little Brown.

Price, D. D. and Meyer, D. J. (1995). Evidence for endogenous Opiate Analgesic Mechanisms Triggered by Somatosensory Stimulation (including Acupuncture) in Humans. *Pain Forum*, **4(1)**, 40–43.

Radloff, L. S. (1977). The CES-D scale: A self-report depression scale for research in the general population. *Applied Psychological Measurement*, **1**, 385–401.

Rainville, P., Duncan, G. H., Price, D. D., Carrier, B. and Bushnell, C. M. (1997). Pain affect encoded in human anterior cingulated gyrus but not somato-sensory cortex. *Science*, **277**, 968–971.

Ramanchandran, V. S. and Rogers-Ramanchandran, D. (2000). Phantom Limbs and Neural Plasticity. *Arch. Neurol.*, **57**, 317–320.

Rosenfeld, J. P., Baehr, E., Gotlib, I. and Rogers, G. (1995). EEG frontal asymmetry measures correlate with mood change scores during asymmetry biofeedback. [Abstract]. *Proceedings of the 26th Annual Meeting of the Association for Applied Psychophysiology and Biofeedback*, 125–128.

Sime, A. (2004). Case study of trigeminal neuralgia using neurofeedback and peripheral biofeedback. *Journal of Neurotherapy*, **8(1)**, 59–71.

Siniatchkin, M., Hierundar, A., Kropp, P., Kuhnert, R., Gerber, W-D. and Stephani, U. (2000). Self-regulation of slow cortical potentials in children with migraine: An exploratory study. *Applied Psychophysiology & Biofeedback*, **25(1)**, 13–32.

Steinberg, M. and Othmer, S. (2004). *ADD – the 20-hour solution.* OR, USA: Robert Reed Publishers.

Sterman, M. B. (1973). Neuro-physiological and clinical studies of sensory-motor EEG biofeedback training: some effects on epilepsy. *Seminars in Psychiatry*, **5(4)**, 507–525.

Sufka, K. J. and Price, D. D. (2002). Gate control theory reconsidered. *Brain and Mind*, **3**, 277–290.

Tansey, M. A. (1991). A neurobiological treatment for migraine: The response of four cases of migraine to EEG biofeedback training. *Headache Quarterly: Current Treatment & Research*, 90–96.

Tansey, M. A. (1993). Ten year stability of EEG biofeedback results for a hyperactive boy who failed the fourth grade perceptually impaired class. *Biofeedback and Self-Regulation*, **18(1)**, 33.

Tolle, T. R., Kaufmann, T., Siessmeier, T., Lautenbacher, S., Berthele, A., Munz, F., Zieggansberger, W., Willoch, F., Schwaiger, M., Conrad, B. and Bartenstein, P. (1999). Region-specific encoding of sensory and affective components of pain in the human brain: a positron emission tomography correlation analysis. *Annals of Neurology*, **45(1)**, 40–47., (http://hendrix.ei.dtu.dk/services/jerne/ brede/WOBIB_79.html)

Toomim, M. K. (1987). EMG Biofeedback and Myofascial Pain Syndrome. *BSC Newsletter*, Vol. **3**.

Treede, R. D., Apkarian, A. V., Bromm, B., Greenspan, J. D. and Lenz, F. A. (2000). Cortical representation of pain: functional characterization of nociceptive areas near the lateral sulcus. *Pain*, **87**, 113–119.

Turk, D. C. and Gatchel, R. J. (1999). Psychosocial factors in pain: Revolution and evolution. In *Psychosocial factors in pain: Critical perspectives* (R. J. Gatchel and D. C. Turk, eds), pp. 481–493. New York: Guilford.

Turk, D. C., Okifuji, A. and Scharf, L. (1995). Chronic pain and depression: Role of perceived impact and perceived control in different age cohorts. *Pain*, **61**, 93–102.

Wayne, J. B. (2005). *MOSBY'S – Dictionary of Complementary & Alternative Medicine.* Elsevier Mosby. St. Louis, MI, USA.

CHAPTER 17

Anxiety, EEG patterns, and neurofeedback

Jane Price, M.A.[1] and Thomas Budzynski, Ph.D.[2]

[1] Sterlingworth Center, Greenville, South Carolina, USA
[2] University of Washington, Washington, USA

Nothing in the affairs of men is worthy of great anxiety.

Plato

I. INTRODUCTION

Plato would decry the world citizens of today for their states of mind. But Plato does not live in the world of today, and the citizens of today respond to their stressful, fast-moving world with great anxieties. Looking into the mental health care system, the most common mental disorders in the United States are the anxiety disorders. Statistics from The World Health Organization indicate that 18% of the adult population in the United States suffers from some type of anxiety disorder. Data collected by the Anxiety Disorders Association of America, and published in the *Journal of Clinical Psychiatry* (Greenberg *et al*, 1999), revealed that anxiety disorders in the United States consume almost one third of the total mental health bill for the nation. The Diagnostic and Statistical Manual of Mental Disorders, 4th edition (DSM-IV) currently recognizes 14 types of anxiety disorders, and notes that these disorders very often co-occur with each other, and with other mental health disorders.

This chapter will briefly review definitions of anxiety and anxiety disorders, identify specific EEG and QEEG patterns which in clinical practice and/or research have been found to be correlates of some anxiety disorders, and cite neurofeedback protocols for treating anxiety as suggested by experienced clinicians and/or by research. Augmenting procedures such as breathwork, muscle relaxation, heart rate variability training, AVE, EMDR, cognitive behavioral therapy, and other psychotherapy forms will be given only a brief mention since most of them are covered in detail in many other publications.

II. THE ANXIETY STATE

The medicalization of anxiety states has undoubtedly contributed to the search for health care, given that the general attitude is that to be in an uncomfortable emotional state is to be mentally disordered. Webster's College Dictionary, 4th edition (2000) defines anxiety as:

1. "A state of being uneasy, apprehensive or worried about what may happen; concern about a possible future event"; and
2. (Psychiatry) "An abnormal state like this, characterized by a feeling of being powerless and unable to cope with threatening events (typically imaginary) and by physical tension, as shown by sweating, trembling, etc."

A question is, should psychiatry/psychology discriminate between the expressions of fear and anxiety? For example, Cromer (2004) notes that fear is the state of alarm elicited by a perceived serious threat to one's well-being, while anxiety more often refers to a vague sense of being in danger, with inability to pinpoint the cause. The distinction between the layman's view and psychiatry's emphasis is that the anxiety disorders described in the DSM-IV possess an element of exaggerated fear. Common symptoms in DSM-IV also include chronic worry, restlessness, muscle tension, sleep disturbance, and subjective feelings of distress. Psychiatry would say that while most, if not all, individuals occasionally experience this distress, to be diagnosed with an anxiety disorder, symptoms must be abnormally severe, disabling, frequent, easily triggered and/or long lasting. How easy it is to slip into a diagnosed status. The therapist or anti-anxiety drugs often are substitutes for our family network, our community catchment, and our churches.

III. ANXIETY TYPES WITH A FOCUS
ON THE EEG PICTURE

The revised DSM-IV describes 14 types of anxiety disorders. While not oblivious of the vast number of behavioral symptom patterns describing anxiety, this chapter on neurofeedback treatment of anxiety necessarily will be oriented to those types of symptom patterns which we know to date to show a discernible repeated EEG picture. Throughout this chapter, as in any discourse on anxiety, we must make treatment plans and goals tempered by a consideration of interaction with such factors as medications and co-morbidity of anxiety with physical illnesses, or mood, or other emotional disorders. All these considerations will affect research findings and treatment outcomes.

A.   Early treatment of anxiety using biofeedback/ neurofeedback

Anxiety as High Muscle Tension

In the years prior to the early 1960s anxiety often was defined, at least in part, as a high level of muscle tension, e.g., increased frontalis muscle readings by an electromyographic (EMG) instrument (Budzynski and Stoyva, 1975). These researchers found that decreasing frontalis EMG levels by EMG biofeedback could alleviate both generalized and specific anxiety patterns, if the EMG was decreased to a low enough level so as to achieve "spillover" into the autonomic nervous system. (Budzynski and Stoyva, 1975; Budzynski *et al.*, 1980). Moreover, Sittenfeld *et al.* (1976) showed that decreasing frontal EMG levels with EMG biofeedback would increase the magnitude of alpha and theta EEG. However, the measuring instruments of the day limited the capability for direct analysis of the relationship of muscle tension with EEG changes. Better ways of analyzing the EEG with Fast Fourier computer chips relegated the use of surface EMG biofeedback more and more to the physical rehabilitation arena. Brain researchers studying anxiety, epilepsy and other disorders turned to measures of spectral analysis of EEG for correlates within various disorders.

The Study of EEG Correlates of Anxiety

During the 1960s there were several published studies concerned with EEG correlates of anxiety. Costa *et al.* (1965) in a study of 72 first-year medical students found a significant negative correlation between alpha amplitude and scores on Welsh's "A" (anxiety) test. Scherzer (1966) examined hospital patients under normal baseline conditions, and then during an insurance claim examination. The EEG showed a lower amplitude and band frequency of alpha rhythm during the insurance claim examination. This finding seems to be similar in terms of EEG activity to that of an earlier study by Cohn (1946) who studied two types of anxiety clients: one group consisted of "reactive types" in which the anxiety was related to specific life situations, and the other group whose anxiety was more severe and chronic. The reactive type showed an intermittent low magnitude alpha which would manifest itself within 20 seconds of the initiation of deep breathing. The chronic group showed a rhythmic, high amplitude beta between 18 and 22 Hz in frontal leads, and these subjects did not respond to deep breathing.

IV.   ALPHA EEG BIOFEEDBACK PRIOR TO QEEG-BASED NEUROTHERAPY

Enhancement of alpha captured the attention of early clinicians, and remains a theme of treatment of anxiety even today. Studies on anxiety published prior to the use of QEEG for determining EEG sub-types of anxiety involved neu-rofeedback training to increase magnitude (and/or relative percentage) of alpha, most often at midline occipital sites (Budzynski and Stoyva, 1972). It was widely believed that anxiety inhibited alpha, and that the training in alpha increase would counter the anxiety.

The alpha feedback procedure (a tone signaled the presence of alpha above a given threshold) was based on the early work of Kamiya (1968) who noted the calming, relaxing quality of the "alpha state." In one study, for example, Alpha increase was intended to desensitize a client with thanataphobia. The client was first trained to increase his alpha at O1 from approximately 10% up to 70–80%. Next, this "high percent-alpha state" was used to counter the anxiety generated by the presentation of an individualized anxiety/fear hierarchy. Between visualizations of the anxiety scenes built into the hierarchy, the client would use the alpha feedback to bring himself back to a high-percent-alpha-state, and thus decrease his anxiety before starting the next visualization of the anxiety scene. When the client could visualize the scene for 20 seconds without anxiety he was progressed to the next scene up the hierarchy. The successful treatment took only four sessions (Budzynski and Stoyva, 1972; Budzynski, 1999). Follow-ups over a 35-year period revealed no return of the phobia. This was quite possibly the first clinical application to a men-tal disorder of what would later be called *neurotherapy* (Budzynski, 1999).

Compilations of early anxiety neurofeedback research by Moore (2000) and Hammond (2005a and b) listed a number of studies which support alpha training. For example, Moore summarized seven studies of anxiety in which the protocol of alpha increase was used with success. Two of the studies also found anxiety decreases with an alpha *suppression* protocol, although the level of anxiety decrease was not as great as that with the alpha increase treatment. Perhaps related to this, later sub-typing of anxious clients has revealed a global alpha patterning in a cer-tain percentage of anxiety clients (Gurnee, 2000; Demos, 2005). Moore (2000, p. 5) concluded that, "EEG-biofeedback was associated with clinical improvement in generalized anxiety, phobic disorder, obsessive-compulsive disorder and PTSD."

Rice *et al.* (1993) studied 45 volunteers with an average of 3.8 years of reported anxiety, of whom 38 met the DSM-III criteria for general anxiety disorder (GAD). Eventually, there were nine clients in each of four protocol groups: a fron-tal EMG, a decrease alpha, an increase alpha, and pseudo-meditation. Four treat-ments were given in two one-hour sessions per week. Each session consisted of only 20 minutes of feedback in an eyes-closed condition. Only the frontal EMG and the alpha increase groups improved significantly on the Welsh anxiety scale. In addition, only the alpha increase group showed reductions of heart rate reactivity to stress. The improvements were maintained 6 weeks after treatment.

Hammond (2005a) suggested that three studies of phobic anxiety by Garrett and Silver (1976) were among the finest. The experiments involved random assignment, alternative treatment controls, and wait-list controls. In one study the group receiving the alpha enhancement treatment produced 33% more alpha post-treatment, and all three feedback groups demonstrated significant reductions in test anxiety. The untreated control group and the relaxation training group showed no significant reduction. Another experiment combined phases of alpha enhancement and EMG feedback. Alpha production improved from 64–78%, and anxiety scores dropped significantly compared to a non-treatment control group.

The extent of use of alpha feedback for mental disorders grew broader over the years. For example, Passini *et al.* (1977) asked, "Could alpha biofeedback help anxious alcoholics?" Passini compared 25 anxious alcoholics to matched controls before and after 10 hours of alpha feedback training spread over 3 weeks. The alpha training produced significant changes in both state and trait anxiety compared with controls. The alpha group increased their eyes-closed alpha EEG from 38–55%, while the controls decreased slightly. In an 18-month follow-up (Watson, Herder, & Passini, 1978), close to identical results were still present.

Peniston and Kulkosky (1991) used relaxation training and an alpha/theta protocol to produce a deeply relaxed state in alcoholics at a VA hospital. Subjects were also given practice at visualizing scenes that had alcoholic abuse themes. During the training the subjects first relaxed and produced the alpha/theta EEG state, and then were given scenes from a hierarchy to be visualized while maintaining the deeply relaxed state. Earlier, Budzynski (1976, 1986) had noted that this deeply relaxed state could loosen the fully conscious brain's defense mechanisms that otherwise would often block the assimilation of such positive words and imagery. Budzynski's "twilight learning" technique involved the shaping of a primarily theta state during which affirmative verbal statements would be "heard," and thus assimilated by the client in this semiconscious state (Budzynski, 1977). The Peniston–Kulkosky Protocol, as it came to be called, appeared to be quite effective for the treatment of addictions, and even PTSD.

PTSD was the focus of two early studies by Peniston and Kulkosky (1991) and Peniston *et al.* (1993) as they applied the same protocol used for addictions to PTSD. In the first randomized control group study they added thirty 30-minute sessions of the alpha–theta training to the typical VA hospital treatment program. Fifteen Vietnam veterans with PTSD given the alpha–theta training were compared to a control group of 14 who only received the traditional treatment. A 30-month follow-up showed all 14 controls had relapsed, but only three of the 15 neurofeedback treated patients had relapsed. Moreover, 14 of the 15 neurofeedback group decreased their medication requirements but only one of the controls did so.

In a second study, Peniston *et al.* (1993) selected 20 chronic PTSD VA patients, who also suffered from alcohol abuse, for the treatment. On a 26-month follow-up, only four of the 20 reported some recurrence of nightmares and/or flashbacks. The other 16 reported no PTSD symptoms. As a result of such findings, Hammond (2005a, p. 133) noted that finally it has been recognized that "according to APA Clinical Psychology Division criteria for efficacious treatments, neurofeedback qualifies for the status of possibly efficacious" for PTSD.

In a more recent anxiety-related study, musical performance was enhanced with alpha/theta feedback. Students at the prestigious London's Royal College of Music were engaged in a randomized, blinded, controlled experiment wherein they had to perform before a group of judges (very stressful) as a baseline, after which they trained with alpha/theta feedback, beta feedback, physical exercise, Alexander Technique, and SMR feedback. They then performed again and were judged. Only the alpha–theta group improved on their musical performances. Not only that but this group experienced a number of other changes, e.g., clothing styles, bonding together, more creative in their musical ability, etc. (Egner and Gruzelier, 2003).

V.   QEEG CORRELATES OF ANXIETY SYMPTOMS

As implied in earlier paragraphs, interest in the EEG correlates of anxiety dates back to at least the middle of the twentieth century. Recently, a number of contemporary scientists have attempted to determine correlates between specific symptom patterns of anxiety and locations of EEG disturbances using QEEG (quantitative EEG) technology. Identifying QEEG sub-types could aid in diagnosis and in design of neurotherapy training protocols.

Several QEEG sub-types have emerged (Demos, 2005; Gurnee, 2000; Hammond, 2005b). Figure 17.1 shows the six anxiety QEEG sub-types seen by Gurnee in a study of 100 anxiety clients. Note the percentages of anxiety clients with particular patterns, indicating that many of these clients show more than one pattern. Gurnee has noted that, "most (anxiety clients) show 3 or 4 of the patterns and they are stable. In some cases you will find one or two patterns in the eyes open and another one or two in eyes closed. All must be trained away for thorough and lasting symptom resolution". (Gurnee, personal communication, 2008)

Anxiety sub-types also have emerged from other recent techniques. The LORETA (Low Resolution Electromagnetic Tomography) technique, which is generated via software from the usual 10/20 19-channel raw EEG information, is now used by neurotherapists to "view" deeper brain structures. According to Sherlin (personal communication, 2008), the most common anxiety pattern using LORETA is beta localized along the anterior cingulate or the midline cortex (more superficially). Sherlin also mentioned a second prominent pattern, and that is the mis-location of alpha (alpha not found where expected). The LORETA as a diagnostic tool and as a form of neurofeedback is discussed in Chapter 4 in this volume.

Amen's SPECT scan sub-types of anxiety. The unique use of the SPECT scan by Amen and Routh (2003) has resulted in a delineation of brain structures both neo- and sub-cortical which have been compromised in function. Amen has identified seven types of anxiety based on his interpretation of single photon emission computed tomography (SPECT) scan data (Amen, 2004). Most of the anxiety SPECT scans reveal heightened activity in the basal ganglia region. When the excessive activity is in the left basal ganglia it is associated with anxiety and irritability, which he calls *expressed anxiety*. When the increased basal ganglia activity is

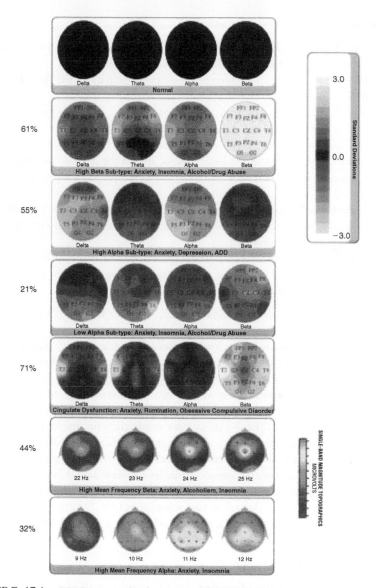

FIGURE 17.1   QEEG/topographic brain maps of generalized anxiety disorder sub-types. (see color plate)

on the right side there is anxiety, social withdrawal and conflict avoidance. Panic attack patients may show excessive activity in both left and right basal ganglia. Increased activity in temporal lobes may also be associated with anxiety. When the increased activity is seen in the anterior cingulate, the individual may have trouble with repetitive thoughts about his or her anxiety.

Here are Amen's seven types of anxiety:

Type 1: Pure Anxiety is characterized by increased bilateral activity in the basal ganglia, seen in both baseline and concentration studies.

Type 2: Pure Depression is characterized by excessive activity in the deep limbic system both at rest and concentration.

Type 3: Mixed Anxiety and Depression—the deep limbic activity is joined by increased activity in the basal ganglia as well.

Type 4: Overfocused Anxiety/ Depression is characterized by excessive activity in the anterior cingulate gyrus, the basal ganglia, and/ or the deep limbic system.

Type 5: Cyclic Anxiety/Depression results from excessive focal activity in the basal ganglia and/or deep limbic system.

Type 6: Temporal Lobe Anxiety/Depression stems from too much or too little activity in the brain's temporal lobes, in addition to excess activity in the basal ganglia and/or deep limbic system.

Type 7: Unfocused Anxiety/Depression occurs when there is too little activity in the brain's prefrontal cortex, in addition to excessive activity in the basal ganglia and/or deep limbic system.

Amen's SPECT images provide a look at deeper levels of brain functioning just as LORETA does.

In the following sections we review samples of more recent research and clinician-based opinions concerning EEG/QEEG correlates of several types of anxiety disorders, and the neurofeedback treatment which is undertaken. Clinicians, confronted upon initial interview only with a history of symptoms of anxiety, may not have ready access to a QEEG to help locate the disrupted EEG areas of the brain. Rather than have a QEEG evaluation completed, some might rely on studies which can provide information about regions of disturbed EEG commonly associated with given patterns of anxiety. Let's take a symptom pattern such as obsessive-compulsive disorder as an example. In a review article on uses of conventional and quantitative electroencephalography in Hughes and John (1999) cite work by Small (1993) who described two sub-types of OCD. One type exhibited increased alpha activity in the EEG, and the other type exhibited increased theta, predominantly in the frontal and frontotemporal areas.

A.   Obsessive-compulsive disorder

Advances in QEEG processing have produced significant understandings about the EEG pathology, and how to approach OCD with neurofeedback treatment today. Research, Tot et al. (2002) compared the EEG data gathered in a resting state and during hyperventilation of 22 unmedicated right-handed OCD patients with 20 right-handed "healthy" control participants matched for age and gender. Members of the experimental group had a wide range of OCD symptoms, but no co-morbid psychiatric disorder. The Yale-Brown obsessive compulsive scale (Y-BOCS) was used to assess severity of symptoms. EEG data were collected from 14 monopolar electrode sites referenced to CZ. QEEG results indicated that the OCD group had significantly higher relative power in delta, and greater theta frequencies at left frontotemporal regions, but only in the resting state. Greater left temporal theta activity correlated positively with higher Y-BCOS scores in the resting condition.

The authors also reported that visual analyses of raw EEG data revealed several instances of irregular theta activity in the OCD group especially at left frontotemporal sites. They note that the latter finding is similar to that of Flor-Henry *et al.* (1979) who reported predominantly left hemisphere temporal and parietal EEG power spectral abnormalities in their sample of individuals with OCD.

Other researchers have examined OCD-EEG patterns in still more detail. Attempts by Karadag *et al.* (2003) to correlate four OCD sub-types with EEG and QEEG abnormalities revealed that in all sub-types dysfunction was found in frontotemporal regions. Karadag used the Maudsley obsessive compulsive questionnaire which defines and rates symptoms within four sub-groups of OCD: checking, doubting, cleaning and slowness. Participants who scored at or above cut-off scores on any of the defined sub-groups were classified as OCD within that sub-group. EEG recordings of participants in each sub-group revealed that those in the checking group showed significantly lower absolute alpha and beta frequency band power at P3, O1, and O2. These patients also had higher relative theta frequency band power at F2, F4, T5, T6, C3, O1, and O2 electrode sites than those in other sub-groups. The doubting sub-group had significantly lower alpha asymmetry scores, and lower absolute alpha frequency band power at all frontal electrode sites (FP1, FP2, F3, F4, F7, F8, FZ,) and at some occipital and central electrode sites (C4, CZ, P3, O1).

Absolute theta band power was significantly higher at electrode sites Fp1, F3, FZ, F4, C3, P3, P4, O1, O2; and relative delta band power at F3, F4, F7, F8, FZ, C3, PZ, O2 sites was significantly higher in the doubting sub-group than in other OCD sub-groups. The cleaning sub-type had higher absolute delta frequency band power at frontotemporal sites F7, F8, T4, T6 than did any other OCD sub-type. Participants of the slowness sub-type exhibited significantly lower absolute beta band powers at temporal electrode sites T3 and T4. When comparing mild OCD to severe OCD, Karadag reported that those suffering from severe OCD exhibited significantly lower relative alpha frequency band power at electrode sites FP2, F3, F4, F7, F8, C3, O2, PZ, and significantly lower alpha band power at PZ. Those with severe OCD also exhibited significantly higher absolute delta and theta band power at sites F7 and FZ compared to those with moderate and mild forms of OCD. In summary, excessive absolute power of lower frequency bands in frontal areas (but not limited to frontal) was a distinguishing feature correlated with obsessive-compulsive behavior.

Several other researchers tend to concur with Karadag about OCD and EEG patterns. Research by Pogarell *et al.* (2006) comparing EEG patterns of mixed

OCD patients with EEG patterns of healthy controls revealed differences in cortical patterns. The EEG data of participants with OCD exhibited greater overall slowing of EEG activity primarily in the frontotemporal and frontal regions. This group also exhibited an increased delta and decreased power in the higher frequency bands of alpha and beta. The participants with OCD were subdivided based on their scores on the Yale-Brown Obsessive Compulsive Scale (Y-BOCS), and their EEG patterns compared. Those who scored high on the Y-BOCS for compulsions were more likely to have low absolute power especially in the lower frequencies, while those who scored high for obsessions were more likely to have higher absolute EEG power especially in the alpha 2 and beta 1 frequency bands.

Because all of the above detail might confuse even the most OC of readers, we offer here an attempted summary of the results. Based on the above research regarding OCD, it is suggested that the disorder involves primarily frontotemporal and frontal EEG and QEEG abnormalities. More specifically: 1) Severe OCD clients showed lower relative alpha in frontal areas and at Pz, along with higher absolute delta and theta at F7, Fz when compared to less severe OCD cases; and 2) More often the slowing was seen in the left frontotemporal area.

B. Trait anxiety

Some of the more complex of the clients presenting with anxiety are the ones who suffer from trait anxiety. According to Spielberger (1983),

> Trait anxiety refers to relatively stable individual differences in anxiety-proneness, that is, to differences between people, in the tendency to perceive stressful situations as dangerous or threatening and to respond to such situations with elevations in the intensity of their state anxiety (S-Anxiety).

In contrast, state anxiety usually refers to an emotional state at a particular moment or relatively brief period of time. Along with long-term physiological symptoms associated with the chronic arousal and stress of trait anxiety is also the unresolved question of causality. No one event may have precipitated the onset of trait anxiety, and symptoms may present as mild to severe.

Studies attempting to correlate EEG patterns to high trait anxiety have found a difference in laterality patterns of regional brain activity at rest and during arousal-provoking states. A behavior activation system (BAS) and behavior inhibition system (BIS) model developed by Gray (cited by Aftanas and Pavlov, 2004) has been used in related research. Goal-directed behavior is controlled by the BAS, and becomes activated when a positive stimulus is a reward, while the BIS is responsible for inhibiting ongoing behavior and for being alert to stimuli in the environment. It has been speculated that anxiety is increased in response to the activation of BIS. Aftanas and Pavlov (2004) examined how trait anxiety influenced EEG asymmetries during arousal and non-arousal states, and how those EEG patterns can be explained by the BAS and BIS theory developed by Gray.

Participants were divided, based on the scores they received on the Spielberger State-Trait Anxiety Inventory (1983), into two groups: a control group and a high trait anxiety group. They were asked to view and self-report on their emotional state for each of several movie film clips that varied in emotional valance. Participants who had high (trait) anxiety exhibited more beta 1 (12–18 Hz) activity in the right hemisphere with eyes open while viewing a neutral film. With eyes closed, and in the presumably lowest arousal state, this group exhibited increased right parieto-temporal theta 1 activity (4–6 Hz) and beta 1 activity (12–18 Hz). When the same high anxiety group viewed a film chosen to elicit more negative emotion, beta 1 power (12–18 Hz) decreased in the right parieto-temporal area. It was suggested that individuals who are anxious scan their environment for potential threats, and that BIS is alert to stimuli in the environment as evidenced by the increased beta 1 power in the right parieto-temporal area.

Aftanas and Pavlov speculated on the mechanisms which may account for these findings. It is believed that when individuals with high anxiety are in an anxious arousal state, they utilize an avoidant response to avoid the aversive stimuli. The BIS becomes more activated, which increases arousal as they recheck behavioral options. This could be observed in the EEG as right parieto-temporal beta 1 desynchronizing, and bilateral alpha continuing to desynchronize. This change in EEG pattern is believed to reflect the activation of the flight or fight response, which involves avoidance behavior. The asymmetrical parietal beta activity that is observed may be related to response and withdrawal behavioral responses.

In another attempt to associate anxiety with distinct types of brain electrical activity, Heller et al. (1997) examined 20 participants who self-reported very high trait anxiety, defined as anxious apprehension and worry (in contrast to anxious arousal). They noted that most former research on anxiety and EEG patterns had found right hemisphere abnormalities, and speculated that this may have been due to research participants more often being in states of anxious arousal (related to panic states or state anxiety) rather than being persons with high trait anxiety. They hypothesized that persons of the latter type may have more left hemisphere abnormalities, and that those relatively few earlier studies which reported left hemisphere abnormalities, or found no hemispheric differences, may have included more persons suffering from high trait anxiety. They compared the brain electrical activity of their high trait anxiety group to that of a control group of 20 participants with low trait anxiety before (resting, eyes closed) and during listening to emotional narratives which had been rated in earlier pilot studies as highly arousing and unpleasant.

Both groups had scored within normal limits on a depression inventory. The dependent variable was EEG alpha measured at scalp sites CZ, F3, F4, P3 and P4 (with decreases in alpha presumably indicating increases in activation). In general, anxious participants had more left than right hemisphere activity as compared to controls. However, when listening to the narratives, anxious participants exhibited a selective increase in right parietal activity. Heller et al. (1997) suggested that, for the anxious participants, a decrease in right hemispheric activity resulted in the increased magnitude of asymmetry in favor of the left hemisphere. They stated that this finding is consistent with other studies of individuals with trait anxiety or anxious apprehension associated with rumination. The greater activation in the right posterior region during reading of the narratives was believed to be associated with anxious arousal associated with physiological hyper-arousal.

VI. THE CONCEPT OF A DEFAULT MODE NETWORK (DMN)

It would seem that searching for the appropriate EEG pattern and selecting a protocol to fit the patient is an intimidating clinical decision. Research on systemic functional networks in EEG involving the concept of "default mode network" (DMN) may ease the decision-making process. The diversified methods for examining subtypes of anxiety through structural and EEG dynamic means may be consolidated in the near future, integrating a spate of studies pioneered by Fox, Raichle and a team of scientists at Washington University School of Medicine, by another team with Baliki, Geha and Apkarian at Northwestern University, and by others at Stanford and Shanghai Universities. This concept of "default mode network" was developed through neuroimaging studies by Posner and Raichle (Posner and Raichle, 1998; Raichle and Snyder, 2007), and emerged through efforts to explain the intrinsic activity of the brain while testing tasking efforts(Raichle and MacLeod, 2001).

In essence, it was found, through fMRI measurements, that observed brain activity decreased (after task activity was subtracted) when subjects were asked to perform various tasks. Not only was an observed brain area of interest shown to decrease, but a network of brain areas showed a decrease during the task efforts. This "control of self-referenced activity" has been called the *default network*, a resting-state mode of brain function noted to be airly impervious to the stimulation of tasking. The belief is that a functionally interconnected default system is required for internally directed mental activity at resting states. This default mode retains the integrity of the brain function when the brain is expected to undertake outside goal tasks (Gusnard *et al.*, 2001; Chen *et al.*, 2008; Fair *et al.*, 2008; Greicius *et al.*, 2008).

The relation of this concept of DMN to chronic disease is another emerging line of research. The research to date supports the consideration that given that a default mode of activity maintains the integrity of the brain's self-referenced activity, under the condition of a disorder such as chronic pain the default mode network dynamics becomes disrupted. Thus, chronic pain patients display changes in the at-rest default mode, and subsequent alterations in the DMN (Baliki *et al.*, 2006; Baliki *et al.*, 2008). The research findings buttressing this relationship arise from studies of chronic pain, one study of which associated the disruption with the medial frontal cortex, including the rostral anterior cingulated (Baliki *et al.*, 2006; Apkarian *et al.*, 2004). Altered DMN activity was also studied with some anxiety disorders, and observed by fMRI to be located in the medial prefrontal cortex, the posterior cingulated cortex, and the medial parietal cortex (Zhao *et al.*, 2007). It seems apparent that neurotherapists are treating a network which can have existing disruptions in differing locations.

VII. FINDINGS FROM CLINICAL EXPERIENCE

Nerves and butterflies are fine – they're a physical sign that you're mentally ready and eager. You have to get the butterflies to fly in formation, that's the trick.

Steve Bull

On speech anxiety: "Learn to love your audience as you prepare to speak"

Tom Budzynski

At this stage in the application of a technology such as neurofeedback to a disorder such as anxiety, which can include a variety of EEG patterning, it is useful to survey the field of clinicians who have obtained successful results with anxiety clients. In preparing this chapter, requests were posted on two of the major on-line QEEG and neurofeedback-related sites asking for comments from experienced clinicians regarding QEEG patterns commonly observed in clients with anxiety disorders, and regarding any specific neurotherapy training protocols found to be especially useful. Results of these personal communications are summarized in this section. It should be noted that most of these experienced clinicians employ, in addition to neurofeedback training, other therapy forms such as cognitive behavior therapy.

Hammond (2007) mentioned the following QEEG patterns often associated with anxiety disorders:

1. Asymmetry of frontal alpha.
2. Excessive power in beta frequencies at parietal sites.
3. Excessive power in beta frequencies at right frontal sites (commonly seen in panic disorder).
4. Excessive power in beta frequencies at midline sites, especially CZ (associated with rumination, obsessing and insomnia).

His recommendations for neurofeedback training protocols for each of these four QEEG pattern types, respectively, were:

1. Use of the "frontal asymmetry protocol" commonly used for depression.
2. Reward increases in higher theta frequencies (6–8 Hz), and inhibit power in beta frequencies (20–34 Hz) at the parietal sites involved.
3. Reward increases in power in alpha frequencies, and inhibit power in beta frequencies, using a bipolar electrode montage at right-side sites T4-F4.
4. With client's eyes closed, strictly inhibit power in the 19–34 Hz range at the relevant midline site(s).

Hammond (2005b) subsequently noted that a frequently overlooked EEG pattern sometimes found associated with anxiety patterns is excessive power in the alpha band at various frontal sites, especially the frontal poles.

McCarthy (2007) reported that he often finds OCD to be accompanied by excessive power in the higher beta frequencies (21–30 Hz) at left frontal sites, especially F3. He noted that this often is accompanied by excessive power at slower frequencies, e.g., delta in the range of 1–4 Hz. In treating clients with this EEG pattern, he uses a training protocol which inhibits 21–30 Hz power at site F3 (and, when indicated, 1–4 Hz power), while concurrently rewarding increases in power in the 8–12 Hz range. He added that in some cases where there also is excessively decreased power at 14–18 Hz, he will try rewarding increases in that range. Finally, he stated that in some cases he has found "standard alpha–theta training" to be effective.

Angelakis (2007) reported a frequently observed pattern where there is excessive power at higher beta frequencies (18–30 Hz) around electrode sites C3, CZ and/or C4, accompanied by client complaints of both anxiety and problems with attention. He notes that this may be seen even when there is a normal theta to beta ratio, and may be accompanied by ADHD-like behaviors. He recommended inhibiting power in the 18–30 Hz range at the central site(s) where the excessive power was noted in the QEEG record.

Arns (2008) emphasized that there is no single QEEG pattern associated uniquely with anxiety. However, he noted three patterns frequently encountered in clients with anxiety disorders and/or high scores on an anxiety scale. These were:

1. Synchronous beta or beta spindles.
2. Increased right frontal activity, e.g., lower alpha or higher beta, or beta spindles usually at site F4 or the dorsolateral prefrontal cortex area.
3. Alpha peak frequency > 11.5 Hz.

Regarding the latter, he cautions that downtraining peak frequency could have adverse effects on memory, given past research which has found an association between low peak frequency and poor memory.

Based on his many years of clinical experience with various types of electrophysiological measures, Natani (2008) concluded that "generalized anxiety disorder produces a 'low voltage fast' EEG, with elevated activity in high alpha through high beta." He also noted that both state and trait anxiety "produce beta blips at 30–32 Hz, and probably higher"; and in those with high trait anxiety there is no rapid habituation as often occurs with state (acute) anxiety. Thompson and Thompson (2007) observed that anxiety usually corresponds to an increase in 19–22 Hz activity found in conjunction with a decrease in 15–18 Hz activity measured at Cz. Rumination they claim is also associated with higher beta frequencies. The range that is elevated can be quite narrow and above 22 Hz, sometimes as high as 32–37 Hz. Bursts of activity in frequencies in the mid-20s to low 30s have what Thompson and Thompson call a "busy brain." Such a pattern also may correspond to worrying and sleep onset insomnia.

Each of these experienced clinicians has reported excessive or otherwise abnormal beta (often with decreased power in alpha), as a common EEG/QEEG accompaniment of anxiety disorders. Frontal and central sites most often were implicated, although midline and parietal sites also were mentioned. All clinicians claimed to have had success treating clients with neurofeedback, usually by using training protocols designed to normalize the EEG or QEEG abnormalities noted. Given that there are several basic types of anxiety disorders, not to mention subtypes of the basic ones, the consistency in these clinician reports was surprising.

VIII. AUGMENTING PROCEDURES FOR ANXIETY CLIENTS

Since anxiety typically manifests as heightened muscle tone and increased arousal in terms of cardiovascular and autonomic activity, biofeedback of these variables as an initial stage of training may be considered. Before neurofeedback became popular these other parameters often were used to counter anxiety, sometimes in a desensitization paradigm. Biofeedback clinicians of that era often worked with a variety of "stand-alone" units, e.g., individual EMG, peripheral temperature, and electrodermal response (EDR) devices. Thus, the anxious client first learned to produce a relaxed musculature, warm hands, and low normal EDR. Most often abdominal breathing was taught as well. In many cases this training was enough to allow the client to wean away from Librium, Valium, or later, Xanax as they began to feel less anxiety.

In more recalcitrant cases these variables were monitored as a systematic desensitization was carried out. Budzynski et al. (1980) designed a systems flow chart for carrying out this sort of training. Homework assignments involved a six-phase cassette tape relaxation training program along with the "reminder dot" approach described below. Today's neurotherapists might well consider using biofeedback training as an initial phase to help insure a faster result with the neurofeedback treatment (see Thompson and Thompson, 2007).

A. Diaphragmatic breathing

Demos 2005 has noted that clients with excessive beta are usually reverse breathers who will benefit from breath-work training. Because anxious clients often breathe rapidly from their thoracic, upper chests, which can actually provoke a panic attack, an initial training protocol should be diaphragmatic breathing to an eventual rate of approximately 6–9 breaths per minute. Clients can be taught to identify this correct pattern by first practicing while standing with their arms held straight overhead. This forces diaphragmatic breathing and most clients quickly assimilate the feelings associated with "belly breathing." A second helpful training procedure is to have the client practice at home by lying on a bed with a heavy book on the abdomen, and making the book rise when inhaling and lowering it on the exhalation. As clients become more comfortable with this breathing style they can gradually learn to slow the rhythm.

B. Becoming aware of "bracing efforts"

Stressed, anxious clients often have acquired a number of maladaptive cognitive and physical habits. The physical forms are: muscle bracing, fast thoracic shallow breathing, moist hands and/or feet, cold extremities, dry mouth, and pounding heart and/or arrhythmic beating. The cognitive habits are essentially the thoughts, however subtle, that evoke anxious feelings. In the case of PTSD and GAD the original evoking stimuli may have generalized over the years to the point where the anxiety-evoking cognitive process is not easily available to consciousness. Various forms of psychotherapy including EMDR (Grand, 2001) may assist in uncovering and neutralizing these stimuli, however generalized they may be.

The training in awareness of muscle bracing and abnormal breathing, however, can assist the client in decreasing the anxiety episodes as they begin to occur. For example, a client who tends to have panic attacks can be taught to produce abdominal, slow breathing and relaxation of key muscles as the symptoms of an oncoming attack manifest. Clients can be instructed to retreat to a place where they can implement these procedures such as pulling off to the side of the road if driving, or retreating to a bathroom stall if available.

Budzynski has long employed "reminder dots" (small stick-on circles of bright colors available at office supply stores) which are placed on wristwatch dials, cell phones, steering wheels, computer monitors, etc. The dots remind the client to check for bracing efforts, improper breathing and negative thought process and, if detected, to change them in a more adaptive direction. Incidentally, the color needs to be changed at least once a week or the client simply adapts to it, and the awareness drops off.

C. Premack principle

High probability events can be used to reinforce lower probability adaptive behaviors and thoughts. Based on conditioning theory which dictates that following a low probability event immediately with a high probability event (HBE) increases the probability of occurrence of the lower probability event (LPE), the act of thinking or doing an adaptive action just before engaging in a high probability behavior (e.g., checking email, going through a doorway, or using a cell phone) will increase the likelihood of engaging in that adaptive behavior more often. Anxious clients can be taught to breathe properly and think a positive thought, e.g., "I can relax" before accomplishing the HPB. Clients will need to remember to do this until it is instilled as a habit. During that time the "reminder dots" will do the trick.

D. Brief guided relaxation technique

As society became more and more hurried, it was evident that many busy clients would simply not take the time to devote 30–45 minutes to relaxation training at home, or especially at work. Consequently, Budzynski developed a 12-minute deep relaxation program, now on CD, that features a blend of effective techniques. Besides a sequencing of soft binaural tones that proceed from a starting beta frequency down through the alpha band to 8 Hz and then, in the last 3 minutes, up to 10 Hz, the CD features left-right "whisper tracks" (softly spoken but not subliminal), an Ericksonian center track induction, and backgrounds of a mountain stream and an ocean. We have found that over the 12 years it has been in use, the CD/tape has seen sufficient utilization by clients to constitute a clinic staple for homework.

The *Revitalizer*, as it is called, was recently compared with Mozart music at Seattle University in an attempt to lower blood pressure in the elderly (Tang *et al.*, in press). Participants attended 12 sessions over 4 weeks during which they listened to either a Mozart sonata (MS), or the audio-guided relaxation training (ATP). Systolic (SBP) and diastolic (DBP) blood pressures were recorded using an automated BP machine pre–post the intervention by assistants blinded to the group. The results showed the Revitalizer group decreased significantly (p = 0.015) in SBP compared with the Mozart group (8.9 mm vs. 6.0 mm) while the reduction in DBP was greater in the Revitalizer group (2.9 mm vs. 1.4 mm) compared with the Mozart subjects, but did not quite reach significance (p = 0.06). The researchers concluded that the decrease in SBP after the intervention is large enough to be clinically significant, and may provide a supplemental method for lowering blood pressure in older adults.

IX. VIRTUAL REALITY THERAPY FOR ANXIETY

While at the University of West Florida in 1993, Budzynski carried out a small (N = 3) unpublished study of the effects of a 3-D shutter glass downhill skiing video vs. the same video viewed in the usual 2-D. The results indicated that the 3-D version increased heart rate, frontalis EMG, and electrodermal response (EDR) as well as lowering hand temperature. It would appear that the visualization in 3-D captures the "interest" of the autonomic nervous system more so than watching a flat 2-D presentation. This shutter glass approach is probably not quite as compelling as true virtual reality but is considerably cheaper to set up.

Wiederhold and Wiederhold (2005) have published a text on the use of virtual reality in desensitization in which they report successful treatment of a variety of phobias and anxieties with their VR system. Perhaps one day the neurotherapy screens, including LORETA's can be produced in a virtual reality world. One can only imagine how this might accelerate the treatment time.

X. SUMMARY

That anxiety states are complex disorders is obvious, not only because of the multiple patterns of differences displayed by QEEG, fMRI and SPECT, but also due to the disparate manifest emotional/behavioral symptoms that may or may not correlate with the above physiological measurements. Despite the diversity of EEG anxiety patterns, clusters of them often occur, constituting an emotional/behavioral clinical picture such as obsessive-compulsive disorder.

There are some QEEG patterns found by research, and/or through clinical experience, to be associated with general or specific anxiety disorders, and there are some neurofeedback training protocols rather consistently cited by expert clinicians as efficacious for treatment of these disorders. For example, given a fairly clear anxiety-related behavioral state, or given one or more specific EEG/QEEG pattern, attention to increasing posterior alpha power and/or decreasing beta power in frontal or temporal sites is a commonly reported approach.

If clinicians cannot clearly pinpoint the area of the brain for treating anxiety, they can take solace from the possibility that the brain does, in fact, appear to operate with a "default mode network" such that neurofeedback might resolve disruptions in a widespread fashion. The brain tends to respond globally to neurofeedback treatment, and patients generally do get better.

REFERENCES

Aftanas, L. I. and Pavlov, S. V. (2004). Trait anxiety impact on posterior activation asymmetries at rest and during evoked negative emotions. *International Journal of Psychophysiology*, **55(1)**, 85–94.

Amen, D. G. and Routh, L. C. (2003). *Healing Anxiety and Depression*. New York: Berkley Books.

Angelakes, E. (2007). Personal communication.

Apkarian, A., Soso, Y., Sonty, S., *et al*. (2004). Chronic back pain is associated with decreased prefrontal and thalamic gray matter density. *Journal of Neuroscience*, **24(46)**, 10410–10415.

Arns, M. (2008). Personal communication.

Baliki, M., Chialvo, D., Geha, P., *et al*. (2006). Chronic pain and the emotional brain: Specific brain activity associated with spontaneous fluctuations of intensity of chronic back pain. *Journal of Neuroscience*, **26(47)**, 12165–12173.

Baliki, M., Geha, P., Apkarian, A and Chialvo, D. (2008). Beyond feeling: Chronic pain hurts the brain, disrupting the default-mode network dynamics. *Journal of Neuroscience*, **28(6)**, 1398–1403.

Budzynski, T. H. (1976). Biofeedback and the twilight states of consciousness. In *Consciousness and Self-Regulation* (G. E. Schwartz and D. Shapiro, eds), **Vol.1**, 261–312. New York: Plenum Press.

Budzynski, T. H. (1977). Tuning in on the Twilight Zone. *Psychology Today*, **111**, 38–44.

Budzynski, T. H. (1986). Clinical applications of non-drug-induced states. In *Handbook of States of Consciousness* (B. B. Wolman and M. Uhllman, eds), pp. 1–2. New York: Van Nostrand Reinhold.

Budzynski, T. H. (1999). From EEG to neurofeedback. In *Quantitative EEG and Neurofeedback, 1st edition* (J. R. Evans and A. Abarbanel, eds), pp. 244–304. San Diego: Academic Press.

Budzynski, T. H. and Stoyva, J. M. (1972). Biofeedback techniques in behavior therapy. In *Die bewaltingung von angst. Beitrage der neuropsychologie zur angstforschung. Reihe Fortschritte der klinischen psychologie, 4th edition* (N. Birbaumer, ed.), Munchen, Vien: Verlag, Urban & Schwarzenberg. Republished in 1973 in *Biofeedback and self-control*. (D. Shapiro *et al.*, eds), Chicago: Aldine-Atherton.

Budzynski, T. H. and Stoyva, J. M. (1975). Biofeedback methods in general and specific anxiety disorders. In *Biofeedback-therapie: Lernmethoden in derpsychosomatics, neurology und rehabilitation. Fortschritt der klinischen psychologie* (H. Legewie and L. Nusselt, eds), **Vol. 6**. Munchen–Berlin: Urban and Schwarzenberg. Republished in 1984 in *Principles and Practice of Stress Management*. (R. Woolfolk and P. Lehrer, eds) pp. New York: Guilford Press.

Budzynski, T. H., Stoyva, J. M. and Peffer, K. E. (1980). Biofeedback techniques in psychosomatic disorders. In *Handbook of Behavioral Interventions* (A. Goldstein and E. B. Foa, eds). New York: John Wiley & Sons.

Chen, A., Feng, W., Zhao, H., Yin, Y. and Wang, P. (2008). EEG default mode network in the human brain: Spectral regional field power. *NeuroImage* (article in press).

Cohn, R. (1946). The influence of emotion on the human electroencephalogram. *Journal of Nervous and Mental Disease*, **104**, 351.

Costa, L. D., Cox, M. and Katzman, R. (1965). Relationship between MMPI variables and percentage and amplitude of EEG alpha activity. *Journal of Consulting Psychology*, **29**, 90.

Cromer, R. J. (2004). *Abnormal Psychology*, 5th edition.. New York: Worth Publishers.

Demos, J. N. (2005). *Getting Started with Neurofeedback*. New York: W.W. Norton & Co.

Egner, T. and Gruzelier, J. H. (2003). Ecological validity of neurofeedback: Modulation of slow wave EEG enhances musical performance. NeuroReport, **14**, 1125–1128.

Fair, D., Cohen, A., Dosenbach, N., *et al.* (2008). The maturing architecture of the brain's default network. *Proceedings of National Academy of Science, USA*, **105(10)**, 4028–4032.

Flor-Henry, P., Yeudall, L. T., Koles, Z. J. and Howard, B. G. (1979). Neuropsychological and power spectral investigation of the obsessive-compulsive syndrome. *Biological Psychiatry*, **14**, 119–130.

Garrette, B. L. and Silver, M. P. (1976). The use of EMG and alpha biofeedback to relieve test anxiety in college students. In *Biofeedback, Behavior Therapy and Hypnosis* (I. Wickramasekera, ed.), Chicago: Nelson-Hall.

Grand, D. (2001). *Emotional Healing at Warp Speed: The Power of EMDR*. New York: Harmony Books.

Greenberg, P. E., Sisitsky, M. A., Kessler, R. C., *et al.* (1999). The economic burden of anxiety disorders in the 1990s. *Journal of Clinical Psychiatry*, **60(7)**, 427–435.

Greicius, M., Supekat, K., Menon, V. and Dougherty, R. (2008). Resting-state functional connectivity reflects structural connectivity in the default mode network. *Cerebral Cortex, advanced access* (Oxford University Press).

Gurnee, R. (2000). QEEG subtypes of anxiety. Presented at the Annual ISNR Conference. St. Paul, MN September, 20–24.

Gurnee, R. (2008). Personal communication.

Gusnard, D., Akbudak, E., Shulman, G. and Raichle, M. (2001). Medial prefrontal cortex and self-referential mental activity: Relation to a default mode of brain function. *Proceedings of National Academy of Sciences, USA*, **98(7)**, 4259–4264.

Hammond, C. (2003). QEEG-guided neurofeedback in the treatment of obsessive-compulsive disorder. *Journal of Neurotherapy*, **7**, 25–52.

Hammond, D. C. (2005a). Neurofeedback treatment of depression and anxiety. *Journal of Adult Development*, **12(2)**, 131–137.

Hammond, C. (2005b). Neurofeedback with anxiety and affective disorders. *Child and Adolescent Psychiatric Clinics of North America*, **14**, 105–123.

Hammond, D. (2007). Personal communication.

Heller, W., Nitchke, J. K., Etienne, M. and Miller, G. (1997). Patterns of regional activity differentiate types of anxiety. *Journal of Abnormal Psychology*, **106(3)**, 376–385.

Hughes, J. R. and John, E. R. (1999). Conventional and quantitative electroencephalography. In. *The Journal of Neuropsychiatry and Clinical Neurosciences*, **11(2)**, 190–208.

Kamiya, J. (1968). Conscious control of brain waves. *Psychology Today*, **1**, 57–60.

Karadag, F., Oguzhanoglu, N., Kurt, T., *et al.* (2003). Quantitative EEG analysis in obsessive-compulsive disorder. *International Journal of Neuroscience*, **113**, 833–847.

McCarthy, R. E. (2007). Personal communication.

Moore, N.C. (2000). A review of EEG biofeedback treatment of anxiety disorders. *Clinical Electroencephalography*, **31(1)**, 1–6.

Natani, K. (2008). Personal communication.

Peniston, E. G. and Kulkosky, P. J. (1991). Alpha–theta brainwave neuro-feedback therapy for Vietnam veterans with combat-related post-traumatic stress disorder. *Medical Psychotherapy*, **4**, 47–60.

Peniston, E. G., Marrinan, D. A., Deming, W. A. and Kulkosky, P. J. (1993). EEG alpha–theta synchronization in Vietnam theater veterans with combat-related post-traumatic stress disorder and alcohol abuse. *Advances in Medical Psychotherapy*, **6**, 37–50.

Pogarell, O., Juckel, G., Mavrogiorgou, P., Mulert, C., Folkerts, M., Hauke, W., Zandig, M., Moller, H.J., and Hegert, U. (2006). *Journal of International Psychophysiology*.

Posner, M. I. and Raichle, M. E. (1998). The neuroimaging of human brain function. Proceedings-National Academy of Sciences USA. **95(3)**, 763–764.

Raichle, M., McLeod, A., Snyder, A., Powers, W., Gusnard, D. and Shulman, G. (2001). A default mode of brain function. *Proceedings of National Academy of Science, USA*, **98**, 676–682.

Raichle, M. and Snyder, A. (2007). A default mode of brain function: A brief history of an evolving idea. *NeuroImage*, **37**, 1083–1090.

Rice, K. M., Blanchard, E.B. and Parcell, M. (1993). Biofeedback treatments of generalized anxiety disorder: Preliminary results. *Biofeedback and Self-Regulation*, **18**, 93–105.

Scherzer, E. (1966). Low voltage EEG's as the bio-electrical measure of tense expectancy (psychogenic alpha reduction). *Psychiatric Neurology*, **152**, 207.

Sherlin, L. (2008). Personal communication.

Sittenfeld, P., Budzynski, T. and Stoyva, J. (1976). Differential shaping of EEG theta rhythms. *Biofeedback and Self-Regulation*, **1**, 31–45.

Small, J. G. (1993). Psychiatric disorders and EEG in electroencephalography: Basic principles, clinical applications and related fields. In *Electroencephalography* 5th ed. (E. Niedermeyer and F. Lopes de Silva, eds) pp. 581–596. Baltimore: Williams & Wilkins.

Speilberger, C.D., Gorusch, G.L. and Luschene, R. (1983). The State-Trait Anxiety Inventory (Test Manual). Palo Alto. CA Consulting Psychological Press.

Tang, H.Y., Harms, V., and Vezeau, T (in press). An audio relaxation tool for blood pressure reduction in older adults. *Journal of Geriatric Nursing*.

Thompson, M. and Thompson, L. (2007). Neurofeedback for stress management. In *Priniciples and Practice of Stress Management, 3rd edition* (P. M. Lehrer, R. L. Woolfolk and W. E. Sime, eds). New York: Guilford Publications. 249–287

Tot, S., Ozge, A., Comolekoglu, U., Yazici, K. *et al.* (2002). Association of QEEG findings with clinical characteristics of OCD: Evidence of left frontotemporal dysfunction. *Canadian Journal of Psychiatry*, **47(6)**, 538–545.

Wiederhold, B. K. and Wiederhold, M. D. (2005). *Virtual Reality Therapy for Anxiety Disorders: Advances in Evaluation and Treatment.* Washington, DC: American Psychological Association.

Zhao, X., Wang, P., Li, C., *et al.* (2007). Altered default mode network activity in patient with anxiety disorders: An fMRI study. *European Journal of Radiology*, **63**, 373–378.

Ethical/Legal Issues

CHAPTER 18

Ethics in neurofeedback practice

Sebastian Striefel, Ph.D.

Professor Emeritus, Utah State University, Logan, Utah, USA

I. INTRODUCTION

During the last 10 years, many changes have occurred in the application of ethics in daily neurofeedback practice. Neurofeedback practice has matured considerably, and is in part due to: more research data being available; the expansion in clinical applications; the availability of efficacy papers; the broader availability of continuing education activities for practitioners; and the greater familiarity with neurofeedback by the general public, third-party payers, and regulatory agencies. These changes have necessitated updates in the application of ethical principles, laws, and in practice guidelines and standard. Practitioners will want to remain current on all of the laws, ethical principles, and practice guidelines and standards that are applicable to their practice activities. Changes often occur yearly in laws, rules, and regulations. Changes in professional ethical principles and practice guidelines and standards occur less frequently. In either case, ignorance is no excuse for violating a law, ethical guideline, or other guidance document. Continuing education, home study, and membership in various professional associations are all ways of remaining current.

Many uses of the electroencephalogram (EEG), hemoencephalography (HEG), light-sound stimulation, quantitative EEGs (QEEG), and some other neurofeedback technologies are not as experimental as they were 7–10 years ago. Several applications have moved into the realm of validated applications because of the amount of research and clinical support available. Of course, some applications are still relatively new, thus insufficient clinical or research support exists to consider them validated. For example, the work by Birbaumer and Cohen on using magnetoencephalographic biofeedback to promote brain reorganization in patients who have had strokes is very new (Birbaumer, 2007). Other newer applications are quite controversial, for example the area of brain fingerprinting which uses the EEG to determine the truth about criminal behavior (Witchalls, 2004; Thornton, 2005).

Also of concern are areas in which many clinicians are active, but research studies have not yet been conducted. For example, many clinicians are sending EEG equipment home with clients so that they can do home training, yet scientific studies to identify potential problems, efficacy, and efficiency are not available. The application of EEG biofeedback in telehealth situations is also in dire need of research studies. Practitioners have an ethical responsibility to remain current on the research and clinical data related to the areas in which they practice. Doing so increases the likelihood that the services that they provide will meet or exceed the expected standard of care.

So what are the ethical, legal, and professional neurofeedback practice issues about which practitioners should be concerned? Clearly neurofeedback has great potential for helping many clients with many different types of problems. The technology available today continues to expand rapidly in both hardware and software. Opportunities are also enhanced by the wide range of brain-related data available in other basic and applied neuroscience research using technologies such as functional magnetic resonance imaging (fMRI). The number of practitioners providing neurofeedback services continues to increase, and can pose a potentially serious problem for the future credibility of neurofeedback if careful attention is not paid to training and verification of practitioner competence via degree and certification programs such as the Biofeedback Certification Program of America (BCIA).

Caution is wise in terms of the claims made about the value of neurofeedback. Exaggerated claims, the provision of incompetent services that result in harm to clients, a lack of treatment progress, and the lack of a good clinical and research foundation can all seriously hinder the growth of this very useful technology and treatment approach in terms of acceptance and uses. All statements verbalized or printed should be accurate and balanced (Striefel, 2004a). All neurofeedback stakeholders need to work cooperatively to ensure that those who are providing neurofeedback services are competent in what they do, behave in an ethical and professional manner, and all need to encourage quality research and the collection of meaningful clinical data to support what practitioners do.

II.   CURRENT STATUS OF ETHICAL AND PROFESSIONAL ISSUES

The purpose of this chapter is to provide information on the current status of some of the ethical, legal and professional issues associated with neurofeedback services. The intent is to help practitioners provide services that meet the expected practice standards (duty of care) that clients, other health care professionals, and third-party payers expect, while simultaneously helping practitioners avoid unnecessary risks. At the outset it must be stated that from an ethical, legal and professional viewpoint, *neurofeedback is more similar to, than different from, other biofeedback applications* (Striefel, 1999a). Many ethical issues encountered by neurofeedback practitioners are the same as those encountered by practitioners using other biofeedback modalities, for example client confidentiality, informed consent, need for clinical and research support, and fees and billing issues. In addition, conservative groups like state licensing boards are accepting more and more neurofeedback applications as being traditional interventions.

As always, newer, non-traditional biofeedback procedures require practitioners to take extra precautions, e.g., during the informed consent process, to avoid unnecessary risks, and to maintain good working relationships with their clients, other practitioners, and third-party payers. It is also important to remember that "The ethical clinician never promises a cure and always makes it clear from the start that not everyone responds." (Demos, 2005, p. 8)

A variety of issues associated with practicing neurofeedback will be discussed in the sections that follow. It is assumed that readers are familiar with the standards of practice and ethical principles for their own discipline, with those of the Biofeedback Certification Institute of America, and with those of professional associations such as the Association of Applied Psychophysiology and Biofeedback (AAPB) and the International Society for Neurofeedback and Research (ISNR), for example. See AAPB (2003) and Striefel (2004a) for copies of the current ethical principles and practice guidelines, and standards of practice adopted by AAPB, and see Hammond *et al.* (2004) for a copy of the standards for the use of the QEEG in neurofeedback. For more background information on professional ethical behavior in applied psychophysiology and biofeedback the reader is referred to Striefel (1995a, 2003a, 2003b, 2004b).

III. THE NECESSITY OF DEFINITIONS

Neurotherapy and *neurofeedback* are terms that are often used synonymously with electroencephalographic (EEG) biofeedback. Demos (2005) often uses the terms *neurofeedback* and *neurotherapy* interchangeably. Yet each term can have different connotations, and there are advantages and disadvantages to the use of each term. Striefel (1999a) discussed many of the advantages and disadvantages of each term, so most of that information will not be repeated herein.

Some third-party payers pay for biofeedback services in general, and some even pay for EEG biofeedback. Because reimbursement codes currently exist for EEG biofeedback, but not for neurotherapy or neurofeedback, it may be useful to use the term *EEG biofeedback* when dealing with insurance companies. One disadvantage of the term *EEG biofeedback* is that it is not broad enough to cover all of the clinical applications and research efforts being used, e.g., hemoencephalography and light-sound interventions. Othmer *et al.* (1999) have argued that EEG biofeedback does not fit the medical model, and that we should move beyond the use of the *Diagnostic and Statistical Manual of Mental Disorders: DSM-IV*, 4th edition (American Psychiatric Association (APA), 1994) of discrete, canonical disorders toward a spectrum theory of mental disorders. A potential problem with doing so is that reimbursement from third-party payers may be even more difficult to obtain than it is when using the medical model. See Othmer *et al.* (1999) for more information on their disregulation model of psychopathology.

Hammond (2006a) summarized some of the research documenting that abnormal brain wave patterns are associated with a variety of medical conditions, and of course each medical condition fits well within the medical model. He also discussed what neurofeedback is and is not (Hammond, 2006b). Gunkelman (2006) reported that many of the EEG abnormalities associated with various diagnoses based on the DSM are more similar than different. He called these similar EEG patterns, *phenotypes*. Furthermore, specific phenotypes that exist across various diagnostic categories may well respond to the same EEG treatment protocol. Research designed to support these positions is needed because, from an ethical viewpoint, it is important to practice in ways that maximize the probability of a client's insurance company paying for needed services. However, doing so requires practitioners to operate within the legal and ethical guidelines that exist.

The term *neurofeedback* easily encompasses both feedback and other applied psychophysiological approaches for modifying brain function. Demos (2005, p. 3) defines it as, "a Comprehensive Training System that promotes growth and change at the cellular level of the brain." However, the term *neurofeedback* is still new enough that it may be unfamiliar to others such as third-party payers, and thus reimbursement issues can and do arise when it is used.

The terms *EEG biofeedback*, *neurotherapy*, and *neurofeedback* do not yet have definitions that are commonly accepted by all stakeholders. It seems important for professional associations like AAPB and ISNR to define these terms before some other group defines them in some restrictive manner, e.g., imagine what would happen if the terms and the practice thereof were defined as the exclusive practice of medicine? At present, care should be taken in deciding what term to use with different stakeholders (e.g., patients, other professional health care providers, and third-party payers), and for different purposes, for example which term or terms are most readily understood by your referral sources, clients/patients, and insurance company representatives?

Perhaps it is easier to educate managed care and other third-party payers by using the term *biofeedback* when discussing EEG treatment applications with them, and to use the term *neurofeedback* when using other brain-related treatment modalities (e.g., hemoencephalography or light-sound stimulation), or when communicating with the clients served. This chapter will generally use the term *neurofeedback* because it is more representative of the broader implications of using EEG technology to train or treat individuals. Other terms will be used as needed in specific contexts.

IV. PROFESSIONAL DECISION-MAKING

Practitioners make decisions daily about whether or not to accept a particular client for treatment. Numerous variables should be considered in such decision-making, including but not limited to the symptoms, likely side effects and abreactions, diagnosis, duration of symptoms, previous treatments and their effectiveness, existing laws, and the client's ability to pay. Practitioners must seriously consider their own demonstratable competence for treating the client's problems, with or without supervision or consultation, whether or not they can legally do so, and if the client's needs would be better met if referred elsewhere. Perhaps the practitioner should work cooperatively with other health care professionals to best meet the client's needs. These are considerations that can produce ethical dilemmas in a clinician's practice. Integration of healthy personal experiences and values, positive emotions, and good judgment serves to establish an ethical practice.

V. CHARACTERISTICS OF AN ETHICAL PRACTICE

Practitioners need certain character traits and skills in order to be successful (Striefel, 1999a). Fowers (2005) defines character as the overall state of a practitioner in regard to virtue (i.e., the kind of person one is). Character strengths equal virtue. "A virtuous life is a life lived well as a whole, with a coherent, integrated set of aims, the strength of character necessary to pursue those ends, and the social bonds that give place and purpose to our activities" (Fowers, 2005, p. 5). Striefel (1999a) provided some definitions for some of the important character traits and skills as follows:

- Confidence—belief in one's ability to succeed or reliance on one's own power to do what is right, proper or effective. It includes the degree of hopefulness or optimism that one has for dealing with a situation.
- Compassion—awareness of another's distress and desire to help overcome it. It includes a concern, empathy, loyalty, sympathy and warmth for others who are in distress.
- Commitment—accepting one's responsibility to carry out an obligation to a client. Degree of assurance that one will do what is right, i.e., doing what you know is right for those you serve. In general, the more committed a provider is to an ethical line of action, the less likely it is that personal and friendship related concerns will negatively influence his or her decision-making or actions in resolving an ethical dilemma.
- Ethical competence—the ability to identify the appropriate ethical intervention when an ethical dilemma occurs, i.e., knowing what to do and how to do it. Ethical knowledge alone is not sufficient for producing ethical behavior. A provider must also be committed to behaving ethically in spite of potential negative repercussions, and that takes character.
- Ethical resoluteness—refers to the likelihood that a provider will intervene ethically when an ethical dilemma occurs. It is the degree of confidence that a provider has that he or she will follow through in doing what is ethically correct.

- Ethical willingness—refers to whether a provider would do what he or she identifies as being what he or she should do when encountering an ethical dilemma. It is a measure of motivation.

"The best practitioners are those who are self-aware, focused on seeking beneficial outcomes for their clients, respectful of client autonomy, respectful of cultural differences, honest, sufficiently courageous to confront difficulties . . ." (Fowers, 2005, p. 21). One might add that practitioners need to be honest, generous, just, loyal, and fair to the interests of those they serve. Two major components of ethical decision-making are ethical competence and commitment. Practitioners need to develop both in order to practice in an ethical manner.

VI. CAUTIONS AND CONTRAINDICATIONS IN USING NEUROFEEDBACK

It can be helpful for practitioners to be aware of issues in which other neurofeedback practitioners have had difficulties with licensing boards, ethics committees, lawsuits, and/or third-party payers. Awareness can lead to proactive rather than reactive activities. There is no one way to become or remain aware. Reading, attending conferences, interacting with other practitioners, and state licensing boards can all be helpful.

For example, at the 2007 ISNR meeting in San Francisco a discussion was held concerning a neurofeedback provider in Maryland who received a "cease and desist order" from the State Medical Board for practicing medicine without a license (Stokes, 2007). Mary Lee Esty, Ph.D., a licensed social worker, was using the Flexyx neurotherapy system (FNS), an early version of the low energy neurofeedback system (LENS) developed by Len Ochs (see Ochs, 2006), and articles by other authors in the same issue of the *Journal of Neurotherapy* for a complete discussion of the LENS). The Maryland State Board of Social Work and the BCIA have both found Dr. Esty innocent of any wrongdoing, but the verdict by the state medical board is still out. The scope of practice for Dr. Esty allows her to diagnose and treat any condition listed in the Diagnostic and Statistical Manual IV (DSM–IV), but the state medical board is taking the position that the small electrical stimulation induced by the FNS is invasive, and therefore practicing medicine without a license.

Defending one's self against a complaint, even if you win, will be expensive in time, dollars, energy, stress, reputation, future referrals, and professional contacts. Proactive behavior can decrease the likelihood of a practitioner having to deal with a licensing board, ethics committee, or the Food and Drug Administration (FDA). Some issues for each neurofeedback practitioner to consider and deal with in order to be in compliance with state licensing laws and the rules of the FDA follow:

1. If you are licensed, what does the scope of practice for your license allow you to do? Are there any other licensing laws (e.g., the law for the practice of medicine) that restrict what you can and cannot do? Hint: In most states

the licensing law for physicians will have restrictions you did not even think about, such as those encountered by Dr. Esty. Can you diagnose and treat specific conditions and/or diseases, e.g., those listed in DSM IV, or can you only treat the symptoms of such conditions? Is all of the written information on your web site, advertising and promotional literature, your informed consent forms, billing forms, policies and procedures, and all of the verbal information you share with patients and others in compliance with what you are allowed to do? If not, take the steps needed to make it so. Use the services of an attorney to help you with this task if needed.

2. If you are not licensed, can you legally practice neurofeedback in the state in which you are practicing? What steps do you have to take to be in compliance with the law? Because the issues of scope of practice and language used in promotional material are even more complex for those who are not licensed in a health care discipline than for those who are, legal consultation is strongly advised.

3. What is the definition of neurofeedback, neurotherapy, applied psychophysiology, biofeedback, and what are the implications of the definitions used? Many states restrict the practice of biofeedback, and therefore neurofeedback and electroencephalographic (EEG) biofeedback, to those licensed in specific health care disciplines or supervised by same. It is risky to assume that one can practice outside the law and get away with it. Sooner or later such a practitioner will be called to task because of a jealous rival practitioner, a client compliant, or a diligent licensing board. Clearly, some equipment used does not fit any of the commonly used definitions of neurofeedback because no physiological measurement is taken, e.g., electrical stimulation using an alpha-stimulation machine. So what is the practitioner doing? Is it within the scope of practice allowed for his or her license, and within the guidelines of practice allowed by the FDA? Perhaps some forms of stimulation, because of the way specific state laws are worded, can be defined as the practice of medicine in those specific states. How would you go about being in compliance with such laws and, if you consider them unjust, how would you go about getting the laws changed?

4. Is the equipment you are using registered with the FDA, and what uses have they approved? According to Rick Jaffe, Dr. Esty's attorney, the use of equipment not registered (approved) by the FDA, is considered by them to be equivalent to the use of street drugs (Stokes, 2007). Do you want to try to defend your self against the wrath of the FDA? Licensed health care practitioners can use FDA approved equipment for "off-label" uses provided that the use is within the scope of practice for that provider's license. If you are not licensed you should probably seek legal advice from an attorney familiar with the FDA way of operating before using equipment "off-label."

Being an active part of the state and national association for their discipline can help in educating the members of the Association and other practitioners concerning neurofeedback practice and issues. Since state licensing board members tend to be selected from the membership of the state association for a discipline, being active therein can also help educate the state licensing board members. In general, because of their gatekeeping functions licensing boards tend to be conservative, thus practitioners should be proactive in terms of how they engage in the practice of neurofeedback. Planning ahead can help avoid problems later. Described below are some areas in which practitioners have been questioned by licensing boards or professional colleagues in the past, but the number of occurrences has decreased as practitioners, third-party payers, and consumers have become better informed.

A.   Efficaciousness of interventions

Have you ever struggled with the idea of whether a neurofeedback intervention is an alternative, complimentary or mainstream intervention? Have you tried to decide which procedures are truly supported by existing research or clinical data? Practitioners engaged in applied psychophysiology- and/or neurofeedback-related activities are daily faced with making decisions about what to tell clients concerning the published and clinical support for the clinical interventions that they are proposing to use to help the client overcome their presenting problem(s). Practitioners are ethically expected to clarify during the informed consent process which procedures are efficacious, which are experimental, and to get written informed consent for procedures that are, or might well be, considered experimental (AAPB, 2003; Striefel, 2004a). Doing so is not an easy task.

Practitioners are advised to be honest, prudent, and to provide all the information that a reasonable person would need in order to make decisions when explaining neurofeedback interventions to clients during the informed consent process. According to Beutler and Davidson (1995) there is no one agreed upon standard for when a treatment approach is considered to be valid and reliable (efficacious), and thus no longer experimental. Hopefully that is changing with the adoption of recommendations of the joint AAPB and ISNR Task Force on Efficacious Treatments to use a template for that purpose (La Vaque et al., 2002). The template adopted is similar to those proposed and/or adopted by the American Psychological Association (APA) (1993), AAPB (Striefel, 1997a), and Striefel (1998). In fact, based on such a template and the number of research studies attesting to the effectiveness of EEG biofeedback, Striefel (1998) concluded that EEG biofeedback per se was no longer an experimental procedure, but rather a validated intervention. Individual EEG biofeedback applications are an entirely separate matter.

The template adopted by the joint task force has an eight point hierarchy ranging from anecdotal evidence to double-blind control studies (La Vaque et al.,

2002). The template is now being used to determine the efficacy status of various areas of neurofeedback interventions. For example, Monastra *et al.* (2005, p. 95) concluded that, "EEG biofeedback was determined to be 'probably efficacious' for the treatment of ADHD." Seventy five percent of clients in the reviewed research studies made clinically significant improvements. How many clinical interventions, including drugs, are you aware of that can make that claim? In addition, in 2004, ISNR published a proposed set of standards for the use of the QEEG in neurofeedback (Hammond *et al.*, 2004). As a practitioner you should be aware of the template, the standards, and the status and efficacy of the interventions you use. If you are not, how can you obtain meaningful informed consent from your clients?

Even neurofeedback interventions that meet the new standards for validation/ efficacy may well not be accepted by conservative groups that use a different standard (Barkley, 1992), or by managed care organizations who have a profit motivated approach to intervention. Managed care organizations do not seem to use any consistent standard for deciding when a treatment is efficacious. Their standard often seems to be one that allows them to refuse to pay for services. Newer treatments are usually held to a higher standard than existing treatments for proving their clinical efficacy. In fact, many existing treatments (biofeedback and otherwise) could not meet the requirement of having been proved in double-blind control studies. There is no one agreed upon standard for making decisions about when a procedure or approach is no longer experimental outside of the neurofeedback practitioner community, but hopefully that is no longer true within the neurofeedback community. Applying a standard, in this case the "efficacy template," to available data and publishing the results is a good place to start.

The ethical principles for many professionals require them to report actual or suspected ethical violations. Some professionals either do not know what neurotherapy is, know of neurotherapy providers who do not explain to clients that a specific neurotherapy intervention is considered to be experimental by many professionals, or know of providers who make what they consider to be exaggerated claims about what neurotherapy can accomplish. They therefore consider such activities to be unethical, and thus they file an ethics complaint.

Trudeau (2001) reviewed the work of several authors that compared the results of randomized controlled trials versus observational studies, and concluded that well designed observational studies are similar in validity to randomized controlled studies. He concluded that observational studies can be as valid as randomized controlled studies in support of the clinical efficacy of neurotherapy. How does such information impact the validation of treatments from your personal perspective?

Not all biofeedback practitioners consider neurofeedback to have enough documented research support for the various interventions to be efficacious. Perhaps an annual symposium could be held to determine what the concerns of these biofeedback practitioners are, and how to address them as part of the approach for educating the public, other professionals not involved in biofeedback, and third-party payers on the validity of different neurofeedback approaches. Newly published reviews using the "efficacy template" could be highlighted at these symposia.

Some neurofeedback interventions may well need to be explained to consumers during the informed consent process as not yet totally validated until:

- Sufficient published research is available to convince most practitioners and other stakeholders that neurofeedback is efficacious. The reviews applying the validation standards adopted by AAPB and ISNR should help in this process.
- Neurofeedback becomes one of the predominant treatment approaches for a particular problem or diagnosis.
- Third-party payers regularly pay for neurofeedback intervention.
- Neurofeedback is accepted by licensing boards, and is written into their state licensing laws and administrative regulations.
- Neurofeedback is regularly requested by consumers as the treatment they prefer for dealing with one or more of their problems (Striefel, 1999a).

B. Informed consent

For practical purposes, neurofeedback practitioners should be familiar with the current literature, so that they can explain to potential clients the efficacy status of various interventions so as not to mislead clients or third-party payers. To protect both the client and practitioner, informed consent should be well documented to make clear what was and what was not explained, including other treatment options, and the pros and cons of each.

Written informed consent is important for several reasons, including: a) the ethical principles of AAPB require that informed consent be obtained for all procedures, and that it be obtained in written form if the procedure is not yet demonstrated to be efficacious (AAPB, 2003); and b) written informed consent provides documentation of what a client was or was not told, and to what they agreed, should later questions be raised by the client, a competitor, or a licensing board. Written informed consent has been very useful for several neurofeedback practitioners in dealing with situations that arose after the fact (Striefel, 1997b).

The informed consent process should:

a) Provide the client with all the information needed to make the required decisions.
b) Provide the information so it is understood by the client as verified by having the client answer questions about the information.
c) Ensure that the client has the capacity to give consent (assumed unless there is evidence to the contrary, e.g., client has obvious mental disability).
d) The consent must be given voluntarily without coercion.

e) The client must actually give consent verbally or in writing (don't assume client consents just because he or she did not verbalize a disagreement).

f) Document the process carefully, using written forms for the components that are the same for all clients e.g., limits of confidentiality, fees, billings, and collections (Striefel, 2004b).

As a general "rule of thumb," the less published literature that exists to support a specific neurofeedback intervention, the more cautious a neurofeedback practitioner should be in their explanation to the client, and the more documentation, supervision and/or consultation a practitioner should seek. Unpublished clinical data is not available for clients, third-party payers, or licensing boards to review.

C. Advertising

The ethical principles for several professional disciplines require members to report actual or suspected ethical violations. Advertisements that members of such disciplines consider to be dishonest or exaggerations can result in a complaint being filed by a well-meaning professional who is trying to protect the public and the reputation of a particular discipline or treatment approach (Striefel, 1997b, 1997c, 1999a). Several neurofeedback practitioners have been questioned by colleagues and/or licensing boards on the basis of what they put in their brochures or other advertisements (Striefel, 1997b, 1999a). Claims that are considered to be exaggerations by others, especially those whose incomes are being impacted because clients are going to a neurofeedback practitioner, have in the past resulted in formal or informal complaints being filed.

Licensing laws often contain statements about dishonest and/or misleading advertisements. Thus, licensing boards have in the past become concerned about neurofeedback advertisements that they considered to be exaggerations or untrue. The actions of such licensing boards have resulted in practitioners being required to "tone down" or reword advertisements to fit what the board considered realistic and honest. Clear, honest and truthful ads that can be supported by the existing published literature can help a practitioner avoid problems, clarify the situation if questions arise, and enhance the credibility of neurofeedback.

One deceptive or exaggerated claim can negatively impact the reputation of neurofeedback per se, and of those who provide such services. It is best to be conservative in what is included in a practitioner's advertisements, and to have ads reviewed by a colleague who has a reputation for being honest in terms of the feedback they give. It is also a good idea to keep on file a copy of all advertisements, brochures, and even radio or television ads in case questions arise. Thankfully, there seems to have been a decrease in the number of complaints during the last 5–10 years concerning advertising. One might conclude that practitioners are being more truthful in their advertisements. Potential clients have many questions about neurofeedback (Demos, 2005), and should not be mislead by advertising.

D. Boundary issues

Practitioners must be aware of the practice boundaries for different groups of licensed professionals. Care should be taken to avoid practicing in an area reserved for practice by those licensed in another professional discipline. Making a medical diagnosis, or discussing with a client changes in medication if one is not a licensed medical practitioner, are fairly clear examples of areas where a practitioner can easily cross the boundary into practicing medicine without a license. Situations such as that encountered by Dr. Esty are not as easy to foresee or to deal with in a proactive manner.

Neurofeedback practitioners need to know not only the boundaries for their own discipline but also those for other professional disciplines. There is nothing wrong with suggesting to a client that they contact their physician to see if a medication adjustment might be appropriate, or obtaining the client's permission to have a discussion with said physician. If one is not an appropriately licensed medical practitioner, it is not appropriate, and is in fact illegal, to suggest to a client that they stop taking a medication. Caution in selecting the words used will help protect one from practicing beyond the boundaries of one's discipline and one's areas of competence. Litigation to counteract a licensing board decision could be extremely expensive.

VII. STANDARD OF CARE

Standards of care consist of federal and state laws, rules and regulations, and guidelines (e.g., ethical principles, practice guidelines and standards) developed by some professional association or organization to help guide the practice activities of its members, to inform third-party payers and consumers of what acceptable practice behavior is, and to preclude unnecessary regulation by other groups such as state legislators. Practitioners must render services that are at least as competent and skillfully applied as they would be by the ordinary practitioner (Zuckerman, 2003). The intent of standards of care is to prevent injury to clients, and thus also to reduce the risk to the practitioner. Failure to meet the relevant standard of care expected of a practitioner can result in a malpractice lawsuit, filing of an ethics complaint, loss of income, damage to one's reputation, a loss of referral, and even the loss of one's livelihood. For more information on malpractice issues the reader is referred to Bennett *et al.* (1990) and Striefel (1995b; 1999a, 2001, 2003a, 2003b).

Many sets of ethical principles are available to help guide the activities of neurofeedback practitioners, e.g., those of AAPB and ISNR. At present, no published set of practice standards exists for neurofeedback per se. A set of practice guidelines and standards of practice do exist for biofeedback in general, and they are very applicable to neurofeedback (Striefel, 2004a). Practitioners should adhere to the practice guidelines of AAPB, and to those of their professional discipline, those of their supervisor, and those used by closely related disciplines as appropriate. Some common standards for practitioners to consider are listed below (Striefel, 1999a; Zuckerman, 2003):

- Adhere to all relevant state and federal laws, guidelines and regulations. The laws may vary from state to state, but generally include:

  1. State licensing laws, title or practice acts. (See Striefel, 1999a, 2000, for a full discussion of the issues not previously covered in this chapter).
  2. Child abuse and neglect reporting laws (most states also have abuse and neglect laws related to people with developmental disabilities, the elderly, etc.).
  3. Records retention laws (Striefel, 2003a, 2004a).
  4. Privileged communications laws (often included in licensing or mental health laws).
  5. Billing, insurance, and fee collection laws (obtain informed consent from clients on your fees before or during the first treatment session whenever possible, or as soon thereafter as is reasonable.) (See Striefel, 2003a, 2003b, 2003c, 2003d; Striefel et al., 2003, and Whitehouse & Striefel, 2003).
  6. Office of Health and Safety Administration regulations concerning prevention of diseases, e.g., in disinfecting electrodes.
  7. Infectious diseases reporting laws.
  8. Duty to warn and/or protect laws.
  9. The Health Insurance Portability and Accountability Act (HIPAA).

Copies of these laws, as relevant to a particular state can be obtained from the Internet since all states now have a web site for their laws. The state office of licensing and the state department of mental health are often familiar with the relevant state laws, and can help one access other relevant laws.

- Adhere to all relevant ethical principles and standards of practice (e.g., AAPB, 2003, Striefel, 2004a).
- Protect the rights and welfare of those you serve by doing no harm through acts of omission or commission.
- Make no exaggerated claims for neurotherapy in either verbal or written form. Be honest in all of your dealings with clients, those you supervise, and with other professionals. Do not exaggerate your qualifications.
- Obtain informed consent, preferably in writing, for all neurofeedback applications. Be cautious in what you tell clients in terms of which treatments you consider validated, and be sure you can support the claims you make with research and/or appropriate clinical data.
- Engage in no sexual activity with current or former clients, and avoid other problematic dual relationships with clients, supervisees, students, and research subjects.

- Know the boundaries of your areas of competence, and practice only within them. The *Ethical Principles* of AAPB state that, "members recognize the boundaries of their competence and operate within their level of competence using only those biofeedback and other psychophysiological self-regulation techniques in which they are competent by training and experience," (AAPB, 2003, p. 2). The AAPB, 2004, Practice Guidelines and Standards (Striefel, 2004a, p. 27) clarifies that, "To be competent means the provider has the knowledge to understand a particular client's problem and to formulate an appropriate treatment plan, has the skills needed to apply that knowledge effectively, and the judgment to use such knowledge and skills appropriately."

   Each neurofeedback provider should be prepared to demonstrate that they are competent by training and experience to provide neurofeedback and related services in general, and also any specific neurofeedback and related services that are or have been provided by that practitioner. They must also be able to demonstrate that they are competent to work with the particular kind of client (e.g., child versus adult) and presenting problem(s). They must also be competent enough to recognize different diagnostic categories and their associated behavioral symptoms, to make the diagnosis if it has not already been made and, if allowed to do so by law, to treat the specific brain wave abnormalities associated with different diagnostic categories. Also, depending on state law, a neurofeedback practitioner may have to be licensed in a specific health care profession, or be supervised by someone who is.

- Participate in ongoing continuing education to both maintain and expand your areas of competence.
- Strive to improve your credentials by becoming certified in specialties relevant to what you do in practice (e.g., BCIA certification in neurofeedback), and by becoming licensed in a relevant health care discipline if not already licensed.
- Refer clients for treatment to another practitioner if you are not competent to provide services that at least meet the expected minimum standard of care with supervision and/or consultation available.
- When a type of client, presenting problem, or treatment approach is new for you, or when in doubt about how to proceed, seek competent supervision and/or consultation (Striefel, 2004d; Zuckerman, 2003).
- Supervise only in those areas in which you are competent unless appropriately supervised. Delegate to supervisees only those responsibilities that they are competent to perform.
- Do not try to treat every problem that comes into your office with neurotherapy. Be sure the treatments that you recommend and/or provide are appropriate for the client in terms of efficacy and cost.

- Practitioners should monitor their own mental states, physical health, and behaviors for signs of fatigue, burn out, and personal and emotional problems that could negatively impact client services.
- Accept your responsibilities for what you do and fail to do. All neurofeedback practitioners are responsible for their own actions and those whom they supervise (Striefel, 1995a, 1999a, 2006a; Zuckerman, 2003).
- Do not abandon a client in need. When and if appropriate, help clients access needed services from other providers.
- Maintain a client support backup system for dealing with after-hour emergencies and your absence.
- Keep good clinical records that adhere to state and federal laws, rules, and regulations. The less supported the treatment approach used, the better your records should be in terms of detail.
- Inform clients of the limits of confidentiality as soon as possible (preferably in the first session), and do not violate confidentiality without a reason recognized by other professionals as acceptable. Obtain a signed release of information before releasing confidential information in all non-emergency situations. Strive to exceed the HIPAA requirements.
- Do not falsify any diagnostic or procedural codes in an effort to collect from third-party payers.
- Do not discriminate against any client on the basis or age, race, gender, nationality, sexual preference, religion, disability, or socioeconomic status.
- Do not engage in sexual harassment.
- Inform all parties concerned of any conflict of interest. Do not exploit clients, supervisees, students, or research subjects.
- Address any potential ethical violation by another by trying to resolve it with the person involved where possible, or by reporting it to the appropriate ethics committee or licensing board if it does not seem appropriate for informal resolution.
- Do not make false statements or complaints about other practitioners.
- Do not intentionally or unintentionally influence a client inappropriately, e.g., imposing your belief system on the client.
- Backup all computer files related to clients and their activities, and ensure that the confidentiality of those backup files is established and maintained.

Practitioners should review this list and add to it in light of their own training and experience.

VIII. CONCLUSION

A vast number of topics were covered in this chapter. Because of space, however, a vast number of other topics were not covered. Some of them may well be covered in some detail in other chapters but in fairness to readers, some guidance will be provided on four topics deemed important enough to warrant further study. Sources for more information include: ethical decision-making models and related information (Haas and Malouf, 1989, Striefel, 1999b, 2004c); contraindications (Hammond and Kirk, 2007, Striefel, 2007a, 2007b); QEEG considerations (e.g., should a pre- and post-QEEG be required?) (Demos, 2005; Duffy *et al.*, 1994; Hammond *et al.*, 2001; Hammond *et al.*, 2004; Hoffman, 2006; Ochs, 2006; Striefel, 1999a, 2006b; Walker and Norman, 2006); and FDA issues (Striefel, 1999a).

REFERENCES

AAPB (Association of Applied Psychophysiology and Biofeedback) (2003). *Ethical principles of applied psychophysiology and biofeedback.* Wheat Ridge, CO: Association for Applied Psychophysiology and Biofeedback.

American Psychiatric Association (1994). *Diagnostic and Statistical Manual of Mental Disorders: DSM-IV.* Washington, DC: American Psychiatric Association.

American Psychological Association (1993). *Promotion and dissemination of psychological procedures.* An unpublished task force report for Division 12. Washington, DC: American Psychological Association.

Barkley, R. A. (1992). Is EEG biofeedback treatment effective for ADHD children?. *ChaADDer Box,* 5–11.

Bennett, B. E., Bryant, B. K., VandenBos, G. R. and Greenwood, A. (1990). *Professional liability and risk management.* Washington, DC: American Psychological Association.

Beutler, L. E. and Davidson, E. H. (1995). What standards should we use?. In *Scientific standards of psychological practice: Issues and recommendations* (S. C. Hayes, V. M. Follette, R. M. Dawes and K. E. Grady, eds), pp. 11–24. Reno, NV: Context Press.

Birbaumer, N. (2007). A brain computer interface for restoration of movement following stroke. *Neuro Connections,* **7(9)**, 11–12.

Demos, J. N. (2005). *Getting started with neurofeedback.* New York: W. W. Norton & Company.

Duffy, F. H., Hughes, J. R., Miranda, F., Bernard, P. and Cook, P. (1994). Status of quantitative EEG (QEEG) in clinical practice: 1994. *Clinical Electroencephalography,* **25(4)**, VI–XXII.

Fowers, B. J. (2005). *Virtue and psychology: Pursuing excellence in ordinary practice.* Washington, DC: American Psychological Association.

Gunkelman, J. (2006). Transcend the DSM using phenotypes. *Biofeedback,* **34(3)**, 95–98.

Haas, L. J. and Malouf, J. L. (1989). *Keeping up the good work: A practitioner's guide to mental health ethics.* Sarasota, FL: Professional Resources Exchange.

Hammond, D. C. (2006a). Quantitative electroencephalography patterns associated with medical conditions. *Biofeedback,* **34(3)**, 87–94.

Hammond, D. C. (2006b). What is Neurofeedback? *Journal of Neurotherapy,* **10(4)**, 25–36.

Hammond, D. C. and Kirk, L. (2007). Negative effects and the need for standards of practice in neurofeedback. *Biofeedback,* **35(4)**, 139–145.

Hammond, D. C., Stockdale, S., Hoffman, D., Ayers, M. E. and Nash, J. (2001). Adverse reactions and potential iatrogenic effects in neurofeedback training. *Journal of Neurotherapy,* **4(4)**, 57–69.

Hammond, D. C., Walker, J., Hoffman, D., *et al.* (2004). Standard for the use of quantitative electroencephalography (QEEG) in neurofeedback: A position paper of the International Society for Neuronal Regulation. *Journal of Neurotherapy,* **8(1)**, 5–27.

Hoffman, D. A. (2006). LORETA: An attempt at a simple answer to a complex controversy. *Journal of Neurotherapy,* **10(1)**, 57–71.

La Vaque, T. J., Hammond, D. C., Trudeau, D., Monastra, V. J., Perry, J. and Lehrer, P. (2002). Template for developing guidelines for the evaluation of the clinical efficacy of psychophysiological interventions. *Applied Psychophysiology and Biofeedback*, **27(4)**, 273–281.

Monastra, V. J., Lynn, S., Linden, M., Lubar, J. F., Gruzelier, J. and La Vaque, T. J. (2005). Electro-encephalographic biofeedback in the treatment of attention-deficit/hyperactive disorder. *Applied Psychophysiology and Biofeedback*, **30(2)**, 95–114.

Ochs, L. (2006). The low energy neurofeedback system (LENS): Theory, background, and introduction. *Journal of Neurotherapy*, **10(2/3)**, 5–40.

Othmer, S., Othmer, S. F. and Kaiser, D. A. (1999). EEG biofeedback: An emerging model for its global efficacy. In *Introduction to Quantitative EEG and Neurofeedback* (J. R. Evans and A. Abarbanel, eds), pp. 244–310. San Diego, CA: Academic Press.

Stokes, D. (2007). A report from the ISNR meeting on the LENS attack. *EEG Info Newsletter*, **Sept. 19**, http://eeginfo.com/newsletter/.

Striefel, S. (1995a). Professional ethical behavior for providers of biofeedback. In *Biofeedback: A practitioner's guide* (M. S. Schwartz, ed.), pp. 685–705. New York, NY: The Guilford Press.

Striefel, S. (1995b). Ethical areas of confusion: Part 2 – Professional competence. *Biofeedback*, **23(1)**, 13–14.

Striefel, S. (1997a). Possible criteria for empirical validation of treatments. *Biofeedback*, **25(3)**, 2A–3A.

Striefel, S. (1997b). Ethical issues in EEG biofeedback. *Biofeedback*, **25(1)**, 6–7.

Striefel, S. (1997c). Response to Fahrion *et al. Biofeedback*, 25(2), 16–17.

Striefel, S. (1998). Is EEG per se experimental? *Biofeedback*, **26(4)**, 4–6 & 12.

Striefel, S. (1999a). Ethical, legal, and professional pitfalls associated with neurofeedback services. In *Introduction to Quantitative EEG and Neurofeedback*, 1st edition. (J. R. Evans and A. Abarbanel, eds), pp. 371–399. San Diego, CA: Academic Press.

Striefel, S. (1999b). Making the right ethical choice is not always easy. *Biofeedback*, **27(2)**, 4–5.

Striefel, S. (2000). The role of aspirational ethics and licensing laws in the practice of neurofeedback. *Journal of Neurotherapy*, **4(1)**, 43–55.

Striefel, S. (2001). Ethics and risk management. In *Applied neurophysiology and brain biofeedback* (An E-Book) (R. Kall, J. Kamiya and G. Schwartz, eds), pp. 483–514. Trevose, PA: Futurehealth.

Striefel, S. (2003a). The application of ethics and law in daily practice. In *Biofeedback: A practitioner's guide* (M. S. Schwartz and F. Andrasik, eds), pp. 813–834. New York, NY: The Guilford Press.

Striefel, S. (2003b). Professional ethics and practice standards in mind-body medicine. In *Handbook of mind-body medicine for primary care* (D. Moss, A. McGrady, T. C. Davies and I. Wickramasekera, eds), pp. 93–106. Thousand Oaks, CA: Sage Publications.

Striefel, S. (2003c). Overview for series of articles on billing, coding, and reimbursement. *Biofeedback*, **31(4)**, 4.

Striefel, S. (2003d). Ethics and other issues in billing, coding, and reimbursement. *Biofeedback*, **31(4)**, 9–12.

Striefel, S. (2004a). *Practice guidelines and standards for providers of biofeedback and applied psychophysiological services*, Wheat Ridge, CO: Association for Applied Psychophysiology and Biofeedback.

Striefel, S. (2004b). Module 8: Professional conduct. In *Introduction to biofeedback* (A. Crider and D. D. Montgomery, eds), Wheat Ridge, CO: Association for Applied Psychophysiology and Biofeedback.

Striefel, S. (2004c). Morality: What kind of professional do I want to be and how do I get there? *Biofeedback*, **32(1)**, 4–7 & 12.

Striefel, S. (2004d). Do I need supervision or consultation? *Biofeedback*, **32(2)**, 4–7.

Striefel, S. (2006a). Ethical responsibility and professional socialization. *Biofeedback*, **34(2)**, 43–47.

Striefel, S. (2006b). Are QEEGs necessary? *Biofeedback*, **31(3)**, 82–86.

Striefel, S. (2007a). Positive aspects of side effects: Part I, an overview. *Biofeedback*, **35(3)**, 75–79.

Striefel, S. (2007b). Positive aspects of side effects: Part II, treating stress. *Biofeedback*, **35(4)**, 115–119.

Striefel, S., Whitehouse, R. and Schwartz, M. S. (2003). Other professional topics and issues. In *Biofeedback: A practitioner's guide* (M. S. Schwartz and F. Andrasik, eds), pp. 835–866. New York, NY: The Guilford Press.

Thornton, K. E. (2005). The qEEG in the lie detection problem: The localization of guilt? *Journal of Neurotherapy*, **9(3)**, 31–43.

Trudeau, D. (2001). The value of observational studies. *Journal of Neurotherapy*, **4(2)**, 1–4.

Walker, J. E. and Norman, C. A. (2006). The neurophysiology of dyslexia: A selective review with implications for neurofeedback remediation and results of treatment in twelve consecutive cases. *Journal of Neurotherapy*, **10(1)**, 45–55.

Whitehouse, R. and Striefel, S. (2003). Billing, coding, and reimbursement issues. *Biofeedback*, **31(4)**, 5–8.

Witchalls, C. (2006). Murder in mind. *The Guardian*, 25 March. www.guardian.co.uk/science/2004/mar/25/crime.uknews.

Zuckerman, E. I. (2003). *The paper office*, 3rd edition. New York: Guilford Press.

Index

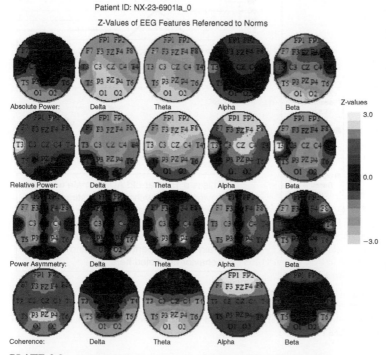

Right Hemispher Hematoma—Maximal in C4 >P4 > O2

C4
P4
O2

FFT Peak at
5–6 Hz

Z-Scores
5–6 Hz—Max. in
C4 > P4 > O2

LORETA Z-Scores
5 Hz—Right
Hemisphere Source
(X=39, Y=−18, Z=15)
Broadmann Area 41
Tramsverse Temporal Gyrus

Left Hemisphere   Right Hemisphere   Postcentral Gyrus

PLATE 2.8 The EEG from a patient with a right hemisphere hematoma where the maximum shows waves are present in C4, P4 and O2 (Top). The FFT power spectrum from 1–30 Hz and the corresponding Z-scores of the surface EEG are shown in the right side of the EEG display. Left and right hemisphere displays of the maximal Z-scores using LORETA (Bottom). It can be seen that only the right hemisphere has statistically significant Z values. Planned comparisons and hypothesis testing based on the frequency and location of maximal deviation from normal on the surface EEG are confirmed by the LORETA Z-score normative analysis. (From Thatcher *et al.*, 2005b.) (see Figure 2.8.)

Patient ID: NX-23-6901la_0

Z-Values of EEG Features Referenced to Norms

| Absolute Power: | Delta | Theta | Alpha | Beta |

| Relative Power: | Delta | Theta | Alpha | Beta |

| Power Asymmetry: | Delta | Theta | Alpha | Beta |

| Coherence: | Delta | Theta | Alpha | Beta |

Z-values
3.0

0.0

−3.0

PLATE 3.2 Univariate Z-scores measures for Case DS (see Figure 3.2).

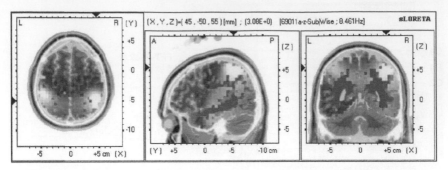

PLATE 3.3   sLORETA source localization for Case DS at 8.64 Hz (see Figure 3.3).

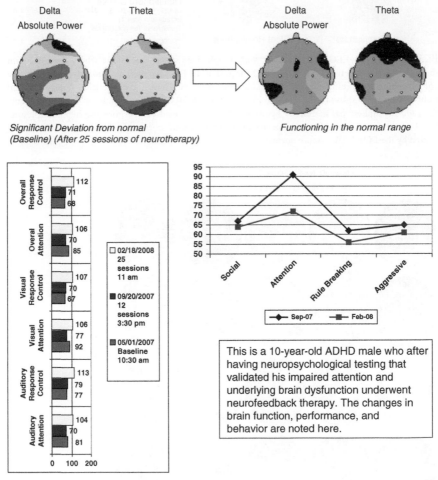

PLATE 3.4   Electrophysiological, performance, and behavior rating measures before and after neurofeedback therapy (see Figure 3.4).

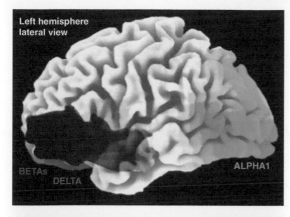

PLATE 4.2 Left hemisphere lateral view of expected current source density distribution (see Figure 4.2).

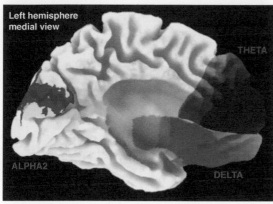

PLATE 4.3 Left hemisphere medial view of expected current source density distribution (see Figure 4.3).

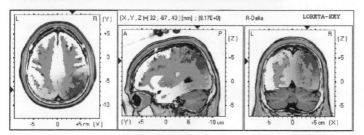

PLATE 4.5 Displayed are the horizontal (left), sagittal (middle), and coronal (right) sections through the voxel with maximal current source density localized to Brodmann area 19; Precuneus in visual processing learning disability case (see Figure 4.5).

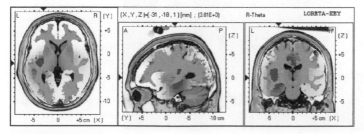

PLATE 4.6 Displayed are the horizontal (left), sagittal (middle), and coronal (right) sections through the voxel with maximal current source density localized to Brodmann area 13; Insula in bi-polar disorder case (see Figure 4.6).

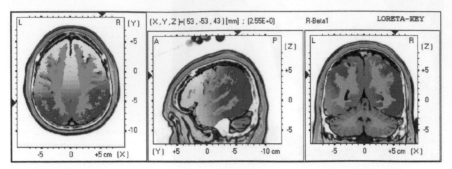

PLATE 4.7 Displayed are the horizontal (left), sagittal (middle), and coronal (right) sections through the voxel with maximal current source density localized to Brodmann area 40; Inferior Parietal Lobule in anxiety and inattention case (see Figure 4.7).

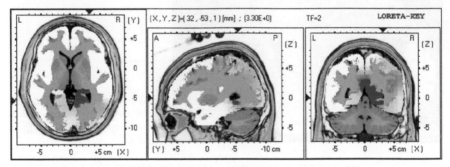

PLATE 4.8 Displayed are the horizontal (left), sagittal (middle), and coronal (right) sections through the voxel with maximal current source density in the theta (4–7.5 Hz) band localized to Brodmann area 30; Parahippocampal Gyrus illustrating slowed alpha generator (see Figure 4.8).

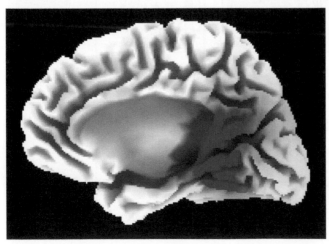

PLATE 4.9 3-D surface sagittal image of theta (4–7.5 Hz) of the left hemisphere with maximal current source density localized to Brodmann area 30; Parahippocampal Gyrus illustrating slowed alpha generator (see Figure 4.9).

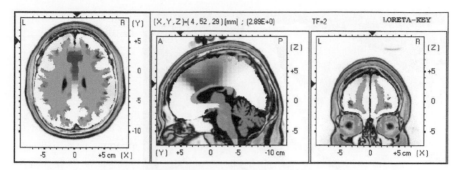

PLATE 4.10 Displayed are the horizontal (left), sagittal (middle), and coronal (right) sections through the voxel with maximal current source density in the theta (4–7.5 Hz) band localized to the Anterior Cingulate post neurofeedback (see Figure 4.10).

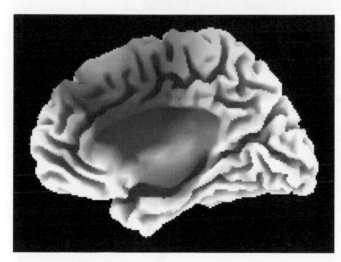

PLATE 4.11 3-D surface sagittal image of theta (4–7.5 Hz) of the left hemisphere with maximal current source density localized to the Anterior Cingulate post neurofeedback (see Figure 4.11).

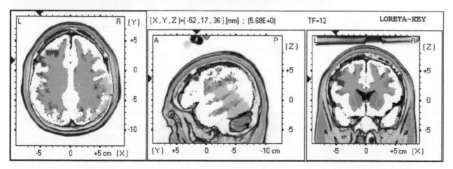

PLATE 4.12 Displayed are the horizontal (left), sagittal (middle), and coronal (right) sections through the voxel with maximal current source density in the beta 4 (24–28 Hz) band localized to Brodmann areas 9 and 24 (see Figure 4.12).

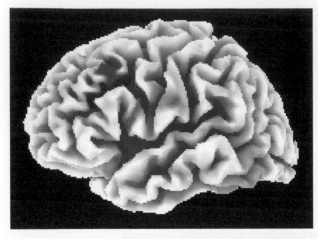

PLATE 4.13 3-D surface sagittal image of beta (24–28 Hz) of the left hemisphere with maximal current source density localized to Brodmann areas 9 and 24 (see Figure 4.13).

Click View > Dynamic JTFA > Color Maps to view instantaneous power, coherence, phase, amplitude asymmetry, derivatives and phase reset

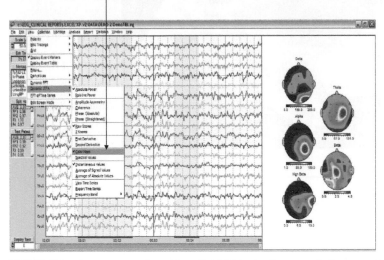

PLATE 5.2 Screen capture from NeuroGuide™ in the Demo mode from a patient with right parietal and right central injury. Instantaneous Z-scores are on the right; EEG traces are on the left. Depress the left mouse button and move the mouse over the traces. Move the mouse to the right border and watch a movie of the dynamic Z-scores. Download the free NeuroGuide™ Demo at www. appliedneuroscience.com (see Figure 5.2)

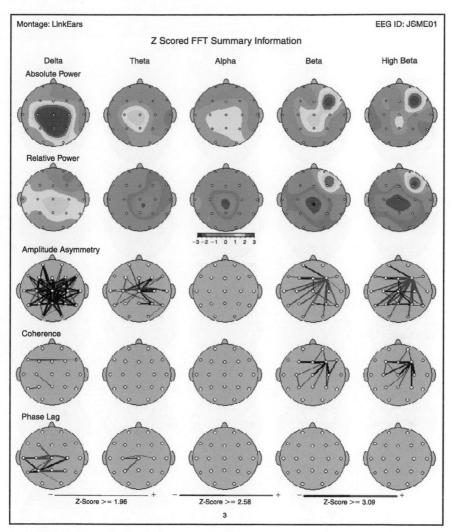

PLATE 5.6 Jack's first QEEG revealing abnormal slow wave activity in central and parietal regions combined with delta and beta coherence abnormalities (see Figure 5.6).

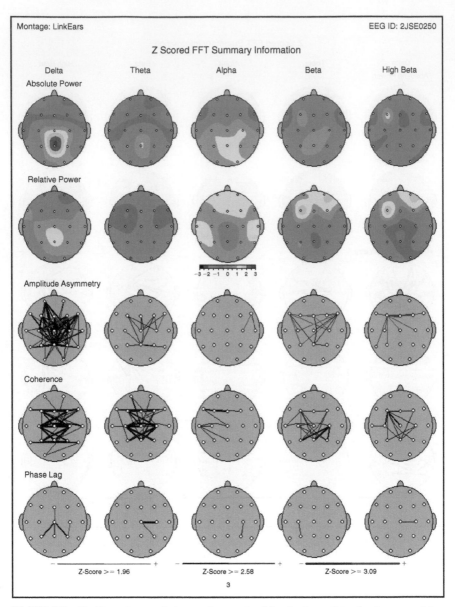

PLATE 5.7 Significant increase in hypo-coherence in all bands after traditional coherence training (see Figure 5.7).

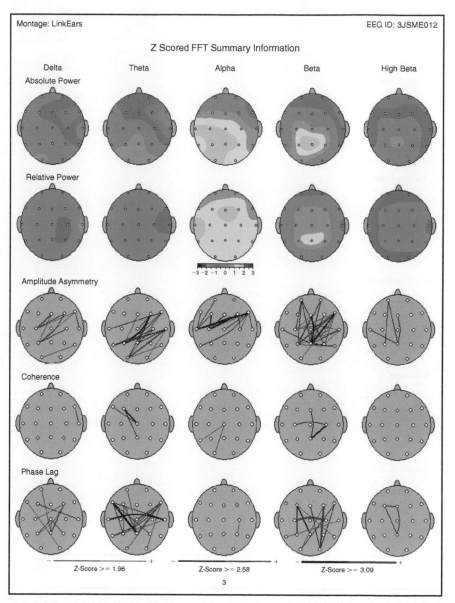

PLATE 5.8 Substantial remediation of abnormal coherence values after Z-score coherence range training (see Figure 5.8).

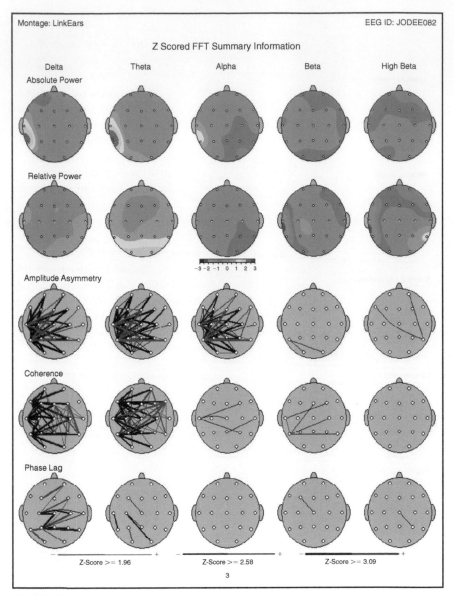

PLATE 5.9   John's first QEEG demonstrating focal slow wave activity over the area of the hemorrhage, and theta abnormalities in occipital, parietal and temporal lobes with left hemisphere hypocoherence and right hemisphere hyper-coherence (see Figure 5.9).

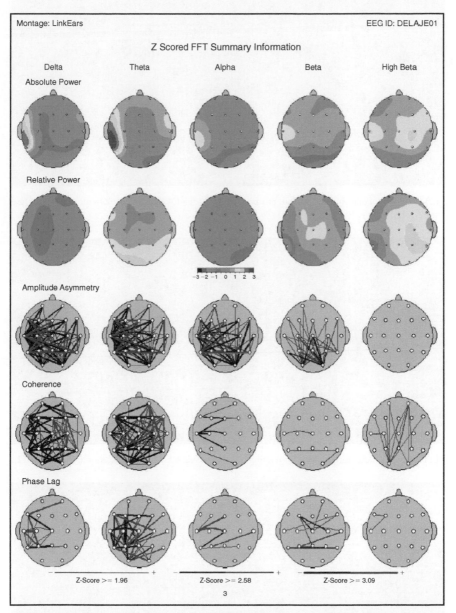

PLATE 5.10 After 60 sessions of traditional inhibit and coherence training. Note the significant increase in hyper-coherence in the right hemisphere (see Figure 5.10).

PLATE 5.11

SITES: O1 Pz (EO)	Abs	Rel	Rat/T	Rat/A	Rat/B	Rat/G	SITES: T4 P4 (EO)	Abs	Rel	Rat/T	Rat/A	Rat/B	Rat/G
Delta (1.0-4.0)	0.6	0.1	-0.4	0.4	0.3	0.5	Delta (1.0-4.0)	1.7	0.2	-0.2	0.5	0.2	0.4
Theta (4.0-8.0)	1.0	0.7		0.8	0.6	0.8	Theta (4.0-8.0)	1.8	0.5		0.8	0.4	0.6
Alpha (8.0-12.5)	-0.0	-0.6			-0.2	0.0	Alpha (8.0-12.5)	0.8	-0.6			-0.4	-0.1
Beta (12.5-25.5)	0.2	0.3				0.0	Beta (12.5-25.5)	1.3	-0.1				0.3
Beta 1 (12.0-15.5)	-0.1	-0.5					Beta 1 (12.0-15.5)	0.9	-0.4				
Beta 2 (15.0-18.0)	0.3	-0.1					Beta 2 (15.0-18.0)	1.4	-0.1				
Beta 3 (18.0-25.5)	0.8	0.4					Beta 3 (18.0-25.5)	1.7	0.3				
Gamma (25.5-30.5)	0.2	-0.2					Gamma (25.5-30.5)	1.1	-0.2				
Delta (1.0-4.0)	1.0	0.3	-0.1	0.5	0.2	0.6	Delta (1.0-4.0)	1.3	0.4	0.0	0.7	0.4	0.8
Theta (4.0-8.0)	1.1	0.4		0.6	0.3	0.7	Theta (4.0-8.0)	1.3	0.4		0.8	0.4	0.8
Alpha (8.0-12.5)	0.2	-0.6			-0.3	0.0	Alpha (8.0-12.5)	0.2	-0.8			-0.4	-0.0
Beta (12.5-25.5)	0.7	-0.1				0.4	Beta (12.5-25.5)	0.8	-0.2				0.4
Beta 1 (12.0-15.5)	0.2	-0.5					Beta 1 (12.0-15.5)	0.2	-0.7				
Beta 2 (15.0-18.0)	0.8	-0.0					Beta 2 (15.0-18.0)	0.9	-0.1				
Beta 3 (18.0-25.5)	0.9	0.2					Beta 3 (18.0-25.5)	1.1	0.1				
Gamma (25.5-30.5)	0.5	-0.2					Gamma (25.5-30.5)	0.7	-0.3				

	O1-Pz ASY	COH	PHA	O1-T4 ASY	COH	PHA	O1-P4 ASY	COH	PHA	Pz-T4 ASY	COH	PHA	Pz-P4 ASY	COH	PHA	T4-P4 ASY	COH	PHA
Delta (1.0-4.0)	-0.4	-0.5	0.4	-0.9	0.4	-0.3	-0.8	-0.1	0.1	-0.6	-0.0	0.1	-0.4	-1.7	1.4	0.4	0.1	0.1
Theta (4.0-8.0)	-0.1	0.5	-0.2	-0.7	1.0	-0.3	-0.3	0.6	-0.3	-0.7	1.1	-0.5	-0.3	0.4	-0.1	0.7	1.1	-0.6
Alpha (8.0-12.5)	-0.3	0.3	-0.2	-0.8	-0.3	-0.1	-0.2	-0.0	-0.0	-0.6	-0.3	-0.0	-0.0	-0.1	0.1	0.7	0.2	-0.2
Beta (12.5-25.5)	-0.5	1.4	-0.4	-0.9	1.0	-0.4	-0.6	1.5	-0.4	-0.6	0.8	-0.3	-0.2	0.7	-0.2	0.5	0.5	-0.2
Beta 1 (12.0-15.5)	-0.3	0.2	-0.1	-0.8	-0.0	-0.0	-0.3	0.5	-0.3	-0.6	-0.3	0.0	-0.1	-0.0	-0.1	0.6	-0.3	-0.1
Beta 2 (15.0-18.0)	-0.5	0.8	-0.4	-0.9	0.2	-0.4	-0.5	0.7	-0.4	-0.5	0.2	-0.3	-0.2	0.4	-0.2	0.4	0.2	-0.1
Beta 3 (18.0-25.5)	-0.2	1.0	-0.6	-0.8	0.6	-0.6	-0.3	1.1	-0.7	-0.7	0.5	-0.4	-0.2	0.5	-0.4	0.6	0.3	-0.2
Gamma (25.5-30.5)	-0.3	1.0	-0.4	-0.7	0.3	-0.3	-0.4	1.1	-0.5	-0.5	0.2	-0.2	-0.2	0.4	-0.2	0.5	0.2	-0.2

PLATE 5.11 Four-channel Z-score protocol based on the QEEG and this Z-score assessment (see Figure 5.11).

PLATE 5.12

SITES: O1 Pz (EO)	Abs	Rel	Rat/T	Rat/A	Rat/B	Rat/G	SITES: T4 P4 (EO)	Abs	Rel	Rat/T	Rat/A	Rat/B	Rat/G
Delta (1.0-4.0)	0.8	0.3	0.0	0.4	0.4	0.6	Delta (1.0-4.0)	1.3	0.5	0.1	0.5	0.6	0.9
Theta (4.0-8.0)	0.8	0.4		0.4	0.4	0.7	Theta (4.0-8.0)	1.2	0.3		0.4	0.5	0.8
Alpha (8.0-12.5)	0.2	-0.3			-0.0	0.0	Alpha (8.0-12.5)	0.6	-0.3			0.1	0.4
Beta (12.5-25.5)	0.3	-0.2				0.0	Beta (12.5-25.5)	0.5	-0.5				0.3
Beta 1 (12.0-15.5)	-0.1	-0.6					Beta 1 (12.0-15.5)	0.1	-0.8				
Beta 2 (15.0-18.0)	0.2	-0.3					Beta 2 (15.0-18.0)	0.6	-0.3				
Beta 3 (18.0-25.5)	0.4	-0.1					Beta 3 (18.0-25.5)	0.6	-0.3				
Gamma (25.5-30.5)	0.2	-0.3					Gamma (25.5-30.5)	0.4	-0.5				
Delta (1.0-4.0)	0.7	0.2	0.1	0.2	0.0	0.4	Delta (1.0-4.0)	0.8	0.3	0.2	0.4	0.3	0.7
Theta (4.0-8.0)	0.5	0.0		0.1	-0.1	0.3	Theta (4.0-8.0)	0.6	0.1		0.3	0.1	0.6
Alpha (8.0-12.5)	0.3	-0.1			-0.2	0.2	Alpha (8.0-12.5)	0.2	-0.4			-0.2	0.2
Beta (12.5-25.5)	0.7	0.2				0.4	Beta (12.5-25.5)	0.5	-0.1				0.5
Beta 1 (12.0-15.5)	0.2	-0.3					Beta 1 (12.0-15.5)	-0.1	-0.7				
Beta 2 (15.0-18.0)	0.5	-0.0					Beta 2 (15.0-18.0)	0.3	-0.3				
Beta 3 (18.0-25.5)	0.8	0.4					Beta 3 (18.0-25.5)	0.7	0.1				
Gamma (25.5-30.5)	0.7	0.2					Gamma (25.5-30.5)	0.5	-0.1				

	O1-Pz ASY	COH	PHA	O1-T4 ASY	COH	PHA	O1-P4 ASY	COH	PHA	Pz-T4 ASY	COH	PHA	Pz-P4 ASY	COH	PHA	T4-P4 ASY	COH	PHA
Delta (1.0-4.0)	0.0	0.4	-0.3	-0.5	0.6	-0.5	-0.1	0.3	-0.3	-0.5	0.4	-0.3	-0.2	0.1	-0.0	0.5	0.3	-0.3
Theta (4.0-8.0)	0.3	0.1	-0.1	-0.4	0.2	-0.1	0.2	-0.0	0.1	-0.6	0.6	-0.2	-0.1	0.2	0.1	0.6	0.9	-0.4
Alpha (8.0-12.5)	-0.2	0.1	-0.2	-0.4	-0.1	-0.0	0.0	-0.1	0.1	-0.2	-0.1	-0.1	0.2	-0.6	0.2	0.4	0.1	-0.2
Beta (12.5-25.5)	-0.4	1.0	-0.4	-0.2	0.5	-0.3	-0.2	0.7	-0.2	0.1	0.5	-0.3	0.3	0.7	0.1	0.1	0.7	-0.3
Beta 1 (12.0-15.5)	-0.2	0.4	-0.3	-0.2	-0.0	0.0	0.0	0.5	-0.3	0.0	-0.4	0.1	0.3	-0.5	0.2	0.2	-0.5	0.2
Beta 2 (15.0-18.0)	-0.3	0.5	-0.3	-0.3	0.1	-0.1	-0.1	0.4	-0.3	-0.1	-0.0	-0.1	0.2	-0.6	0.3	0.3	0.1	-0.0
Beta 3 (18.0-25.5)	-0.5	0.6	-0.4	-0.2	0.2	-0.4	-0.2	0.5	-0.4	0.2	0.1	-0.1	0.3	-0.8	0.4	-0.0	0.3	-0.3
Gamma (25.5-30.5)	-0.6	0.9	-0.4	-0.1	0.4	-0.5	-0.2	0.7	-0.4	0.3	0.5	-0.4	0.4	-0.5	0.1	-0.0	0.7	-0.5

PLATE 5.12 After three sessions of training, Z-scores reveal substantial remediation (see Figure 5.12).

PLATE 5.13

SITES: F3 P3 (EO)	Abs	Rel	Rat/T	Rat/A	Rat/B	Rat/G	SITES: F7 T5 (EO)	Abs	Rel	Rat/T	Rat/A	Rat/B	Rat/G
Delta (1.0-4.0)	0.6	-0.1	-0.3	0.1	-0.2	0.7	Delta (1.0-4.0)	0.5	-0.2	-0.3	0.1	-0.3	0.7
Theta (4.0-8.0)	1.0	0.4		0.4	0.1	1.0	Theta (4.0-8.0)	1.0	0.4		0.5	0.0	1.0
Alpha (8.0-12.5)	0.4	-0.2			-0.3	0.6	Alpha (8.0-12.5)	0.3	-0.3			0.4	0.6
Beta (12.5-25.5)	0.7	0.2				1.0	Beta (12.5-25.5)	0.9	0.4				1.1
Beta 1 (12.0-15.5)	-0.4	-1.0					Beta 1 (12.0-15.5)	-0.4	-1.0				
Beta 2 (15.0-18.0)	0.8	0.2					Beta 2 (15.0-18.0)	1.0	0.4				
Beta 3 (18.0-25.5)	1.3	0.8					Beta 3 (18.0-25.5)	1.5	0.9				
Gamma (25.5-30.5)	0.4	-0.1					Gamma (25.5-30.5)	0.6	-0.0				
Delta (1.0-4.0)	0.1	-0.6	-0.7	-0.3	-0.5	0.2	Delta (1.0-4.0)	1.0	-0.6	-1.0	-0.5	-0.0	0.7
Theta (4.0-8.0)	0.9	0.5		0.3	0.2	0.8	Theta (4.0-8.0)	2.2	0.8		0.4	0.9	1.5
Alpha (8.0-12.5)	0.4	-0.1			-0.2	0.5	Alpha (8.0-12.5)	1.4	0.2			0.4	1.1
Beta (12.5-25.5)	0.7	0.2				0.7	Beta (12.5-25.5)	1.0	-0.5				0.8
Beta 1 (12.0-15.5)	-0.2	-0.7					Beta 1 (12.0-15.5)	0.0	-1.4				
Beta 2 (15.0-18.0)	0.9	0.3					Beta 2 (15.0-18.0)	1.3	-0.1				
Beta 3 (18.0-25.5)	1.1	0.6					Beta 3 (18.0-25.5)	1.5	0.0				
Gamma (25.5-30.5)	0.6	0.1					Gamma (25.5-30.5)	0.8	-0.7				

	F3-P3: ASY	COH	PHA	F3-F7: ASY	COH	PHA	F3-T5: ASY	COH	PHA	P3-F7: ASY	COH	PHA	P3-T5: ASY	COH	PHA	F7-T5: ASY	COH	PHA
Delta (1.0-4.0)	0.4	0.0	0.4	-0.1	-0.3	0.6	-0.4	-0.2	0.9	-0.3	-0.3	0.4	-1.0	-1.6	1.1	-0.4	-0.0	0.4
Theta (4.0-8.0)	-0.0	-0.4	0.4	-0.0	-0.5	0.1	-1.1	0.1	0.7	0.0	-0.2	0.6	-1.5	-0.9	0.3	-1.0	0.3	0.5
Alpha (8.0-12.5)	-0.1	-0.4	0.3	0.1	0.1	-0.1	-1.1	0.2	0.4	0.1	0.2	0.2	-1.3	-0.4	0.2	-1.0	0.1	0.3
Beta (12.5-25.5)	0.0	0.9	-0.3	-0.1	1.7	-0.7	-0.2	0.6	-0.3	-0.2	1.7	-0.5	-0.4	0.4	-0.1	-0.1	1.2	-0.5
Beta 1 (12.0-15.5)	-0.2	-0.1	0.0	-0.0	0.7	-0.5	-0.4	0.2	0.1	0.2	-0.2	-0.1	-0.2	-0.5	0.2	-0.4	0.1	-0.1
Beta 2 (15.0-18.0)	-0.1	0.2	-0.3	-0.2	0.9	-0.5	-0.5	0.0	-0.2	-0.1	0.5	-0.4	-0.6	0.2	-0.1	-0.3	0.5	-0.3
Beta 3 (18.0-25.5)	0.2	0.7	-0.5	-0.2	1.1	-0.8	-0.1	0.8	-0.4	-0.3	1.0	-0.7	-0.4	0.5	-0.3	-0.0	0.9	-0.5
Gamma (25.5-30.5)	-0.1	0.8	-0.5	-0.1	1.5	-0.7	-0.3	0.4	-0.3	-0.0	1.5	-0.7	-0.2	0.2	-0.1	-0.2	0.8	-0.5

PLATE 5.13 First Z-score training of F3/P3/F7/T5. Note the damage in the temporal area at T5 reflected in abnormal absolute power Z-scores, and the significant deviation in connectivity measures (see Figure 5.13).

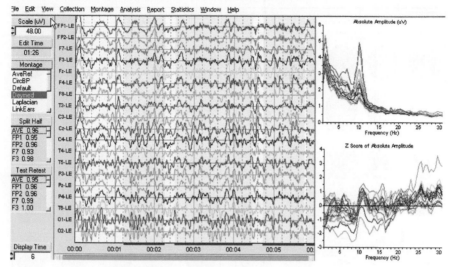

PLATE 5.14A Q1, FFT frequency distribution, eyes–closed (see Figure 5.14A).

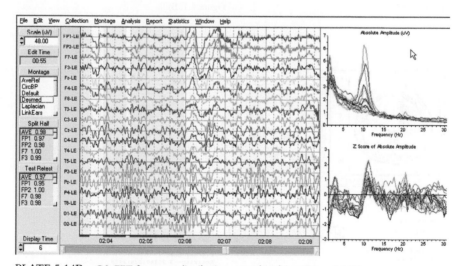

PLATE 5.14B Q2, FFT frequency distribution, eyes–closed (see Figure 5.14B).

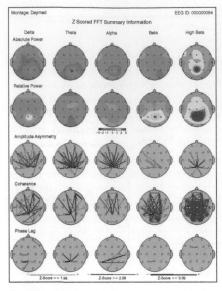
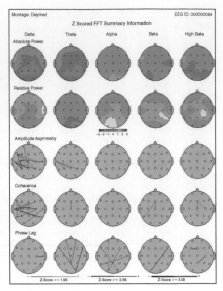

PLATE 5.15A   Q1, FFT summary EC (see Figure 5.15A).

PLATE 5.15B   Q2, FFT summary EC (see Figure 5.15B).

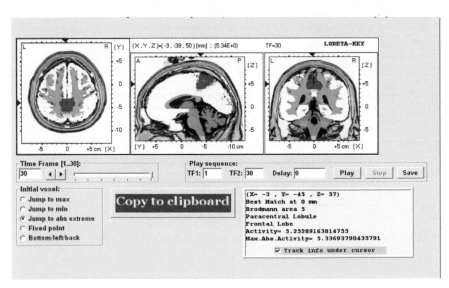

PLATE 5.16A   Q1, LORETA @ 30 EC (see Figure 5.16A).

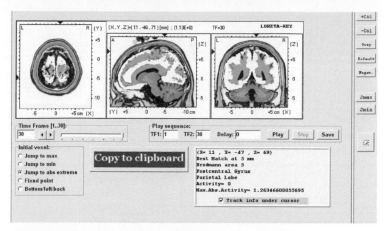

PLATE 5.16B   Q2, LORETA @ 30 Hz EC (see Figure 5.16B).

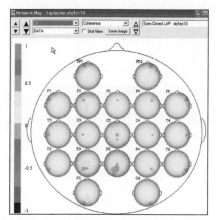

PLATE 5.17A   Q1, coherence @ 30 EC
(see Figure 5.17A).

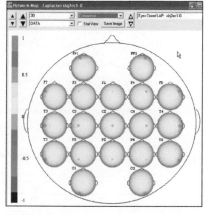

PLATE 5.17B   Q2, coherence @ 30 EC
(see Figure 5.17B).

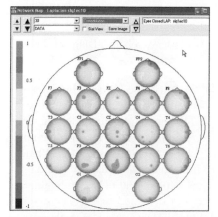

PLATE 5.18A   Q1, comod @ 30 EC (see
Figure 5.18A).

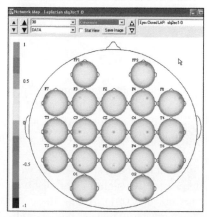

PLATE 5.18B   Q2, comod @ 30 EC (see
Figure 5.18B).

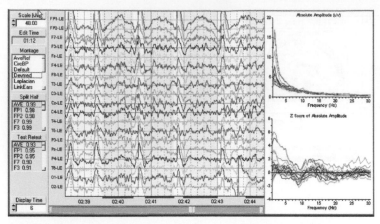

PLATE 5.19A   Q1, FFT frequency distribution, eyes-open (see Figure 5.19A).

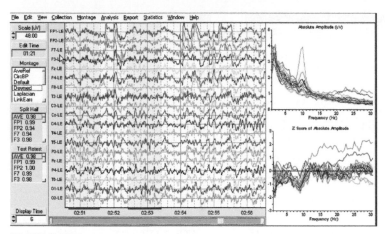

PLATE 5.19B   Q2, FFT frequency distribution, eyes-open (see Figure 5.19B).

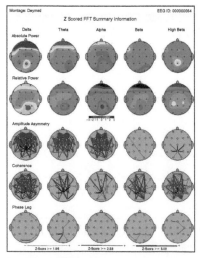

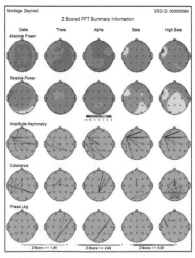

PLATE 5.20A   Q1, FFT summary EO
(see Figure 5.20A).

PLATE 5.20B   Q2, FFT summary EO
(see Figure 5.20B).

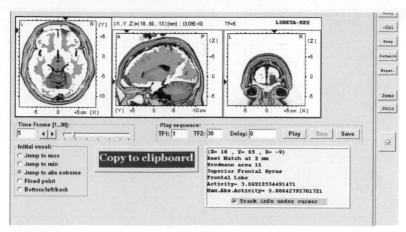

PLATE 5.21A   Q1, LORETA @ 5 Hz EC (see Figure 5.21A).

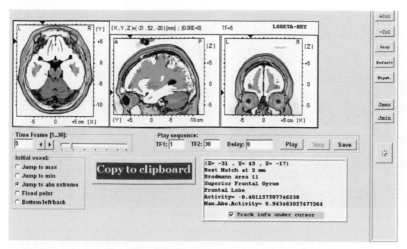

PLATE 5.21B   Q2, LORETA @ 5 Hz EC (see Figure 5.21B).

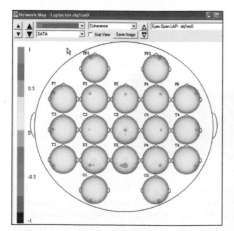

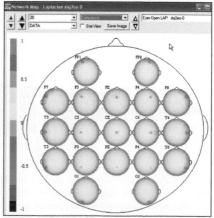

PLATE 5.22A   Q1, coherence @ 20 EO (see Figure 5.22A).

PLATE 5.22B   Q2, coherence @ 20 EO (see Figure 5.22B).

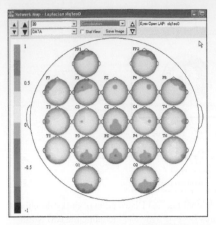

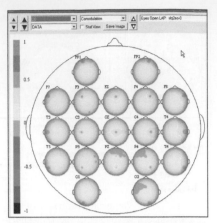

PLATE 5.23A Q1, comod @ 20 EO. (see Figure 5.23A)

PLATE 5.23B Q2, comod @ 20 EO (see Figure 5.23B).

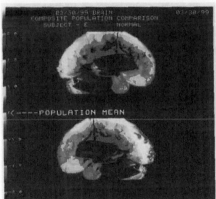

Before HEG

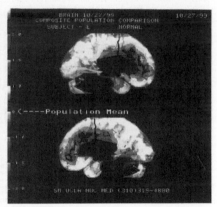

After HEG

PLATE 7.4 Hypoperfused (blue) area shrinks after 23 sessions of HEG training at Fp1 and Fp2. Illustrated here is the remote effect. In this SPECT study, a measure of abnormal blood flow, one can see the posterior cingulate gyrus becomes more normal even though the training was at the prefrontal cortex (see Figure 7.4).

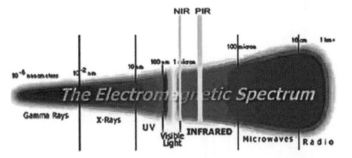

PLATE 7.7 The wavelengths used in the NIR system are shorter than those used in the PIR system. The primary difference between short wavelength infrared and long wavelength infrared is that the longer wavelengths are sensitive to heat in the range of human body temperature whereas short wavelength infrared is insensitive to heat in that range. Both systems are based on photon detection, making them immune to electrical signal artifacts. By contrast, EEG neurofeedback is based on electron detection (see Figure 7.7).

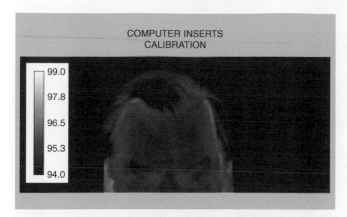

PLATE 7.9   Calibration gives all images a common thermal reference (see Figure 7.9).

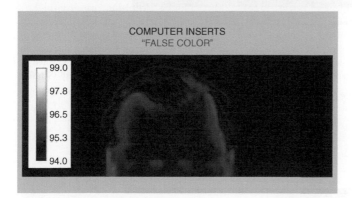

PLATE 7.10   The final step in the sequence is the introduction of *false color*. This is called *false color* because wavelengths in this frequency have no color. The computer injects the color to make it easier for human interpretation of the image. This is an image of a "normal forehead." (see Figure 7.10)

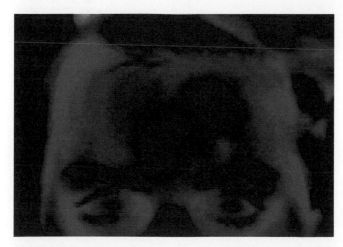

PLATE 7.11   This is an example of a pre-session image captured with infrared camera. This image is of a 16-year-old male with severe concentration problems and severe word finding problems (see Figure 7.11).

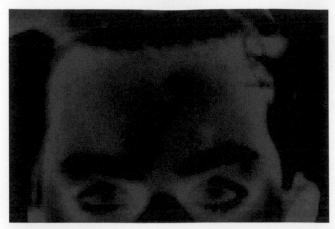

PLATE 7.12   Post-session image. Previously dark areas on the forehead are lighter. Previously light areas on the forehead are less intense. There is less variability across the forehead. In this post-session image, the pinna of the left ear has a large increase in thermal output. Sometimes it is seen on the non-language side instead. Research on temperature changes of the pinna has not confirmed its meaning, although the general consensus is that it is probably related to language activity (Schiffer, 1998) (see Figure 7.12).

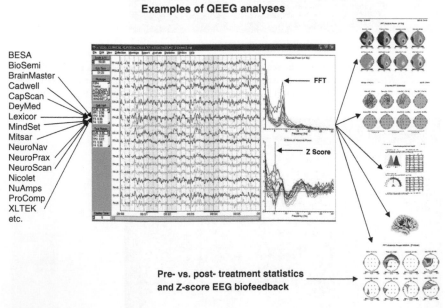

PLATE 11.1   Example of QEEG analyses in which calibrated EEG digital data are imported; test–retest and split half reliabilities are computed; spectral analyses are performed (FFT) and compared to a normative database (e.g., Z Scores); discriminant analyses and color topographic maps are produced; three-dimensional source localization is measured; and objective pre-treatment vs. post-treatment, or pre-mediation vs. post-medication, statistics within a few minutes using the same computer program (see Figure 11.1).

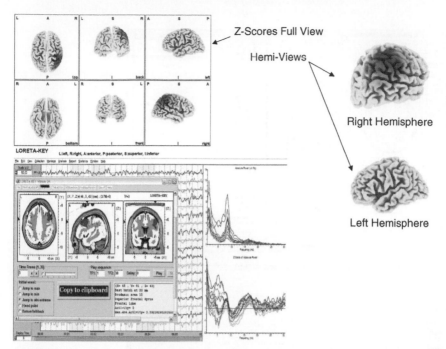

PLATE 11.5 Example of the use of Low Resolution Electromagnetic Tomography (LORETA) to evaluate the effects of TBI involving a patient hit with a bat on the near right parietal lobe. The lower left panel is the digital EEG and QEEG that are simultaneously available for the evaluation of the EEG with the Key Institute LORETA control panel superimposed on the EEG. The upper and right panels are examples of the location of Z-score deviations from normal, which were confined to the right parietal and right central regions and are consistent with the location of impact (see Figure 11.5).

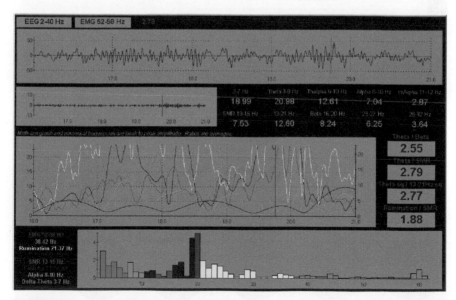

PLATE 15.1 Beta spindling, 20 Hz; eyes-open is seen using the Infiniti instrument (Thought Technology) and the "Clinical Success" assessment screen (Thompson and Thompson, 1995) (see Figure 15.1).

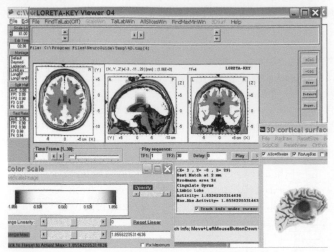

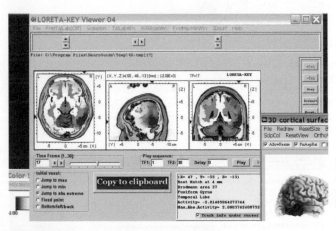

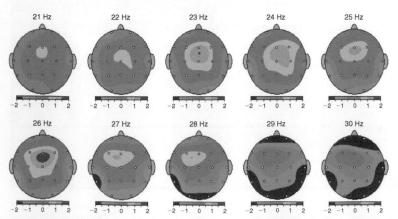

PLATE 15.7 Brain map, linked-ear reference, eyes-open, showing standard deviations (SD) (see Figure 15.7).

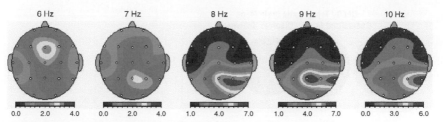

PLATE 15.8   Brain map, absolute power, linked-ear reference, eyes-open (see Figure 15.8).

Before Training:

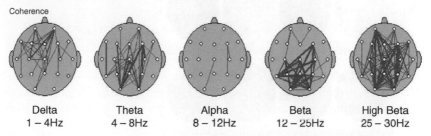

PLATE 15.12   Coherence map before training: Coherence, eyes-open, linked-ears showing hyper-coherence between many sites (see Figure 15.12).

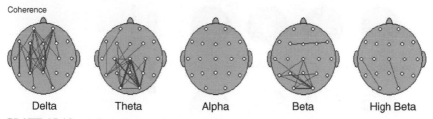

PLATE 15.13   Coherence map after 40 sessions (see Figure 15.13).

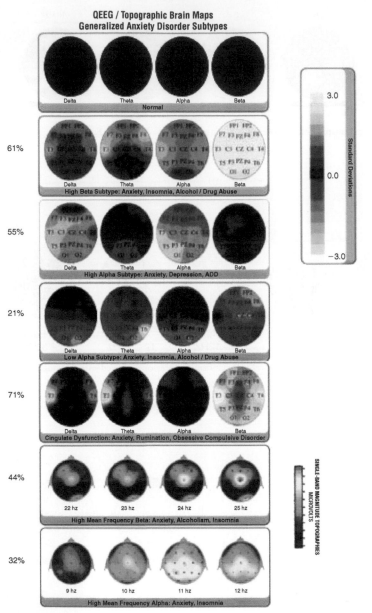

PLATE 17.1   QEEG/topographic brain maps of generalized anxiety disorder sub-types. (see Figure 17.1)

Printed and bound by CPI Group (UK) Ltd, Croydon, CR0 4YY

03/10/2024

01040412-0012